Secondary Analysis of Electronic Health Records

MIT Critical Data

Secondary Analysis of Electronic Health Records

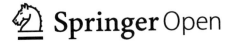

MIT Critical Data
Massachusetts Institute of Technology
Cambridge, MA
USA

Additional material to this book can be downloaded from http://link.springer.com/978-3-319-43740-8.

ISBN 978-3-319-43740-8   ISBN 978-3-319-43742-2   (eBook)
DOI 10.1007/978-3-319-43742-2

Library of Congress Control Number: 2016947212

© The Editor(s) (if applicable) and The Author(s) 2016 This book is published open access.
Open Access This book is distributed under the terms of the Creative Commons Attribution-NonCommercial 4.0 International License (http://creativecommons.org/licenses/by-nc/4.0/), which permits any noncommercial use, duplication, adaptation, distribution and reproduction in any medium or format, as long as you give appropriate credit to the original author(s) and the source, a link is provided to the Creative Commons license and any changes made are indicated.
The images or other third party material in this book are included in the work's Creative Commons license, unless indicated otherwise in the credit line; if such material is not included in the work's Creative Commons license and the respective action is not permitted by statutory regulation, users will need to obtain permission from the license holder to duplicate, adapt or reproduce the material.
The use of general descriptive names, registered names, trademarks, service marks, etc. in this publication does not imply, even in the absence of a specific statement, that such names are exempt from the relevant protective laws and regulations and therefore free for general use.
The publisher, the authors and the editors are safe to assume that the advice and information in this book are believed to be true and accurate at the date of publication. Neither the publisher nor the authors or the editors give a warranty, express or implied, with respect to the material contained herein or for any errors or omissions that may have been made.

Printed on acid-free paper

This Springer imprint is published by Springer Nature
The registered company is Springer International Publishing AG
The registered company address is: Gewerbestrasse 11, 6330 Cham, Switzerland

Preface

Diagnostic and therapeutic technologies continue to evolve rapidly, and both individual practitioners and clinical teams face increasingly complex decisions. Unfortunately, the current state of medical knowledge does not provide the guidance to make the majority of clinical decisions on the basis of evidence. According to the 2012 Institute of Medicine Committee Report, only 10–20 % of clinical decisions are evidence based. The problem even extends to the creation of clinical practice guidelines (CPGs). Nearly 50 % of recommendations made in specialty society guidelines rely on expert opinion rather than experimental data. Furthermore, the creation process of CPGs is "marred by weak methods and financial conflicts of interest," rendering current CPGs potentially less trustworthy.

The present research infrastructure is inefficient and frequently produces unreliable results that cannot be replicated. Even randomized controlled trials (RCTs), the traditional gold standards of the research reliability hierarchy, are not without limitations. They can be costly, labor-intensive, slow, and can return results that are seldom generalizable to every patient population. It is impossible for a tightly controlled RCT to capture the full, interactive, and contextual details of the clinical issues that arise in real clinics and inpatient units. Furthermore, many pertinent but unresolved clinical and medical systems issues do not seem to have attracted the interest of the research enterprise, which has come to focus instead on cellular and molecular investigations and single-agent (e.g., a drug or device) effects. For clinicians, the end result is a "data desert" when it comes to making decisions.

Electronic health record (EHR) data are frequently digitally archived and can subsequently be extracted and analyzed. Between 2011 and 2019, the prevalence of EHRs is expected to grow from 34 to 90 % among office-based practices, and the majority of hospitals have replaced or are in the process of replacing paper systems with comprehensive, enterprise EHRs. The power of scale intrinsic to this digital transformation opens the door to a massive amount of currently untapped information. The data, if properly analyzed and meaningfully interpreted, could vastly improve our conception and development of best practices. The possibilities for quality improvement, increased safety, process optimization, and personalization of clinical decisions range from impressive to revolutionary. The National Institutes of

Health (NIH) and other major grant organizations have begun to recognize the power of big data in knowledge creation and are offering grants to support investigators in this area.

This book, written with support from the National Institute for Biomedical Imaging and Bioengineering through grant R01 EB017205-01A1, is meant to serve as an illustrative guide for scientists, engineers, and clinicians that are interested in performing retrospective research using data from EHRs. It is divided into three major parts.

The first part of the book paints the current landscape and describes the body of knowledge that dictates clinical practice guidelines, including the limitations and the challenges. This sets the stage for presenting the motivation behind the secondary analysis of EHR data. The part also describes the data landscape, who the key players are, and which types of databases are useful for which kinds of questions. Finally, the part outlines the political, regulatory and technical challenges faced by clinical informaticians, and provides suggestions on how to navigate through these challenges.

In the second part, the process of parsing a clinical question into a study design and methodology is broken down into five steps. The first step explains how to formulate the right research question, and bring together the appropriate team. The second step outlines strategies for identifying, extracting, Oxford, and preprocessing EHR data to comprehend and address the research question of interest. The third step presents techniques in exploratory analysis and data visualization. In the fourth step, a detailed guide on how to choose the type of analysis that best answers the research question is provided. Finally, the fifth and final step illustrates how to validate results, using cross validation, sensitivity analyses, testing of falsification hypotheses, and other common techniques in the field.

The third, and final part of the book, provides a comprehensive collection of case studies. These case studies highlight various aspects of the research pipeline presented in the second part of the book, and help ground the reader in real world data analyses.

We have written the book so that a reader at different levels may easily start at different parts. For the novice researcher, the book should be read from start to finish. For individuals who are already acquainted with the challenges of clinical informatics, but would like guidance on how to most effectively perform the analysis, the book should be read from the second part onward. Finally, the part on case studies provides project-specific practical considerations on study design and methodology and is recommended for all readers.

The time has come to leverage the data we generate during routine patient care to formulate a more complete lexicon of evidence-based recommendations and support shared decision making with patients. This book will train the next generation of scientists, representing different disciplines, but collaborating to expand the knowledge base that will guide medical practice in the future.

We would like to take this opportunity to thank Professor Roger Mark, whose vision to create a high resolution clinical database that is open to investigators around the world, inspired us to write this textbook.

Cambridge, USA   MIT Critical Data

MIT Critical Data

MIT Critical Data consists of data scientists and clinicians from around the globe brought together by a vision to engender a data-driven healthcare system supported by *clinical informatics without walls*. In this ecosystem, the creation of evidence and clinical decision support tools is initiated, updated, honed, Oxford, and enhanced by scaling the access to and meaningful use of clinical data.

Leo Anthony Celi has practiced medicine in three continents, giving him broad perspectives in healthcare delivery. His research is on secondary analysis of electronic health records and global health informatics. He founded and co-directs Sana at the Institute for Medical Engineering and Science at the Massachusetts Institute of Technology. He also holds a faculty position at Harvard Medical School as an intensivist at the Beth Israel Deaconess Medical Center and is the clinical research director for the Laboratory of Computational Physiology at MIT. Finally, he is one of the course directors for HST.936 at MIT—innovations in global health informatics and HST.953—secondary analysis of electronic health records.

Peter Charlton gained the degree of M.Eng. in Engineering Science in 2010 from the University of Oxford. Since then he held a research position, working jointly with Guy's and St Thomas' NHS Foundation Trust, and King's College London. Peter's research focuses on physiological monitoring of hospital patients, divided into three areas. The first area concerns the development of signal processing techniques to estimate clinical parameters from physiological signals. He has focused on unobtrusive estimation of respiratory rate for use in ambulatory settings, invasive estimation of cardiac output for use in critical care, and novel techniques for analysis of the pulse oximetry (photoplethysmogram) signal. Secondly, he is investigating the effectiveness of technologies for the acquisition of continuous and intermittent physiological measurements in ambulatory and intensive care settings. Thirdly, he is developing techniques to transform continuous monitoring data into measurements that are appropriate for real-time alerting of patient deteriorations.

Mohammad Mahdi Ghassemi is a doctoral candidate at the Massachusetts Institute of Technology. As an undergraduate, he studied Electrical Engineering and graduated as both a Goldwater scholar and the University's "Outstanding

Engineer". In 2011, Mohammad received an MPhil in Information Engineering from the University of Cambridge where he was also a recipient of the Gates-Cambridge Scholarship. Since arriving at MIT, he has pursued research at the interface of machine learning and medical informatics. Mohammad's doctoral focus is on signal processing and machine learning techniques in the context of multi-modal, multiscale datasets. He has helped put together the largest collection of post-anoxic coma EEGs in the world. In addition to his thesis work, Mohammad has worked with the Samsung Corporation, and several entities across campus building "smart devices" including: a multi-sensor wearable that passively monitors the physiological, audio and video activity of a user to estimate a latent emotional state.

Alistair Johnson received his B.Eng. in Biomedical and Electrical Engineering at McMaster University, Canada, and subsequently read for a DPhil in Healthcare Innovation at the University of Oxford. His thesis was titled "Mortality and acuity assessment in critical care", and its focus included using machine learning techniques to predict mortality and develop new severity of illness scores for patients admitted to intensive care units. Alistair also spent a year as a research assistant at the John Radcliffe hospital in Oxford, where he worked on building early alerting models for patients post-ICU discharge. Alistair's research interests revolve around the use of data collected during routine clinical practice to improve patient care.

Matthieu Komorowski holds board certification in anesthesiology and critical care in both France and the UK. A former medical research fellow at the European Space Agency, he completed a Master of Research in Biomedical Engineering at Imperial College London focusing on machine learning. Dr Komorowski now pursues a Ph.D. at Imperial College and a research fellowship in intensive care at Charing Cross Hospital in London. In his research, he combines his expertise in machine learning and critical care to generate new clinical evidence and build the next generation of clinical tools such as decision support systems, with a particular interest in septic shock, the number one killer in intensive care and the single most expensive condition treated in hospitals.

Dominic Marshall is an Academic Foundation doctor in Oxford, UK. Dominic read Molecular and Cellular biology at the University of Bath and worked at Eli Lilly in their Alzheimer's disease drug hunting research program. He pursued his medical training at Imperial College London where he was awarded the Santander Undergraduate scholarship for academic performance and ranked first overall in his graduating class. His research interests range from molecular biology to analysis of large clinical data sets and he has received non-industry grant funding to pursue the development of novel antibiotics and chemotherapeutic agents. Alongside clinical training, he is involved in a number of research projects focusing on analysis of electronic health care records.

Tristan Naumann is a doctoral candidate in Electrical Engineering and Computer Science at MIT working with Dr. Peter Szolovits in CSAIL's Clinical Decision Making group. His research includes exploring relationships in complex, unstructured data using data-informed unsupervised learning techniques, and the application of natural language processing techniques in healthcare data. He has been an organizer for workshops and "datathon" events, which bring together participants with diverse backgrounds in order to address biomedical and clinical questions in a manner that is reliable and reproducible.

Kenneth Paik is a clinical informatician democratizing access "to healthcare" through technology innovation, with his multidisciplinary background in medicine, artificial intelligence, business management, and technology strategy. He is a research scientist at the MIT Laboratory for Computational Physiology investigating the secondary analysis of health data and building intelligent decision support system. As the co-director of Sana, he leads programs and projects driving quality improvement and building capacity in global health. He received his MD and MBA degrees from Georgetown University and completed fellowship training in biomedical informatics at Harvard Medical School and the Massachusetts General Hospital Laboratory for Computer Science.

Tom Joseph Pollard is a postdoctoral associate at the MIT Laboratory for Computational Physiology. Most recently he has been working with colleagues to release MIMIC-III, an openly accessible critical care database. Prior to joining MIT in 2015, Tom completed his Ph.D. at University College London, UK, where he explored models of health in critical care patients in an interdisciplinary project between the Mullard Space Science Laboratory and University College Hospital. Tom has a broad interest in improving the way clinical data is managed, shared, and analyzed for the benefit of patients. He is a Fellow of the Software Sustainability Institute.

Jesse Raffa is a research scientist in the Laboratory for Computational Physiology at the Massachusetts Institute of Technology in Cambridge, USA. He received his Ph.D. in biostatistics from the University of Waterloo (Canada) in 2013. His primary methodological interests are related to the modeling of complex longitudinal data, latent variable models and reproducible research. In addition to his methodological contributions, he has collaborated and published over 20 academic articles with colleagues in a diverse set of areas including: infectious diseases, addiction and critical care, among others. Jesse was the recipient of the distinguished student paper award at the Eastern North American Region International Biometric Society conference in 2013, and the new investigator of the year for the Canadian Association of HIV/AIDS Research in 2004.

Justin Salciccioli is an Academic Foundation doctor in London, UK. Originally from Toronto, Canada, Justin completed his undergraduate and graduate studies in the United States before pursuing his medical studies at Imperial College London. His research pursuits started as an undergraduate student while completing a biochemistry degree. Subsequently, he worked on clinical trials in emergency medicine and intensive care medicine at Beth Israel Deaconess Medical Center in Boston and completed a Masters degree with his thesis on vitamin D deficiency in critically ill patients with sepsis. During this time he developed a keen interest in statistical methods and programming particularly in SAS and R. He has co-authored more than 30 peer-reviewed manuscripts and, in addition to his current clinical training, continues with his research interests on analytical methods for observational and clinical trial data as well as education in data analytics for medical students and clinicians.

Contents

Part I Setting the Stage: Rationale Behind and Challenges to Health Data Analysis

1 Objectives of the Secondary Analysis of Electronic Health Record Data 3
    1.1   Introduction 3
    1.2   Current Research Climate 3
    1.3   Power of the Electronic Health Record 4
    1.4   Pitfalls and Challenges 5
    1.5   Conclusion 6
    References 7

2 Review of Clinical Databases 9
    2.1   Introduction 9
    2.2   Background 9
    2.3   The Medical Information Mart for Intensive Care (MIMIC) Database 10
        2.3.1   Included Variables 11
        2.3.2   Access and Interface 12
    2.4   PCORnet 12
        2.4.1   Included Variables 12
        2.4.2   Access and Interface 13
    2.5   Open NHS 13
        2.5.1   Included Variables 13
        2.5.2   Access and Interface 13
    2.6   Other Ongoing Research 14
        2.6.1   eICU—Philips 14
        2.6.2   VistA 14
        2.6.3   NSQUIP 15
    References 16

3 Challenges and Opportunities in Secondary Analyses of Electronic Health Record Data ... 17
- 3.1 Introduction ... 17
- 3.2 Challenges in Secondary Analysis of Electronic Health Records Data ... 17
- 3.3 Opportunities in Secondary Analysis of Electronic Health Records Data ... 20
- 3.4 Secondary EHR Analyses as Alternatives to Randomized Controlled Clinical Trials ... 21
- 3.5 Demonstrating the Power of Secondary EHR Analysis: Examples in Pharmacovigilance and Clinical Care ... 22
- 3.6 A New Paradigm for Supporting Evidence-Based Practice and Ethical Considerations ... 23
- References ... 25

4 Pulling It All Together: Envisioning a Data-Driven, Ideal Care System ... 27
- 4.1 Use Case Examples Based on Unavoidable Medical Heterogeneity ... 28
- 4.2 Clinical Workflow, Documentation, and Decisions ... 29
- 4.3 Levels of Precision and Personalization ... 32
- 4.4 Coordination, Communication, and Guidance Through the Clinical Labyrinth ... 35
- 4.5 Safety and Quality in an ICS ... 36
- 4.6 Conclusion ... 39
- References ... 41

5 The Story of MIMIC ... 43
- 5.1 The Vision ... 43
- 5.2 Data Acquisition ... 44
  - 5.2.1 Clinical Data ... 44
  - 5.2.2 Physiological Data ... 45
  - 5.2.3 Death Data ... 46
- 5.3 Data Merger and Organization ... 46
- 5.4 Data Sharing ... 47
- 5.5 Updating ... 47
- 5.6 Support ... 48
- 5.7 Lessons Learned ... 48
- 5.8 Future Directions ... 49
- References ... 49

6 Integrating Non-clinical Data with EHRs ... 51
- 6.1 Introduction ... 51
- 6.2 Non-clinical Factors and Determinants of Health ... 51
- 6.3 Increasing Data Availability ... 53
- 6.4 Integration, Application and Calibration ... 54

	6.5	A Well-Connected Empowerment.........................	57
	6.6	Conclusion	58
	References...		59
7	**Using EHR to Conduct Outcome and Health Services**		
	Research...		61
	7.1	Introduction	61
	7.2	The Rise of EHRs in Health Services Research	62
		7.2.1 The EHR in Outcomes and Observational	
		Studies..	62
		7.2.2 The EHR as Tool to Facilitate Patient Enrollment	
		in Prospective Trials	63
		7.2.3 The EHR as Tool to Study and Improve Patient	
		Outcomes......................................	64
	7.3	How to Avoid Common Pitfalls When Using EHR to	
		Do Health Services Research	64
		7.3.1 Step 1: Recognize the Fallibility of the EHR........	65
		7.3.2 Step 2: Understand Confounding, Bias, and	
		Missing Data When Using the EHR	
		for Research	65
	7.4	Future Directions for the EHR and Health Services	
		Research	67
		7.4.1 Ensuring Adequate Patient Privacy Protection......	67
	7.5	Multidimensional Collaborations.........................	67
	7.6	Conclusion	68
	References...		68
8	**Residual Confounding Lurking in Big Data:**		
	A Source of Error...		71
	8.1	Introduction	71
	8.2	Confounding Variables in Big Data	72
		8.2.1 The Obesity Paradox...........................	72
		8.2.2 Selection Bias	73
		8.2.3 Uncertain Pathophysiology	74
	8.3	Conclusion	77
	References...		77
Part II	**A Cookbook: From Research Question Formulation**		
	to Validation of Findings		
9	**Formulating the Research Question**...........................		81
	9.1	Introduction	81
	9.2	The Clinical Scenario: Impact of Indwelling Arterial	
		Catheters..	82
	9.3	Turning Clinical Questions into Research Questions.........	82
		9.3.1 Study Sample	82

		9.3.2	Exposure	83
		9.3.3	Outcome	84
	9.4	Matching Study Design to the Research Question		85
	9.5	Types of Observational Research		87
	9.6	Choosing the Right Database		89
	9.7	Putting It Together		90
	References			91
10	**Defining the Patient Cohort**			93
	10.1	Introduction		93
	10.2	PART 1—Theoretical Concepts		94
		10.2.1	Exposure and Outcome of Interest	94
		10.2.2	Comparison Group	95
		10.2.3	Building the Study Cohort	95
		10.2.4	Hidden Exposures	97
		10.2.5	Data Visualization	97
		10.2.6	Study Cohort Fidelity	98
	10.3	PART 2—Case Study: Cohort Selection		98
	References			100
11	**Data Preparation**			101
	11.1	Introduction		101
	11.2	Part 1—Theoretical Concepts		102
		11.2.1	Categories of Hospital Data	102
		11.2.2	Context and Collaboration	103
		11.2.3	Quantitative and Qualitative Data	104
		11.2.4	Data Files and Databases	104
		11.2.5	Reproducibility	107
	11.3	Part 2—Practical Examples of Data Preparation		109
		11.3.1	MIMIC Tables	109
		11.3.2	SQL Basics	109
		11.3.3	Joins	112
		11.3.4	Ranking Across Rows Using a Window Function	113
		11.3.5	Making Queries More Manageable Using WITH	113
	References			114
12	**Data Pre-processing**			115
	12.1	Introduction		115
	12.2	Part 1—Theoretical Concepts		116
		12.2.1	Data Cleaning	116
		12.2.2	Data Integration	118
		12.2.3	Data Transformation	119
		12.2.4	Data Reduction	120

	12.3	PART 2—Examples of Data Pre-processing in R	121
		12.3.1 R—The Basics	121
		12.3.2 Data Integration	129
		12.3.3 Data Transformation	132
		12.3.4 Data Reduction	136
	12.4	Conclusion	140
	References		141
13	**Missing Data**		**143**
	13.1	Introduction	143
	13.2	Part 1—Theoretical Concepts	144
		13.2.1 Types of Missingness	144
		13.2.2 Proportion of Missing Data	146
		13.2.3 Dealing with Missing Data	146
		13.2.4 Choice of the Best Imputation Method	152
	13.3	Part 2—Case Study	153
		13.3.1 Proportion of Missing Data and Possible Reasons for Missingness	153
		13.3.2 Univariate Missingness Analysis	154
		13.3.3 Evaluating the Performance of Imputation Methods on Mortality Prediction	159
	13.4	Conclusion	161
	References		161
14	**Noise Versus Outliers**		**163**
	14.1	Introduction	163
	14.2	Part 1—Theoretical Concepts	164
	14.3	Statistical Methods	165
		14.3.1 Tukey's Method	166
		14.3.2 Z-Score	166
		14.3.3 Modified Z-Score	166
		14.3.4 Interquartile Range with Log-Normal Distribution	167
		14.3.5 Ordinary and Studentized Residuals	167
		14.3.6 Cook's Distance	167
		14.3.7 Mahalanobis Distance	168
	14.4	Proximity Based Models	168
		14.4.1 k-Means	169
		14.4.2 k-Medoids	169
		14.4.3 Criteria for Outlier Detection	169
	14.5	Supervised Outlier Detection	171
	14.6	Outlier Analysis Using Expert Knowledge	171
	14.7	Case Study: Identification of Outliers in the Indwelling Arterial Catheter (IAC) Study	171
	14.8	Expert Knowledge Analysis	172

	14.9	Univariate Analysis	172
	14.10	Multivariable Analysis	177
	14.11	Classification of Mortality in IAC and Non-IAC Patients	179
	14.12	Conclusions and Summary	181
	Code Appendix	182
	References	183
15	**Exploratory Data Analysis**	185
	15.1	Introduction	185
	15.2	Part 1—Theoretical Concepts	186
		15.2.1 Suggested EDA Techniques	186
		15.2.2 Non-graphical EDA	187
		15.2.3 Graphical EDA	191
	15.3	Part 2—Case Study	199
		15.3.1 Non-graphical EDA	199
		15.3.2 Graphical EDA	200
	15.4	Conclusion	202
	Code Appendix	202
	References	203
16	**Data Analysis**	205
	16.1	Introduction to Data Analysis	205
		16.1.1 Introduction	205
		16.1.2 Identifying Data Types and Study Objectives	206
		16.1.3 Case Study Data	209
	16.2	Linear Regression	210
		16.2.1 Section Goals	210
		16.2.2 Introduction	210
		16.2.3 Model Selection	213
		16.2.4 Reporting and Interpreting Linear Regression	220
		16.2.5 Caveats and Conclusions	223
	16.3	Logistic Regression	224
		16.3.1 Section Goals	224
		16.3.2 Introduction	225
		16.3.3 2×2 Tables	225
		16.3.4 Introducing Logistic Regression	227
		16.3.5 Hypothesis Testing and Model Selection	232
		16.3.6 Confidence Intervals	233
		16.3.7 Prediction	234
		16.3.8 Presenting and Interpreting Logistic Regression Analysis	235
		16.3.9 Caveats and Conclusions	236
	16.4	Survival Analysis	237
		16.4.1 Section Goals	237
		16.4.2 Introduction	237

		16.4.3	Kaplan-Meier Survival Curves.	238

- 16.4.3 Kaplan-Meier Survival Curves... 238
- 16.4.4 Cox Proportional Hazards Models... 240
- 16.4.5 Caveats and Conclusions... 243
- 16.5 Case Study and Summary... 244
  - 16.5.1 Section Goals... 244
  - 16.5.2 Introduction... 244
  - 16.5.3 Logistic Regression Analysis... 250
  - 16.5.4 Conclusion and Summary... 259
- References... 261

17 Sensitivity Analysis and Model Validation... 263
- 17.1 Introduction... 263
- 17.2 Part 1—Theoretical Concepts... 264
  - 17.2.1 Bias and Variance... 264
  - 17.2.2 Common Evaluation Tools... 265
  - 17.2.3 Sensitivity Analysis... 265
  - 17.2.4 Validation... 266
- 17.3 Case Study: Examples of Validation and Sensitivity Analysis... 267
  - 17.3.1 Analysis 1: Varying the Inclusion Criteria of Time to Mechanical Ventilation... 267
  - 17.3.2 Analysis 2: Changing the Caliper Level for Propensity Matching... 268
  - 17.3.3 Analysis 3: Hosmer-Lemeshow Test... 269
  - 17.3.4 Implications for a 'Failing' Model... 269
- 17.4 Conclusion... 270
- Code Appendix... 270
- References... 271

Part III Case Studies Using MIMIC

18 Trend Analysis: Evolution of Tidal Volume Over Time for Patients Receiving Invasive Mechanical Ventilation... 275
- 18.1 Introduction... 275
- 18.2 Study Dataset... 277
- 18.3 Study Pre-processing... 277
- 18.4 Study Methods... 277
- 18.5 Study Analysis... 278
- 18.6 Study Conclusions... 280
- 18.7 Next Steps... 280
- 18.8 Connections... 281
- Code Appendix... 282
- References... 282

19 Instrumental Variable Analysis of Electronic Health Records 285
19.1 Introduction 285
19.2 Methods 287
19.2.1 Dataset 287
19.2.2 Methodology 287
19.2.3 Pre-processing 290
19.3 Results 291
19.4 Next Steps 292
19.5 Conclusions 293
Code Appendix 293
References 293

20 Mortality Prediction in the ICU Based on MIMIC-II Results from the Super ICU Learner Algorithm (SICULA) Project 295
20.1 Introduction 295
20.2 Dataset and Pre-preprocessing 297
20.2.1 Data Collection and Patients Characteristics 297
20.2.2 Patient Inclusion and Measures 297
20.3 Methods 299
20.3.1 Prediction Algorithms 299
20.3.2 Performance Metrics 301
20.4 Analysis 302
20.4.1 Discrimination 302
20.4.2 Calibration 303
20.4.3 Super Learner Library 305
20.4.4 Reclassification Tables 305
20.5 Discussion 308
20.6 What Are the Next Steps? 309
20.7 Conclusions 309
Code Appendix 310
References 311

21 Mortality Prediction in the ICU 315
21.1 Introduction 315
21.2 Study Dataset 316
21.3 Pre-processing 317
21.4 Methods 318
21.5 Analysis 319
21.6 Visualization 319
21.7 Conclusions 321
21.8 Next Steps 321
21.9 Connections 322
Code Appendix 323
References 323

22 Data Fusion Techniques for Early Warning of Clinical Deterioration ... 325
- 22.1 Introduction ... 325
- 22.2 Study Dataset ... 326
- 22.3 Pre-processing ... 327
- 22.4 Methods ... 328
- 22.5 Analysis ... 330
- 22.6 Discussion ... 333
- 22.7 Conclusions ... 335
- 22.8 Further Work ... 335
- 22.9 Personalised Prediction of Deteriorations ... 336
- Code Appendix ... 337
- References ... 337

23 Comparative Effectiveness: Propensity Score Analysis ... 339
- 23.1 Incentives for Using Propensity Score Analysis ... 339
- 23.2 Concerns for Using Propensity Score ... 340
- 23.3 Different Approaches for Estimating Propensity Scores ... 340
- 23.4 Using Propensity Score to Adjust for Pre-treatment Conditions ... 341
- 23.5 Study Pre-processing ... 343
- 23.6 Study Analysis ... 346
- 23.7 Study Results ... 346
- 23.8 Conclusions ... 347
- 23.9 Next Steps ... 347
- Code Appendix ... 348
- References ... 348

24 Markov Models and Cost Effectiveness Analysis: Applications in Medical Research ... 351
- 24.1 Introduction ... 351
- 24.2 Formalization of Common Markov Models ... 352
  - 24.2.1 The Markov Chain ... 352
  - 24.2.2 Exploring Markov Chains with Monte Carlo Simulations ... 353
  - 24.2.3 Markov Decision Process and Hidden Markov Models ... 355
  - 24.2.4 Medical Applications of Markov Models ... 356
- 24.3 Basics of Health Economics ... 356
  - 24.3.1 The Goal of Health Economics: Maximizing Cost-Effectiveness ... 356
  - 24.3.2 Definitions ... 357
- 24.4 Case Study: Monte Carlo Simulations of a Markov Chain for Daily Sedation Holds in Intensive Care, with Cost-Effectiveness Analysis ... 359

24.5	Model Validation and Sensitivity Analysis for Cost-Effectiveness Analysis	364
24.6	Conclusion	365
24.7	Next Steps	366
Code Appendix		366
References		366

25 Blood Pressure and the Risk of Acute Kidney Injury in the ICU: Case-Control Versus Case-Crossover Designs ... 369

25.1	Introduction	369
25.2	Methods	370
	25.2.1 Data Pre-processing	370
	25.2.2 A Case-Control Study	370
	25.2.3 A Case-Crossover Design	372
25.3	Discussion	374
25.4	Conclusions	374
Code Appendix		375
References		375

26 Waveform Analysis to Estimate Respiratory Rate ... 377

26.1	Introduction	377
26.2	Study Dataset	378
26.3	Pre-processing	380
26.4	Methods	381
26.5	Results	384
26.6	Discussion	385
26.7	Conclusions	386
26.8	Further Work	386
26.9	Non-contact Vital Sign Estimation	387
Code Appendix		388
References		389

27 Signal Processing: False Alarm Reduction ... 391

27.1	Introduction	391
27.2	Study Dataset	393
27.3	Study Pre-processing	394
27.4	Study Methods	395
27.5	Study Analysis	397
27.6	Study Visualizations	398
27.7	Study Conclusions	399
27.8	Next Steps/Potential Follow-Up Studies	400
References		401

28 Improving Patient Cohort Identification Using Natural Language Processing ... 405
- 28.1 Introduction ... 405
- 28.2 Methods ... 407
  - 28.2.1 Study Dataset and Pre-processing ... 407
  - 28.2.2 Structured Data Extraction from MIMIC-III Tables ... 408
  - 28.2.3 Unstructured Data Extraction from Clinical Notes ... 409
  - 28.2.4 Analysis ... 410
- 28.3 Results ... 410
- 28.4 Discussion ... 413
- 28.5 Conclusions ... 414
- Code Appendix ... 414
- References ... 415

29 Hyperparameter Selection ... 419
- 29.1 Introduction ... 419
- 29.2 Study Dataset ... 420
- 29.3 Study Methods ... 420
- 29.4 Study Analysis ... 423
- 29.5 Study Visualizations ... 424
- 29.6 Study Conclusions ... 425
- 29.7 Discussion ... 425
- 29.8 Conclusions ... 426
- References ... 427

Erratum to: Secondary Analysis of Electronic Health Records ... E1

Part I
Setting the Stage: Rationale Behind and Challenges to Health Data Analysis

Introduction

While wonderful new medical discoveries and innovations are in the news every day, healthcare providers continue to struggle with using information. Uncertainties and unanswered clinical questions are a daily reality for the decision makers who provide care. Perhaps the biggest limitation in making the best possible decisions for patients is that the information available is usually not focused on the specific individual or situation at hand.

For example, there are general clinical guidelines that outline the ideal target blood pressure for a patient with a severe infection. However, the truly best blood pressure levels likely differ from patient to patient, and perhaps even change for an individual patient over the course of treatment. The ongoing computerization of health records presents an opportunity to overcome this limitation. By analyzing electronic data from many providers' experiences with many patients, we can move ever closer to answering the age-old question: What is truly best for each patient?

Secondary analysis of routinely collected data—contrasted with the primary analysis conducted in the process of caring for the individual patient—offers an opportunity to extract more knowledge that will lead us towards the goal of optimal care. Today, a report from the National Academy of Medicine tells us, most doctors base most of their everyday decisions on guidelines from (sometimes biased) expert opinions or small clinical trials. It would be better if they were from multi-center, large, randomized controlled studies, with tightly controlled conditions ensuring the results are as reliable as possible. However, those are expensive and difficult to perform, and even then often exclude a number of important patient groups on the basis of age, disease and sociological factors.

Part of the problem is that health records are traditionally kept on paper, making them hard to analyze en masse. As a result, most of what medical professionals might have learned from experiences is lost, or is inaccessible at least. The ideal digital system would collect and store as much clinical data as possible from as many patients as possible. It could then use information from the past—such as blood pressure, blood sugar levels, heart rate, and other measurements of patients' body functions—to guide future providers to the best diagnosis and treatment of similar patients.

But "big data" in healthcare has been coated in "Silicon Valley Disruptionese", the language with which Silicon Valley spins hype into startup gold and fills it with grandiose promises to lure investors and early users. The buzz phrase "precision medicine" looms large in the public consciousness with little mention of the failures of "personalized medicine", its predecessor, behind the façade.

This part sets the stage for secondary analysis of electronic health records (EHR). Chapter 1 opens with the rationale behind this type of research. Chapter 2 provides a list of existing clinical databases already in use for research. Chapter 3 dives into the opportunities, and more importantly, the challenges to retrospective analysis of EHR. Chapter 4 presents ideas on how data could be systematically and more effectively employed in a purposefully engineered healthcare system. Professor Roger Mark, the visionary who created the Medical Information Mart for Intensive Care or MIMIC database that is used in this textbook, narrates the story behind the project in Chap. 5. Chapter 6 steps into the future and describes integration of EHR with non-clinical data for a richer representation of health and disease. Chapter 7 focuses on the role of EHR in two important areas of research—outcome and health services. Finally, Chap. 8 tackles the bane of observational studies using EHR: residual confounding.

We emphasize the importance of bringing together front-line clinicians such as nurses, pharmacists and doctors with data scientists to collaboratively identify questions and to conduct appropriate analyses. Further, we believe this research partnership of practitioner and researcher gives caregivers and patients the best individualized diagnostic and treatment options in the absence of a randomized controlled trial. By becoming more comfortable with the data available to us in the hospitals of today, we can reduce the uncertainties that have hindered healthcare for far too long.

Chapter 1
Objectives of the Secondary Analysis of Electronic Health Record Data

Sharukh Lokhandwala and Barret Rush

Take Home Messages

- Clinical medicine relies on a strong research foundation in order to build the necessary evidence base to inform best practices and improve clinical care, however, large-scale randomized controlled trials (RCTs) are expensive and sometimes unfeasible. Fortunately, there exists expansive data in the form of electronic health records (EHR).
- Data can be overwhelmingly complex or incomplete for any individual, therefore we urge multidisciplinary research teams consisting of clinicians along with data scientists to unpack the clinical semantics necessary to appropriately analyze the data.

1.1 Introduction

The healthcare industry has rapidly become computerized and digital. Most healthcare delivered in America today relies on or utilizes technology. Modern healthcare informatics generates and stores immense amounts of detailed patient and clinical process data. Very little real-world patient data have been used to further advance the field of health care. One large barrier to the utilization of these data is inaccessibility to researchers. Making these databases easier to access as well as integrating the data would allow more researchers to answer fundamental questions of clinical care.

1.2 Current Research Climate

Many treatments lack proof in their efficacy, and may, in fact, cause harm [1]. Various medical societies disseminate guidelines to assist clinician decision-making and to standardize practice; however, the evidence used to formulate these guidelines is inadequate. These guidelines are also commonly derived from RCTs with limited patient cohorts and with extensive inclusion and exclusion criteria resulting in reduced generalizability. RCTs, the gold standard in clinical research, support only 10–20 % of medical decisions [2] and most clinical decisions have never been supported by RCTs [3]. Furthermore, it would be impossible to perform randomized trials for each of the extraordinarily large number of decisions clinicians face on a daily basis in caring for patients for numerous reasons, including constrained financial and human resources. For this reason, clinicians and investigators must learn to find clinical evidence from the droves of data that already exists: the EHR.

1.3 Power of the Electronic Health Record

Much of the work utilizing large databases in the past 25 years have relied on hospital discharge records and registry databases. Hospital discharge databases were initially created for billing purposes and lack the patient level granularity of clinically useful, accurate, and complete data to address complex research questions. Registry databases are generally mission-limited and require extensive extracurricular data collection. The future of clinical research lies in utilizing big data to improve the delivery of care to patients.

Although several commercial and non-commercial databases have been created using clinical and EHR data, their primary function has been to analyze differences in severity of illness, outcomes, and treatment costs among participating centers. Disease specific trial registries have been formulated for acute kidney injury [4], acute respiratory distress syndrome [5] and septic shock [6]. Additionally, databases such as the Dartmouth Atlas utilize Medicare claims data to track discrepancies in costs and patient outcomes across the United States [7]. While these coordinated databases contain a large number of patients, they often have a narrow scope (i.e. for severity of illness, cost, or disease specific outcomes) and lack other significant clinical data that is required to answer a wide range of research questions, thus obscuring many likely confounding variables.

For example, the APACHE Outcomes database was created by merging APACHE (Acute Physiology and Chronic Health Evaluation) [8] with Project IMPACT [9] and includes data from approximately 150,000 intensive care unit (ICU) stays since 2010 [1]. While the APACHE Outcomes database is large and has contributed significantly to the medical literature, it has incomplete physiologic and laboratory measurements, and does not include provider notes or waveform data. The Phillips eICU [10], a telemedicine intensive care support provider, contains a database of over 2 million ICU stays. While it includes provider documentation entered into the software, it lacks clinical notes and waveform data. Furthermore, databases with different primary objectives (i.e., costs, quality improvement, or research) focus on different variables and outcomes, so caution must be taken when interpreting analyses from these databases.

1.3 Power of the Electronic Health Record

Since 2003, the Laboratory for Computational Physiology at the Massachusetts Institute of Technology partnered in a joint venture with Beth Israel Deaconess Medical Center and Philips Healthcare, with support from the National Institute of Biomedical Imaging and Bioinformatics (NIBIB), to develop and maintain the Medical Information Mart for Intensive Care (MIMIC) database [11]. MIMIC is a public-access database that contains comprehensive clinical data from over 60,000 inpatient ICU admissions at Beth Israel Deaconess Medical Center. The de-identified data are freely shared, and nearly 2000 investigators from 32 countries have utilized it to date. MIMIC contains physiologic and laboratory data, as well as waveform data, nurse verified numerical data, and clinician documentation. This high resolution, widely accessible, database has served to support research in critical care and assist in the development of novel decision support algorithms, and will be the prototype example for the majority of this textbook.

1.4 Pitfalls and Challenges

Clinicians and data scientists must apply the same level of academic rigor when analyzing research from clinical databases as they do with more traditional methods of clinical research. To ensure internal and external validity, researchers must determine whether the data are accurate, adjusted properly, analyzed correctly, and presented cogently [12]. With regard to quality improvement projects, which frequently utilize hospital databases, one must ensure that investigators are applying rigorous standards to the performance and reporting of their studies [13].

Despite the tremendous value that the EHR contains, many clinical investigators are hesitant to use it to its full capacity partly due to its sheer complexity and the inability to use traditional data processing methods with large datasets. As a solution to the increased complexity associated with this type of research, we suggest that investigators work in collaboration with multidisciplinary teams including data scientists, clinicians and biostatisticians. This may require a shift in financial and academic incentives so that individual research groups do not compete for funding or publication; the incentives should promote joint funding and authorship. This would allow investigators to focus on the fidelity of their work and be more willing to share their data for discovery, rather than withhold access to a dataset in an attempt to be "first" to a solution.

Some have argued that the use of large datasets may increase the frequency of so-called "p-hacking," wherein investigators search for significant results, rather than seek answers to clinically relevant questions. While it appears that p-hacking is widespread, the mean effect size attributed to p-hacking does not generally undermine the scientific consequences from large studies and meta-analyses. The use of large datasets may, in fact, reduce the likelihood of p-hacking by ensuring that researchers have suitable power to answer questions with even small effect sizes, making the need for selective interpretation and analysis of the data to obtain significant results unnecessary. If significant discoveries are made utilizing big databases, this work can be used as a foundation for more rigorous clinical trials to confirm these findings. In the future, once comprehensive databases become more accessible to researchers, it is hoped that these resources can be used as hypothesis generating and testing ground for questions that will ultimately undergo RCT. If there is not a strong signal observed in a large preliminary retrospective study, proceeding to a resource-intensive and time-consuming RCT may not be advisable.

1.5 Conclusion

With advances in data collection and technology, investigators have access to more patient data than at any time in history. Currently, much of these data are inaccessible and underused. The ability to harness the EHR would allow for continuous learning systems, wherein patient specific data are able to feed into a population-based database and provide real-time decision support for individual patients based on data from similar patients in similar scenarios. Clinicians and patients would be able to make better decisions with those resources in place and the results would feed back into the population database [14].

The vast amount of data available to clinicians and scientists poses daunting challenges as well as a tremendous opportunity. The National Academy of Medicine has called for clinicians and researchers to create systems that "foster continuous learning, as the lessons from research and each care experience are systematically captured, assessed and translated into reliable care" [2]. To capture, assess, and translate these data, we must harness the power of the EHR to create data repositories, while also providing clinicians as well as patients with data-driven decision support tools to better treat patients at the bedside.

Open Access This chapter is distributed under the terms of the Creative Commons Attribution-NonCommercial 4.0 International License (http://creativecommons.org/licenses/by-nc/4.0/), which permits any noncommercial use, duplication, adaptation, distribution and reproduction in any medium or format, as long as you give appropriate credit to the original author(s) and the source, a link is provided to the Creative Commons license and any changes made are indicated.

The images or other third party material in this chapter are included in the work's Creative Commons license, unless indicated otherwise in the credit line; if such material is not included in the work's Creative Commons license and the respective action is not permitted by statutory regulation, users will need to obtain permission from the license holder to duplicate, adapt or reproduce the material.

References

1. Celi LA, Mark RG, Stone DJ, Montgomery RA (2013) "Big data" in the intensive care unit. Closing the data loop. Am J Respir Crit Care Med 187:1157–1160
2. Smith M, Saunders R, Stuckhardt L, McGinnis JM (2013) Best care at lower cost: the path to continuously learning health care in America. National Academies Press
3. Mills EJ, Thorlund K, Ioannidis JP (2013) Demystifying trial networks and network meta-analysis. BMJ 346:f2914
4. Mehta RL, Kellum JA, Shah SV, Molitoris BA, Ronco C, Warnock DG, Levin A, Acute Kidney Injury N (2007) Acute Kidney Injury Network: report of an initiative to improve outcomes in acute kidney injury. Crit Care 11:R31
5. The Acute Respiratory Distress Syndrome Network (2000) Ventilation with lower tidal volumes as compared with traditional tidal volumes for acute lung injury and the acute respiratory distress syndrome. N Engl J Med 342:1301–1308
6. Dellinger RP, Levy MM, Rhodes A, Annane D, Gerlach H, Opal SM, Sevransky JE, Sprung CL, Douglas IS, Jaeschke R, Osborn TM, Nunnally ME, Townsend SR, Reinhart K, Kleinpell RM, Angus DC, Deutschman CS, Machado FR, Rubenfeld GD, Webb SA, Beale RJ, Vincent JL, Moreno R, Surviving Sepsis Campaign Guidelines Committee including the Pediatric S (2013) Surviving sepsis campaign: international guidelines for management of severe sepsis and septic shock: 2012. Crit Care Med 41:580–637
7. The Dartmouth Atlas of Health Care. Lebanon, NH. The Trustees of Dartmouth College 2015. Accessed 10 July 2015. Available from http://www.dartmouthatlas.org/
8. Zimmerman JE, Kramer AA, McNair DS, Malila FM, Shaffer VL (2006) Intensive care unit length of stay: Benchmarking based on Acute Physiology and Chronic Health Evaluation (APACHE) IV. Crit Care Med 34:2517–2529
9. Cook SF, Visscher WA, Hobbs CL, Williams RL, Project ICIC (2002) Project IMPACT: results from a pilot validity study of a new observational database. Crit Care Med 30:2765–2770
10. eICU Program Solution. Koninklijke Philips Electronics N.V, Baltimore, MD (2012)
11. Saeed M, Villarroel M, Reisner AT, Clifford G, Lehman L-W, Moody G, Heldt T, Kyaw TH, Moody B, Mark RG (2011) Multiparameter Intelligent Monitoring in Intensive Care II (MIMIC-II): a public-access intensive care unit database. Crit Care Med 39:952
12. Meurer S (2008) Data quality in healthcare comparative databases. MIT Information Quality Industry symposium
13. Davidoff F, Batalden P, Stevens D, Ogrinc G, Mooney SE, group Sd (2009) Publication guidelines for quality improvement studies in health care: evolution of the SQUIRE project. BMJ 338:a3152
14. Celi LA, Zimolzak AJ, Stone DJ (2014) Dynamic clinical data mining: search engine-based decision support. JMIR Med Informatics 2:e13

Chapter 2
Review of Clinical Databases

Jeff Marshall, Abdullah Chahin and Barret Rush

Take Home Messages

- There are several open access health datasets that promote effective retrospective comparative effectiveness research.
- These datasets hold a varying amount of data with representative variables that are conducive to specific types of research and populations. Understanding these characteristics of the particular dataset will be crucial in appropriately drawing research conclusions.

2.1 Introduction

Since the appearance of the first EHR in the 1960s, patient driven data accumulated for decades with no clear structure to make it meaningful and usable. With time, institutions began to establish databases that archived and organized data into central repositories. Hospitals were able to combine data from large ancillary services, including pharmacies, laboratories, and radiology studies, with various clinical care components (such as nursing plans, medication administration records, and physician orders). Here we present the reader with several large databases that are publicly available or readily accessible with little difficulty. As the frontier of healthcare research utilizing large datasets moves ahead, it is likely that other sources of data will become accessible in an open source environment.

2.2 Background

Initially, EHRs were designed for archiving and organizing patients' records. They then became coopted for billing and quality improvement purposes. With time, EHR driven databases became more comprehensive, dynamic, and interconnected.

However, the medical industry has lagged behind other industries in the utilization of big data. Research using these large datasets has been drastically hindered by the poor quality of the gathered data and poorly organised datasets. Contemporary medical data evolved to more than medical records allowing the opportunity for them to be analyzed in greater detail. Traditionally, medical research has relied on disease registries or chronic disease management systems (CDMS). These repositories are a priori collections of data, often specific to one disease. They are unable to translate data or conclusions to other diseases and frequently contain data on a cohort of patients in one geographic area, thereby limiting their generalizability.

In contrast to disease registries, EHR data usually contain a significantly larger number of variables enabling high resolution of data, ideal for studying complex clinical interactions and decisions. This new wealth of knowledge integrates several datasets that are now fully computerized and accessible. Unfortunately, the vast majority of large healthcare databases collected around the world restrict access to data. Some possible explanations for these restrictions include privacy concerns, aspirations to monetize the data, as well as a reluctance to have outside researchers direct access to information pertaining to the quality of care delivered at a specific institution. Increasingly, there has been a push to make these repositories freely open and accessible to researchers.

2.3 The Medical Information Mart for Intensive Care (MIMIC) Database

The MIMIC database (http://mimic.physionet.org) was established in October 2003 as a Bioengineering Research Partnership between MIT, Philips Medical Systems, and Beth Israel Deaconess Medical Center. The project is funded by the National Institute of Biomedical Imaging and Bioengineering [1].

This database was derived from medical and surgical patients admitted to all Intensive Care Units (ICU) at Beth Israel Deaconess Medical Center (BIDMC), an academic, urban tertiary-care hospital. The third major release of the database, MIMIC-III, currently contains more than 40 thousand patients with thousands of variables. The database is de-identified, annotated and is made openly accessible to the research community. In addition to patient information driven from the hospital, the MIMIC-III database contains detailed physiological and clinical data [2]. In addition to big data research in critical care, this project aims to develop and evaluate advanced ICU patient monitoring and decision support systems that will improve the efficiency, accuracy, and timeliness of clinical decision-making in critical care.

2.3 The Medical Information Mart ...

Through data mining, such a database allows for extensive epidemiological studies that link patient data to clinical practice and outcomes. The extremely high granularity of the data allows for complicated analysis of complex clinical problems.

2.3.1 Included Variables

There are essentially two basic types of data in the MIMIC-III database; clinical data driven from the EHR such as patients' demographics, diagnoses, laboratory values, imaging reports, vital signs, etc (Fig. 2.1). This data is stored in a relational database of approximately 50 tables. The second primary type of data is the bedside monitor waveforms with associated parameters and events stored in flat binary files (with ASCII header descriptors). This unique library includes high-resolution data driven from tracings recorded from patients' electroencephalograms (EEGs), electrocardiograms (EKGs or ECGs), and real-time, second to second tracings of vital signs of patients in the intensive care unit. IRB determined the requirement for individual patient consent was waived, as all public data were de-identified.

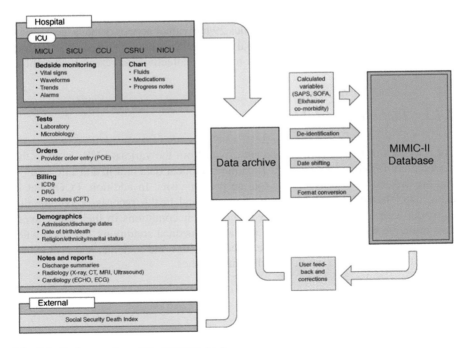

Fig. 2.1 Basic overview of the MIMIC database

2.3.2 Access and Interface

MIMIC-III is an open access database available to any researchers around the globe who are appropriately trained to handle sensitive patient information. The database is maintained by PhysioNet (http://physionet.org), a diverse group of computer scientists, physicists, mathematicians, biomedical researchers, clinicians, and educators around the world. The third release was published in 2015 and is anticipated to continually be updated with additional patients as time progresses.

2.4 PCORnet

PCORnet, the National Patient-Centered Clinical Research Network, is an initiative of the Patient-Centered Outcomes Research Institute (PCORI). PCORI involves patients as well as those who care for them in a substantive way in the governance of the network and in determining what questions will be studied. This PCORnet initiative was started in 2013, hoping to integrate data from multiple Clinical Data Research Networks (CDRNs) and Patient-Powered Research Networks (PPRNs) [3]. Its coordinating center bonds 9 partners: Harvard Pilgrim Health Care Institute, Duke Clinical Research Institute, AcademyHealth, Brookings Institution, Center for Medical Technology Policy, Center for Democracy & Technology, Group Health Research Institute, Johns Hopkins Berman Institute of Bioethics, and America's Health Insurance Plans. PCORnet includes 29 individual networks that together will enable access to large amounts of clinical and healthcare data. The goal of PCORnet is to improve the capacity to conduct comparative effectiveness research efficiently.

2.4.1 Included Variables

The variables in PCORnet database are driven from the various EHRs used in the nine centers forming this network. It captures clinical data and health information that are created every day during routine patient visits. In addition, PCORNet is using data shared by individuals through personal health records or community networks with other patients as they manage their conditions in their daily lives. This initiative will facilitate research on various medical conditions, engage a wide range of patients from all types of healthcare settings and systems, and provide an excellent opportunity to conduct multicenter studies.

2.4.2 Access and Interface

PCORnet is envisioned as a national research resource that will enable teams of health researchers and patients to work together on questions of shared interest. These teams will be able to submit research queries and receive to data conduct studies. Current PCORnet participants (CDRNs, PPRNs and PCORI) are developing the governance structures during the 18-month building and expansion phase [4].

2.5 Open NHS

The National Health Services (NHS England) is an executive non-departmental public body of the Department of Health, a governmental entity. The NHS retains one of the largest repositories of data on people's health in the world. It is also one of only a handful of health systems able to offer a full account of health across care sectors and throughout lives for an entire population.

Open NHS is one branch that was established in October of 2011. The NHS in England has actively moved to open the vast repositories of information used across its many agencies and departments. The main objective of the switch to an open access dataset was to increase transparency and trace the outcomes and efficiency of the British healthcare sector [5]. High quality information is hoped to empower the health and social care sector in identifying priorities to meet the needs of local populations. The NHS hopes that by allowing patients, clinicians, and commissioners to compare the quality and delivery of care in different regions of the country using the data, they can more effectively and promptly identify where the delivery of care is less than ideal.

2.5.1 Included Variables

Open NHS is an open source database that contains publicly released information, often from the government or other public bodies.

2.5.2 Access and Interface

Prior to the creation of Open NHS platform, SUS (Secondary Uses Service) was set up as part of the National Programme for IT in the NHS to provide data for planning, commissioning, management, research and auditing. Open NHS has now replaced SUS as a platform for accessing the national database in the UK.

The National Institute of Health Research (NIHR) Clinical Research Network (CRN) has produced and implemented an online tool known as the Open Data Platform.

In addition to the retrospective research that is routinely conducted using such databases, another form of research is already under way to compare the data quality derived from electronic records with that collected by research nurses. Clinical Research Network staff can access the Open Data Platform and determine the number of patients recruited into research studies in a given hospital as well as the research being done at that hospital. They then determine which hospitals are most successful at recruiting patients, the speed with which they recruit, and in what specialty fields.

2.6 Other Ongoing Research

The following are other datasets that are still under development or have more restrictive access limitations:

2.6.1 eICU—Philips

As part of its collaboration with MIT, Philips will be granting access to data from hundreds of thousands of patients that have been collected and anonymized through the Philips Hospital to Home eICU telehealth program. The data will be available to researchers via PhysioNet, similar to the MIMIC database.

2.6.2 VistA

The **Veterans Health Information Systems and Technology Architecture (VistA)** is an enterprise-wide information system built around the Electronic Health Record (EHR), used throughout the United States Department of Veterans Affairs (VA) medical system. The VA health care system operates over 125 hospitals, 800 ambulatory clinics and 135 nursing homes. All of these healthcare facilities utilize the VistA interface that has been in place since 1997. The VistA system amalgamates hospital, ambulatory, pharmacy and ancillary services for over 8 million US veterans. While the health network has inherent research limitations and biases due to its large percentage of male patients, the staggering volume of high fidelity records available outweighs this limitation. The VA database has been used by numerous medical researchers in the past 25 years to conduct landmark research in many areas [6, 7].

The VA database has a long history of involvement with medical research and collaboration with investigators who are part of the VA system. Traditionally the dataset access has been limited to those who hold VA appointments. However, with the recent trend towards open access of large databases, there are ongoing discussions to make the database available to more researchers. The vast repository of information contained in the database would allow a wide range of researchers to improve clinical care in many domains. Strengths of the data include the ability to track patients across the United States as well as from the inpatient to outpatient settings. As all prescription drugs are covered by the VA system, the linking of this data enables large pharmacoepidemiological studies to be done with relative ease.

2.6.3 NSQUIP

The National Surgical Quality Improvement Project is an international effort spearheaded by the American College of Surgeons (ACS) with a goal of improving the delivery of surgical care worldwide [8]. The ACS works with institutions to implement widespread interventions to improve the quality of surgical delivery in the hospital. A by-product of the system is the gathering of large amounts of data relating to surgical procedures, outcomes and adverse events. All information is gathered from the EHR at the specific member institutions.

The NSQUIP database is freely available to members of affiliated institutions, of which there are over 653 participating centers in the world. This database contains large amounts of information regarding surgical procedures, complications, and baseline demographic and hospital information. While it does not contain the granularity of the MIMIC dataset, it contains data from many hospitals across the world and thus is more generalizable to real-world surgical practice. It is a particularly powerful database for surgical care delivery and quality of care, specifically with regard to details surrounding complications and adverse events from surgery.

Open Access This chapter is distributed under the terms of the Creative Commons Attribution-NonCommercial 4.0 International License (http://creativecommons.org/licenses/by-nc/4.0/), which permits any noncommercial use, duplication, adaptation, distribution and reproduction in any medium or format, as long as you give appropriate credit to the original author(s) and the source, a link is provided to the Creative Commons license and any changes made are indicated.

The images or other third party material in this chapter are included in the work's Creative Commons license, unless indicated otherwise in the credit line; if such material is not included in the work's Creative Commons license and the respective action is not permitted by statutory regulation, users will need to obtain permission from the license holder to duplicate, adapt or reproduce the material.

References

1. Lee J, Scott DJ, Villarroel M, Clifford GD, Saeed M, Mark RG (2011) Open-access MIMIC-II database for intensive care research. In: Annual international conference of the IEEE engineering in medicine and biology society, pp 8315–8318
2. Scott DJ, Lee J, Silva I et al (2013) Accessing the public MIMIC-II intensive care relational database for clinical research. BMC Med Inform Decis Mak 13:9
3. Fleurence RL, Curtis LH, Califf RM, Platt R, Selby JV, Brown JS (2014) Launching PCORnet, a national patient-centered clinical research network. J Am Med Inform Assoc JAMIA 21 (4):578–582
4. Califf RM (2014) The patient-centered outcomes research network: a national infrastructure for comparative effectiveness research. N C Med J 75(3):204–210
5. Open data at the NHS [Internet]. Available from: http://www.england.nhs.uk/ourwork/tsd/data-info/open-data/
6. Maynard C, Chapko MK (2004) Data resources in the department of veterans affairs. Diab Care 27(Suppl 2):B22–B26
7. Smith BM, Evans CT, Ullrich P et al (2010) Using VA data for research in persons with spinal cord injuries and disorders: lessons from SCI QUERI. J Rehabil Res Dev 47(8):679–688
8. NSQUIP at the American College of Surgeons [Internet]. Available from: https://www.facs.org/quality-programs/acs-nsqip

Chapter 3
Challenges and Opportunities in Secondary Analyses of Electronic Health Record Data

Sunil Nair, Douglas Hsu and Leo Anthony Celi

Take Home Messages

- Electronic health records (EHR) are increasingly useful for conducting secondary observational studies with power that rivals randomized controlled trials.
- Secondary analysis of EHR data can inform large-scale health systems choices (e.g., pharmacovigilance) or point-of-care clinical decisions (e.g., medication selection).
- Clinicians, researchers and data scientists will need to navigate numerous challenges facing big data analytics—including systems interoperability, data sharing, and data security—in order to utilize the full potential of EHR and big data-based studies.

3.1 Introduction

The increased adoption of EHR has created novel opportunities for researchers, including clinicians and data scientists, to access large, enriched patient databases. With these data, investigators are in a position to approach research with statistical power previously unheard of. In this chapter, we present and discuss challenges in the secondary use of EHR data, as well as explore the unique opportunities provided by these data.

3.2 Challenges in Secondary Analysis of Electronic Health Records Data

Tremendous strides have been made in making pooled health records available to data scientists and clinicians for health research activities, yet still more must be done to harness the full capacity of big data in health care. In all health related fields, the data-holders—i.e., pharmaceutical firms, medical device companies, health systems, and now burgeoning electronic health record vendors—are simultaneously facing pressures to protect their intellectual capital and proprietary platforms, ensure data security, and adhere to privacy guidelines, without hindering research which depends on access to these same databases. Big data success stories are becoming more common, as highlighted below, but the challenges are no less daunting than they were in the past, and perhaps have become even more demanding as the field of data analytics in healthcare takes off.

Data scientists and their clinician partners have to contend with a research culture that is highly competitive—both within academic circles, and among clinical and industrial partners. While little is written about the nature of data secrecy within academic circles, it is a reality that tightening budgets and greater concerns about data security have pushed researchers to use such data as they have on-hand, rather than seek integration of separate databases. Sharing data in a safe and scalable manner is extremely difficult and costly or impossible even within the same institution. With access to more pertinent data restricted or impeded, statistical power and the ability for longitudinal analysis are reduced or lost. None of this is to say researchers have hostile intentions—in fact, many would appreciate the opportunity for greater collaboration in their projects. However, the time, funding, and infrastructure for these efforts are simply deficient. Data is also often segregated into various locales and not consistently stored in similar formats across clinical or research databases. For example, most clinical data is kept in a variety of unstructured formats, making it difficult to query directly via digital algorithms [1]. Within many hospitals, emergency department or outpatient clinical data may exist separately from the hospital and the Intensive Care Unit (ICU) electronic health records, so that access to one does not guarantee access to the other. Images from Radiology and Pathology are typically stored separately in yet other different systems and therefore are not easily linked to outcomes data. The Medical Information Mart for Intensive Care (MIMIC) database described later in this chapter, which contains ICU EHR data from the Beth Israel Deaconess Medical Center (BIDMC), addresses and resolves these artificial divisions, but requires extensive engineering and support staff not afforded to all institutions.

After years of concern about data secrecy, the pharmaceutical industry has recently turned a corner, making detailed trial data available to researchers outside their organizations. GlaxoSmithKline was among the first in 2012 [2], followed by a larger initiative—the Clinical Trial Data Request—to which other large pharmaceutical firms have signed-on [3]. Researchers can apply for access to large-scale information, and integrate datasets for meta-analysis and other systematic reviews. The next frontier will be the release of medical records held at the health system level. The 2009 Health Information Technology for Economic and Clinical Health (HITECH) Act was a boon to the HIT sector [4], but standards for interoperability between record systems continue to lag [5]. The gap has begun to be resolved by government sponsored health information exchanges, as well as the creation of novel research networks [6, 7], but most experts, data scientists, and working clinicians continue to struggle with incomplete data.

Many of the commercial and technical roadblocks alluded to above have their roots in the privacy concerns held by vendors, providers and their patients. Such concerns are not without merit—data breaches of large health systems are becoming distressingly common [8]. Employees of Partners Healthcare in Boston were recently targeted in a "phishing" scheme, unwittingly providing personal information that allowed hackers unauthorized access to patient information [9]; patients of Seton Healthcare in Texas suffered a similar breach just a few months prior [10]. Data breaches aren't limited to healthcare providers—80 million Anthem enrollees may have suffered loss of their personal information to a cyberattack, the largest of its kind to-date [11]. Not surprisingly in the context of these breaches, healthcare companies have some of the lowest scores of all industries in email security and privacy practices [12]. Such reports highlight the need for prudence amidst exuberance when utilizing pooled electronic health records for big data analytics—such use comes with an ethical responsibility to protect population- and personal-level data from criminal activity and other nefarious ends. For this purpose, federal agencies have convened working groups and public hearings to address gaps in health information security, such as the de-identification of data outside HIPAA-covered entities, and consensus guidelines on what constitutes "harm" from a data breach [13].

Even when issues of data access, integrity, interoperability, security and privacy have been successfully addressed, substantial infrastructure and human capital costs will remain. Though the marginal cost of each additional big data query is small, the upfront cost to host a data center and employ dedicated data scientists can be significant. No figures exist for the creation of a healthcare big data center, and these figures would be variable anyway, depending on the scale and type of data. However, it should not be surprising that commonly cited examples of pooled EHRs with overlaid analytic capabilities—MIMIC (BIDMC), STRIDE (Stanford), the MemorialCare data mart (Memorial Health System, California, $2.2 Billion annual revenue), and the High Value Healthcare Collaborative (hosted by Dartmouth, with 16 other members and funding from the Center for Medicare and Medicaid Services) [14]—come from large, high revenue healthcare systems with regional big-data expertise.

In addition to the above issues, the reliability of studies published using big data methods is of significant concern to experts and physicians. The specific issue is whether these studies are simply amplifications of low-level signals that do not have clinical importance, or are generalizable beyond the database from which they are derived. These are genuine concerns in a medical and academic atmosphere already saturated with innumerable studies of variable quality. Skeptics are concerned that big data analytics will only, "add to the noise," diverting attention and resources from other venues of scientific inquiry, such as the traditional randomized controlled clinical trial (RCT). While the limitations of RCTs, and the favorable comparison of large observational study results to RCT findings are discussed below, these sentiments nevertheless have merit and must be taken seriously as secondary analysis of EHR data continues to grow. Thought leaders have suggested expounding on the big data principles described above to create open, collaborative learning environments, whereby de-identified data can be shared between researchers—in this manner, data sets can be pooled for greater power, or similar inquiries run on different data sets to see if similar conclusions are reached [15]. The costs for such transparency could be borne by a single institution—much of the cost of creating MIMIC has already been invested, for instance, so the incremental cost of making the data open to other researchers is minimal—or housed within a dedicated collaborative—such as the High Value Healthcare Collaborative funded by its members [16] or PCORnet, funded by the federal government [7]. These collaborative ventures would have transparent governance structures and standards for data access, permitting study validation and continuous peer review of published and unpublished works [15], and mitigating the effects of selection bias and confounding in any single study [17].

As pooled electronic health records achieve even greater scale, data scientists, researchers and other interested parties expect that the costs of hosting, sorting, formatting and analyzing these records are spread among a greater number of stakeholders, reducing the costs of pooled EHR analysis for all involved. New standards for data sharing may have to come into effect for institutions to be truly comfortable with records-sharing, but within institutions and existing research collaboratives, safe practices for data security can be implemented, and greater collaboration encouraged through standardization of data entry and storage. Clear lines of accountability for data access should be drawn, and stores of data made commonly accessible to clarify the extent of information available to any institutional researcher or research group. The era of big data has arrived in healthcare, and only through continuous adaptation and improvement can its full potential be achieved.

3.3 Opportunities in Secondary Analysis of Electronic Health Records Data

The rising adoption of electronic health records in the U.S. health system has created vast opportunities for clinician scientists, informaticians and other health researchers to conduct queries on large databases of amalgamated clinical information to answer questions both large and small. With troves of data to explore, physicians and scientists are in a position to evaluate questions of clinical efficacy and cost-effectiveness—matters of prime concern in 21st century American health care—with a qualitative and statistical power rarely before realized in medical research. The commercial APACHE Outcomes database, for instance, contains physiologic and laboratory measurements from over 1 million patient records across 105 ICUs since 2010 [18]. The Beth Israel Deaconess Medical Center—a tertiary care hospital with 649 licensed beds including 77 critical care beds—provides an open-access single-center database (MIMIC) encompassing data from over 60,000 ICU stays [19].

Single- and multi-center databases such as those above permit large-scale inquiries without the sometimes untenable expense and difficulty of a randomized clinical trial (RCT), thus answering questions previously untestable in RCTs or prospective cohort studies. This can also be done with increased precision in the evaluation of diagnostics or therapeutics for select sub-populations, and for the detection of adverse events from medications or other interventions with greater expediency, among other advantages [20]. In this chapter, we offer further insight into the utility of secondary analysis of EHR data to investigate relevant clinical questions and provide useful decision support to physicians, allied health providers and patients.

3.4 Secondary EHR Analyses as Alternatives to Randomized Controlled Clinical Trials

The relative limitations of RCTs to inform real-world clinical decision-making include the following: many treatment comparisons of interest to clinicians have not been addressed by RCTs; when RCTs have been performed and appraised, half of systemic reviews of RCTs report insufficient evidence to support a given medical intervention; and, there are realistic cost and project limitations that prevent RCTs from exploring specific clinical scenarios. The latter include rare conditions, clinically uncommon or disparate events, and a growing list of combinations of recognized patient sub-groups, concurrent conditions (genetic, chronic, acute and healthcare-acquired), and diagnostic and treatment options [20, 21].

Queries on EHR databases to address clinical questions are essentially large, nonrandomized observational studies. Compared to RCTs, they are relatively more efficient and less expensive to perform [22], the majority of the costs having been absorbed by initial system installation and maintenance, and the remainder consisting primarily of research personnel salaries, server or cloud space costs. There is literature to suggest a high degree of correlation between treatment effects reported in nonrandomized studies and randomized clinical trials. Ioannidis et al. [23] found significant correlation (Spearman coefficient of 0.75, $p < 0.001$) between the treatment effects reported in randomized trials versus nonrandomized studies across 45 diverse topics in general internal medicine, ranging from anticoagulation in myocardial infarction to low-level laser therapy for osteoarthritis. Of particular interest, significant variability in reported treatment outcome "was seen as frequently among the randomized trials as between the randomized and nonrandomized studies," and they observed that variability was common among *both* randomized trials and nonrandomized studies [23]. It is worth pointing out that larger treatment effects were more frequently reported in nonrandomized studies than randomized trials (exact $p = 0.009$) [23]; however, this need not be evidence of publication bias, as relative study size and conservative trial protocol could also cause this finding. Ioannidis et al.'s [24] results are echoed by a more recent Cochrane meta-analysis, which found no significant difference in effect estimates between RCTs and observational studies regardless of the observational study design or heterogeneity.

To further reduce confounding in observational studies, researchers have employed propensity scoring [25], which allows balancing of numerous covariates between treatment groups as well as stratification of samples by propensity score for more nuanced analysis [26]. Kitsios and colleagues matched 18 unique propensity score studies in the ICU setting with at least one RCT evaluating the same clinical question and found a high degree of agreement between their estimates of relative risk and effect size. There was substantial difference in the magnitude of effect sizes in a third of comparisons, reaching statistical significance in one case [27]. Though the RCT remains atop the hierarchy of evidence-based medicine, it is hard to ignore the power of large observational studies that include adequate adjusting for covariates, such as carefully performed studies derived from review of EHRs. The scope of pooled EHR data—whether sixty thousand or one million records—affords insight into small treatment effects that may be under-reported or even missed in underpowered RCTs. Because costs are small compared to RCTs, it is also possible to investigate questions where realistically no study-sponsor will be found. Finally, in the case of databased observational studies, it becomes much more feasible to improve and repeat, or simply repeat, studies as deemed necessary to investigate accuracy, heterogeneity of effects, and new clinical insights.

3.5 Demonstrating the Power of Secondary EHR Analysis: Examples in Pharmacovigilance and Clinical Care

The safety of pharmaceuticals is of high concern to both patients and clinicians. However, methods for ensuring detection of adverse events post-release are less robust than might be desirable. Pharmaceuticals are often prescribed to a large, diverse patient population that may have not been adequately represented in pre-release clinical trials. In fact, RCT cohorts may deliberately be relatively homogeneous in order to capture the intended effect(s) of a medication without "noise" from co-morbidities that could modulate treatment effects [28]. Humphreys and colleagues (2013) reported that in highly-cited clinical trials, 40 % of identified patients with the condition under consideration were not enrolled, mainly due to restrictive eligibility criteria [29]. Variation in trial design (comparators, endpoints, duration of follow-up) as well as trial size limit their ability to detect low-frequency or long-term side-effects and adverse events [28]. Post-market surveillance reports are imperfectly collected, are not regularly amalgamated, and may not be publically accessible to support clinical-decision making by physicians or inform decision-making by patients.

Queries on pooled EHRs—essentially performing secondary observational studies on large study populations—could compensate for these gaps in pharmacovigilance. Single-center approaches for this and similar questions regarding medication safety in clinical environments are promising. For instance, the highly publicized findings of the Kaiser Study on Vioxx® substantiated prior suspicions of an association between celecoxib and increased risk of serious coronary heart disease [30]. These results were made public in April 2004 after presentation at an international conference; Vioxx® was subsequently voluntarily recalled from the market in September of the same year. Graham and colleagues were able to draw on *2,302,029* person-years of follow-up from the Kaiser Permanente database, to find 8143 cases of coronary heart disease across all NSAIDs under consideration, and subsequently drill-down to the appropriate odds ratios [31].

Using the MIMIC database mentioned above, researchers at the Beth Israel Deaconess Medical Center were able to describe for the first time an increased mortality risk for ICU patients who had been on selective serotonin reuptake inhibitors prior to admission [32]. A more granular analysis revealed that mortality varied by specific SSRI, with higher mortality among patients taking higher-affinity SSRIs (i.e., those with greater serotonin inhibition); on the other hand, mortality could not be explained by common SSRI adverse effects, such as impact on hemodynamic variables [32].

The utility of secondary analysis of EHR data is not limited to the discovery of treatment effects. Lacking published studies to guide their decision to potentially anticoagulate a pediatric lupus patient with multiple risk factors for thrombosis, physicians at Stanford turned to their own EHR-querying platform (the Stanford Translational Research Integrated Database Environment—STRIDE) to create an electronic cohort of pediatric lupus patients to study complications from this illness [33]. In four hours' time, a single clinician determined that patients with similar lupus complications had a high relative risk of thrombosis, and the decision was made to administer anticoagulation [33].

3.6 A New Paradigm for Supporting Evidence-Based Practice and Ethical Considerations

Institutional experiences such as those above, combined with evidence supporting the efficacy of observational trials to adequately inform clinical practice, validate the concept of pooled EHRs as large study populations possessing copious amounts of information waiting to be tapped for clinical decision support and patient safety. One can imagine a future clinician requesting a large or small query such as those described above. Such queries might relate to the efficacy of an intervention across a subpopulation, or for a single complicated patient whose circumstances are not satisfactorily captured in any published trial. Perhaps this is sufficient for the clinician to recommend a new clinical practice; or maybe they will design a pragmatic observational study for more nuance—evaluating dose-responsiveness, or adverse effect profiles across subpopulations. As clinical decisions are made and the patient's course of care shaped, this intervention and outcomes information is entered into the electronic health record, effectively creating a feedback loop for future inquiries [34].

Of course, the advantages of secondary analysis of electronic health records must always be balanced with ethical considerations. Unlike traditional RCTs, there is no explicit consent process for the use of demographic, clinical and other potentially sensitive data captured in the EHR. Sufficiently specific queries could yield very narrow results—theoretically specific enough to re-identify an individual patient. For instance, an inquiry on patients with a rare disease, within a certain age bracket, and admitted within a limited timeframe, could include someone who may be known to the wider community. Such an extreme example highlights the need for compliance with federal privacy laws as well as ensuring high institutional standards of data security such as secured servers, limited access, firewalls from the internet, and other data safety methods.

Going further, data scientists should consider additional measures intentionally designed to protect patient anonymity, e.g. date shifting as implemented in the MIMIC database (see Sect. 5.1, Chap. 5). In situations where queries might potentially re-identify patients, such as in the investigation of rare diseases, or in the course of a contagious outbreak, researchers and institutional research boards should seek accommodation with this relatively small subset of potentially affected patients and their advocacy groups, to ensure their comfort with secondary analyses. Disclosure of research intent and methods by those seeking data access might be required, and a patient option to embargo one's own data should be offered.

It is incumbent on researchers and data scientists to explain the benefits of participation in a secondary analysis to patients and patient groups. Such sharing allows the medical system to create a clinical database of sufficient magnitude and quality to benefit individual- and groups of patients, in real-time or in the future. Also, passive clinical data collection allows the patient to contribute, at relatively very low risk and no personal cost, to the ongoing and future care of others. We believe that people are fundamentally sufficiently altruistic to consider contributions their data to research, provided the potential risks of data usage are small and well-described.

Ultimately, secondary analysis of EHR will only succeed if patients, regulators, and other interested parties are assured and reassured that their health data will be kept safe, and processes for its use are made transparent to ensure beneficence for all.

Open Access This chapter is distributed under the terms of the Creative Commons Attribution-NonCommercial 4.0 International License (http://creativecommons.org/licenses/by-nc/4.0/), which permits any noncommercial use, duplication, adaptation, distribution and reproduction in any medium or format, as long as you give appropriate credit to the original author(s) and the source, a link is provided to the Creative Commons license and any changes made are indicated.

The images or other third party material in this chapter are included in the work's Creative Commons license, unless indicated otherwise in the credit line; if such material is not included in the work's Creative Commons license and the respective action is not permitted by statutory regulation, users will need to obtain permission from the license holder to duplicate, adapt or reproduce the material.

References

1. Riskin D (2012) Big data: opportunity and challenge. HealthcareITNews, 12 June 2012. URL: http://www.healthcareitnews.com/news/big-data-opportunity-and-challenge
2. Harrison C (2012) GlaxoSmithKline opens the door on clinical data sharing. Nat Rev Drug Discov 11(12):891–892. doi:10.1038/nrd3907 [Medline: 23197021]
3. Clinical Trial Data Request. URL: https://clinicalstudydatarequest.com/. Accessed 11 Aug 2015. [WebCite Cache ID 6TFyjeT7t]
4. Adler-Milstein J, Jha AK (2012) Sharing clinical data electronically: a critical challenge for fixing the health care system. JAMA 307(16):1695–1696
5. Verdon DR (2014) ONC's plan to solve the EHR interoperability puzzle: an exclusive interview with National Coordinator for Health IT Karen B. DeSalvo. Med Econ. URL: http://medicaleconomics.modernmedicine.com/medical-economics/news/onc-s-plan-solve-ehr-interoperability-puzzle?page=full
6. Green M (2015) 10 things to know about health information exchanges. Becker's Health IT CIO Rev. URL: http://www.beckershospitalreview.com/healthcare-information-technology/10-things-to-know-about-health-information-exchanges.html
7. PCORnet. URL: http://www.pcornet.org/. Accessed 11 Aug 2015
8. Dvorak K (2015) Big data's biggest healthcare challenge: making sense of it all. FierceHealthIT, 4 May 2015. URL: http://www.fiercehealthit.com/story/big-datas-biggest-healthcare-challenge-making-sense-it-all/2015-05-04
9. Bartlett J (2015) Partners healthcare reports data breach. Boston Bus J. URL: http://www.bizjournals.com/boston/blog/health-care/2015/04/partners-healthcare-reports-potential-data-breach.html
10. Dvorak K (2015) Phishing attack compromises info of 39 K at Seton healthcare family. FierceHealthIT, 28 April 2015. URL: http://www.fiercehealthit.com/story/phishing-attack-compromises-info-39k-seton-healthcare-family/2015-04-28
11. Bowman D (2015) Anthem hack compromises info for 80 million customers. FierceHealthPayer, 5 February 2015. URL: http://www.fiercehealthpayer.com/story/anthem-hack-compromises-info-80-million-customers/2015-02-05
12. Dvorak K (2015) Healthcare industry 'behind by a country mile' in email security. FierceHealthIT, 20 February 2015. URL: http://www.fiercehealthit.com/story/healthcare-industry-behind-country-mile-email-security/2015-02-20
13. White house seeks to leverage health big data, safeguard privacy. HealthData Manage. URL: http://www.healthdatamanagement.com/news/White-House-Seeks-to-Leverage-Health-Big-Data-Safeguard-Privacy-50829-1.html
14. How big data impacts healthcare. Harv Bus Rev. URL: https://hbr.org/resources/pdfs/comm/sap/18826_HBR_SAP_Healthcare_Aug_2014.pdf. Accessed 11 Aug 2015
15. Moseley ET, Hsu DJ, Stone DJ, Celi LA (2014) Beyond open big data: addressing unreliable research. J Med Internet Res 16(11):e259

16. High value healthcare collaborative. URL: http://highvaluehealthcare.org/. Accessed 14 Aug 2015
17. Badawi O, Brennan T, Celi LA et al (2014) Making big data useful for health care: a summary of the inaugural mit critical data conference. JMIR Med Inform 2(2):e22
18. APACHE Outcomes. Available at: https://www.cerner.com/Solutions/Hospitals_and_Health_Systems/Critical_Care/APACHE_Outcomes/. Accessed Nov 2014
19. Saeed M, Villarroel M, Reisner AT et al (2011) Multiparameter intelligent monitoring in intensive care II (MIMIC-II): a public-access intensive care unit database. Crit Care Med 39:952
20. Ghassemi M, Celi LA, Stone DJ (2015) State of the art review: the data revolution in critical care. Crit Care 19:118
21. Mills EJ, Thorlund K, Ioannidis J (2013) Demystifying trial networks and network meta-analysis. BMJ 346:f2914
22. Angus DC (2007) Caring for the critically ill patient: challenges and opportunities. JAMA 298:456–458
23. Ioannidis JPA, Haidich A-B, Pappa M et al (2001) Comparision of evidence of treatment effects in randomized and nonrandomized studies. JAMA 286:7
24. Anglemyer A, Horvath HT, Bero L (2014) Healthcare outcomes assess with observational study designs compared with those assessed in randomized trials. Cochrane Database Syst Rev 29:4
25. Gayat E, Pirracchio R, Resche-Rigon M et al (2010) Propensity scores in intensive care and anaesthesiology literature: a systematic review. Intensive Care Med 36:1993–2003
26. Glynn RJ, Schneeweiss S, Stürmer T (2006) Indications for propensity scores and review of their use in pharmacoepidemiology. Basic Clin Pharmacol Toxicol 98:253–259
27. Kitsios GD, Dahabreh IJ, Callahan S et al (2015) Can we trust observational studies using propensity scores in the critical care literature? A systematic comparison with randomized clinical trials. Crit Care Med (Epub ahead of print)
28. Celi LA, Moseley E, Moses C et al (2014) from pharmacovigilance to clinical care optimization. Big Data 2(3):134–141
29. Humphreys K, Maisel NC, Blodgett JC et al (2013) Extent and reporting of patient nonenrollment in influential randomized clinical trials, 2001 to 2010. JAMA Intern Med 173:1029–1031
30. Vioxx and Drug Safety. Statement of Sandra Kweder M.D. (Deputy Director, Office of New Drugs, US FDA) before the Senate Committee on Finance. Available at: http://www.fda.gov/NewsEvents/Testimony/ucm113235.htm. Accessed July 2015
31. Graham DJ, Campen D, Hui R et al (2005) Risk of acute myocardial infarction and sudden cardiac death in patients treated with cyclo-oxygenase 2 selective and non-selective non-steroidal anti-inflammatory drugs: nested case-control study. Lancet 365(9458):475–481
32. Ghassemi M, Marshall J, Singh N et al (2014) Leveraging a critical care database: selective serotonin reuptake inhibition use prior to ICU admission is associated with increased hospital mortality. Chest 145(4):1–8
33. Frankovich J, Longhurst CA, Sutherland SM (2011) Evidence-based medicine in the EMR era. New Engl J Med 365:19
34. Celi LA, Zimolzak AJ, Stone DJ (2014) Dynamic clinical data mining: search engine-based decision support. JMIR Med Inform 2(1):e13

Chapter 4
Pulling It All Together: Envisioning a Data-Driven, Ideal Care System

David Stone, Justin Rousseau and Yuan Lai

Take Home Messages

- An Ideal Care System should incorporate fundamental elements of control engineering, such as effective and data-driven sensing, computation, actuation, and feedback.
- These systems must be carefully and intentionally designed to support clinical decision-making, rather than being allowed to evolve based on market pressures and user convenience.

This chapter presents ideas on how data could be systematically more effectively employed in a purposefully engineered healthcare system. We have previously written on potential components of such a system—e.g. dynamic clinical data mining, closing the loop on ICU data, optimizing the data system itself, crowdsourcing, etc., and will attempt to 'pull it all together' in this chapter, which we hope will inspire and encourage others to think about and move to create such a system [1–10]. Such a system, in theory, would support clinical workflow by [1] leveraging data to provide both accurate personalized, or 'precision,' care for individuals while ensuring optimal care at a population level; [2] providing coordination and communication among the users of the system; and [3] defining, tracking, and enhancing safety and quality. While health care is intrinsically heterogeneous at the level of individual patients, encounters, specialties, and clinical settings, we also propose some general systems-based solutions derived from contextually defined use cases. This chapter describes the fundamental infrastructure of an Ideal Care System (ICS) achieved through identifying, organizing, capturing, analyzing, utilizing and appropriately sharing the data.

4.1 Use Case Examples Based on Unavoidable Medical Heterogeneity

The intrinsic heterogeneities inherent in health care at the level of individual patients, encounters, specialties, and clinical settings has rendered the possibility of a single simple systems solution impossible. We anticipate requirements in an ICS

Table 4.1 Clinical use cases with pertinent clinical and data objectives

Clinical use case	Clinical objective(s)	Data objectives
Outpatient in state of good health	Provide necessary preventive care; address mild intermittent acute illnesses	Health maintenance documentation: vaccination records, cancer screening records, documentation of allergies; data on smoking and obesity
Outpatient with complex chronic medical problems	Connect and coordinate care among diverse systems and caregivers	Ensure accurate and synchronized information across care domains without need for oversight by patient and/or family; targeted monitors to prevent admission, readmission
Inpatient—elective surgery	Provide a safe operative and perioperative process	Track processes relevant to safety and quality; track outcomes, complication rates, including safety related outcomes
Inpatient (emergency department, inpatient wards, intensive care units)	Identify and predict ED patients who require ICU care; ICU safety and quality; Identify and predict adverse events	Track outcomes of ED patients including ICU transfers and mortality; Track adverse events; Track usual and innovative ICU metrics
Nursing home patient	Connect and coordinate care among diverse locations and caregivers for a patient who may not be able to actively participate in the process	Ensure accurate and synchronized information across care domains without need for oversight by patient and/or family
Recent discharge from hospital	Prevent re-admission	Data mining for predictors associated with re-admission and consequent interventions based on these determinations; Track functional and clinical outcomes
Labor and delivery	Decision and timing for caesarian section; Lower rates of intervention and complications	Data mining for predictors associated with c-section or other interventions; track complication rates and outcomes
Palliative care/end of life	Decision and timing for palliative care; Ensure comfort and integrity	Data mining to determine characteristics that indicate implementation of palliative care

of identifying common core elements that apply to the medical care of all patients (e.g. safety principles, preventive care, effective end of life care, accurate and up-to-date problem list and medication list management), and subsequently formulating pathways based on specific context. One should note that an individual patient can cross over multiple categories. Any complex outpatient will also have the baseline requirements of meeting objectives of an outpatient in good health and may at some point have an inpatient encounter. Table 4.1 identifies a variety of use cases including abbreviated forms of the pertinent clinical and data issues associated with them.

4.2 Clinical Workflow, Documentation, and Decisions

The digitalization of medicine has been proceeding with the wide adoption of electronic health records, thanks in part to meaningful use as part of the Health Information Technology for Economic and Clinical Health (HITECH) Act [11], but has received varying responses by clinicians. An extensive degree of digitalization is a fundamental element for creating an ICS. Defined at the highest level, a system is a collection of parts and functions (a.k.a. components and protocols) that accepts inputs and produces outputs [3]. In healthcare, the inputs are the patients in various states of health and disease, and the outputs are the outcomes of these patients. Figure 4.1 provides a simple control loop describing the configuration of a data driven health system.

The practice of medicine has a long history of being data driven, with diagnostic medicine dating back to ancient times [12]. Doctors collect and assemble data from histories, physical exams, and a large variety of tests to formulate diagnoses, prognoses, and subsequent treatments. However, this process has not been optimal in the sense that these decisions, and the subsequent actuations based on these decisions, have been made in relative isolation. The decisions depend on the prior experience and current knowledge state of the involved clinician(s), which may or may not be based appropriately on supporting evidence. In addition, these decisions have, for the most part, not been tracked and measured to determine their impact on safety and quality. We have thereby lost much of what has been done that was good and failed to detect much of what was bad [1]. The digitization of medicine provides an opportunity to remedy these issues. In spite of the suboptimal usability of traditional paper documentation, the entries in physicians' notes in natural language constitute the core data required to fuel an ideal care system. While data items such as lab values and raw physiological vital signs may be reasonably reliable and quantitative, they generally do not represent the decision-making and the diagnoses that are established or being considered, which are derived from the analysis and

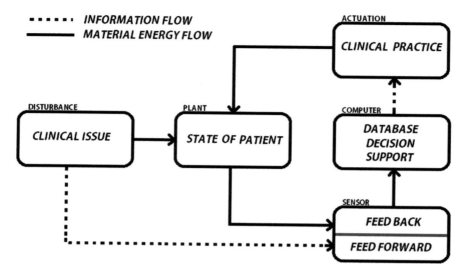

Fig. 4.1 Control loop depicting a data-driven care system. A clinical issue such as an infection or vascular occlusion affects the state of the patient. Subsequently, the system sensor detects this change and submits the relevant data to the computer for storage and analysis. This may or may not result in actuation of a clinical practice intervention that further affects the state of the patient, which feeds back into the system for further analysis. Feed-forward control involves the transmission of disturbances directly to the sensor without first affecting the state of the patient. The detection of a risk factor for venous thromboembolism that triggers prophylaxis in a protocol-based manner represents a clinical example of feed-forward control [3]

synthesis of the available data (the assessment with differential diagnosis) as well as the data to be acquired in the diagnostic workup (the plan).

The digitalization of medicine has encountered two key issues: [1] How does one develop a digitally based workflow that supports rapid, accurate documentation so that the clinician feels enlightened rather than burdened by the process? [2] How can the documentation process of data entry support and enhance the medical decision-making process? The first iteration of electronic health records (EHRs) has simply attempted to replicate the traditional paper documentation in a digital format. In order to address the first issue, smarter support of the documentation process will require innovative redesigns to improve the EHR as it evolves. Rather than requiring the clinician to sit at a keyboard facing away from a patient, the process needs to capture real-time input from the patient encounter in such potential modes as voice and visual recognition. This must be done so that the important details are captured without unduly interfering with personal interactions or without erroneous entries due to delayed recall. The receiving system must 'consider' the patient's prior information in interpreting new inputs in order to accurately recognize and

4.2 Clinical Workflow, Documentation, and Decisions

assimilate the essential information from the current encounter. Furthermore, the data that is collected should not be functionally lost as the patient advances through time and moves between geographic locales. A critical issue is one that has been perpetuated in the current practice of medicine from one encounter to another—the physician and patient should not need to 'reinvent the informational wheel' with every encounter. While each physician should provide a fresh approach to the patient, this should not require refreshing the patient's entire medical story with each single encounter, wasting time and effort. Furthermore, what is documented should be transparent to the patient in contrast to the physician beneficence model that has been practiced for most of the history of medicine where it was considered beneficial to restrict patients' access to their own records. Steps are being taken toward this goal of transparency with the patient with the OpenNotes movement that began in 2010. The effects of this movement are being recognized nationally with significant potential benefits in many areas relating to patient safety and quality of care [13].

Regarding the second issue, we have written of how quality data entry can support medical decision-making [14]. Future iterations of an innovatively redesigned EHR in an ideal care system should assist in the smart assembly and presentation of the data as well as presentation of decision support in the form of evidence and education. The decision-maker is then able to approach each encounter with the advantage of prior knowledge and supporting evidence longitudinally for the individual patient as well as comparisons of their states of health with patients with similar data and diagnoses (Fig. 4.2). Patterns and trends in the data can be recognized, particularly in the context of that patient's prior medical history and evolving current state (Fig. 4.3).

Population data should be leveraged to optimize decisions for individuals, with information from individual encounters captured, stored and utilized to support the care of others as we have described as 'dynamic clinical data mining [2].' This also is similar to what has been described as a 'learning healthcare system' or by a 'green button' for consulting such population data for decision support [15, 16].

In summary, an ICS must have tools (e.g. enhanced versions of current EHRs) to capture and utilize the data in ways that make documentation and decision-making effective and efficient rather than isolated and burdensome. While we realize that individual clinicians function brilliantly in spite of the technical and systems-level obstacles and inefficiencies with which they are faced, we have reached a point of necessity, one recognized by the Institute of Medicine threatening the quality and safety of healthcare, requiring the development of digital tools that facilitate necessary data input and decisions as well as tools that can interact with and incorporate other features of an integrated digitally-based ICS [17]. This will require close interactions and collaborations among health care workers, engineers including software and hardware experts, as well as patients, regulators, policy-makers, vendors and hospital business and technical administrators [5].

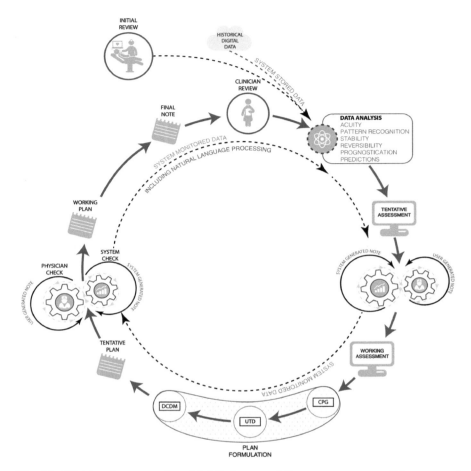

Fig. 4.2 Clinician documentation with fully integrated data systems support. Prior notes and data are input for future notes and decisions. The digital system analyzes input and displays suggested diagnoses and problem list, and then diagnostic test and treatment recommendations hierarchically based on various levels of evidence: CPG—clinical practice guidelines, UTD—Up to Date®, DCDM—Dynamic clinical data mining [14]

4.3 Levels of Precision and Personalization

Many of the tools available to clinicians have become fantastically sophisticated, including technical devices and molecular biological and biochemical knowledge. However, other elements, including those used intensively on a daily basis, are more primitive and would be familiar to clinicians of the distant past. These elements include clinical data such as the heart rates and blood pressures recorded in a

4.3 Levels of Precision and Personalization

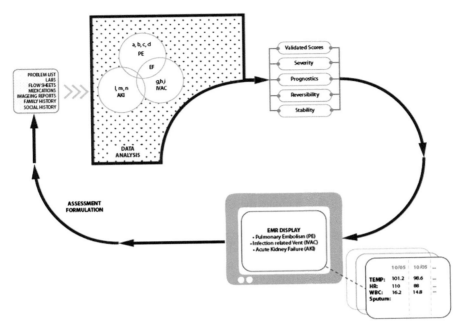

Fig. 4.3 Mock screenshot for the Assessment screen with examples of background data analytics. Based on these analytics that are constantly being performed by the system and are updated as the user begins to enter a note, a series of problems are identified and suggested to the user by EMR display. After consideration of these suggestions in addition to their own analysis, the user can select or edit the problems that are suggested or input entirely new problems. The final selection of problems is considered with ongoing analytics for future assessments [14]

nursing flowsheet. Patient monitoring is not generally employed on a data driven basis, particularly decisions regarding who gets monitored with what particular signals, the duration of monitoring, and whether the data are stored, analyzed, and utilized beyond the current time. Furthermore, it is questionable whether the precedent of setting common numeric thresholds for abnormally high or low values extracts maximal clinical information from those signals. This recognition of abnormal values has become a significant problem of excessive false alarms and alarm fatigue [18]. Data analysis should provide clinicians with personalized and contextualized characterizations of individual vital signs (e.g. heart and respiratory rate variability patterns, subtle ECG waveform shapes, etc.) so that truly important changes can be recognized quickly and effectively while not overwhelming the cognitive load of the clinician. This would constitute 'personalized data driven monitoring' in which the raw data on the monitor screen is analyzed in real time to provide more information regarding the state of the patient. This will become more important and pressing as monitoring becomes more ubiquitous both in the hospital and in outpatient settings, which is not far from a reality with the exponential development of mobile health monitors and applications. A potential approach to this issue would be to treat monitors as specialized component of the EHR rather than standalone devices that display the heart rate and beep frequently, at times even when there is no good reason. In fact, this has occurred to some functional extent as monitors have become networked and in many cases can import data into the EHR. The loop will be closed when information flows bi-directionally so that the EHR (and other elements such as infusion pumps) can assist in providing clinical contexts and personalized information to enhance the performance potential of the monitors [14]. Whereas the user interface of the monitor is currently solely one of adjusting the monitored channels and the alarm settings, the user interface will also be increasingly rich so that the user could, for instance with the proper credentials, access, edit and annotate the EHR from a bedside or central monitor, or add information directly to the monitor to calibrate the monitoring process.

The data from monitors is beginning to be used for prospective analytic purposes in terms of predicting neonatal sepsis and post cardiac surgery problems [19, 20]. The HeRO neonatal alert focuses on diminution in heart rate variability and increase in decelerations to identify potential sepsis, whereas the Etiometry alert employs a sophisticated statistical analysis of those monitored elements reflecting cardiac function to detect and define problems earlier than humans could ordinarily do. The HeRO team is now working to develop predictive analytics for respiratory deterioration, significant hemorrhage, and sepsis in adults [21]. The essential point is that monitors employing such predictive analytics, as well as streaming and retrospective analytics, can leverage large amounts of personal data to improve the monitoring process as well as the healthcare encounter experience, particularly in areas of quality and safety. However, it is essential that such individual applications, exponentially growing in complexity and sophistication, not be introduced as unrelated bits into an already data-overburdened and under-engineered health care system. In the current state of the healthcare system, there is already plenty of data. However, it is not being systematically handled, utilized and leveraged. It is essential that such new applications be embedded thoughtfully into workflows. They must also be systematically interfaced and interoperable with the core care system, represented by the next generation of EHRs, so that the information can be used in a coordinated fashion, audited in terms of its impact on workflows, and tracked in terms of its impact on patient outcomes, quality, and safety. The addition of further system elements should be planned, monitored, and evaluated in a data-driven fashion. New elements should contribute to the system that uses data in a targeted, well-managed fashion rather than simply collecting it. The introduction of elements outside the core EHR requires communication and coordination among all system elements, just as effectively using the EHR alone requires communication and coordination among caregivers and patients.

4.4 Coordination, Communication, and Guidance Through the Clinical Labyrinth

Coordination and communication would be fundamental properties of an ICS contrasted with the enormous individual efforts required to achieve these goals in the current state. Patients and caregivers should be able to assume that the system captures, stores, and shares their information where and when it is needed. When the patient leaves her nursing home to be seen in a local emergency room or by her neurologist, the clinicians should have all previously available information necessary to treat her. This should also be the case when she returns to the nursing home with the system updating her record with events from her previous encounter as well as implementing new orders reflecting that encounter. This seamless communication and coordination is especially important for the kinds of patients who cannot provide this support themselves: people who are elderly, cognitively impaired, acutely ill, etc. Unfortunately, the current system was developed as a tool to aid in billing and reimbursement of interventions and the challenge that we face with transforming and continuing to develop it into an ICS is to transition its focus to patient care. Currently, patients and their advocates must battle with unrelenting challenges of opacity and obstruction facing immense frustration and threats to patient safety and quality of care where such risks would not be tolerated in any other industry.

Data and the efficient transmission of information where and when it is needed are at the core of an ICS. Information networks that permeate all the relevant locales must be created employing all the interoperability, privacy, and security features necessary. The system must maintain its focus on the patient and must instantly (or sufficiently quickly to meet clinical needs) update, synchronize, and transmit the information to all those who need to know, including qualified and permitted family members and the patients themselves relevant to the care of the patient. Many clinicians may be misinterpreted as being unresponsive, or even uncaring, in response to their continuing frustration with the difficulty of obtaining timely and accurate information. The current state of siloed healthcare systems makes obtaining information from other locales prohibitively challenging with no particular reward for continuing to struggle to obtain pertinent information for the continued care of patients, evoking reactions from caregivers including rudeness, neglect, hostility, or burnout. This challenge to obtain information from outside sources also leads to repeat diagnostic testing exposing patients to unnecessary risks and exposures such as is seen when a patient is transferred from one institution to another but the imaging obtained at the first institution is not able to be transferred appropriately [22]. Unfortunately, the Health Insurance Portability and Accountability Act of 1996 (HIPAA), the very legislation designed to enable the portability of information relevant to patient care, has further hindered this transmission of information. An efficient system of communication and coordination would benefit the caregiver experience in addition to the patients by providing them with the tools and information that they need to carry out their jobs.

The scope of those affected by the challenges inherent in the current healthcare system is broad. Not only does it affect those that are cognitively impaired, but also those with limited education or resources. It affects those that have complicated medical histories as well as those without previous histories. Even when patients are capable of contributing to the management of their own clinical data, there is potential to be overwhelmed and incapacitated through the complexities of the system when affected by illness, no matter the acuity, severity, or complexity. Interoperable EHRs focused on patients rather than locations or brands would provide the necessary and updated information as a patient moves from office A to hospital system B to home and back to emergency room C. When people are sick, they and their caregivers should be supported by the system rather than forced to battle it.

The sharing of data among patients and caregivers in a safe and efficient manner is not primarily a technical problem at this time, although there are many technical challenges to achieving such seamless interoperability. It is also a business as well as a political problem. This complex interaction can be seen in efforts toward healthcare architecture and standards supporting interoperability described in the JASON report, "A Robust Health Data Infrastructure" with responses from industry and EHR vendors in the development and adoption of HL7 Fast Healthcare Interoperability Resources (FHIR) standards [23, 24]. In an ICS, all parties must cooperate to interconnect EHRs among caregivers and locals so that the accurate and reliable data essential for healthcare can be coordinated, synchronized, and communicated across practice domains but within each patient's domain. As we have seen on individual patient levels, an overabundance of data is not useful if it is not processed, analyzed, placed into the appropriate context, and available to the right people at the right places and times.

4.5 Safety and Quality in an ICS

There are many examples in healthcare, such as with bloodletting with leeches, where what was thought to be best practice, based on knowledge or evidence at the time, was later found to be harmful to patients. Our knowledge and its application must be in a continual state of assessment and re-assessment so that unreliable elements can be identified and action taken before, or at least minimal, harm is done [4]. There is currently no agreement on standard metrics for safety and quality in healthcare and we are not going to attempt to establish standard definitions in this chapter [25]. However, in order to discuss these issues, it is important to establish a common understanding of the terminologies and their meaning.

At a conceptual level, we conceive clinical **safety** as a strategic optimization problem in which the maximum level of permissible actuation must be considered and implemented in the simultaneous context of allowing the minimal degree of care-related harm. The objective is to design and implement a care system that minimizes safety risks to approach a goal of zero. The digitization of medicine

4.5 Safety and Quality in an ICS

affords a realistic chance of attaining this goal in an efficient and effective manner. The application of systems engineering principles also provides tools to design these kinds of systems.

The overall **quality** of healthcare is a summation of the experience of individuals, and for these individuals, there may be varying degrees of quality for different periods of their experience. Similar to safety, we also think of quality as a strategic optimization problem in which outcomes and benefits are maximized or optimized, while the costs and risks involved in the processes required to achieve them, are minimized. The provision of quality via optimized outcomes in clinical care is, to a large extent, a problem in engineering information reliability and flow, providing the best evidence at the right times to assist in making the best decisions [3]. The concepts of the 'best evidence' and 'best decisions' themselves depend on input sources that range from randomized control trials to informed expert opinion to local best practices. To provide actual actuation, information flows must be supplemented by chemical (medications), mechanical (surgery, physical therapy, injections, human touch) and electromagnetic (imaging, ultrasound, radiation therapy, human speech) modalities, which can institute the processes indicated by those information flows.

Furthermore, quality may also be defined with respect to the degree of success in treatment of the disease state. Diseases addressed in modern medicine are, to a surprisingly large and increasingly recognized extent, those of control problems in bioengineering [10]. These diseases may stem from control problems affecting inflammation, metabolism, physiological homeostasis, or the genome. However, these all represent failure in an element or elements of a normally well-controlled biological system. The quality of the clinical response to these failures is best improved by understanding them sufficiently and thoroughly enough so that targeted and tolerable treatments can be developed that control and/or eliminate the systems dysfunction represented by clinical disease. This should be accomplished in a way that minimizes undue costs in physical, mental, or even spiritual suffering. Ultimately, medical quality is based primarily on outcomes, but the nature of the processes leading to those outcomes must be considered. Optimal outcomes are desirable, but not at any cost, in the broad definition of the term. For example, prolonging life indefinitely is not an optimal outcome in some circumstances that are contextually defined by individual, family, and cultural preferences.

Having defined safety and quality in our context, the next step is to develop systems that capture, track and manage these concepts in retrospective, real-time, and predictive manners. It is only when we know precisely what static and dynamic elements of safety and quality we wish to ensure that we can design the systems to support these endeavors. These systems will involve the integration of hardware and software systems such as physiologic monitors with the EHR (including Computerized Provider Order Entry, Picture Archiving and Communication System, etc.), and will require a variety of specialized, domain-specific data analytics as well as technical innovations such as wireless body sensor networks to capture patient status in real time. The system will connect and communicate pertinent information among caregivers by populating standardized, essential access and alert nodes with timely and accurate information. It is also necessary that information flows bi-directionality (from the records of individuals to the population record, and from the population record to individuals) so that both can benefit from the data [2, 14]. Clearly, this will require an overall monitoring and information system that is interoperable, interactive both with its own components and its users, and actively but selectively informative. Future generations of clinicians will receive their education in an environment in which these systems are ubiquitous, selectively modifiable based on inputs such as crowdsourcing, and intrinsic to the tasks at hand, in contrast to the siloed and apparently arbitrarily imposed applications current clinicians may resist and resent [5, 8].

We noted the importance of control problems in disease, and control will also represent a fundamental component in the design of future safety and quality systems. The detection and prevention of adverse events is a significant challenge when depending on self-reporting methods or chart review and this issue is of high importance in the US [26, 27]. Predictive analytics can be developed as elements of the system to prospectively inform users of threats to safety and quality [19–21]. Carefully designed feed-forward components will inform participants in real time that an high risk activity is occurring so that it can be rectified without requiring retroactive analysis (Fig. 4.4—safety control loop below). Retrospective data analytics will track the factors affecting quality and safety so that practice,

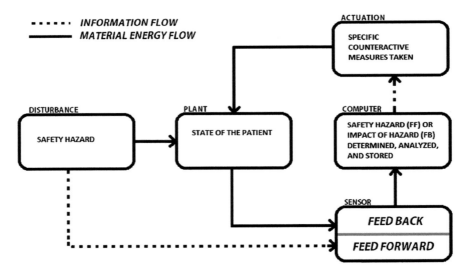

Fig. 4.4 Control loop depicting a data-driven safety system. A clinical safety issue affects the state of the patient. Subsequently, the system sensor detects this change and submits the relevant data to the computer for storage and analysis. This may or may not result in actuation of a counteractive intervention that further affects the state of the patient, which feeds back into the system for further analysis. Feed-forward control involves the transmission of disturbances directly to the sensor without first affecting the state of the patient. An example of such a feed-forward control includes a faulty device or a biohazard

4.5 Safety and Quality in an ICS

workflow, and technological systems can be accordingly modified. Such an ICS will be capable of monitoring medical errors, adverse events, regulatory and safety agency concerns and metrics, and compliance with best practice as well as meaningful use in parallel with costs and outcomes.

4.6 Conclusion

The basic systems solutions to the health care data problem rest on fully and inclusively addressing the axes of patient, care giver and care system considerations, which at times are apparently independent, but are ultimately interactive and interdependent. The required systems design will also greatly benefit from basic incorporation of the fundamental elements of control engineering such as effective and data-driven sensing, computation, actuation, and feedback. An Ideal Care System must be carefully and intentionally designed rather than allowed to evolve based on market pressures and user convenience.

The patient's data should be accurate, complete, and up-to-date. As patients progress in time, their records must be properly and timely updated with new data while concurrently, old data are modified and/or deleted as the latter become irrelevant or no longer accurate. New entry pipelines such as patient-generated and remotely generated data, as well as genomic data, must be taken into consideration and planned for. These data should be securely, reliably, and easily accessible to the designated appropriate users including the patient. The caregiver should have access to these data via a well-designed application that positively supports the clinical documentation process and includes reasonable and necessary decision support modalities reflecting best evidence, historical data of similar cases in the population, as well as the patient's own longitudinal data. All should have access to the data so far as it is utilized to construct the current and historical patterns of safety and quality. In addition to the data of individuals, access to the data of populations is required for the above purposes as well as to provide effective interventions in emergency situations such as epidemics. The creation of this kind of multimodal systems solution (Fig. 4.5—Ideal Care System Architecture below) will require the input of a great variety of experts including those from the EHR, monitoring devices, data storage, and data analytic industries along with leaders in healthcare legislation, policy makers, regulation, and administration.

Many important engineering, economic, and political questions remain that are not addressed in this chapter. What and who will provide the infrastructure and who will pay for it? Will this kind of system continue to work with current hardware and software or require fundamental upgrades to function at the required level of reliability and security? How and where will the controls be embedded in the system?

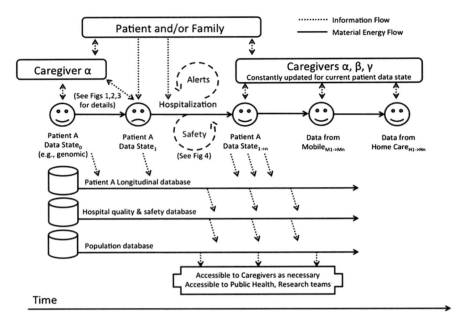

Fig. 4.5 Information Architecture of an Ideal Care System. This diagram integrates the concepts described in this chapter depicting data driven care systems, safety systems, along with connection and coordination of patient data across multiple modalities to achieve an Ideal Care System. Patients move through time and interact with the ICS in different contexts. Parallel databases are integrated with the patient data states in time including an individual patient's longitudinal database, hospital quality and safety database, and a population database. Data from the patient, mobile technologies and from the home care entities keep caregivers informed of the most current patient data state

For example, will they be at the individual smart monitoring level or at a statewide public health level? How will the metadata obtained be handled for the good of individuals and populations? It is critical that the addition of new modalities and devices be fully integrated into the system rather than adding standalone components that may contribute more complexity and confusion than benefit. These goals will require cooperation previously unseen among real and potential competitors and those who have previously been able to work in relative isolation.

Open Access This chapter is distributed under the terms of the Creative Commons Attribution-NonCommercial 4.0 International License (http://creativecommons.org/licenses/by-nc/4.0/), which permits any noncommercial use, duplication, adaptation, distribution and reproduction in any medium or format, as long as you give appropriate credit to the original author(s) and the source, a link is provided to the Creative Commons license and any changes made are indicated.

The images or other third party material in this chapter are included in the work's Creative Commons license, unless indicated otherwise in the credit line; if such material is not included in the work's Creative Commons license and the respective action is not permitted by statutory regulation, users will need to obtain permission from the license holder to duplicate, adapt or reproduce the material.

References

1. Celi LA, Mark RG, Stone DJ, Montgomery R (2013) "Big data" in the ICU: closing the data loop. Am J Respir Crit Care Med 187(11):1157–1160
2. Celi LA, Zimolzak AJ, Stone DJ (2014) Dynamic clinical data mining: search engine-based clinical decision support. J Med Internet Res Med Inform 2(1):e13. doi:10.2196/medinform.3110
3. Celi LA, Csete M, Stone D (2014) Optimal data systems: the future of clinical predictions and decision support. Curr Opin Crit Care 20:573–580
4. Moseley ET, Hsu D, Stone DJ, Celi LA (2014) Beyond data liberation: addressing the problem of unreliable research. J Med Internet Res 16(11):e259
5. Celi LA, Ippolito A, Montgomery R, Moses C, Stone DJ (2014) Crowdsourcing knowledge discovery and innovations in medicine. J Med Internet Res 16(9):e216. doi:10.2196/jmir.3761
6. Celi LA, Moseley E, Moses C, Ryan P, Somai M, Stone DJ, Tang K (2014) From pharmacovigilance to clinical care optimization. Big Data 2(3):134–141. doi:10.1089/big.2014.0008
7. Badawi O, Brennan T, Celi LA, Feng M, Ghassemi M, Ippolito A, Johnson A, Mark RG, Mayaud L, Moody G, Moses C, Naumann T, Pimentel M, Pollard TJ, Santos M, Stone DJ, Zimolzak AJ (2014) Making big data useful for health care: a summary of the inaugural MIT critical data conference. J Med Internet Res Med Inform 2(2):e22. doi:10.2196/medinform.3447
8. Moskowitz A, McSparron J, Stone DJ, Celi LA (2015) Preparing a new generation of clinicians for the era of big data. Harvard Med Student Rev 2(1):24–27
9. Ghassemi M, Celi LA, Stone DJ (2015) The data revolution in critical care. Ann Update Intensive Care Emerg Med 2015(2015):573–586
10. Stone DJ, Csete ME, Celi LA (2015) Engineering control into medicine. J Crit Care. Published Online: January 29, 2015. doi:10.1016/j.jcrc.2015.01.019
11. Health Information Technology for Economic and Clinical Health (HITECH) Act, Title XIII of Division A and Title IV of Division B of the American Recovery and Reinvestment Act of 2009 (ARRA), Pub. L. No. 111-5, 123 Stat. 226 (Feb. 17, 2009), codified at 42 U.S.C. §§300jj et seq.; §§17901 et seq
12. Horstmanshoff HFJ, Stol M, Tilburg C (2004) Magic and rationality in ancient near Eastern and Graeco-Roman medicine, pp 97–99. Brill Publishers. ISBN 978-90-04-13666-3
13. Bell SK, Folcarelli PH, Anselmo MK, Crotty BH, Flier LA, Walker J (2014) Connecting Patients and Clinicians: The Anticipated Effects of Open Notes on Patient Safety and Quality of Care. Jt Comm J Qual Patient Saf 41(8):378–384(7)
14. Celi LA, Marshall JD, Lai Y, Stone DJ, Physician documentation and decision making in the digital era. J Med Internet Res Med Inform (Forthcoming)
15. Longhurst CA, Harrington RA, Shah NH (2014) A 'green button' for using aggregate patient data at the point of care. Health Aff 33(7):1229–1235
16. Friedman C, Rubin J, Brown J et al (2014) J Am Med Inform Assoc 0:1–6. doi:10.1136/amiajnl-2014-002977
17. Institute of Medicine (2012) Best care at lower cost: the path to continuously learning health care in America. Retrieved from: http://iom.nationalacademies.org/Reports/2012/Best-Care-at-Lower-Cost-The-Path-to-Continuously-Learning-Health-Care-in-America.aspx
18. The Joint Commission (2014) National Patient safety goal on alarm management 2013
19. www.etiometry.com
20. www.heroscore.com
21. Personal communication, Randall Moorman, MD
22. Sodickson A, Opraseuth J, Ledbetter S (2011) Outside imaging in emergency department transfer patients: CD import reduces rates of subsequent imaging utilization. Radiology 260(2):408–413

23. A Robust Health Data Infrastructure. (Prepared by JASON at the MITRE Corporation under Contract No. JSR-13-700). Agency for Healthcare Research and Quality, Rockville, MD. April 2014. AHRQ Publication No. 14-0041-EF
24. Health Level Seven® International. HL7 Launches Joint Argonaut Project to Advance FHIR. N.p., 4 Dec. 2014. Web. 31 Aug. 2015. http://www.hl7.org/documentcenter/public_temp_32560CB2-1C23-BA17-0CBD5D492A8F70CD/pressreleases/HL7_PRESS_20141204.pdf
25. Austin JM et al (2015) National hospital ratings systems share few common scores and may generate confusion instead of clarity. Health Aff 34(3):423–430. doi:10.1377/hlthaff.2014.0201
26. Elton GEBM, Ripcsak GEH (2005) Automated detection of adverse events using natural language processing of discharge summaries. J Am Med Inform Assoc 12:448–458
27. Kohn LT, Corrigan JM, Donaldson MS (eds) (2000) To err is human: building a safer health system, vol 2. National Academy Press, Washington, DC

Chapter 5
The Story of MIMIC

Roger Mark

Take Home Messages

- MIMIC is a Medical Information Mart for Intensive Care and consists of several comprehensive data streams in the intensive care environment, in high levels of richness and detail, supporting complex signal processing and clinical querying that could permit early detection of complex problems, provide useful guidance on therapeutic interventions, and ultimately lead to improved patient outcomes.
- This complicated effort required a committed and coordinated collaboration across academic, industry, and clinical institutions to provide a radically open access data platform accessible by researchers around the world.

5.1 The Vision

Patients in hospital intensive care units (ICUs) are physiologically fragile and unstable, generally have life-threatening conditions, and require close monitoring and rapid therapeutic interventions. They are connected to an array of equipment and monitors, and are carefully attended by the clinical staff. Staggering amounts of data are collected daily on each patient in an ICU: multi-channel waveform data sampled hundreds of times each second, vital sign time series updated each second or minute, alarms and alerts, lab results, imaging results, records of medication and fluid administration, staff notes and more. In early 2000, our group at the Laboratory of Computational Physiology at MIT recognized that the richness and detail of the collected data opened the feasibility of creating a new generation of monitoring systems to track the physiologic state of the patient, employing the power of modern signal processing, pattern recognition, computational modeling, and knowledge-based clinical reasoning. In the long term, we hoped to design monitoring systems that not only synthesized and reported all relevant measurements to clinicians, but also formed pathophysiologic hypotheses that best explained the observed data. Such systems would permit early detection of complex problems, provide useful guidance on therapeutic interventions, and ultimately lead to improved patient outcomes.

It was also clear that although petabytes of data are captured daily during care delivery in the country's ICUs, most of these data were not being used to generate evidence or to discover new knowledge. The challenge, therefore, was to employ existing technology to collect, archive and organize finely detailed ICU data, resulting in a research resource of enormous potential to create new clinical knowledge, new decision support tools, and new ICU technology. We proposed to develop and make public a "substantial and representative" database gathered from complex medical and surgical ICU patients.

5.2 Data Acquisition

In 2003, with colleagues from academia (Massachusetts Institute of Technology), industry (Philips Medical Systems), and clinical medicine (Beth Israel Deaconess Medical Center, BIDMC) we received NIH (National Institutes of Health) funding to launch the project "Integrating Signals, Models and Reasoning in Critical Care", a major goal of which was to build a massive critical care research database. The study was approved by the Institutional Review Boards of BIDMC (Boston, MA) and MIT (Cambridge, MA). The requirement for individual patient consent was waived because the study would not impact clinical care and all protected health information was to be de-identified.

We set out to collect comprehensive clinical and physiologic data from all ICU patients admitted to the multiple adult medical and surgical ICUs of our hospital (BIDMC). Each patient record began at ICU admission and ended at final discharge from the hospital. The data acquisition process was continuous and invisible to staff. It did not impact the care of patients or methods of monitoring. Three categories of data were collected: *clinical data*, which were aggregated from ICU information systems and hospital archives; high-resolution *physiological data* (waveforms and time series of vital signs and alarms obtained from bedside monitors); and *death data* from Social Security Administration Death Master Files (See Fig. 5.1).

5.2.1 Clinical Data

Bedside clinical data were downloaded from archived data files of the CareVue Clinical Information System (Philips Healthcare, Andover, MA) used in the ICUs. Additional clinical data were obtained from the hospital's extensive digital archives. The data classes included:

5.2 Data Acquisition

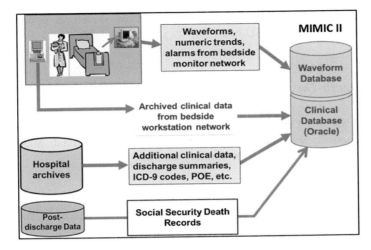

Fig. 5.1 MIMIC II data sources

- **Patient demographics**
- **Hospital administrative data**: admission/discharge/death dates, room tracking, billing codes, etc.
- **Physiologic**: hourly vital signs, clinical severity scores, ventilator settings, etc.
- **Medications**: IV medications, physician orders
- **Lab tests**: chemistry, hematology, ABGs, microbiology, etc.
- **Fluid balance data**
- **Notes and reports**: Discharge summaries; progress notes; ECG, imaging and echo reports.

5.2.2 Physiological Data

Physiological data were obtained with the technical assistance of the monitoring system vendor. Patient monitors were located at every ICU patient bed. Each monitor acquired and digitized multi-parameter physiological waveform data, processed the signals to derive time series (trends) of clinical measures such as heart rate, blood pressures, and oxygen saturation, etc., and also produced bedside monitor alarms. The waveforms (such as electrocardiogram, blood pressures, pulse plethysmograms, respirations) were sampled at 125 Hz, and trend data were updated each minute. The data were subsequently stored temporarily in a central database server that typically supported several ICUs. A customized archiving agent created and stored permanent copies of the physiological data. The data were physically transported from the hospital to the laboratory every 2–4 weeks where they were de-identified, converted to an open source data format, and incorporated into the MIMIC II waveform database. Unfortunately, limited capacity and intermittent failures of the archiving agents limited waveform collection to a fraction of the monitored ICU beds.

5.2.3 Death Data

The Social Security Death Master files were used to document subsequent dates of death for patients who were discharged alive from the hospital. Such data are important for 28-day and 1-year mortality studies.

5.3 Data Merger and Organization

A major effort was required in order to organize the diverse collected data into a well-documented relational database containing integrated medical records for each patient. Across the hospital's clinical databases, patients are identified by their unique Medical Record Numbers and their Fiscal Numbers (the latter uniquely identifies a particular hospitalization for patients who might have been admitted multiple times), which allowed us to merge information from many different hospital sources. The data were finally organized into a comprehensive relational database. More information on database merger, in particular, how database integrity was ensured, is available at the MIMIC-II web site [1]. The database user guide is also online [2].

An additional task was to convert the patient waveform data from Philips' proprietary format into an open-source format. With assistance from the medical equipment vendor, the waveforms, trends, and alarms were translated into WFDB, an open data format that is used for publicly available databases on the National Institutes of Health-sponsored *PhysioNet* web site [3].

All data that were integrated into the MIMIC-II database were de-identified in compliance with Health Insurance Portability and Accountability Act standards to facilitate public access to MIMIC-II. Deletion of protected health information from structured data sources was straightforward (e.g., database fields that provide the patient name, date of birth, etc.). We also removed protected health information from the discharge summaries, diagnostic reports, and the approximately 700,000 free-text nursing and respiratory notes in MIMIC-II using an automated algorithm that has been shown to have superior performance in comparison to clinicians in detecting protected health information [4]. This algorithm accommodates the broad spectrum of writing styles in our data set, including personal variations in syntax, abbreviations, and spelling. We have posted the algorithm in open-source form as a general tool to be used by others for de-identification of free-text notes [5].

5.4 Data Sharing

MIMIC-II is an unprecedented and innovative open research resource that grants researchers from around the world free access to highly granular ICU data and in the process substantially accelerates knowledge creation in the field of critical care medicine. The MIMIC Waveform Database is freely available to all via the PhysioNet website, and no registration is required. The MIMIC Clinical Database is also available without cost. To restrict users to legitimate medical researchers, access to the clinical database requires completion of a simple data use agreement (DUA) and proof that the researcher has completed human subjects training [6].

The MIMIC-II clinical database is available in two forms. In the first form, interested researchers can obtain a flat-file text version of the clinical database and the associated database schema that enables them to reconstruct the database using a database management system of their choice. In the second form, interested researchers can gain limited access to the database through QueryBuilder, a password-protected web service. Database searches using QueryBuilder allow users to familiarize themselves with the database tables and to program database queries using the Structured Query Language. Query output, however, is limited to 1000 rows because of our laboratory's limited computational resources. Accessing and processing data from MIMIC-II is complex. It is recommended that studies based on the MIMIC-II clinical database be conducted as collaborative efforts that include clinical, statistical, and relational database expertise. Detailed documentation and procedures for obtaining access to MIMIC-II are available at the MIMIC-II web site [1]. The current release of MIMIC-II is version 2.6, containing approximately 36,000 patients, including approximately 7000 neonates, and covering the period 2001–2008. At the present time approximately 1700 individuals worldwide in academia, industry, and medicine have been credentialed to access MIMIC-II and are producing research results in physiologic signal processing, clinical decision support, predictive algorithms in critical care, pharmacovigilance, natural language processing, and more.

5.5 Updating

In 2008 the hospital made a major change in the ICU information system technology and in ICU documentation procedures. The Philips CareVue system was replaced with iMDsoft's MetaVision technology. In 2013 we began a major update to MIMIC to incorporate adult ICU data for the period 2008–2012. The effort required learning the entirely new data schema of MetaVision, and merging the new data format with the existing MIMIC design. The new MetaVision data included new data elements such as physician progress notes, oral and bolus medication administration records, etc. Updated data were extracted from hospital archives and from the SSA death files for the newly added patients. Almost two years of effort was invested to acquire, organize, debug, normalize and document the new database before releasing it.

MIMIC-III includes 20,000 new adult ICU admissions, bringing the total to approximately 60,000. The new database is known as MIMIC-III, and the acronym has been recast as "Medical Information Mart for Intensive Care" [7].

5.6 Support

Support of the MIMIC databases includes: credentialing new users, administration of the authorized user list (i.e. users who have signed the DUA and have been granted permission to access MIMIC-II), user account creation, password resets and granting/revoking permissions. The servers providing MIMIC-II include authentication, application, database and web servers. All systems must be monitored, maintained, upgraded and backed up; the maintenance burden continues to increase as the number of database users grows. The engineering staff at LCP attempt to answer user queries as needed. Common questions are added to list of frequently asked questions on the MIMIC website and we regularly update our online documentation.

5.7 Lessons Learned

Building and distributing MIMIC-like databases is challenging, complex, and requires the cooperation and support of a number of individuals and institutions. A list of some of the more important requirements follows (Table 5.1).

Table 5.1 Health data requirements

1. The availability of digitized ICU and hospital data including structured and unstructured clinical data and high resolution waveform and vital sign data
2. A cooperative and supportive hospital IT department to assist in data extraction
3. A supportive IRB and hospital administration to assure both protection of patient privacy and release of de-identified data to the research community
4. Adequate engineering and data science capability to design and implement the database schema and to de-identify the data (including the unstructured textual data)
5. Sophisticated signal processing expertise to reformat and manage proprietary waveform data streams
6. Cooperation and technical support of equipment vendors
7. Adequate computational facilities for data archiving and distribution
8. Adequate technical and administrative personnel to provide user support and credentialing of users
9. Adequate financial support

5.8 Future Directions

The MIMIC-III database is a powerful and flexible research resource, but the generalizability of MIMIC-based studies is somewhat limited by the fact that the data are collected from a single institution. Multi-center data would have the advantages of including wider practice variability, and of course a larger number of cases. Data from international institutions would add still greater strength to the database owing to the even larger variations in practice and patient populations.

Our long-term goal is to create a public, multi-center, international data archive for critical care research. We envisage a massive, detailed, high-resolution ICU data archive containing complete medical records from patients around the world. The difficulty of such a project cannot be understated; nevertheless we propose to lay the foundation for such a system by developing a scalable framework that can readily incorporate data from multiple institutions, capable of supporting research on cohorts of critically ill patients from around the world.

Acknowledgments The development and maintenance of the MIMIC and PhysioNet resources have been funded by the National Institute of Biomedical Imaging and Bioengineering (NIBIB) and the National Institute of General Medical Sciences (NIGMS) over the period 2003 to present. Grants R01EB1659, R01EB017205, R01GM104987, and U01EB008577.

Open Access This chapter is distributed under the terms of the Creative Commons Attribution-NonCommercial 4.0 International License (http://creativecommons.org/licenses/by-nc/4.0/), which permits any noncommercial use, duplication, adaptation, distribution and reproduction in any medium or format, as long as you give appropriate credit to the original author(s) and the source, a link is provided to the Creative Commons license and any changes made are indicated.

The images or other third party material in this chapter are included in the work's Creative Commons license, unless indicated otherwise in the credit line; if such material is not included in the work's Creative Commons license and the respective action is not permitted by statutory regulation, users will need to obtain permission from the license holder to duplicate, adapt or reproduce the material.

References

1. MIMIC-II Web Site. http://physionet.org/mimic2
2. MIMIC User Guide. http://physionet.org/mimic2/UserGuide/
3. WaveForm DataBase Data Format. http://www.physionet.org/physiotools/wfdb.shtml
4. Neamatullah I, Douglass M, Lehman LH, Reisner A, Villarroel M, Long WJ, Szolovits P, Moody GB, Mark RG, Clifford GD (2008) Automated de-identification of free-text medical records. BMC Med Inform Decis Mak 8:32. doi:10.1186/1472-6947-8-327
5. Deidentification Software. http://www.physionet.org/physiotools/deid/
6. Accessing MIMIC. http://www.physionet.org/mimic2/mimic2_access.shtml
7. MIMIC-III Website. http://mimic.physionet.org/

Chapter 6
Integrating Non-clinical Data with EHRs

Yuan Lai, Edward Moseley, Francisco Salgueiro and David Stone

Take Home Messages

- Non-clinical factors make a significant contribution to an individual's health and providing this data to clinicians could inform context, counseling, and treatments.
- Data stewardship will be essential to protect confidential health information while still yielding the benefits of an integrated health system.

6.1 Introduction

The definition of "clinical" data is expanding, as a datum becomes clinical once it has a relation to a disease process. For example: the accessibility of one's home would classically be defined as non-clinical data, but in the context of a patient with a disability, this fact may become clinically relevant, and entered into the encounter note much like the patient's blood pressure and body temperature. However, even with this simple example, we can envision some of the problems with traditional non-clinical data being re-classified as clinical data, particularly due to its complexity.

6.2 Non-clinical Factors and Determinants of Health

Non-clinical factors are already significantly linked to health. Many public health policies focusing on transportation, recreation, food systems and community development are based on the relation between health and non-clinical determinants

---

The original version of this chapter was revised: A chapter author's name Edward Moseley was added. The erratum to this chapter is available at 10.1007/978-3-319-43742-2_30

© The Author(s) 2016
MIT Critical Data, *Secondary Analysis of Electronic Health Records*,
DOI 10.1007/978-3-319-43742-2_6

such as behavioral, social and environmental factors [1]. Behavioral factors such as physical activity, diet, smoking and alcohol consumption are highly related to epidemic of obesity [2]. Some of this information, such as alcohol and tobacco use, is regularly documented by clinicians. Other information, such as dietary behaviors and physical activity, isn't typically captured, but may be tracked by new technology (such as wearable computers commonly referred to as "wearables") and integrated into electronic health records (EHRs). Such efforts may provide clinicians with additional context with which to counsel patients in an effort to increase their physical activity and reach a desired health outcome.

From a public health perspective, the same data obtained from these devices may be aggregated and used to guide decisions on public health policies. Continuing the prior example, proper amounts of physical activity will contribute to lower rates of mortality and chronic disease including coronary heart disease, hypertension, diabetes, breast cancer and depression across an entire population. Such data can be used to guide public health interventions in an evidence-based, cost-effective manner.

Both social and environmental factors are highly related to health. Social Determinants of Health (SDH) are non-clinical factors that affect the social and economic status of individuals and communities, including such items as their birthplace, living conditions, working conditions and demographic attributes [3]. Also included are social stressors such as crime, violence, and physical disorders, as well as others [4].

Environmental factors (i.e., air pollution, extreme weather, noise and poor indoor environmental quality) are highly related to an individual's health status. Densely built urban regions create air pollution, heat islands and high levels of noise, which have been implicated in causing or worsening a variety of health issues. For example, a study in New York City showed that asthma-related emergency admissions in youth from 5 to 17 years old were highly related to ambient ozone exposure. This annual NYC Community Health Survey also reveals that self-reported chronic health problems are related to extreme heat, suggesting that temperature can effect, or exacerbate, the symptoms of an individual's chronic illness. Social factors such as age and poverty levels also impact health. A study in New York City shows that fine particles ($PM_{2.5}$, a surrogate marker for pollution) attributable asthma hospital admissions are 4.5 times greater in high-poverty neighborhoods [5].

While outdoor environmental conditions merit public health attention, the average American spends only an hour of each day outdoors, and most individuals live, work and rest in an indoor environment, where other concerns reside. Poor indoor quality can cause building related illness and "sick building syndrome" (SBS)—where occupants experience acute health issues and discomfort, while no diagnosable illness can be readily identified [6]. Again in New York City, housing data was combined from multiple agencies in an effort to address indoor pollution concerns—using predictive analytics, the city was able to increase the rate of detection of buildings considered dangerous, as well as improve the timeliness in locating apartments with safety concerns or health hazards [7].

6.3 Increasing Data Availability

For many years scientists and researchers have had to deal with very limited available data to study behavioral, social and environmental factors that exist in cities, as well as the difficulty in evaluating their model with a large pool of urban data [8]. The big data revolution is bringing vast volumes of data and paradigmatic transformations to many industries within urban services and operations. This is particularly true in commerce, security and health care, as more data are systematically gathered, stored, and analyzed. The emergence of urban informatics also coincides with a transition from traditionally closed and fragmented data systems to more fully connected and open data networks that include mass communications, citizen involvement (e.g. social media), and informational flow [9].

In 2008, 3.3 billion of the world's inhabitants lived in cities, representing, for the first time in history the majority of the human population [10]. In 2014, 54 % of population lives in urban area and it is expected to increase to 66 % by 2050 [11]. With the growth of cities, there are rising concerns in public health circles regarding the impact of associated issues such as aging populations, high population densities, inadequate sanitation, environmental degradation, climate change factors, an increasing frequency of natural disasters, as well as current and looming resource shortages. A concomitantly large amount of information is required to plan and provide for the public health of these urban entities, as well as to prevent and react to adverse public events of all types (e.g. epidemiological, natural, criminal and politico-terroristic disasters).

The nature of the city as an agglomeration of inhabitants, physical objects and activities makes it a rich source of urban data. Today, billions of individuals are generating the digital data through their cellphones and use of the Internet including social networks. Hardware like global positioning systems (GPS) and other sensors are also becoming ubiquitous as they become more affordable, resulting in diverse types of data being collected in new and unique ways [12]. This is especially true in cities due to their massive populations, creating hotspots of data generation and hubs of information flow. Such extensive data availability may also provide the substrate for more statistically robust models across multiple disciplines.

An overview of the volume, variety, and format of open urban data is essential to further integration with electronic health records. As more cities begin building their informational infrastructure, the volume of city data increases rapidly. The majority of urban data are in tabular format with location-based information [8]. Data source and collection processes vary based on the nature of urban data. Passive sensors continuously collect environmental data such as temperature, air quality, solar radiation, and noise, and construct an urban sensing infrastructure along with ubiquitous computing [13]. There is also a large amount of city data generated by citizens such as service requests and complaints. Some pre-existing data, like those in the appropriate tabular format, are immediately ready for integration, while other data contained in more complex file types, like Portable

Document Format (PDF) or others, are more difficult to parse. This problem can be compounded if the data are encoded in uncommon character languages.

The fact that many non-clinical data, especially urban data, is geo-located enables clinicians to consider patient health within a broader view. Many environmental, social and behavioral factors link together spatially, and such spatial correlation is a key measurement in epidemiology, as it allows for the facilitation of data integration based on location. Connections and solutions become more visible by linking non-clinical data with EHR on a public health and city planning level. Recently, IBM announced that, by teaming supercomputer Watson's cognitive computing with data from CVS Health (a pharmacy chain with locations across the U.S.), we will have better predictions regarding the prevalence of chronic conditions such as heart disease and diabetes in different cities and locations [14].

6.4 Integration, Application and Calibration

In a summary of all cities in the United States that published open data sets as of 2013, it was found that greater than 75 % of datasets were prepared in tabular format [8]. Tabular data is most amenable for automated integration, as it is already in the final format prior to being integrated into most relational databases (as long as the dataset contains a meaningful attribute, or variable, with which to relate to other data entries). Furthermore, data integration occurs most easily when the dataset is "tidy", or follows the rule of "one observation per row and one variable per column." Any data manipulation process resulting in a dataset that is aggregated or summarized could remove a great deal of utility from that data [15].

For instance, a table that is familiar within one working environment may not be easily decipherable to another individual and may be nearly impossible for a machine to parse without proper context given for what is within the table. An example could be a table of blood pressure over time and in different locations for a number of patients, which may look like (Table 6.1).

Here we see two patients, Patient 1 and Patient 2, presenting to two locations, Random and Randomly, RA, on two different dates. While this table may be easily read by someone familiar with the format, such that an individual would understand that Patient 1 on the 1st of January, 2015, presented to a healthcare setting in Random, RA with a systolic blood pressure of 130 mmHg and a diastolic pressure of 75 mmHg, it may be rather difficult to manipulate these data to a tidy format without understanding the context of the table.

Table 6.1 Example of a table requiring proper context to read

Patient blood pressure chart	Random, RA		Randomly, RA	
	1-Jan-15	7-Jan-15	1-Jan-15	7-Jan-15
Patient 1	130/75	139/83	141/77	146/82
Patient 2	158/95	151/91	150/81	141/84

6.4 Integration, Application and Calibration

If this table were to be manipulated in a manner that would make it easily analyzed by a machine (as well as other individuals without requiring an explanation of the context), it would follow the rule of one column per variable and one row per observation, as below (Table 6.2).

There are further limitations imparted due to data resolutions, which refers to the detail level of data in space, time or theme, especially the spatial dimension of the data [16]. Examples include: MM/DD/YY time formats compared to YYYY; or zip codes compared to geographic coordinates. Even with these limitations, one may still be able to draw relevant information from these spatial and temporal data.

One method to provide spatial orientation to a clinical encounter has recently been adopted by the administrators of the Medical Information Mart for Intensive Care (MIMIC) database, which currently contains data from over 37,000 intensive care unit admissions [17]. Researchers utilize the United States Zip Code system to approximate the patients' area of residence. This method reports the first three digits of the patient's zip code, while omitting the last two digits [18]. The first three digits of a zip code contain two pieces of information: the first integer in the code refers to a number of states, the following two integers refer to a U.S. Postal Service Sectional Center Facility, through which the mail for that state's counties is processed [19]. The first three digits of the zip code are sufficient to find all other zip codes serviced by the Sectional Center Facility, and population level data of many types are available by zip code as per the U.S. Government's census [20].

Table 6.2 A tidy dataset that contains a readily machine-readable format of the data in Table 6.1

Patient ID	Place	Date (MM/DD/YYYY)	Pressure (mmHg)	Cycle
1	Random, RA	1/1/2015	130	Systole
1	Random, RA	1/1/2015	75	Diastole
1	Random, RA	1/7/2015	139	Systole
1	Random, RA	1/7/2015	83	Diastole
1	Randomly, RA	1/1/2015	141	Systole
1	Randomly, RA	1/1/2015	77	Diastole
1	Randomly, RA	1/7/2015	146	Systole
1	Randomly, RA	1/7/2015	82	Diastole
2	Random, RA	1/1/2015	158	Systole
2	Random, RA	1/1/2015	95	Diastole
2	Random, RA	1/7/2015	151	Systole
2	Random, RA	1/7/2015	91	Diastole
2	Randomly, RA	1/1/2015	150	Systole
2	Randomly, RA	1/1/2015	81	Diastole
2	Randomly, RA	1/7/2015	141	Systole
2	Randomly, RA	1/7/2015	84	Diastole

Connections and solutions become more visible by linking non-clinical data with EHRs on a public health and city planning level. Although many previous studies show the correlation between air pollution and asthma, it is only recently individuals became able to trace PM2.5, SO_2 and Nickel (Ni) in the air back to the generators in buildings with aged boilers and heating systems, which is due in large part to increasing data collection and integration across multiple agencies and disciplines [21]. As studies reveal additional links between our environment and pathological processes, our ability to address potential health threats will be limited by our ability to measure these environmental factors in sufficient resolution to be able to apply it to patient level, creating truly personalized medicine.

For instance, two variables, commonly captured in many observations, are geo-spatiality and temporality. Since all actions share these conditions, integration is possible among a variety of data otherwise loosely utilized in the clinical encounter. When engaged in an encounter, a clinician can determine, from data collected during the examination and history taking, the precise location of the patient over a particular period of time within some spatial resolution. As a case example, a patient may present with an inflammatory process of the respiratory tract. The individual may live in random, RA, and work as an administrator in Randomly, RA; one can plot these variables over time, and separate them to represent both the individuals' work and home environment—as well as other travel (Fig. 6.1).

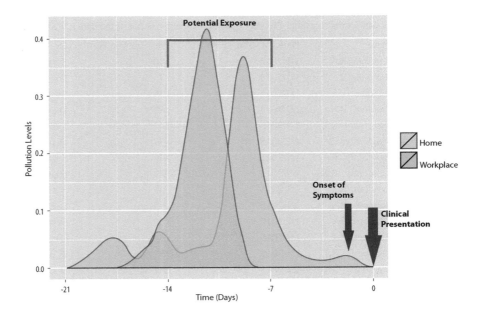

Fig. 6.1 Example of pollution levels over time for a patient's "work" and "home" environment with approximate labels that may provide clinically relevant decision support

6.4 Integration, Application and Calibration

This same method may be applied to other variables that could be determined to have statistical correlates of significance during the timeframe prior to the onset of symptoms and then the clinical encounter.

With the increasing availability of information technology, there is less need for centralized information networks, and the opportunity is open for the individual to participate in data collection, creating virtual sensor networks of environmental and disease measurement. Mobile and social web have created powerful opportunities for urban informatics and disaster planning particularly in public health surveillance and crisis response [13]. There are geo-located mobile crowdsourcing applications such as Health Map's Outbreaks Near Me [22] and Sickweather [23] collecting data on a real-time social network.

In the 2014 Ebola Virus Disease outbreak, self-reporting and close contact reporting was essential to create accurate disease outbreak maps [24]. The emergence of wearables is pushing both EHR manufacturers to develop frameworks that integrate data from wearable devices, and third party companies to provide cloud storage and integration of data from different wearables for greater analytic power.

Attention and investment in digital health and digital cities continues to grow rapidly. In digital health care, investors' funding has soared from $1.1 Billion in 2011 to $5.0 Billion in 2014, and big data analytics ranks as the #1 most active subsector of digital healthcare startups in both amount of investment and number of deals [25]. Integration will be a long process requiring digital capabilities, new policies, collaboration between the public and private sectors, and innovations from both industry leaders and research institutions [26]. Yet we believe with more interdisciplinary collaborations in data mining and analytics, we will gain new knowledge on the health-associated non-clinical factors and indicators of disease outcomes [27]. Furthermore, such integration creates a feedback loop, pushing cities to collect better and larger amounts of data. Integrating non-clinical information into health records remains challenging. Ideally the information obtained from the patient would flow into the larger urban pool and vice versa. Challenges remain on protecting confidentiality at a single patient level and determining applicability of macroscopic data to the single patient.

6.5 A Well-Connected Empowerment

Disease processes can result and be modified by interactions of the patient and his or her environment. Understanding this environment is of importance to clinicians, hospitals, public health policy makers and patients themselves. With this information we can preempt patients at risk for disease (primary prevention), act earlier in minimizing morbidity from disease (secondary prevention) and optimize therapeutics.

A good example of the use of non-clinical data for disease prevention is the use of geographical based information systems (GIS) for preemptive screening of populations at risk for sexually transmitted diseases (STDs). Geographical information systems are used for STD surveillance in about 50 % of state STD surveillance programs is the U.S. [28]. In Baltimore (Maryland, U.S.) a GIS based study identified core groups of repeat gonococcal (an STD) infection that showed geographical clustering [29]. The authors hinted at the possibility of increased yield when directing prevention to geographically restricted populations.

A logical next step is the interaction between public health authority systems and electronic medical records. As de-identified geographical health information becomes publically available, an electronic medical record would be able to download this information from the cloud, apply it to the patient's zip code, sex, age and sexual preference (if documented) and warn/cue the clinician that would decide if an intervention is required based on a calculated risk to acquire a STD.

6.6 Conclusion

Good data stewardship will be essential for protecting confidential health information from unintended and illegal disclosure. For patients, the idea of increasing empowerment in their health is essential [8]. Increasing sensor application and data visualization make our own behavior and surroundings more visible and tangible, and alert us about potential environmental risks. More importantly, it will help us to better understand and gain power over our own lives.

The dichotomy of addressing population health versus individual health must be addressed. Researchers should ask: what information is relevant to the target which I'm addressing, and what data do we feed from this patient's record into the public health realm? The corollary to that question is: how can we balance the individual's right to privacy with the benefit of non-clinical data applicable to the individual and to the large populations? Finally: how can we create systems that select relevant data from a single patient and present it to the clinician in a population-health context? In this chapter, we have attempted to provide an overview of the potential use of traditionally non-clinical data in electronic health records, in addition to mapping some of the pitfalls and strategies to using such data, as well as highlighting practical examples of the use of these data in a clinical environment.

Open Access This chapter is distributed under the terms of the Creative Commons Attribution-NonCommercial 4.0 International License (http://creativecommons.org/licenses/by-nc/4.0/), which permits any noncommercial use, duplication, adaptation, distribution and reproduction in any medium or format, as long as you give appropriate credit to the original author(s) and the source, a link is provided to the Creative Commons license and any changes made are indicated.

The images or other third party material in this chapter are included in the work's Creative Commons license, unless indicated otherwise in the credit line; if such material is not included in the work's Creative Commons license and the respective action is not permitted by statutory regulation, users will need to obtain permission from the license holder to duplicate, adapt or reproduce the material.

References

1. Barton H, Grant M (2013) Urban planning for health cities, a review of the progress of the european healthy cities program. J Urban Health Bull NY Acad Med 90:129–141
2. Badland HM, Schofield GM, Witten K, Schluter PJ, Mavoa S, Kearns RA, Hinckson EA, Oliver M, Kaiwai H, Jensen VG, Ergler C, McGrath L, McPhee J (2009) Understanding the relationship between activity and neighborhoods (URBAN) study: research design and methodology. BMC Pub Health 9:244
3. Osypuk TL, Joshi P, Geronimo K, Acevedo-Garcia D (2014) Do social and economic policies influence health? Rev Curr Epidemiol Rep 1:149–164
4. Shmool JLC, Kubzansky LD, Newman OD, Spengler J, Shepard P, Clougherty JE (2014) Social stressors and air pollution across New York City communities: a spatial approach for assessing correlations among multiple exposures. Environ Health 13:91
5. Kheirbek I, Wheeler K, Walters S, Kass D, Matte T (2013) PM2.5 and ozone health impacts and disparities in New York City: sensitivity to spatial and temporal resolution. Air Qual Atmos Health 6:473–486
6. Indoor Air Facts No. 4 sick building syndrome. United States Environmental Protection Agency, Research and Development (MD-56) (1991)
7. Goldstein B, Dyson L (2013) Beyond transparency: open data and the future of civic innovation. Code for America Press, San Francisco
8. Barbosa L, Pham K, Silva C, Vieira MR, Freire J (2014) Structured open urban data: understanding the landscape. Big Data 2:144–154
9. Shane DG (2011) Urban design since 1945—a global perspective. Wiley, New York, p 284
10. National Intelligence Council (2012) Global trends 2030: alternative worlds. National Intelligence Council
11. World Urbanization Prospects, United Nations (2014)
12. Goldsmith S, Crawford S (2014) The responsive city: engaging communities through data-smart governance. Wiley, New York
13. Boulos M, Resch B, Crowley D, Breslin J, Sohn G, Burtner R, Pike W, Jezierski E, Chuang K (2011) Crowdsourcing, citizen sensing and sensor web technologies for public and environmental health surveillance and crisis management: trends, OGC standards and application examples. Int J Health Geographic 10:67
14. McMullan T. Dr Watson: IBM plans to use Big Data to manage diabetes and obesity. URL: http://www.alphr.com/life-culture/1001303/dr-watson-ibm-plans-to-use-big-data-to-manage-diabetes-and-obesity
15. Wickham H (2014) Tidy data. J Stat Softw 10:59
16. Haining R (2004) Spatial data analysis—theory and practice. Cambridge University Press, Cambridge, p 67
17. MIMIC II Databases. Available from: http://physionet.org/mimic2. Accessed 02 Aug 2015
18. Massachusetts Institute of Technology, Laboratory of Computational Physiology. mimic2 v3.0 D_PATIENTS table. URL: https://github.com/mimic2/v3.0/blob/ad9c045a5a778c6eb283bdad310594484cca873c/_posts/2015-04-22-dpatients.md. Accessed 02 Aug 2015 (Archived by WebCite® at http://www.webcitation.org/6aUNzhW6g)
19. http://pe.usps.com/businessmail101/glossary.htm
20. http://factfinder.census.gov/
21. Jeffery N, McKelvey W, Matte T (2015) using tracking infrastructure to support public health programs, policies, and emergency response in New York City. Pub Health Manag Pract 21(2 Supp):S102–S106
22. http://www.healthmap.org/outbreaksnearme/
23. http://www.sickweather.com

24. Kouadio KI, Clement P, Bolongei J, Tamba A, Gasasira AN, Warsame A, Okeibunor JC, Ota MO, Tamba B, Gumede N, Shaba K, Poy A, Salla M, Mihigo R, Nshimirimana D (2015) Epidemiological and surveillance response to Ebola virus disease outbreak in Lofa County, Liberia (Mar–Sept 2014); lessons learned, edn 1. PLOS Currents Outbreaks. 6 May 2015. doi: 10.1371/currents.outbreaks.9681514e450dc8d19d47e1724d2553a5
25. The re-imagination of healthcare. StartUp Health Insights. www.startuphealth.com/insights
26. Ericsson Networked Society City Index (2014)
27. Corti B, Badland H, Mavoa S, Turrell G, Bull F, Boruff B, Pettit C, Bauman A, Hooper P, Villanueva K, Burt T, Feng X, Learnihan V, Davey R, Grenfell R, Thackway S (2014) Reconnecting urban planning with health: a protocol for the development and validation of national livability indicators associated with non-communicable disease risk behaviors and health outcomes. Pub Health Res Pract 25(1):e2511405
28. Bissette JM, Stover JA, Newman LM, Delcher PC, Bernstein KT, Matthews L (2009) Assessment of geographic information systems and data confidentiality guidelines in STD programs. Pub Health Rep 124(Suppl 2):58–64
29. Bernstein TK, Curriero FC, Jennings JM et al (2004) Defining core gonorrhea transmission utilizing spatial data. Am J Epidemiol 160:51–58

Chapter 7
Using EHR to Conduct Outcome and Health Services Research

Laura Myers and Jennifer Stevens

Take Home Messages

- Electronic Health Records have become an essential tool in clinical research, both as a supplement to existing methods, but also in the growing domains of outcomes research and analytics.
- While EHR data is extensive and analytics are powerful, it is essential to fully understand the biases and limitations introduced when used in health services research.

7.1 Introduction

Data from electronic health records (EHR) can be a powerful tool for research. However, researchers must be aware of the fallibility of data collected for clinical purposes and of biases inherent to using EHR data to conduct sound health outcomes and health services research. Innovative methods are currently being developed to improve the quality of data and thus our ability to draw conclusions from studies that use EHR data.

The United States devotes a large share of the Gross Domestic Product (17.6 % in 2009) to health care [1]. With such a huge financial and social investment in healthcare, important questions are fundamental to evaluating this investment:

> How do we know what treatment works and for which patients?
> How much should health care cost? When is too much to pay? In what type of care should we invest more or less resources?
> How does the health system work and how could it function better?

Health services research is a field of research that lives at the intersection of health care policy, management, and clinical care delivery and seeks to answer these questions. Fundamentally, health services research places the health system under the microscope as the organism of study.

To begin to address these questions, researchers need large volumes of data across multiple patients, across different types of health delivery structures, and across time. The simultaneous growth of this field of research in the past 15 years has coincided with the development of the electronic health record and the increasing number of providers who make use of them in their workspace [2]. The EHR provides large quantities of raw data to fuel this research, both at the granular level of the patient and provider and at the aggregated level of the hospital, state, or nation.

Conducting research with EHR data has many challenges. EHR data are riddled with biases, collected for purposes other than research, inputted by a variety of users for the same patient, and difficult to integrate across health systems [See previous chapter "Confounding by Indication"]. This chapter will focus on the attempts to capitalize on the promise of the EHR for health services research with careful consideration of the challenges researchers must address to derive meaningful and valid conclusions.

7.2 The Rise of EHRs in Health Services Research

7.2.1 The EHR in Outcomes and Observational Studies

Observational studies, either retrospective or prospective, attempt to draw inferences about the effects of different exposures. Within health services research, these exposures include both different types of clinical exposures (e.g., does hormone replacement therapy help or hurt patients?) and health care delivery exposures (e.g., does admission to a large hospital for cardiac revascularization improve survival from myocardial infarction over admission to a small hospital). The availability of the extensive health data in electronic health records has fueled this type of research, as data extraction and transcription from paper records has ceased to be a barrier to research. These studies capitalize on the demographic and clinical elements that are routinely recorded as part of an encounter with the health system (e.g., age, sex, race, procedures performed, length of stay, critical care resources used).

We have highlighted a number of examples of this type of research below. Each one is an example of research that has made use of electronic health data, either at the national or hospital level, to draw inferences about health care delivery and care.

Does health care delivery vary? The researchers who compile and examine the Dartmouth Atlas have demonstrated substantial geographic variation in care. In their original article in *Science*, Wennberg and Gittlesohn noted wide variations in the use of health services in Vermont [3]. These authors employed data derived from the use of different types of medical services—home health services, inpatient discharges, etc.—to draw these inferences. Subsequent investigations into national variation in care have been able to capitalize on the availability of such data electronically [4].

Do hospitals with more experience in a particular area perform better? Birkmeyer and colleagues studied the intersection of hospital volume and surgical outcomes with absolute differences in adjusted mortality rates between low volume hospitals and high volume hospitals ranging from 12 % for pancreatic resection to 0.2 % for carotid endarterectomy [5]. Kahn et al. also used data available in over 20,000 patients to demonstrate that mortality associated with mechanical ventilation was 37 % lower in high volume hospitals compared with low volume hospitals [6]. Both of these research groups made use of large volumes of clinical and claims data—Medicare claims data in the case of Birkmeyer and colleagues and the APACHE database from Cerner for Kahn et al.—to ask important questions about where patients should seek different types of care.

How can we identify harm to patients despite usual care? Herzig and colleagues made use of the granular EHR at a single institution and found that the widely-prescribed medications that suppress acid production were associated with an increased risk of pneumonia [7]. Other authors have similarly looked at the EHR found that these types of medications are often continued on discharge from the hospital [8, 9].

To facilitate appropriate modeling and identification of confounders in observational studies, researchers have had to devise methods to extract markers of diagnoses, severity of illness, and patient comorbidities using only the electronic fingerprint. Post et al. [10] developed an algorithm to search for patients who had diuretic-refractory hypertension by querying for patients who had a diagnosis of hypertension despite 6 months treatment with a diuretic. Previously validated methods for reliably measuring the severity of a patient's illness, such as APACHE or SAPS scores [11, 12], have data elements that are not easily extracted in the absence of manual inputting of data. To meet these challenges, researchers such as Escobar and Elixhauser have proposed alternative, electronically derived methods for both severity of illness measures [13, 14] and identification of comorbidities [14]. Escobar's work, with a severity of illness measure with an area under the curve of 0.88, makes use of highly granular electronic data including laboratory values; Elixhauser's comorbidity measure is publically available through the Agency for Healthcare Research and Quality and solely requires billing data [15].

Finally, researchers must develop and employ appropriate mathematical models that can accommodate the short-comings of electronic health data or else they risk drawing inaccurate conclusions. Examples of such modeling techniques are extensive have included propensity scores, causal methods such as marginal structural models and inverse probability weights, and designs from other fields such as instrumental variable analysis [16–19]. The details of these methods are discussed elsewhere in this text.

7.2.2 The EHR as Tool to Facilitate Patient Enrollment in Prospective Trials

Despite the power of the EHR to conduct health services and outcomes research retrospectively, the gold standard in research remains prospective and randomized trials. The EHR has functioned as a valuable tool to screen patients at a large scale for eligibility. In this instance, research staff uses the data available through the electronic record as a high-volume screening technique to target recruitment efforts to the most appropriate patients. Clinical trials that develop electronic strategies for patient identification and recruitment are at an even greater advantage, although such robust methods have been described as sensitive but not specific, and frequently require coupling screening efforts with manual review of individual records [20]. Embi et al. [21] have proposed using the EHR to simultaneously generate Clinical Trial Alerts, particularly in commercial EHRs such as Epic to leverage the EHR in a point of care strategy. This strategy could expedite enrollment although it must be weighed against the risk of losing patient confidentiality, an ongoing tension between patient care and clinical trial enrollment [22].

7.2.3 The EHR as Tool to Study and Improve Patient Outcomes

Quality can also be tracked and reported through EHRs, either for internal quality improvement or for national benchmarking; the Veterans' Affairs' (VA) healthcare system highlights this. Byrne et al. [23] reported that in the 1990s, the VA spent more money on information technology infrastructure and achieved higher rates of adoption compared to the private sector. Their home-grown EHR, which is called VistA, provided a way to track preventative care processes such as cancer and diabetes screening through electronic pop up messages. Between 2004 and 2007, they found that the VA system achieved better glucose and lipid control for diabetics compared to a Medicare HMO benchmark [23]. While much capital investment was needed during the initial implementation of VistA, it is estimated that adopting this infrastructure saved the VA system $3.09 billion in the long term. It also continues to be a source of quality improvement as quality metrics evolve over time [23].

7.3 How to Avoid Common Pitfalls When Using EHR to Do Health Services Research

We would propose the following hypothetical research study as a case study to highlight common challenges to conducting health services research with electronic health data:

> Proposed research study: Antipsychotic medications (e.g. haloperidol) are prescribed frequently in the intensive care unit to treat patients with active delirium. However, these medications have been associated with their own potential risk of harm [24] that is separate from the overall risk of harm from delirium. The researchers are interested in whether treatment with antipsychotics increases the risk of in-hospital death and increases the cost of care and use of resources in the hospital.

7.3.1 Step 1: Recognize the Fallibility of the EHR

The EHR is rarely complete or correct. Hogan et al. [25] tried to estimate how complete and accurate data are in studies that are conducted on an EHR, finding significant variability in both. Completeness ranged from 31 to 100 % and correctness ranged from 67 to 100 % [25]. Table 7.1 highlights examples of different diagnoses and possible sources of data, which may or may not be present for all patients.

> Proposed research study: The researchers will need to extract which patients were exposed to antipsychotics and which were not. However, there is unlikely to be one single place where this information is stored. Should they use pharmacy dispensing data? Nursing administration data? Should they look at which patients were charged for the medications? What if they need these data from multiple hospitals with different electronic health records?

Additionally, even with a robust data extraction strategy, the fidelity of different types of data is variable [26–33]. For example, many EHR systems have the option of entering free text for a medical condition, which may be spelled wrong or be worded unconventionally. As another example, the relative reimbursement of a particular billing code may influence the incidence of that code in the electronic health record so billing may not reflect the true incidence and prevalence of the disease [34, 35].

7.3.2 Step 2: Understand Confounding, Bias, and Missing Data When Using the EHR for Research

We would highlight the following methodological issues inherent in conducting research with electronic health records: selection bias, confounding, and missing data. These are explored in greater depth in other chapters of this text.

Table 7.1 Examples of the range of data elements that may be used to identify patients with either ischemic heart disease or acute lung injury through the electronic health record

Disease state	Data source	Example
Ischemic heart disease	Billing data	ICD-9 code 410 [48]
	Laboratory data	Positive troponin during admission
	Physician documentation	In the discharge summary: "the patient was noted to have ST elevations on ECG and was taken to the cath lab"…
Acute lung injury	Billing data	ICD-9 code 518.5 and 518.82 with the procedural codes 96.70, 96.71 and 96.72 for mechanical ventilation [49]
	Radiology data	"Bilateral" and "infiltrates" on chest x-ray reads [50]
	Laboratory data	PaO2/FiO2 < 300 mmHg

Selection bias, or the failure of the population of study to represent the generalizable population, can occur if all the patients, including controls, are already seeking medical care within an EHR-based system. For example, in EHR-based studies comparing medical versus surgical approaches to the same condition may not be comparing equivalent patients in each group; patients seeking a surgical correction may fundamentally differ from those seeking a more conservative approach. Hripcsak et al. [36] used a large clinical data set from a tertiary center in 2007 to compare mortality from pneumonia to a hand-collected data set that had been published previously; the different search criteria altered the patient population and the subsequent risk of death. While it is not eliminated entirely, selection bias is reduced when prospective randomization takes place [37].

Confounding bias represents the failure to appropriately account for an additional variable that influences both the dependent and independent variable. In research with electronic health records, confounding represents a particular challenge, as identification of all possible confounding variables is nearly impossible.

Proposed research study: The researchers in this study are interested in the patient-level outcomes of what happens to those patients exposed to antipsychotics during their stay. But patients who are actively delirious while in the ICU are likely to be sicker than those who are not actively delirious and sicker patients require more hospital resources. As a result, antipsychotics will appear to be associated with a higher risk of in-hospital mortality and use of hospital resources not due to the independent effect of the drug but rather as a result of confounding by indication.

Missing data or unevenly sampled data collected as part of the EHR creates its own complex set of challenges for health services research. For example, restricting the analysis to patients with only a complete set of data may yield very different (and poorly generalizable) inferences. The multidimentionality of this problem often goes unexamined and underestimated. Nearly all conventional analytic software presumes completeness of the matrix of data, leading many researchers to fail to fully address these issues. For example, data can be misaligned due to lack of sampling, missing data, or simple misalignment. In other words, the data could not be measured during a period of time for an intentional reason (e.g., a patient was extubated and therefore no values for mechanical ventilation were documented) and should not be imputed or the data was measured but was unintentionally not recorded and therefore can be imputed. Rusanov et al. studied 10,000 outpatients at a tertiary center who underwent general anesthesia for elective procedures. Patients with a higher risk of adverse outcome going into surgery had more data points including laboratory values, medication orders and possibly admission orders compared to less sick patients [38], making the missing data for less sick patients intentional. Methods for handling missing data have included omitting cases are note complete, pairwise deletion, mean substitution, regression substitution, or using modeling techniques for maximum likelihood and multiple imputation [39].

7.4 Future Directions for the EHR and Health Services Research

7.4.1 Ensuring Adequate Patient Privacy Protection

It is controversial whether using EHR for research goes against our national privacy standard. In large cohorts, many patients may be present with the same health information, thereby rendering the data sufficiently deidentified. Further, Ingelfinger et al. acknowledge that countries with healthcare registries such as Scandinavia have a distinct research advantage [40]. However, health information is a protected class of information under the Health Insurance Portability and Accountability Act, so there is significant awareness among U.S. healthcare professionals and researchers about its proper storage and dissemination. Some argue that patients should be consented (versus just notified) that their information could be used for research purposes in the future. Ingelfinger et al. [40] recommends IRB approval of registries and a rigorous deidentification process.

Public perception on the secondary use of EHR may not be as prohibitive as policymakers may have believed. In a survey of 3300 people, they were more willing to have their information used for research by university hospitals, compared to public health departments or for quality improvement purposes [41]. They were much less willing to contribute to marketing efforts or have the information used by pharmaceutical companies [41].

With the growing amount of information being entered into EHRs across the country, the American Medical Informatics Association convened a panel to make recommendations for how best to use EHR securely for purposes other than direct patient care. In 2006, the panel called for a national standard to deal with the issue of privacy. They described complex situations where there were security breaches due to problems with deidentification or data was being sold by physicians for profit [42]. While the panel demanded that the national framework be transparent, comprehensive and publicly accepted, they did not propose a particular standard at that time [42]. Other groups such as the Patient-Centered Outcomes Research Institute have since addressed the same conflict in a national forum in 2012. Similarly, while visions were discussed, no explicit recommendation was set forth [PCORI]. Controversy continues in this area.

7.5 Multidimensional Collaborations

Going forward, the true power of integrated data can only be harnessed by forming more collaborations, both within institutions and between them. Research on a national scale in the U.S. has been shown to be feasible. The FDA implemented a pilot program in 2009 called the Mini-Sentinel program. It brought together 31 academic and private organizations to monitor for safety events related to medications and devices currently on the market [43]. Admittedly, merging databases may require significant financial resources, especially if the datasets need to be coded and/or validated, but researchers like Bradley et al. [44] believe this is a cost-effective use of grant money because of the vast potential to make advances in the way we deliver care. Fundamental to the feasibility of multidimensional collaborations is the ability to ensure accuracy of large-scale data and integrate it across multiple health record technologies and platforms. Efforts to ensure data quality and accessibility must be promoted alongside patient privacy.

7.6 Conclusion

Researchers continue to ask fundamental questions of our health system, making use of the deluge of data generated by EHRs. Unfortunately, that deluge is messy and problematic. As the field of health services research with EHRs continues to evolve, we must hold researchers to rigorous standards [45] and encourage more investment in research-friendly clinical databases as well as cross-institutional collaborations. Only then will the discoveries in health outcomes and health services research be one click away [46, 47]. It is time for healthcare to reap the same reward from a rich data source that is already in existence.

Open Access This chapter is distributed under the terms of the Creative Commons Attribution-NonCommercial 4.0 International License (http://creativecommons.org/licenses/by-nc/ 4.0/), which permits any noncommercial use, duplication, adaptation, distribution and reproduction in any medium or format, as long as you give appropriate credit to the original author(s) and the source, a link is provided to the Creative Commons license and any changes made are indicated.

The images or other third party material in this chapter are included in the work's Creative Commons license, unless indicated otherwise in the credit line; if such material is not included in the work's Creative Commons license and the respective action is not permitted by statutory regulation, users will need to obtain permission from the license holder to duplicate, adapt or reproduce the material.

References

1. Center for Medicare and Medicaid Services (2015) National health expenditure data fact sheet
2. Jha AK, DesRoches CM, Campbell EG, Donelan K, Rao SR et al (2009) Use of electronic health records in U.S. hospitals. N Engl J Med 360:1628–1638
3. Wennberg J, Gittelsohn (1973) Small area variations in health care delivery. Science 182:1102–1108
4. Stevens JP, Nyweide D, Maresh S, Zaslavsky A, Shrank W et al (2015) Variation in inpatient consultation among older adults in the United States. J Gen Intern Med 30:992–999
5. Birkmeyer JD (2000) Relation of surgical volume to outcome. Ann Surg 232:724–725
6. Kahn JM, Goss CH, Heagerty PJ, Kramer AA, O'Brien CR et al (2006) Hospital volume and the outcomes of mechanical ventilation. N Engl J Med 355:41–50

References

7. Herzig SJ, Howell MD, Ngo LH, Marcantonio ER (2009) Acid-suppressive medication use and the risk for hospital-acquired pneumonia. JAMA 301:2120–2128
8. Murphy CE, Stevens AM, Ferrentino N, Crookes BA, Hebert JC et al (2008) Frequency of inappropriate continuation of acid suppressive therapy after discharge in patients who began therapy in the surgical intensive care unit. Pharmacotherapy 28:968–976
9. Zink DA, Pohlman M, Barnes M, Cannon ME (2005) Long-term use of acid suppression started inappropriately during hospitalization. Aliment Pharmacol Ther 21:1203–1209
10. Post AR, Kurc T, Cholleti S, Gao J, Lin X et al (2013) The analytic information warehouse (AIW): a platform for analytics using electronic health record data. J Biomed Inform 46:410–424
11. Zimmerman JE, Kramer AA, McNair DS, Malila FM (2006) Acute physiology and chronic health evaluation (APACHE) IV: hospital mortality assessment for today's critically ill patients. Crit Care Med 34:1297–1310
12. Moreno RP, Metnitz PG, Almeida E, Jordan B, Bauer P et al (2005) SAPS 3—from evaluation of the patient to evaluation of the intensive care unit. Part 2: development of a prognostic model for hospital mortality at ICU admission. Intensive Care Med 31:1345–1355
13. Escobar GJ, Greene JD, Scheirer P, Gardner MN, Draper D et al (2008) Risk-adjusting hospital inpatient mortality using automated inpatient, outpatient, and laboratory databases. Med Care 46:232–239
14. Elixhauser A, Steiner C, Harris DR, Coffey RM (1998) Comorbidity measures for use with administrative data. Med Care 36:8–27
15. Project HCaU (2015) Comorbidity software, Version 3.7
16. Rubin DB, Thomas N (1996) Matching using estimated propensity scores: relating theory to practice. Biometrics 52:249–264
17. Rubin DB (1997) Estimating causal effects from large data sets using propensity scores. Ann Intern Med 127:757–763
18. Howell MD, Novack V, Grgurich P, Soulliard D, Novack L et al (2010) Iatrogenic gastric acid suppression and the risk of nosocomial Clostridium difficile infection. Arch Intern Med 170:784–790
19. Hernan MA, Brumback B, Robins JM (2000) Marginal structural models to estimate the causal effect of zidovudine on the survival of HIV-positive men. Epidemiology 11:561–570
20. Thadani SR, Weng C, Bigger JT, Ennever JF, Wajngurt D (2009) Electronic screening improves efficiency in clinical trial recruitment. J Am Med Inform Assoc 16:869–873
21. Embi PJ, Jain A, Clark J, Harris CM (2005) Development of an electronic health record-based clinical trial alert system to enhance recruitment at the point of care. AMIA Annu Symp Proc, 231–235
22. PCORnet (2015) Rethinking clinical trials: a living textbook of pragmatic clinical trials
23. Byrne CM, Mercincavage LM, Pan EC, Vincent AG, Johnston DS et al (2010) The value from investments in health information technology at the U.S. Department of Veterans Affairs. Health Aff (Millwood) 29:629–638
24. Ray WA, Chung CP, Murray KT, Hall K, Stein CM (2009) Atypical antipsychotic drugs and the risk of sudden cardiac death. N Engl J Med 360:225–235
25. Hogan WR, Wagner MM (1997) Accuracy of data in computer-based patient records. J Am Med Inform Assoc 4:342–355
26. Lee DS, Donovan L, Austin PC, Gong Y, Liu PP et al (2005) Comparison of coding of heart failure and comorbidities in administrative and clinical data for use in outcomes research. Med Care 43:182–188
27. Iwashyna TJ, Odden A, Rohde J, Bonham C, Kuhn L et al (2014) Identifying patients with severe sepsis using administrative claims: patient-level validation of the angus implementation of the international consensus conference definition of severe sepsis. Med Care 52:e39–e43
28. Jones G, Taright N, Boelle PY, Marty J, Lalande V et al (2012) Accuracy of ICD-10 codes for surveillance of clostridium difficile infections, France. Emerg Infect Dis 18:979–981
29. Kramer JR, Davila JA, Miller ED, Richardson P, Giordano TP et al (2008) The validity of viral hepatitis and chronic liver disease diagnoses in Veterans Affairs Administrative databases. Aliment Pharmacol Ther 27:274–282

30. van de Garde EM, Oosterheert JJ, Bonten M, Kaplan RC, Leufkens HG (2007) International classification of diseases codes showed modest sensitivity for detecting community-acquired pneumonia. J Clin Epidemiol 60:834–838
31. Movig KL, Leufkens HG, Lenderink AW, Egberts AC (2003) Validity of hospital discharge International classification of diseases (ICD) codes for identifying patients with hyponatremia. J Clin Epidemiol 56:530–535
32. Sickbert-Bennett EE, Weber DJ, Poole C, MacDonald PD, Maillard JM (2010) Utility of international classification of diseases, ninth revision, clinical modification codes for communicable disease surveillance. Am J Epidemiol 172:1299–1305
33. Jhung MA, Banerjee SN (2009) Administrative coding data and health care-associated infections. Clin Infect Dis 49:949–955
34. O'Malley KJ, Cook KF, Price MD, Wildes KR, Hurdle JF et al (2005) Measuring diagnoses: ICD code accuracy. Health Serv Res 40:1620–1639
35. Richesson RL, Rusincovitch SA, Wixted D, Batch BC, Feinglos MN et al (2013) A comparison of phenotype definitions for diabetes mellitus. J Am Med Inform Assoc 20:e319–e326
36. Hripcsak G, Knirsch C, Zhou L, Wilcox A, Melton G (2011) Bias associated with mining electronic health records. J Biomed Discov Collab 6:48–52
37. Hernan MA, Alonso A, Logan R, Grodstein F, Michels KB et al (2008) Observational studies analyzed like randomized experiments: an application to postmenopausal hormone therapy and coronary heart disease. Epidemiology 19:766–779
38. Rusanov A, Weiskopf NG, Wang S, Weng C (2014) Hidden in plain sight: bias towards sick patients when sampling patients with sufficient electronic health record data for research. BMC Med Inform Decis Mak 14:51
39. Allison PD (2001) Missing data. Sage Publishers, Thousand Oaks
40. Ingelfinger JR, Drazen JM (2004) Registry research and medical privacy. N Engl J Med 350:1452–1453
41. Grande D, Mitra N, Shah A, Wan F, Asch DA (2013) Public preferences about secondary uses of electronic health information. JAMA Intern Med 173:1798–1806
42. Safran C, Bloomrosen M, Hammond WE, Labkoff S, Markel-Fox S et al (2007) Toward a national framework for the secondary use of health data: an American medical informatics association white paper. J Am Med Inform Assoc 14:1–9
43. Platt R, Carnahan RM, Brown JS, Chrischilles E, Curtis LH et al (2012) The U.S. food and drug administration's mini-sentinel program: status and direction. Pharmacoepidemiol Drug Saf 21(Suppl 1):1–8
44. Bradley CJ, Penberthy L, Devers KJ, Holden DJ (2010) Health services research and data linkages: issues, methods, and directions for the future. Health Serv Res 45:1468–1488
45. Kahn MG, Raebel MA, Glanz JM, Riedlinger K, Steiner JF (2012) A pragmatic framework for single-site and multisite data quality assessment in electronic health record-based clinical research. Med Care 50(Suppl):S21–S29
46. Weber GM, Mandl KD, Kohane IS (2014) Finding the missing link for big biomedical data. JAMA 311:2479–2480
47. Murdoch TB, Detsky AS (2013) The inevitable application of big data to health care. JAMA 309:1351–1352
48. Birman-Deych E, Waterman AD, Yan Y, Nilasena DS, Radford MJ et al (2005) Accuracy of ICD-9-CM codes for identifying cardiovascular and stroke risk factors. Med Care 43:480–485
49. Reynolds HN, McCunn M, Borg U, Habashi N, Cottingham C et al (1998) Acute respiratory distress syndrome: estimated incidence and mortality rate in a 5 million-person population base. Crit Care 2:29–34
50. Herasevich V, Tsapenko M, Kojicic M, Ahmed A, Kashyap R et al (2011) Limiting ventilator-induced lung injury through individual electronic medical record surveillance. Crit Care Med 39:34–39

Chapter 8
Residual Confounding Lurking in Big Data: A Source of Error

John Danziger and Andrew J. Zimolzak

Take Home Messages

- Any observational study may have unidentified confounding variables that influence the effects of the primary exposure, therefore we must rely on research transparency along with thoughtful and careful examination of the limitations to have confidence in any hypotheses.
- Pathophysiology is complicated and often obfuscates the measured data with many observations being mere proxies for a physiological process and many different factors progressing to similar dysfunction.

8.1 Introduction

Nothing is more dangerous than an idea, when you have only one…

—Emile Chartier

Big Data is defined by its vastness, often with large highly granular datasets, which when combined with advanced analytical and statistical approaches, can power very convincing conclusions [1]. Herein perhaps lies the greatest challenge with using big data appropriately: understanding what is not available. In order to avoid false inferences of causality, it is critical to recognize the influences that might affect the outcome of interest, yet are not readily measurable.

Given the difficulty in performing well-designed prospective, randomized studies in clinical medicine, Big Data resources such as the Medical Information Mart for Intensive Care (MIMIC) database [2] are highly attractive. They provide a powerful resource to examine the strength of potential associations and to test whether assumed physiological principles remain robust in clinical medicine. However, given their often observational nature, causality can not be established, and great care should be taken when using observational data to influence practice patterns. There are numerous examples [3, 4] in clinical medicine where observational data had been used to determine clinical decision making, only to eventually be disproven, and in the meantime, potentially causing harm. Although associations may be powerful, missing the unseen connections leads to false inferences. The unrecognized effect of an additional variable associated with the primary exposure that influences the outcome of interest is known as confounding.

8.2 Confounding Variables in Big Data

Confounding is often referred to as a "mixing of effects" [5] wherein the effects of the exposure on a particular outcome are associated with an additional factor, thereby distorting the true relationship. In this manner, confounding may falsely suggest an apparent association when no real association exists. Confounding is a particular threat in observational data, as is often the case with Big Data, due to the inability to randomize groups to the exposure. The process of randomization essentially mitigates the influence of unrecognized influences, because these influences should be nearly equally distributed to the groups. However, more frequently observational data is composed of patient groups that have been distinguished based on clinical factors. For example, with critical care observational data, such as MIMIC, such "non-random allocation" has occurred simply by reaching the intensive care unit (ICU). There has been some decision process by an admitting team, perhaps in the Emergency Department, that the patient is ill enough for the ICU. That decision process is likely influenced by a host of factors, some of which are identifiable, as in blood pressure and severity of illness, and others that are not, as in "the patient just looks sick" intuition of the provider.

8.2.1 The Obesity Paradox

As an example of the subtlety of this confounding influence, let's tackle the question of obesity as a predictor of mortality. In most community-based studies [6, 7], obesity is associated with poorer outcomes: obese patients have a higher risk of dying than normal weighted individuals likely mediated by an increased incidence of diabetes, hypertension, and cardiovascular disease. However, amongst patients admitted to the ICU, obesity is a strong survival benefit [8, 9], with multiple studies elucidated better outcomes amongst obese critically ill patients than normal weighted critical ill patients.

8.2 Confounding Variables in Big Data

There are potentially many explanations for this paradoxical association. On one hand, it is plausible that critically ill obese patients have higher nutritional stores and are better able to withstand the prolonged state of cachexia associated with critical illness than normal weighted patients. However, let's explore some other possibilities. Since obesity is typically defined by the body mass index (BMI) upon admission to the ICU, it is possible that unrecognized influences on body weight prior to hospitalization that independently affect outcome might be the true reason for this paradoxical association. For example, fluid accumulation, as might occur with congestive heart failure, will increase body weight, but not fat mass, resulting in an inappropriately elevated BMI. This fluid accumulation, when resulting in pulmonary edema, is generally considered a marker of illness severity and a warrants a higher level of care, such as the ICU. Thus, this fluid accumulation would prompt the emergency room team to admit the patient to the ICU rather than to the general medicine ward. Now, heart failure is typically a reasonably treatable disease process. Diuretics are an effective widely used treatment, and likely can resolve the specific factor (i.e. fluid overload) that leads to ICU care. Thus, such a patient would seem obese, but might not be, and would have a reasonable chance of survival. Compare that to another such patient, who developed cachexia from metastatic cancer, and lost thirty pounds prior to presenting to the emergency room. That patient's BMI would have dropped significantly over the few weeks prior to illness, and his poor prognosis and illness might lead to an ICU admission, where his prognosis would be poor. In the latter scenario, concluding that a low BMI was associated with a poor outcome may not be strictly correct, since it is often rather the complications of the underlying cancer that lead to mortality.

8.2.2 Selection Bias

Let's explore one last possibility relating to how the obesity paradox in critical care might be confounded. Imagine two genetically identical fraternal twins with the exact same comorbidities and exposures, presenting with cellulitis, weakness, and diarrhea, both of whom will need frequent cleaning and dressing changes. The only difference is that one twin has a normal weight, whereas the other is morbidly obese. Now, the emergency room team must decide which level of care these patients require. Given the challenges of caring for morbidly obese patient (lifting a heavy leg, turning to change), it is plausible that obesity itself might influence the emergency room's choice regarding disposition. In that case, there would be a tremendous selection bias. In essence, the obese patient who would have been generally healthy enough for a general ward ends up in the ICU due to obesity alone, where the observational data begins. Not surprisingly, that patient will do better than other ICU patients, since he was healthier in the first place and was admitted simply because he was obese.

Such selection bias, which can be quite subtle, is a challenging problem in non-randomly allocated studies. Patients groups are often differentiated by their illness severity, and thus any observational study assessing the effects of related treatments may fail to address underlying associated factors. For example, a recent observational Big Data study attempted to examine whether exposure to proton pump inhibitors (PPI) was associated with hypomagnesemia [10]. Indeed, in many thousands of examined patients, PPI users had lower admission serum magnesium concentrations. Yet, the indication for why the patients were prescribed PPIs in the first place was not known. Plausibly, patients who present with dyspepsia or other related gastrointestinal symptoms, which are major indications for PPI prescription, might have lower intake of magnesium-containing foods. Thus, the conclusion that PPI was responsible for lower magnesium concentrations would be conjecture, since lower dietary intake would be an equally reasonable explanation.

8.2.3 Uncertain Pathophysiology

In addition to selection bias, as illustrated in the obesity paradox and PPI associated hypomagnesemia examples, there is another important source of confounding, particularly in critical care studies. Given that physiology and pathophysiology are such strong determinants of outcomes in critical illness, the ability to fully account for the underlying pathophysiologic pathways is extraordinarily important, but also notoriously difficult. Consider that clinicians caring for patients, standing at the patient's bedside in direct examination of all the details, sometimes cannot explain the physiologic process. Recognizing diastolic heart failure remains challenging. Accurately characterizing organ function is not straightforward. And if the caring physician can't delineate the underlying processes, how can observational data, so removed from the patient? It can't, and this is a huge source of potential mistakes. Let's consider some examples.

In critical care, the frequent laboratory studies that are easily measured with precise reproducibility make a welcoming target for cross sectional analysis. In the literature, almost every common laboratory abnormality has been associated with a poor outcome, including abnormalities of sodium, potassium, chloride, bicarbonate, blood urea nitrogen, creatinine, glucose, hemoglobin, etc. Many of these cross sectional studies have led to management guidelines. The important question however is whether the laboratory abnormality itself leads to a poor patient outcome, or whether instead, the underlying patient pathophysiology that leads to the laboratory abnormality is the primary cause.

Take for example hyponatremia. There is extensive observational data linking hyponatremia to mortality. In response, there have been extensive treatment guidelines on how to correct hyponatremia through a combination of water restriction and sodium administration [11]. However, the mechanistic explanation for how chronic and/or mild hyponatremia might cause a poor outcome is not totally convincing. Some data might suggest that potential subtle cerebral edema might lead to imbalance and falls, but this is not a completely convincing explanation for the association of admission hyponatremia with in-hospital death.

8.2 Confounding Variables in Big Data

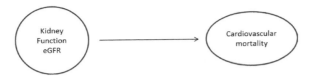

Fig. 8.1 Concept map of the association of kidney function, as determined by the glomerular filtration rate, as a determinant of cardiovascular morality

Many cross-sectional studies have not addressed the underlying reason for hyponatremia in the first place. Most often, hyponatremia is caused by sensed volume depletion, as might occur in liver disease and heart disease. Sensed volume is a concept describing the body's internal measure of intravascular volume, which directly affects the body's sodium avidity, and which under certain conditions affects its water avidity. Sensed volume is quite difficult to determine clinically, and there are no billing or diagnostic codes to describe it. Therefore, even though sensed volume is the strongest determinant of serum sodium concentrations in large population studies, it is not a capturable variable, and thus it cannot be included as a covariate in adjusted analyses. Its absence likely leads to false conclusions. As of now, despite a plethora of studies showing that hyponatremia is associated with poor outcomes, we collectively can not conclude whether it is the water excess itself, or the underlying cardiac or liver pathophysiologic abnormalities that cause the hyponatremia, that is of greater importance.

Let us consider another very important example. There have been a plethora of studies in the critical care literature linking renal function to a myriad of outcomes [12, 13]. One undisputed conclusion is that impaired renal function is associated with increased cardiovascular mortality, as illustrated in Fig. 8.1.

However, this association is really quite complex, with a number of important confounding issues that undermine this conclusion. The first issue is how accurately a serum creatinine measurement reflects the glomerular filtration rate (GFR). Calculations such as the Modification of Diet in Renal Disease (MDRD) equation were developed as epidemiologic tools to estimate GFR [14] but do not accurately define underlying renal physiology. Furthermore, even if one considers the serum creatinine as a measure of GFR, there are multiple other aspects of kidney functions beyond the GFR, including sodium and fluid balance, erythropoietin and activated vitamin D production, and tubular function, none of which are easily measurable, and thus cannot be accounted for.

However, in addition to confounding due to an inability to accurately characterize "renal function," significant residual confounding due to unaccounted pathophysiology is equally problematic. In relation to the association of renal function with cardiovascular mortality, there are many determinants of cardiac function that simultaneously and independently influence both the serum creatinine

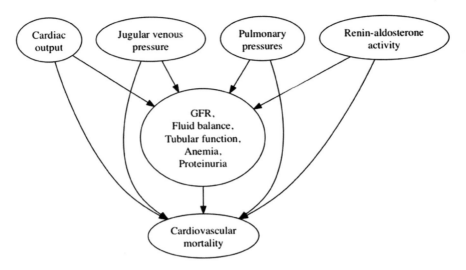

Fig. 8.2 Concept map of the association of renal function and cardiovascular mortality revealing more of the confounding influences

concentration and cardiovascular outcomes. For example, increased jugular venous pressures are a strong determinant of cardiac outcome and influence renal function through renal vein congestion. Cardiac output, pulmonary artery pressures, and activation of the renin-angiotensin-aldosterone axis also likely influence both renal function and cardiac outcomes. The concept map is likely more similar to Fig. 8.2.

Since many of these variables are rarely measured or quantified in large epidemiologic studies, significant residual confounding likely exists, and potential bias by failing to appreciate the complexity of the underlying pathophysiology is likely.

Multiple statistical techniques have been developed to account for residual confounding to non-randomization and to underlying severity of illness in critical care. Propensity scores, which attempt to better capture the factors that lead to the non-randomized allocation (i.e. the factors which influence the decision to admit to the ICU or to expose to a PPI) are used widely to minimize selection bias [15]. Adjustment using variables that attempt to capture severity of illness, such as the Simplified Acute Physiology Score (SAPS) [16], or the Sequential/ Sepsis-related Organ Failure Assessment (SOFA) score [17], or comorbidity adjustment scores, such as Charlson or Elixhauser [18, 19], remain imprecise, as does risk adjustment with area under the receiver operating characteristic curve (AUROC). Ultimately, significant confounding cannot be adjusted away by the most sophisticated statistical techniques, and thoughtful and careful examination of the limitations of any observational study must be transparent.

8.3 Conclusion

In summary, tread gently when harvesting the power of Big Data, for what is not seen is exactly what may be of most interest. Be clear about the limitations of using observational data, and suggest that most observational studies are hypothesis generating and require more well designed studies to better address the question at hand.

Open Access This chapter is distributed under the terms of the Creative Commons Attribution-NonCommercial 4.0 International License (http://creativecommons.org/licenses/by-nc/4.0/), which permits any noncommercial use, duplication, adaptation, distribution and reproduction in any medium or format, as long as you give appropriate credit to the original author(s) and the source, a link is provided to the Creative Commons license and any changes made are indicated.

The images or other third party material in this chapter are included in the work's Creative Commons license, unless indicated otherwise in the credit line; if such material is not included in the work's Creative Commons license and the respective action is not permitted by statutory regulation, users will need to obtain permission from the license holder to duplicate, adapt or reproduce the material.

References

1. Bourne PE (2014) What big data means to me. J Am Med Inf Assoc. 21(2):194–194
2. Saeed M, Villarroel M, Reisner AT, Clifford G, Lehman L-W, Moody G et al (2011) Multiparameter intelligent monitoring in intensive care II: a public-access intensive care unit database. Crit Care Med 39(5):952–960
3. Patel CJ, Burford B, Ioannidis JPA (2015) Assessment of vibration of effects due to model specification can demonstrate the instability of observational associations. J Clin Epidemiol 68 (9):1046–1058
4. Tzoulaki I, Siontis KCM, Ioannidis JPA (2011) Prognostic effect size of cardiovascular biomarkers in datasets from observational studies versus randomised trials: meta-epidemiology study. BMJ 343:d6829
5. Greenland S (2005) Confounding. In: Armitage P, Colton T (eds) Encyclopedia of biostatistics, 2nd edn.
6. National Task Force on the Prevention and Treatment of Obesity (2000) Overweight, obesity, and health risk. Arch Intern Med 160(7):898–904
7. Berrington de Gonzalez A, Hartge P, Cerhan JR, Flint AJ, Hannan L, MacInnis RJ et al (2010) Body-mass index and mortality among 1.46 million white adults. N Engl J Med 363 (23):2211–2219
8. Hutagalung R, Marques J, Kobylka K, Zeidan M, Kabisch B, Brunkhorst F et al (2011) The obesity paradox in surgical intensive care unit patients. Intensive Care Med 37(11):1793–1799
9. Pickkers P, de Keizer N, Dusseljee J, Weerheijm D, van der Hoeven JG, Peek N (2013) Body mass index is associated with hospital mortality in critically ill patients: an observational cohort study. Crit Care Med 41(8):1878–1883
10. Danziger J, William JH, Scott DJ, Lee J, Lehman L-W, Mark RG et al (2013) Proton-pump inhibitor use is associated with low serum magnesium concentrations. Kidney Int 83(4): 692–699
11. Verbalis JG, Goldsmith SR, Greenberg A, Korzelius C, Schrier RW, Sterns RH et al (2013) Diagnosis, evaluation, and treatment of hyponatremia: expert panel recommendations. Am J Med 126(10 Suppl 1):S1–S42

12. Apel M, Maia VPL, Zeidan M, Schinkoethe C, Wolf G, Reinhart K et al (2013) End-stage renal disease and outcome in a surgical intensive care unit. Crit Care 17(6):R298
13. Matsushita K, van der Velde M, Astor BC, Woodward M, Levey AS et al (2010) Chronic kidney disease prognosis consortium. Association of estimated glomerular filtration rate and albuminuria with all-cause and cardiovascular mortality in general population cohorts: a collaborative meta-analysis. Lancet 375(9731):2073–2081
14. Levey AS, Bosch JP, Lewis JB, Greene T, Rogers N, Roth D (1999) A more accurate method to estimate glomerular filtration rate from serum creatinine: a new prediction equation. Modification of diet in renal disease study group. Ann Intern Med 130(6):461–470
15. Gayat E, Pirracchio R, Resche-Rigon M, Mebazaa A, Mary J-Y, Porcher R (2010) Propensity scores in intensive care and anaesthesiology literature: a systematic review. Intensive Care Med 36(12):1993–2003
16. Le Gall JR, Lemeshow S, Saulnier F (1993) A new simplified acute physiology score (SAPS II) based on a European/North American multicenter study. JAMA 270(24):2957–2963
17. Vincent JL, Moreno R, Takala J, Willatts S, De Mendonça A, Bruining H et al (1996) The SOFA (sepsis-related organ failure assessment) score to describe organ dysfunction/failure. On behalf of the working group on sepsis-related problems of the European society of intensive care medicine. Intensive Care Med 22(7):707–710
18. Charlson ME, Pompei P, Ales KL, MacKenzie CR (1987) A new method of classifying prognostic comorbidity in longitudinal studies: development and validation. J Chronic Dis 40(5):373–383
19. Elixhauser A, Steiner C, Harris DR, Coffey RM (1998) Comorbidity measures for use with administrative data. Med Care 36(1):8–27

Part II
A Cookbook: From Research Question Formulation to Validation of Findings

The first part of this textbook has given the reader a general perspective about Electronic Health Records (EHRs), their potential for medical research and use for retrospective data analyses. Part II focuses on the use of one particular EHR, the Medical Information Mart for Intensive Care (MIMIC) database, curated by the Laboratory for Computational Physiology at MIT. The readers will have an opportunity to develop their analytical skills for clinical data mining while following a complete research project, from the initial definition of a research question to the assessment of the final results' robustness. This part is designed like a cookbook, with each chapter comprising some theoretical concepts, followed by worked examples using MIMIC. Part III of this book will be dedicated to a variety of different case studies to further your understanding of more advanced analysis methods.

This part is subdivided into nine chapters that follow the common process of generating new medical evidence using clinical data mining. In Chap. 9, the reader will learn how to transform a clinical question into a pertinent research question, which includes defining an appropriate study design and select the exposure and outcome of interest. In Chap. 10, the researcher will learn how to define which patient population is most relevant for investigating the research question. Owing to the essential and often challenging aspect of analysis of EHRs, it will be described in the following four chapters elaborately. Chapters 11 and 12 deal with the essential task of data preparation and pre-processing, which is mandatory before any data can be fed into a statistical analysis tool. Chapter 11 explains how a database is structured, what type of data they can contain and how to extract the variables of interest using queries; Chap. 12 presents some common methods of data pre-processing, which usually implies cleaning, integrating, then reducing the data; Chap. 13 provides various methods for dealing with missing data; Chap. 14 discusses techniques to identify and handle outliers. In Chap. 15, common methods for exploring the data are presented, both numerical and graphical. Exploration data analysis gives the researcher some invaluable insight into the features and potential issues of a dataset, and can help with generating further hypotheses. Chapter 16, "data analysis", presents the theory and methods for model development (Sect. 16.1) as well as common data analysis techniques in clinical studies, namely linear regression (Sect. 16.2), logistic regression (Sect. 16.3) and survival analysis including Cox proportional hazards models (Sect. 16.4). Finally, Chap. 17 discusses the principles of model validation and sensitivity analyses, where the results of a particular research are tested for robustness in the face of varying model assumptions.

Each chapter includes worked examples inspired from a unique study, published in Chest in 2015 by Hsu et al., which addressed a key question in clinical practice in intensive care medicine: "is the placement of an indwelling arterial catheter (IAC) associated with reduced mortality, in patients who are mechanically ventilated but do not require vasopressor support?" IACs are used extensively in the intensive care unit for continuous monitoring of blood pressure and are thought to be more accurate and reliable than standard, non-invasive blood pressure monitoring. They also have the added benefit of allowing for easier arterial blood gas collection which can reduce the need for repeated arterial punctures. Given their invasive nature, however, IACs carry risks of bloodstream infection and vascular injury, so the evidence of a beneficial effect requires evaluation. The primary outcome of interest selected was 28-day mortality with secondary outcomes that included ICU and hospital length-of-stay, duration of mechanical ventilation, and mean number of blood gas measurements made. The authors identified the encounter-centric 'arterial catheter placement' as their exposure of interest and carried out a propensity score analysis to test the relationship between the exposure and outcomes using MIMIC. The result in this particular dataset (spoiler alert) is that the presence of an IAC is not associated with a difference in 28-day mortality, in hemodynamically stable patients who are mechanically ventilated. This case study provides a basic foundation to apply the above theory to a working example, and will give the reader first-hand perspective on various aspects of data mining and analytical techniques. This is in no way a comprehensive exploration of EHR analytics and, where the case lacks the necessary detail, we have attempted to include additional relevant information for common analytical techniques. For the interested reader, references are provided for more detailed readings.

Chapter 9
Formulating the Research Question

Anuj Mehta, Brian Malley and Allan Walkey

Learning Objectives

- Understand how to turn a clinical question into a research question.
- Principles of choosing a sample.
- Approaches and potential pitfalls.
- Principles of defining the exposure of interest.
- Principles of defining the outcome.
- Selecting an appropriate study design.

9.1 Introduction

The clinical question arising at the time of most health-care decisions is: "will this help my patient?" Before embarking on an investigation to provide data that may be used to inform the clinical question, the question must be modified into a research query. The process of developing a research question involves defining several components of the study and also what type of study is most suited to utilize these components to yield valid and reliable results. These components include: in whom is this research question relevant? The population of subjects defined by the researcher is referred to as the sample. The drug, maneuver, event or characteristic that we are basing our alternative hypothesis on is called the exposure of interest. Finally, the outcome of interest must be defined. With these components in mind the researcher must decide which study design is best or most feasible for answering the question. If an observational study design is chosen, then the choice of a database is also crucial.

In this chapter, we will explore how researchers might work through converting a clinical question into a research question using the clinical scenario of indwelling arterial catheters (IAC) use during mechanical ventilation (MV). Furthermore, we will discuss the strengths and weaknesses of common study designs including randomized controlled trials as well as observational studies.

9.2 The Clinical Scenario: Impact of Indwelling Arterial Catheters

Patients who require MV because they are unable to maintain adequate breathing on their own (e.g. from severe pneumonia or asthma attack) are often the sickest patients in the hospital, with mortality rates exceeding 30 % [1–3]. Multiple options are available to monitor the adequacy of respiratory support for critically ill patients requiring MV, ranging from non-invasive trans-cutaneous measures to invasive, indwelling monitoring systems. IACs are invasive monitoring devices that allow continuous real time blood pressure monitoring and facilitate access to arterial blood sampling to assess arterial blood pH, oxygen and carbon dioxide levels, among others [4–6]. While closer monitoring of patients requiring MV with IACs may appear at face value to be beneficial, IACs may result in severe adverse events, including loss of blood flow to the hand and infection [7, 8]. Currently, data is lacking whether benefits may outweigh risks of more intensive monitoring using IACs. Examining factors associated with the decision to use IACs, and outcomes in patients provided IACs as compared to non-invasive monitors alone, may provide information useful to clinicians facing the decision as to whether to place an IAC.

9.3 Turning Clinical Questions into Research Questions

The first step in the process of transforming a clinical question into research is to carefully define the **study sample (or patient cohort)**, the **exposure** of interest, and the **outcome** of interest. These 3 components—sample, exposure, and outcome—are essential parts of every research question. Slight variations in each component can dramatically affect the conclusions that can be drawn from any research study, and whether the research will appropriately address the overarching clinical question.

9.3.1 Study Sample

In the case of IAC use, one might imagine many potential study samples of interest: for example, one might include all ICU patients, all patients receiving MV, all patients receiving intravenous medications that strongly affect blood pressure, adults only, children only, etc. Alternatively, one could define samples based on specific diseases or syndrome, such as shock (where IACs may be used to closely monitor blood pressure) or severe asthma (where IAC may be used to monitor oxygen or carbon dioxide levels).

The choice of study sample will affect both the internal and the external validity (generalizability) of the study. A study focusing only on a pediatric population may not apply to the adult population. Similarly, a study focused on patients receiving MV may not be applicable to non-ventilated patients. Furthermore, a study including patients with different reasons for using an IAC, with different outcomes related to the reason for IAC use, may lack internal validity due to bias called 'confounding'. Confounding is a type of study bias in which an exposure variable is associated with both the exposure and the outcome.

For instance, if the benefits of IACs on mortality are studied in all patients receiving MV, researchers must take into account the fact that IAC placement may actually be indicative of greater severity of illness. For example, imagine a study with a sample of MV patients in which those with septic shock received an IAC to facilitate vasoactive medications and provide close blood pressuring monitoring while patients with asthma did not receive an IAC as other methods were used to monitor their ventilation (such as end-tidal CO_2 monitoring). Patients with septic shock tend to have a much higher severity of illness compared to patients with asthma regardless of whether an IAC is placed. In such a study, researchers may conclude that IACs are associated with higher mortality only because IACs were used in sicker patients with a higher risk of dying. The variable "diagnosis" is therefore a confounding factor, associated with both the exposure (decision to insert an IAC) and the outcome (death). Careful sample selection is one method of attempting to address issues of confounding related to severity of illness. Restricting study samples to exclude groups that may strongly confound results (i.e. no patients on vasoactive medications) is one strategy to reduce bias. However, the selection of homogeneous study samples to increase internal validity should be balanced with the desire to generalize study findings to broader patient populations. These principles are discussed more extensively in the Chap. 10—"Cohort Selection".

9.3.2 Exposure

The exposure in our research question appears to be fairly clear: placement of an IAC. However, careful attention should be paid as to how each exposure or variable of interest is defined. Misclassifying exposures may bias results. How should IAC be measured? For example, investigators may use methods ranging from direct review of the medical chart to use of administrative claims data (i.e. International Classification of Diseases—ICD-codes) to identify IAC use. Each method of ascertaining the exposure of interest may have pros (improved accuracy of medical chart review) and cons (many person-hours to perform manual chart review).

Defining the time window during which an exposure of interest is measured may also have substantial implications that must be considered when interpreting the research results. For the purposes of our IAC study, the presence of an IAC was defined as having an IAC placed after the initiation of MV. The time-dependent nature of the exposure is critical for answering the clinical question; some IACs placed prior to MV are for monitoring of low-risk surgical patients in the operating room. Including all patients with IACs regardless of timing may bias the results towards a benefit for IACs by including many otherwise healthy patients who had an IAC placed for surgical monitoring. Alternatively, if the exposure group is defined as patients who had an IAC at least 48 h after initiation of MV, the study is at risk for a type of confounding called "immortal time bias": only patients who were alive could have had an IAC placed, whereas patients dying prior to 48 h (supposedly sicker) could not have had an IAC.

Equally important to defining the group of patients who received or experienced an exposure is to define the "unexposed" or control group. While not all research requires a control group (e.g. epidemiologic studies), a control group is needed to assess the effectiveness of healthcare interventions. In the case of the IAC study, the control group is fairly straightforward: patients receiving MV who did not have an IAC placed. However, there are important nuances when defining control groups. In our study example, an alternate control group could be all ICU patients who did not receive an IAC. However, the inclusion of patients not receiving MV results in a control group with a lower severity of illness and expected mortality than patients receiving MV, which would bias in favor of not using IACs. Careful definition of the control group is needed to properly interpret any conclusions from research; defining an appropriate control group is as important as defining the exposure.

9.3.3 Outcome

Finally, the investigator needs to determine the outcome of interest. Several different types of outcomes can be considered, including intermediate or mechanistic outcomes (informs etiological pathways, but may not immediately impact patients), patient-centered outcomes (informs outcomes important to patients, but may lack mechanistic insights: e.g. comfort scales, quality of life indices, or mortality), or healthcare-system centered outcomes (e.g. resource utilization, or costs). In our example of IAC use, several outcomes could be considered including intermediate outcomes (e.g. number of arterial blood draws, ventilator setting changes, or vasoactive medication changes), patient-centered outcomes (e.g. 28-day or 90-day mortality, adverse event rates), or healthcare utilization (e.g. hospitalization costs, added clinician workload). As shown in our example, outcome(s) may build upon each other to yield a constellation of findings that provides a more complete picture to address the clinical question of interest.

After clearly defining the study sample, exposure of interest, and outcome of interest, a research question can be formulated. A research question using our example may be formulated as follows:

"*In the population of interest (**study cohort**), is the exposure to the **variable of interest** associated with a different **outcome** than in the **control group**?*", which becomes, in our example:

"*Among mechanically ventilated, adult ICU patients who are not receiving vasoactive medications (i.e., the study sample) is placement of an IAC after initiation of MV (as compared with not receiving an IAC) (i.e. the exposure and control patients) associated with improved 28-day mortality rates (primary outcome, patient-centered) and the number of blood gas measurements per day (supporting secondary outcome, intermediate/mechanistic)?*"

9.4 Matching Study Design to the Research Question

Once the research question has been defined, the next step is to choose the optimal study design given the question and resources available. In biomedical research, the gold-standard for study design remains the double-blinded, randomized, placebo-controlled trial (RCT) [9, 10]. In a RCT, patients with a given condition (e.g. all adults receiving MV) would be randomized to receive a drug or intervention of interest (e.g. IAC) or randomized to receive the control (e.g. no IAC), with careful measurement of pre-determined outcomes (e.g. 28-day mortality). In ideal conditions, the randomization process eliminates all measured and unmeasured confounding and allows for causal inferences to be drawn, which cannot generally be achieved without randomization. As shown above, confounding is a threat to valid inferences from study results. Alternatively, in our example of septic shock verses asthma, severity of illness associated with the underlying condition may represent another confounder. Randomization solely based on the exposure of interest attempts to suppress issues of confounding. In our examples, proper randomization in a large sample would theoretically create equal age distributions and equal numbers of patients with septic shock and asthma in both the exposure and the control group.

However, RCTs have several limitations. Although the theoretical underpinnings of RCTs are fairly simple, the complex logistics of patient enrollment and retention, informed consent, randomization, follow up, and blinding may result in RCTs deviating from the 'ideal conditions' necessary for unbiased, causal inference. Additionally, RCTs carry the highest potential for patient harm and require intensive monitoring because the study dictates what type of treatment a patient receives (rather than the doctor) and may deviate from routine care. Given the logistic complexity, RCTs are often time- and cost-intensive, frequently taking many years and millions of dollars to complete. Even when logistically feasible, RCTs often 'weed out' multiple groups of patients in order to minimize potential harms and maximize detection of associations between interventions and outcomes of interest. As a result, RCTs can consist of homogeneous patients meeting narrow criteria, which may reduce the external validity of the studies' findings. Despite much effort and cost, an RCT may miss relevance to the clinical question as to whether the intervention of interest is helpful for your particular patient or not. Finally, some clinical questions may not ethically be answered with RCTs. For instance, the link between smoking and lung cancer has never been shown in a RCT, as it is unethical to randomize patients to start smoking in a smoking intervention group, or randomize patients to a control group in a trial to investigate the efficacy of parachutes [11]!

Observational research differs from RCTs. Observational studies are non-experimental; researchers record routine medical practice patterns and derive conclusions based on correlations and associations without active interventions [9, 12]. Observational studies can be retrospective (based on data that has already been collected), prospective (data is actively collected over time), or ambi-directional (a mix). Unlike RCTs, researchers in observational studies have no role in deciding what types of treatments or interventions patients receive. Observational studies tend to be logistically less complicated than RCTs as there is no active intervention, no randomization, no data monitoring boards, and data is often collected retrospectively. As such, observational studies carry less risk of harm to patients (other than loss of confidentiality of data that has been collected) than RCTs, and tend to be less time- and cost-intensive. Retrospective databases like MIMIC-II [13] or the National Inpatient Sample [14] can also provide much larger study samples (tens of thousands in some instances) than could be enrolled in an RCT, thus providing larger statistical power. Additionally, broader study samples are often included in observational studies, leading to greater generalizability of the results to a wider range of patients (external validity). Finally, certain clinical questions that would be unethical to study in an RCT can be investigated with observational studies. For example, the link between lung cancer and tobacco use has been demonstrated with multiple large prospective epidemiological studies [15, 16] and the life-saving effects of parachutes have been demonstrated mostly through the powers of observation.

Although logistically simpler than RCTs, the theoretical underpinnings of observational studies are generally more complex than RCTs. Obtaining causal estimates of the effect of a specific exposure on a specific outcome depends on the philosophical concept of the 'counterfactual' [17]. The counterfactual is the situation in which, all being equal, the same research subject at the same time would receive the exposure of interest and (the counterfactual) not receive the exposure of interest, with the same outcome measured in the exposed and unexposed research subject. Because we cannot create cloned research subjects in the real-world, we rely on creating groups of patients similar to the group that receives an intervention of interest. In the case of an ideal RCT with a large enough number of subjects, the randomization process used to select the intervention and control groups creates two alternate 'universes' of patients that will be similar except as related to the exposure of interest. Because observational studies cannot intervene on study subjects, observational studies create natural experiments in which the counterfactual group is defined by the investigator and by clinical processes occurring in the real-world. Importantly, real-world clinical processes often occur for a reason, and these reasons can cause deviation from counterfactual ideals in which exposed and unexposed study subjects differ in important ways. In short, observational studies may be more prone to bias (problems with internal validity) than RCTs due to difficulty obtaining the counterfactual control group.

Several types of biases have been identified in observational studies. Selection bias occurs when the process of selecting exposed and unexposed patients introduces a bias into the study. For example, the time between starting MV and receiving IAC may introduce a type of "survivor treatment selection bias" since patients who received IAC could not have died prior to receiving IACs. Information bias stems from mismeasurement or misclassification of certain variables. For retrospective studies, the data has already been collected and sometimes it is difficult to evaluate for errors in the data. Another major bias in observational studies is confounding. As stated, confounding occurs when a third variable is correlated with both the exposure and outcome. If the third variable is not taken into consideration, a spurious relationship between the exposure and outcome may be inferred. For example, smoking is an important confounder in several observational studies as it is associated with several other behaviors such as coffee and alcohol consumption. A study investigating the relationship between coffee consumption and incidence of lung cancer may conclude that individuals who drink more coffee have higher rates of lung cancer. However, as smoking is associated with both coffee consumption and lung cancer, it is confounder in the relationship between coffee consumption and lung cancer if unmeasured and unaccounted for in analysis. Several methods have been developed to attempt to address confounding in observational research such as adjusting for the confounder in regression equations if it is known and measured, matching cohorts by known confounders, and using instrumental variables—methods that will be explained in-depth in future chapters. Alternatively, one can restrict the study sample (e.g. excluding patients with shock from a study evaluating the utility of IACs). For these reasons, while powerful, an individual observational study can, at best, demonstrate associations and correlations and cannot prove causation. Over time, a cumulative sum of multiple high quality observational studies coupled with other mechanistic evidence can lead to causal conclusions, such as in the causal link currently accepted between smoking and lung cancer established by observational human studies and experimental trials in animals.

9.5 Types of Observational Research

There are multiple different types of questions that can be answered with observational research (Table 9.1). Epidemiological studies are one major type of observational research that focuses on the burden of disease in predefined populations. These types of studies often attempt to define incidence, prevalence, and risk factors for disease. Additionally, epidemiological studies also can investigate changes to healthcare or diseases over time. Epidemiological studies are the cornerstone of public health and can heavily influence policy decisions, resource

Table 9.1 Major types of observational research, and their purpose

Type of observational research	Purpose
Epidemiological	Define incidence, prevalence, and risk factors for disease
Predictive modeling	Predict future outcomes
Comparative effectiveness	Identify intervention associated with superior outcomes
Pharmacovigilance	Detect rare drug adverse events occurring in the long-term

allocation, and patient care. In the case of lung cancer, predefined groups of patients without lung cancer were monitored for years until some patients developed lung cancer. Researchers then compared numerous risk factors, like smoking, between those who did and did not develop lung cancer which led to the conclusion that smoking increased the risk of lung cancer [15, 16].

There are other types of epidemiological studies that are based on similar principles of observational research but differ in the types of questions posed. Predictive modeling studies develop models that are able to accurately predict future outcomes in specific groups of patients. In predictive studies, researchers define an outcome of interest (e.g. hospital mortality) and use data collected on patients such as labs, vital signs, and disease states to determine which factors contributed to the outcome. Researchers then validate the models developed from one group of patients in a separate group of patients. Predictive modeling studies developed many common prediction scores used in clinical practice such as the Framingham Cardiovascular Risk Score [18], APACHE IV [19], SAPS II [20], and SOFA [21].

Comparative effectiveness research is another form of observational research which involves the comparison of existing healthcare interventions in order to determine effective methods to deliver healthcare. Unlike descriptive epidemiologic studies, comparative effectiveness research compares outcomes between similar patients who received different treatments in order to assess which intervention may be associated with superior outcomes in real-world conditions. This could involve comparing drug A to drug B or could involve comparing one intervention to a control group who did not receive that intervention. Given that there are often underlying reasons why one patient received treatment A versus B or an intervention versus no intervention, comparative effectiveness studies must meticulously account for potential confounding factors. In the case of IACs, the research question comparing patients who had an IAC placed to those who did not have an IAC placed would represent a comparative effectiveness study.

Pharmacovigilance studies are yet another form of observational research. As many drug and device trials end after 1 or 2 years, observational methods are used to evaluate if there are patterns of rarer adverse events occurring in the long-term. Phase IV clinical studies are one form of pharmacovigilance studies in which long-term information related to efficacy and harm are gathered after the drug has been approved.

9.6 Choosing the Right Database

A critical part of the research process is deciding what types of data are needed to answer the research question. Administrative/claims data, secondary use of clinical trial data, prospective epidemiologic studies, and electronic health record (EHR) systems (both from individual institutions and those pooled from multiple institutions) are several sources from which databases can be built. Administrative or claims databases, such as the National Inpatient Sample and State Inpatient Databases complied by the Healthcare Cost and Utilization Project or the Medicare database, contain information on patient and hospital demographics as well as billing and procedure codes. Several techniques have been developed to translate these billing and procedure codes to more clinically useful disease descriptions. Administrative databases tend to provide very large sample sizes and, in some cases, can be representative of an entire population. However, they lack granular patient-level data from the hospitalization such as vital signs, laboratory and microbiology data, timing data (such as duration of MV or days with an IAC) or pharmacology data, which are often important in dealing with possible confounders.

Another common source of data for observational research is large epidemiologic studies like the Framingham Heart Study as well as large multicenter RCTs such as the NIH ARDS Network. Data that has already been can be analyzed retrospectively with new research questions in mind. As the original data was collected for research purposes, these types of databases often have detailed, granular information not available in other clinical databases. However, researchers are often bound by the scope of data collection from the original research study which limits the questions that may be posed. Importantly, generalizability may be limited in data from trials.

The advent of Electronic Health Records (EHR) has resulted in the digitization of medical records from their prior paper format. The resulting digitized medical records present opportunities to overcome some of the shortcomings of administrative data, yielding granular data with laboratory results, medications, and timing of clinical events [13]. These "big databases" take advantage of the fact many EHRs collect data from a variety of sources such as patient monitors, laboratory systems, and pharmacy systems and coalesce them into one system for clinicians. This information can then be translated into de-identified databases for research purposes that contain detailed patient demographics, billing and procedure information, timing data, hospital outcomes data, as well as patient-level granular data and provider notes which can searched using natural language processing tools. "Big data" approaches may attenuate confounding by providing detailed information needed to assess severity of illness (such as lab results and vital signs). Furthermore, the granular nature of the data can provide insight as to the reason why one patient received an intervention and another did not which can partly address confounding by indication. Thus, the promise of "big data" is that it contains small, very detailed data. "Big data" databases, such as MIMIC-III, have the potential to expand the scope of what had previously been possible with observational research.

9.7 Putting It Together

Fewer than 10 % of clinical decisions are supported by high level evidence [22]. Clinical questions arise approximately in every other patient [23] and provide a large cache of research questions. When formulating a research question, investigators must carefully select the appropriate sample of subjects, exposure variable, outcome variable, and confounding variables. Once the research question is clear, study design becomes the next pivotal step. While RCTs are the gold standard for establishing causal inference under ideal conditions, they are not always practical, cost-effective, ethical or even possible for some types of questions. Observational research presents an alternative to performing RCTs, but is often limited in causal inference by unmeasured confounding.

Our clinical scenario gave rise to the question of whether IACs improved the outcomes of patients receiving MV. This translated into the research question: "Among mechanically ventilated ICU patients not receiving vasoactive medications (study sample) is use of an IAC after initiation of MV (exposure) associated with improved 28-day mortality (outcome)?" While an RCT could answer this question, it would be logistically complex, costly, and difficult. Using comparative effectiveness techniques, one can pose the question using a granular retrospective database comparing patients who received an IAC to measurably similar patients who did not have an IAC placed. However, careful attention must be paid to unmeasured confounding by indication as to why some patients received IAC and others did not. Factors such as severity of illness, etiology of respiratory failure, and presence of certain diseases that make IAC placement difficult (such as peripheral arterial disease) may be considered as possible confounders of the association between IAC and mortality. While an administrative database could be used, it could lack important information related to possible confounders. As such, EHR databases like MIMIC-III, with detailed granular patient-level data, may allow for measurement of a greater number of previously unmeasured confounding variables and allow for greater attenuation of bias in observational research.

Take Home Messages

- Most research questions arise from clinical scenarios in which the proper course of treatment is unclear or unknown.
- Defining a research question requires careful consideration of the optimal study sample, exposure, and outcome in order to answer a clinical question of interest.
- While observational research studies can overcome many of the limitations of randomized controlled trials, careful consideration of study design and database selection is needed to address bias and confounding.

9.7 Putting It Together

Open Access This chapter is distributed under the terms of the Creative Commons Attribution-NonCommercial 4.0 International License (http://creativecommons.org/licenses/by-nc/4.0/), which permits any noncommercial use, duplication, adaptation, distribution and reproduction in any medium or format, as long as you give appropriate credit to the original author(s) and the source, a link is provided to the Creative Commons license and any changes made are indicated.

The images or other third party material in this chapter are included in the work's Creative Commons license, unless indicated otherwise in the credit line; if such material is not included in the work's Creative Commons license and the respective action is not permitted by statutory regulation, users will need to obtain permission from the license holder to duplicate, adapt or reproduce the material.

References

1. Esteban A, Frutos-Vivar F, Muriel A, Ferguson ND, Peñuelas O, Abraira V, Raymondos K, Rios F, Nin N, Apezteguía C, Violi DA, Thille AW, Brochard L, González M, Villagomez AJ, Hurtado J, Davies AR, Du B, Maggiore SM, Pelosi P, Soto L, Tomicic V, D'Empaire G, Matamis D, Abroug F, Moreno RP, Soares MA, Arabi Y, Sandi F, Jibaja M, Amin P, Koh Y, Kuiper MA, Bülow H-H, Zeggwagh AA, Anzueto A (2013) Evolution of mortality over time in patients receiving mechanical ventilation. Am J Respir Crit Care Med 188(2):220–230
2. Mehta A, Syeda SN, Wiener RS, Walkey AJ (2014) Temporal trends in invasive mechanical ventilation: severe sepsis/pneumonia, heart failure and chronic obstructive pulmonary disease. In: B23. Clinical trials and outcomes, vols 271. American Thoracic Society, pp. A2537–A2537
3. Stefan MS, Shieh M-S, Pekow PS, Rothberg MB, Steingrub JS, Lagu T, Lindenauer PK (2013) Epidemiology and outcomes of acute respiratory failure in the United States, 2001 to 2009: a national survey. J Hosp Med 8(2):76–82
4. Traoré O, Liotier J, Souweine B (2005) Prospective study of arterial and central venous catheter colonization and of arterial- and central venous catheter-related bacteremia in intensive care units. Crit Care Med 33(6):1276–1280
5. Gershengorn HB, Garland A, Kramer A, Scales DC, Rubenfeld G, Wunsch H (2014) Variation of arterial and central venous catheter use in United States intensive care units. Anesthesiology 120(3):650–664
6. Gershengorn HB, Wunsch H, Scales DC, Zarychanski R, Rubenfeld G, Garland A (2014) Association between arterial catheter use and hospital mortality in intensive care units. JAMA Intern Med 174(11):1746–1754
7. Maki DG, Kluger DM, Crnich CJ (2006) The risk of bloodstream infection in adults with different intravascular devices: a systematic review of 200 published prospective studies. Mayo Clin Proc 81(9):1159–1171
8. Scheer BV, Perel A, Pfeiffer UJ (2002) Clinical review: complications and risk factors of peripheral arterial catheters used for haemodynamic monitoring in anaesthesia and intensive care medicine. Crit Care 6(3):199–204
9. Concato J, Shah N, Horwitz RI (2000) Randomized, controlled trials, observational studies, and the hierarchy of research designs. N Engl J Med 342(25):1887–1892
10. Ho PM, Peterson PN, Masoudi FA (2008) Evaluating the evidence is there a rigid hierarchy? Circulation 118(16):1675–1684
11. Smith GCS, Pell JP (2003) Parachute use to prevent death and major trauma related to gravitational challenge: systematic review of randomised controlled trials. BMJ 327(7429):1459–1461
12. Booth CM, Tannock IF (2014) Randomised controlled trials and population-based observational research: partners in the evolution of medical evidence. Br J Cancer 110(3):551–555

13. Scott DJ, Lee J, Silva I, Park S, Moody GB, Celi LA, Mark RG (2013) Accessing the public MIMIC-II intensive care relational database for clinical research. BMC Med Inform Decis Mak 13(1):9
14. Healthcare Cost and Utilization Project and Agency for Healthcare Research and Quality. Overview of the National (Nationwide) Inpatient Sample (NIS)
15. Doll R, Hill AB (1954) The mortality of doctors in relation to their smoking habits; a preliminary report. Br Med J 1(4877):1451–1455
16. Alberg AJ, Samet JM (2003) Epidemiology of lung cancer. Chest 123(1 Suppl):21S–49S
17. Maldonado G, Greenland S (2002) Estimating causal effects. Int J Epidemiol 31(2):422–429
18. Wilson PWF, D'Agostino RB, Levy D, Belanger AM, Silbershatz H, Kannel WB (1998) Prediction of coronary heart disease using risk factor categories. Circulation 97(18):1837–1847
19. Zimmerman JE, Kramer AA, McNair DS, Malila FM (2006) Acute physiology and chronic health evaluation (APACHE) IV: hospital mortality assessment for today's critically ill patients. Crit Care Med 34(5):1297–1310
20. Le Gall JR, Lemeshow S, Saulnier F (1993) A new simplified acute physiology score (SAPS II) based on a European/North American multicenter study. JAMA 270(24):2957–2963
21. Vincent JL, Moreno R, Takala J, Willatts S, De Mendonça A, Bruining H, Reinhart CK, Suter PM, Thijs LG (1996) The SOFA (sepsis-related organ failure assessment) score to describe organ dysfunction/failure. On behalf of the working group on sepsis-related problems of the European society of intensive care medicine. Intensive Care Med 22(7):707–710
22. Tricoci P, Allen JM, Kramer JM, Califf RM, Smith SC (2009) Scientific evidence underlying the ACC/AHA clinical practice guidelines. JAMA 301(8):831–841
23. Del Fiol G, Workman TE, Gorman PN (2014) Clinical questions raised by clinicians at the point of care: a systematic review. JAMA Intern Med 174(5):710–718

Chapter 10
Defining the Patient Cohort

Ari Moskowitz and Kenneth Chen

Learning Objectives

- Understand the process of cohort selection using large, retrospective databases.
- Learn about additional specific skills in cohort building including data visualization and natural language processing (NLP).

10.1 Introduction

A critical first step in any observational study is the selection of an appropriate patient cohort for analysis. The importance of investing considerable time and effort into selection of the study population cannot be overstated. Failure to identify areas of potential bias, confounding, and missing data up-front can lead to considerable downstream inefficiencies. Further, care must be given to selecting a population of patients tailored to the research question of interest in order to properly leverage the tremendous amount of data captured by Electronic Health Records (EHRs).

In the following chapter we will focus on selection of the study cohort. Specifically, we will review the basics of observational study design with a focus on types of data often encountered in EHRs. Commonly used instrumental variables will be highlighted—they are variables used to control for confounding and measurement error in observational studies. Further, we will discuss how to utilize a combination of data-driven techniques and clinical reasoning in cohort selection. The chapter will conclude with a continuation of the worked example started in part

---

Electronic supplementary material The online version of this chapter (doi:10.1007/978-3-319-43742-2_10) contains supplementary material, which is available to authorized users.

© The Author(s) 2016
MIT Critical Data, *Secondary Analysis of Electronic Health Records*,
DOI 10.1007/978-3-319-43742-2_10

one of this section where we will discuss how the cohort of patients was selected for the study of arterial line placement in the intensive care unit [1].

10.2 PART 1—Theoretical Concepts

10.2.1 Exposure and Outcome of Interest

These notions are discussed in detail in Chap. 9—"Formulating the Research Question". Data mining in biomedical research utilizes a retrospective approach wherein the exposure and outcome of interest occur prior to patient selection. It is critically important to tailor the exposure of interest sought to the clinical question at hand. Selecting an overly broad exposure may allow for a large patient cohort, but at the expense of result accuracy. Similarly, being too specific in the choice of exposure may allow for accuracy but at the expense of sample size and generalizability.

The selection of an exposure of interest is the first step in determining the patient cohort. In general, the exposure of interest can be thought of as patient-centric, episode-centric, or encounter centric. This terminology was developed by the data warehousing firm Health Catalyst for their Cohort Builder tool and provides a reasonable framework for identifying an exposure of interest. Patient-centric exposures focus on traits intrinsic to a group of patients. These can include demographic traits (e.g. gender) or medical comorbidities (e.g. diabetes). In contrast, episode-centric exposures are transient conditions requiring a discrete treatment course (e.g. sepsis). Encounter-centric exposures refer to a single intervention (e.g. arterial line placement) [2]. Although encounter-specific exposures tend to be simpler to isolate, the choice of exposure should be determined by the specific hypothesis under investigation.

The outcome of interest should be identified a priori. The outcome should relate naturally to the exposure of interest and be as specific as possible to answer the clinical question at hand. Care must be taken to avoid identifying spurious correlations that have no pathophysiologic underpinnings (see for instance the examples of spurious correlations shown on http://tylervigen.com). The relationship sought must be grounded in biologic plausibility. Broad outcome measures, such as mortality and length-of-stay, may be superficially attractive but ultimately confounded by too many variables. Surrogate outcome measures (e.g. change in blood pressure, duration of mechanical ventilation) can be particularly helpful as they relate more closely to the exposure of interest and are less obscured by confounding.

As EHRs are not frequently oriented towards data mining and analysis, identifying an exposure of interest can be challenging. Structured numerical data, such as laboratory results and vital signs, are easily searchable with standard querying techniques. Leveraging unstructured data such as narrative notes and radiology reports can be more difficult and often requires the use of natural language processing (NLP) tools. In order to select a specific patient phenotype from a large, heterogeneous group of patients, it can be helpful to leverage both structured and unstructured data forms.

Once an exposure of interest is selected, the investigator must consider how to utilize one or a combination of these data types to isolate the desired study cohort for analysis. This can be done using a combination of data driven techniques and clinical reasoning as will be reviewed later in the chapter.

10.2.2 Comparison Group

In addition to isolating patients mapping to the exposure of interest, the investigator must also identify a comparison group. Ideally, this group should be comprised of patients phenotypically similar to those in the study cohort but who lack the exposure of interest. The selected comparison cohort should be at equal risk of developing the study outcome. In observational research, this can be accomplished notably via propensity score development (Chap. 23—"Propensity Score Analysis"). In general, the comparison group ought to be as large as or larger than the study cohort to maximize the power of the study. It is possible to select too many features on which to 'match' the comparison and study cohorts thereby reducing the number of patients available for the comparison cohort. Care must be taken to prevent over-matching.

In select cases, investigators can take advantage of natural experiments in which circumstances external to the EHR readily establish a study cohort and a comparison group. These so called 'instrumental variables' can include practice variations between care units, hospitals, and even geographic regions. Temporal relationships (i.e. before-and-after) relating to quality improvement initiatives or expert guideline releases can also be leveraged as instrumental variables. Investigators should be on the lookout for these highly useful tools.

10.2.3 Building the Study Cohort

Isolating specific patient phenotypes for inclusion in the study and comparison cohorts requires a combination of clinical reasoning and data-driven techniques. A close working relationship between clinicians and data scientists is an essential component of cohort selection using EHR data.

The clinician is on the frontline of medical care and has direct exposure to complex clinical scenarios that exist outside the realm of the available evidence-base. According to a 2011 Institute of Medicine Committee Report, only 10–20 % of clinical decisions are evidence based [3]. Nearly 50 % of clinical practice guidelines rely on expert opinion rather than experimental data [4]. In this 'data desert' it is the role of the clinician to identify novel research questions important for direct clinical care [5]. These questions lend themselves naturally to the isolation of an exposure of interest.

Once a clinical question and exposure of interest have been identified, the clinician and data scientist will need to set about isolating a patient cohort. Phenotype querying of structured and unstructured data can be complex and requires frequent tuning of the search criteria. Often multiple, complementary queries are required in order to isolate the specific group of interest. In addition, the research team must consider patient 'uniqueness' in that some patients have multiple ICU admissions both during a single hospitalization and over repeat hospital visits. If the same patient is included more than once in a study cohort, the assumption of independent measures is lost.

Researchers must pay attention to the necessity to exclude some patients on the grounds of their background medical history or pathological status, such as pregnancy for example. Failing to do so could introduce confounders and corrupt the causal relationship of interest.

In one example from a published MIMIC-II study, the investigators attempted to determine whether proton pump inhibitor (PPI) use was associated with hypomagnesaemia in critically-ill patients in the ICU [6]. The exposure of interest in this study was 'PPI use.' A comparison group of patients who were exposed to an alternative acid-reducing agent (histamine-2 receptor antagonists) and a comparison group not receiving any acid reducing medications were identified. The outcome of interest was a low magnesium level. In order to isolate the study cohort in this case, queries had to be developed to identify:

1. First ICU admission for each patient
2. PPI use as identified through NLP analysis of the 'Medication' section of the admission History and Physical
3. Conditions likely to influence PPI use and/or magnesium levels (e.g. diarrheal illness, end-stage renal disease)
4. Patients who were transferred from other hospitals as medications received at other hospitals could not be accounted for (patients excluded)
5. Patients who did not have a magnesium level within 36-h of ICU admission (patients excluded)
6. Patients missing comorbidity data (patients excluded)
7. Potential confounders including diuretic use

The SQL queries corresponding to this example are provided under the name "SQL_cohort_selection".

Maximizing the efficiency of data querying from EHRs is an area of active research and development. As an example, the Informatics for Integrating Biology and the Bedside (i2b2) network is an NIH funded program based at Partner's Health Center (Boston, MA) that is developing a framework for simplifying data querying and extraction from EHRs. Software tools developed by i2b2 are free to download and promise to simplify the isolation of a clinical phenotype from raw EHR data https://www.i2b2.org/about/index.html. This and similar projects should help simplify the large number of queries necessary to develop a study cohort [7].

10.2.4 Hidden Exposures

Not all exposures of interest can be identified directly from data contained within EHRs. In these circumstances, investigators need to be creative in identifying recorded data points that track closely with the exposure of interest. Clinical reasoning in these circumstances is important.

For instance, a research team using the MIMIC II database selected 'atrial fibrillation with rapid ventricular response receiving a rate control agent' as the exposure of interest. Atrial fibrillation is a common tachyarrhythmia in critically-ill populations that has been associated with worse clinical outcomes. Atrial fibrillation with rapid ventricular response is often treated with one of three rate control agents: metoprolol, diltiazem, or amiodarone. Unfortunately, 'atrial fibrillation with rapid ventricular response' is not a structured variable in the EHR system connected to the MIMIC II database. Performing an NLP search for the term 'atrial fibrillation with rapid ventricular response' in provider notes and discharge summaries is feasible however would not provide the temporal resolution needed with respect to drug administration.

To overcome this obstacle, investigators generated an algorithm to indirectly identify the 'hidden' exposure. A query was developed to isolate the first dose of an intravenous rate control agent (metoprolol, diltiazem, or amiodarone) received by a unique patient in the ICU. Next, it was determined whether the heart rate of the patient within one-hour of recorded drug administration was >110 beats per minute. Finally, an NLP algorithm was used to search the clinical chart for mention of atrial fibrillation. Those patients meeting all three conditions were included in the final study cohort. Examples of the Matlab code used to identify the cohort of interest is provided (function "Afib"), as well as Perl code for NLP (function "NLP").

10.2.5 Data Visualization

Graphic representation of alphanumeric EHR data can be particularly helpful in establishing the study cohort. Data visualization makes EHR data more accessible and allows for the rapid identification of trends otherwise difficult to identify. It also promotes more effective communication both amongst research team members and between the research team and a general audience not accustomed to 'Big Data' investigation. These principles are discussed more extensively in Chap. 15 of this textbook "Exploratory Data Analysis".

In the above mentioned project exploring the use of rate control agents for atrial fibrillation with rapid ventricular response, one outcome of interest was time until control of the rapid ventricular rate. Unfortunately, the existing literature does not provide specific guidance in this area. Using data visualization, a group consensus was reached that rate control would be defined as a heart <110 for at least 90 % of the time over a 4-h period. Although some aspects of this definition are arbitrary, data visualization allowed for all team members to come to an agreement on what definition was the most statistically and clinically defensible.

10.2.6 Study Cohort Fidelity

Query algorithms are generally unable to boast 100 % accuracy for identifying the sought patient phenotype. False positives and false negatives are expected. In order to guarantee the fidelity of the study cohort, manually reviewing a random subset of selected patients can be helpful. Based on the size of the study cohort, 5–10 % of clinical charts should be reviewed to ensure the presence or absence of the exposure of interest. This task should be accomplished by a clinician. If resources permit, two clinician reviewers can be tasked with this role and their independent results compared using a Kappa statistic.

Ultimately, the investigators can use the 'gold standard' of manual review to establish a Receiver Operating Characteristic (ROC). An area-under the ROC curve of >0.80 indicates 'good' accuracy of the algorithm and should be used as an absolute minimum of algorithm fidelity. If the area under the ROC curve is <0.80, a combination of data visualization techniques and clinical reasoning should be used to better tune the query algorithm to the exposure of interest.

10.3 PART 2—Case Study: Cohort Selection

In the case study presented, the authors analyzed the effect of indwelling arterial catheters (IACs) in hemodynamically stable patients with respiratory failure using multivariate data. They identified the encounter-centric 'arterial catheter placement' as their exposure of interest. IACs are used extensively in the intensive care unit for beat-to-beat measuring of blood pressure and are thought to be more accurate and reliable than standard, non-invasive blood pressure monitoring. They also have the added benefit of allowing for simpler arterial blood gas collection which can reduce the need for repeated venous punctures. Given their invasive nature, however, IACs carry risks of bloodstream infection and vascular injury. The primary outcome of interest selected was 28-day mortality with secondary outcomes that included ICU and hospital length-of-stay, duration of mechanical ventilation, and mean number of blood gas measurements made.

The authors elected to focus their study on patients requiring mechanical ventilation that did not require vasopressor and were not admitted for sepsis. In patients requiring mechanical ventilation, the dual role of IACs to allow for beat-to-beat blood pressure monitoring and to simplify arterial blood gas collection is thought to be particularly important. Patients with vasopressor requirements and/or sepsis were excluded as invasive arterial catheters are needed in this population to assist with the rapid titration of vasoactive agents. In addition, it would be difficult to identify enough patients requiring vasopressors or admitted for sepsis, who did not receive an IAC.

The authors began their cohort selection with all 24,581 patients included in the MIMIC II database. For patients with multiple ICU admissions, only the first ICU admission was used to ensure independence of measurements. The function "cohort1" contains the SQL query corresponding to this step. Next, the patients who required mechanical ventilation within the first 24-h of their ICU admission and received mechanical ventilation for at least 24-h stay were isolated (function "cohort2"). After identifying a cohort of patients requiring mechanical ventilation, the authors queried for placement of an IAC sited after initiation of mechanical ventilation (function "cohort3"). As a majority of patients in the cardiac surgery recovery unit had an IAC placed prior to ICU admission, all patients from the cardiac surgical ICU were excluded from the analysis (function "cohort4"). In order to exclude patients admitted to the ICU with sepsis, the authors utilized the Angus criteria (function "cohort5"). Finally, patients requiring vasopressors during their ICU admission were excluded (function "cohort6").

The comparison group of patients who received mechanical ventilation for at least 24-h within the first 24-h of their ICU admission but did not have an IAC placed was identified. Ultimately, there were 984 patients in the group who received an IAC and 792 patients who did not. These groups were compared using propensity matching techniques described in the Chap. 23—"Propensity Score Analysis".

Ultimately, this cohort consists of unique identifiers of patients meeting the inclusion criteria. Other researchers may be interested in accessing this particular cohort in order to replicate the study results or address a different research questions. The MIMIC website will in the future provide the possibility for investigators to share cohorts of patients, thus allowing research teams to interact and build upon other's work.

Take Home Messages

- Take time to characterize the exposure and outcomes of interest pre-hoc
- Utilize both structured and unstructured data to isolate your exposure and outcome of interest. NLP can be particularly helpful in analyzing unstructured data
- Data visualization can be very helpful in facilitating communication amongst team members

Open Access This chapter is distributed under the terms of the Creative Commons Attribution-NonCommercial 4.0 International License (http://creativecommons.org/licenses/by-nc/4.0/), which permits any noncommercial use, duplication, adaptation, distribution and reproduction in any medium or format, as long as you give appropriate credit to the original author(s) and the source, a link is provided to the Creative Commons license and any changes made are indicated.

The images or other third party material in this chapter are included in the work's Creative Commons license, unless indicated otherwise in the credit line; if such material is not included in the work's Creative Commons license and the respective action is not permitted by statutory regulation, users will need to obtain permission from the license holder to duplicate, adapt or reproduce the material.

References

1. Hsu DJ, Feng M, Kothari R, Zhou H, Chen KP, Celi LA (2015) The association between indwelling arterial catheters and mortality in hemodynamically stable patients with respiratory failure: a propensity score analysis. Chest 148(6):1470–1476
2. Merkley K (2013) Defining patient populations using analytical tools: cohort builder and risk stratification. Health Catalyst, 21 Aug 2013
3. Institute of Medicine (US) Committee on Standards for Developing Trustworthy Clinical Practice Guidelines (2011) Clinical practice guidelines we can trust. National Academies Press (US), Washington (DC)
4. Committee on the Learning Health Care System in America and Institute of Medicine (2013) Best care at lower cost: the path to continuously learning health care in America. National Academies Press (US), Washington (DC)
5. Moskowitz A, McSparron J, Stone DJ, Celi LA (2015) Preparing a new generation of clinicians for the era of big data. Harv Med Stud Rev 2(1):24–27
6. Danziger J, William JH, Scott DJ, Lee J, Lehman L, Mark RG, Howell MD, Celi LA, Mukamal KJ (2013) Proton-pump inhibitor use is associated with low serum magnesium concentrations. Kidney Int 83(4):692–699
7. Jensen PB, Jensen LJ, Brunak S (2012) Mining electronic health records: towards better research applications and clinical care. Nat Rev Genet 13(6):395–405

Chapter 11
Data Preparation

Tom Pollard, Franck Dernoncourt, Samuel Finlayson
and Adrian Velasquez

Learning Objectives

- Become familiar with common categories of medical data.
- Appreciate the importance of collaboration between caregivers and data analysts.
- Learn common terminology associated with relational databases and plain text data files.
- Understand the key concepts of reproducible research.
- Get practical experience in querying a medical database.

11.1 Introduction

Data is at the core of all research, so robust data management practices are important if studies are to be carried out efficiently and reliably. The same can be said for the management of the software used to process and analyze data. Ensuring good practices are in place at the beginning of a study is likely to result in significant savings further down the line in terms of time and effort [1, 2].

While there are well-recognized benefits in tools and practices such as version control, testing frameworks, and reproducible workflows, there is still a way to go before these become widely adopted in the academic community. In this chapter we discuss some key issues to consider when working with medical data and highlight some approaches that can make studies collaborative and reproducible.

11.2 Part 1—Theoretical Concepts

11.2.1 Categories of Hospital Data

Data is routinely collected from several different sources within hospitals, and is generally optimized to support clinical activities and billing rather than research. Categories of data commonly found in practice are summarized in Table 11.1 and discussed below:

- Billing data generally consists of the codes that hospitals and caregivers use to file claims with their insurance providers. The two most common coding systems are the International Statistical Classification of Diseases and Related

Table 11.1 Overview of common categories of hospital data and common issues to consider during analysis

Category	Examples	Common issues to consider
Demographics	Age, gender, ethnicity, height, weight	Highly sensitive data requiring careful de-identification. Data quality in fields such as ethnicity may be poor
Laboratory	Creatinine, lactate, white blood cell count, microbiology results	Often no measure of sample quality. Methods and reagents used in tests may vary between units and across time
Radiographic images and associated reports	X-rays, computed tomography (CT) scans, echocardiograms	Protected health information, such as names, may be written on slides. Templates used to generate reports may influence content
Physiologic data	Vital signs, electrocardiography (ECG) waveforms, electroencephalography (EEG) waveforms	Data may be pre-processed by proprietary algorithms. Labels may be inaccurate (for example, "fingerstick glucose" measurements may be made with venous blood)
Medication	Prescriptions, dose, timing	May list medications that were ordered but not given. Time stamps may describe point of order not administration
Diagnosis and procedural codes	International Classification of Diseases (ICD) codes, Diagnosis Related Groups (DRG) codes, Current Procedural Terminology (CPT) codes	Often based on a retrospective review of notes and not intended to indicate a patient's medical status. Subject to coder biases. Limited by suitability of codes
Caregiver and procedural notes	Admission notes, daily progress notes, discharge summaries, Operative reports	Typographical errors. Context is important (for example, diseases may appear in discussion of family history). Abbreviations and acronyms are common

Health Problems, commonly abbreviated the International Classification of Disease (ICD), which is maintained by the World Health Organization, and the Current Procedural Terminology (CPT) codes maintained by the American Medical Association. These hierarchical terminologies were designed to provide standardization for medical classification and reporting.
- Charted physiologic data, including information such as heart rate, blood pressure, and respiratory rate collected at the bedside. The frequency and breadth of monitoring is generally related to the level of care. Data is often archived at a lower rate than it is sampled (for example, every 5–10 min) using averaging algorithms which are frequently proprietary and undisclosed.
- Notes and reports, created to record patient progress, summaries a patient stay upon discharge, and provide findings from imaging studies such as x-rays and echocardiograms. While the fields are "free text", notes are often created with the help of a templating system, meaning they may be partially structured.
- Images, such as those from x-rays, computerized axial tomography (CAT/CT) scans, echocardiograms, and magnetic resonance imaging.
- Medication and laboratory data. Orders for drugs and laboratory studies are entered by the caregiver into a physician order entry system, which are then fulfilled by laboratory or nursing staff. Depending on the system, some timestamps may refer to when the physician placed the order and others may refer to when the drug was administered or the lab results were reported. Some drugs may be administered days or weeks after first prescribed while some may not be administered at all.

11.2.2 Context and Collaboration

One of the greatest challenges of working with medical data is gaining knowledge of the context in which data is collected. For this reason we cannot emphasize enough the importance of collaboration between both hospital staff and research analysts. Some examples of common issues to consider when working with medical data are outlined in Table 11.1 and discussed below:

- Billing codes are not intended to document a patient's medical status or treatment from a clinical perspective and so may not be reliable [3]. Coding practices may be influenced by issues such as financial compensation and associated paperwork, deliberately or otherwise.
- Timestamps may differ in meaning for different categories of data. For example, a timestamp may refer to the point when a measurement was made, when the measurement was entered into the system, when a sample was taken, or when results were returned by a laboratory.
- Abbreviations and misspelled words appear frequently in free text fields. The string "pad", for example, may refer to either "peripheral artery disease" or to an

absorptive bed pad, or even a diaper pad. In addition, notes frequently mention diseases that are found in the patient's family history, but not necessarily the patient, so care must be taken when using simple text searches.
- Labels that describe concepts may not be accurate. For example, during preliminary investigations for an unpublished study to assess accuracy of fingertip glucose testing, it was discovered that caregivers would regularly take "fingerstick glucose" measurements using vascular blood where it was easily accessible, to avoid pricking the finger of a patient.

Each hospital brings its own biases to the data too. These biases may be tied to factors such as the patient populations served, the local practices of caregivers, or to the type of services provided. For example:

- Academic centers often see more complicated patients, and some hospitals may tend to serve patients of a specific ethnic background or socioeconomic status.
- Follow up visits may be less common at referral centers and so they may be less likely to detect long-term complications.
- Research centers may be more likely to place patients on experimental drugs not generally used in practice.

11.2.3 Quantitative and Qualitative Data

Data is often described as being either quantitative or qualitative. Quantitative data is data that can be measured, written down with numbers and manipulated numerically. Quantitative data can be discrete, taking only certain values (for example, the integers 1, 2, 3), or continuous, taking any value (for example, 1.23, 2.59). The number of times a patient is admitted to a hospital is discrete (a patient cannot be admitted 0.7 times), while a patient's weight is a continuous (a patient's weight could take any value within a range).

Qualitative data is information which cannot be expressed as a number and is often used interchangeably with the term "categorical" data. When there is not a natural ordering of the categories (for example, a patient's ethnicity), the data is called nominal. When the categories can be ordered, these are called ordinal variables (for example, severity of pain on a scale). Each of the possible values of a categorical variable is commonly referred to as a level.

11.2.4 Data Files and Databases

Data is typically made available through a database or as a file which may have been exported from a database. While there are many different kinds of databases and data files in use, relational databases and comma separated value (CSV) files are perhaps the most common.

11.2 Part 1—Theoretical Concepts

Comma Separated Value (CSV) Files

Comma separated value (CSV) files are a plain text format used for storing data in a tabular, spreadsheet-style structure. While there is no hard and fast rule for structuring tabular data, it is usually considered good practice to include a header row, to list each variable in a separate column, and to list observations in rows [4].

As there is no official standard for the CSV format, the term is used somewhat loosely, which can often cause issues when seeking to load the data into a data analysis package. A general recommendation is to follow the definition for CSVs set out by the Internet Engineering Task Force in the RFC 4180 specification document [5]. Summarized briefly, RFC 4180 specifies that:

- files may optionally begin with a header row, with each field separated by a comma;
- Records should be listed in subsequent rows. Fields should be separated by commas, and each row should be terminated with a line break;
- fields that contain numbers may be optionally enclosed within double quotes;
- fields that contain text ("strings") should be enclosed within double quotes;
- If a double quote appears inside a string of text then it must be escaped with a preceding double quote.

The CSV format is popular largely because of its simplicity and versatility. CSV files can be edited with a text editor, loaded as a spreadsheet in packages such as Microsoft Excel, and imported and processed by most data analysis packages. Often CSV files are an intermediate data format used to hold data that has been extracted from a relational database in preparation for analysis. Figure 11.1 shows an annotated example of a CSV file formatted to the RFC 4180 specification.

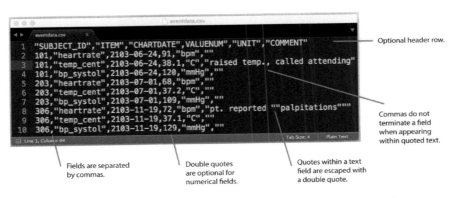

Fig. 11.1 Comma separated value (CSV) file formatted to the RFC 4180 specification

Relational Databases

There are several styles of database in use today, but probably the most widely implemented is the "relational database". Relational databases can be thought of as a collection of tables which are linked together by shared keys. Organizing data across tables can help to maintain data integrity and enable faster analysis and more efficient storage.

The model that defines the structure and relationships of the tables is known as a "database schema". Giving a simple example of a hospital database with four tables, it might comprise of: Table 1, a list of all patients; Table 2, a log of hospital admissions; Table 3, a list of vital sign measurements; Table 4, a dictionary of vital sign codes and associated labels. Figure 11.2 demonstrates how these tables can be linked with primary and foreign keys. Briefly, a primary key is a unique identifier within a table. For example, subject_id is the primary key in the patients table,

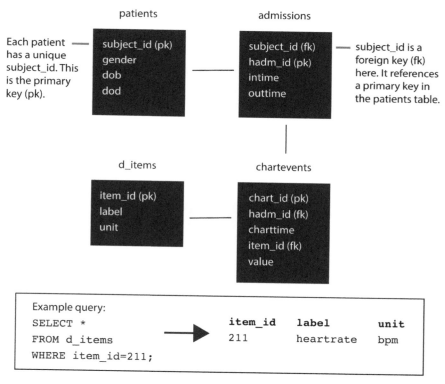

Fig. 11.2 Relational databases consist of multiple data tables linked by primary and foreign keys. The patients table lists unique patients. The admissions table lists unique hospital admissions. The chartevents table lists charted events such as heart rate measurements. The d_items table is a dictionary that lists item_ids and associated labels, as shown in the example query. *pk* is primary key. *fk* is foreign key

because each patient is listed only once. A foreign key in one table points to a primary key in another table. For example, subject_id in the admissions table is a foreign key, because it references the primary key in the patients table.

Extracting data from a database is known as "querying" the database. The programming language commonly used to create a query is known as "Structured Query Language" or SQL. While the syntax of SQL is straightforward, queries are at times challenging to construct as a result of the conceptual reasoning required to join data across multiple tables.

There are many different relational database systems in regular use. Some of these systems such as Oracle Database and Microsoft SQL Server are proprietary and may have licensing costs. Other systems such as PostgreSQL and MySQL are open source and free to install. The general principle behind the databases is the same, but it is helpful to be aware that programming syntax varies slightly between systems.

11.2.5 Reproducibility

Alongside a publishing system that emphasizes interpretation of results over detailed methodology, researchers are under pressure to deliver regular "high-impact" papers in order to sustain their careers. This environment may be a contributor to the widely reported "reproducibility crisis" in science today [6, 7].

Our response should be to ensure that studies are, as far as possible, reproducible. By making data and code accessible, we can more easily detect and fix inevitable errors, help each other to learn from our methods, and promote better quality research.

When practicing reproducible research, the source data should not be modified. Editing the raw data destroys the chain of reproducibility. Instead, code is used to process the data so that all of the steps that take an analysis from source to outcome can be reproduced.

Code and data should be well documented and the terms of reuse should be made clear. It is typical to provide a plain text "README" file that gives an introduction to the analysis package, along with a "LICENSE" file describing the terms of reuse. Tools such as Jupyter Notebook, Sweave, and Knitr can be used to interweave code and text to produce clearly documented, reproducible studies, and are becoming increasingly popular in the research community (Fig. 11.3).

Version control systems such as Git can be used to track the changes made to code over time and are also becoming an increasingly popular tool for researchers [8]. When working with a version control system, a commit log provides a record of changes to code by contributor, providing transparency in the development process and acting as a useful tool for uncovering and fixing bugs.

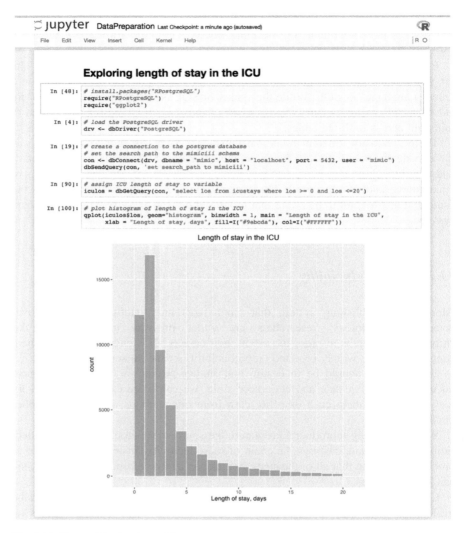

Fig. 11.3 Jupyter Notebooks enable documentation and code to be combined into a reproducible analysis. In this example, the length of ICU stay is loaded from the MIMIC-III (v1.3) database and plotted as a histogram [11]

Collaboration is also facilitated by version control systems. Git provides powerful functionality that facilitates distribution of code and allows multiple people to work together in synchrony. Integration with Git hosting services such as Github provide a simple mechanism for backing up content, helping to reduce the risk of data loss, and also provide tools for tracking issues and tasks [8, 9].

11.3 Part 2—Practical Examples of Data Preparation

11.3.1 MIMIC Tables

In order to carry out the study on the effect of indwelling arterial catheters as described in the previous chapter, we use the following tables in the MIMIC-III clinical database:

- The **chartevents** table, the largest table in the database. It contains all data charted by the bedside critical care system, including physiological measurements such as heart rate and blood pressure, as well as the settings used by the indwelling arterial catheters.
- The **patients** table, which contains the demographic details of each patient admitted to an intensive care unit, such as gender, date of birth, and date of death.
- The **icustays** table, which contains administrative details relating to stays in the ICU, such as the admission time, discharge time, and type of care unit.

Before continuing with the following exercises, we recommend familiarizing yourself with the MIMIC documentation and in particular the table descriptions, which are available on the MIMIC website [10].

11.3.2 SQL Basics

An SQL query has the following format:

```
SELECT [columns]
FROM [table_name]
WHERE [conditions];
```

The result returned by the query is a list of rows. The following query lists the unique patient identifiers (**subject_ids**) of all female patients:

```
SELECT subject_id
FROM patients
WHERE gender = 'F';

-- returns:
 subject_id
------------
        654
        655
        656
        ...
```

We often need to specify more than one condition. For instance, the following query lists the **subject_ids** whose first or last care unit was a coronary care unit (CCU):

```
SELECT subject_id
FROM icustays
WHERE first_careunit = 'CCU' OR last_careunit = 'CCU';

-- returns:
 subject_id
------------
        109
        109
        111
        ...
```

Since a patient may have been in several ICUs, the same patient ID sometimes appears several times in the result of the previous query. To return only distinct rows, use the **DISTINCT** keyword:

```
SELECT DISTINCT subject_id
FROM icustays
WHERE first_careunit = 'CCU' OR last_careunit = 'CCU';

-- returns:
 subject_id
------------
      25949
       6158
      27223
        ...
```

To count how many patients there are in the **icustays** table, combine **DISTINCT** with the **COUNT** keyword. As you can see, if there is no condition, we simply don't use the keyword **WHERE**:

```
SELECT COUNT(DISTINCT subject_id)
FROM icustays;

-- returns:
 count
-------
 46476
```

11.3 Part 2—Practical Examples of Data Preparation

Taking a similar approach, we can count how many patients went through the CCU using the query:

```
SELECT COUNT(DISTINCT subject_id)
FROM icustays
WHERE first_careunit = 'CCU' OR last_careunit = 'CCU';

-- returns:
 count
-------
  7314
```

The operator * is used to display all columns. The following query displays the entire **icustays** table:

```
SELECT *
FROM icustays;

-- returns
subject_id | hadm_id | icustay_id | ...
       109 |  139061 |     257358 | ...
       109 |  172335 |     262652 | ...
       109 |  126055 |     236124 | ...
...
```

The results can be sorted based on one or several columns with **ORDER BY**. To add a comment in a SQL query, use:

```
SELECT subject_id, hadm_id, icustay_id
FROM icustays
ORDER BY subject_id ASC; -- ASC sorts by ascending number

-- returns:
 subject_id | hadm_id | icustay_id
------------+---------+------------
          2 |  163353 |     243653
          3 |  145834 |     211552
          4 |  185777 |     294638
...
```

11.3.3 Joins

Often we need information coming from multiple tables. This can be achieved using SQL joins. There are several types of join, including **INNER JOIN, OUTER JOIN, LEFT JOIN, and RIGHT JOIN**. It is important to understand the difference between these joins because their usage can significantly impact query results. Detailed guidance on joins is widely available on the web, so we will not go into further details here. We will however provide an example of an **INNER JOIN** which selects all rows where the joined key appears in both tables.

Using the **INNER JOIN** keyword, let's count how many adult patients went through the coronary care unit. To know whether a patient is an adult, we need to use the **dob** (date of birth) attribute from the **patients** table. We can use the **INNER JOIN** to indicate that two or more tables should be combined based on a common attribute, which in our case is **subject_id**:

```
-- INNER JOIN will only return rows where subject_id
-- appears in the patients table and the icustays table
SELECT p.subject_id
FROM patients p
INNER JOIN icustays i
ON p.subject_id = i.subject_id
WHERE (i.first_careunit = 'CCU' OR i.last_careunit = 'CCU')
   AND (i.intime - p.dob) >= INTERVAL '18' year
ORDER BY subject_id ASC;

-- returns:
 subject_id
 ------------
         13
         18
         21
        ...
```

Note that:

- we assign an alias to a table to avoid writing its full name throughout the query. In our 0 given the alias 'p'.
- in the **SELECT** clause, we wrote **p.subject_id** instead of simply **subject_id** since both the **patients** and **icustays** tables contain the attribute **subject_id**. If we don't specify from which table **subject_id** comes from, we would get a "column ambiguously defined" error.
- to identify whether a patient is an adult, we look for differences between **intime** and **dob** of 18 years or greater using the **INTERVAL** keyword.

11.3.4 Ranking Across Rows Using a Window Function

We now focus on the case study. One of the first steps is identifying the first ICU admission for each patient. To do so, we can use the **RANK** () function to order rows sequentially by intime. Using the **PARTITION BY** expression allows us to perform the ranking across subject_id windows:

```
SELECT subject_id, icustay_id, intime,
    RANK() OVER (PARTITION BY subject_id ORDER BY intime asc)
FROM icustays;

-- returns:
 subject_id | icustay_id |       intime        | rank
------------+------------+---------------------+------
          6 |     228232 | 2175-05-30 21:30:54 |    1
          7 |     278444 | 2121-05-23 15:35:29 |    1
          7 |     236754 | 2121-05-25 03:26:01 |    2
        ...
```

11.3.5 Making Queries More Manageable Using WITH

To keep SQL queries reasonably short and simple, we can use the **WITH** keyword. **WITH** allows us to break a large query into smaller, more manageable chunks. The following query creates a temporary table called "rankedstays" that lists the order of stays for each patient. We then select only the rows in this table where the rank is equal to one (i.e. the first stay) and the patient is aged 18 years or greater:

```
WITH rankedstays AS (
    SELECT subject_id, icustay_id, intime,
        RANK() OVER (PARTITION BY subject_id ORDER BY intime asc)
    FROM icustays
)
SELECT r.subject_id, r.icustay_id, r.intime, r.rank
FROM rankedstays r
INNER JOIN patients p
ON r.subject_id = p.subject_id
WHERE r.rank = 1
AND (r.intime - p.dob) >= INTERVAL '18' year;

-- returns:
 subject_id | icustay_id |       intime        | rank
------------+------------+---------------------+------
          3 |     211552 | 2101-10-20 19:10:11 |    1
          4 |     294638 | 2191-03-16 00:29:31 |    1
          6 |     228232 | 2175-05-30 21:30:54 |    1
        ...
```

Open Access This chapter is distributed under the terms of the Creative Commons Attribution-NonCommercial 4.0 International License (http://creativecommons.org/licenses/by-nc/4.0/), which permits any noncommercial use, duplication, adaptation, distribution and reproduction in any medium or format, as long as you give appropriate credit to the original author(s) and the source, a link is provided to the Creative Commons license and any changes made are indicated.

The images or other third party material in this chapter are included in the work's Creative Commons license, unless indicated otherwise in the credit line; if such material is not included in the work's Creative Commons license and the respective action is not permitted by statutory regulation, users will need to obtain permission from the license holder to duplicate, adapt or reproduce the material.

References

1. Wilson G, Aruliah DA, Brown CT, Chue Hong NP, Davis M, Guy RT et al (2014) Best practices for scientific computing. PLoS Biol 12(1):e1001745. doi:10.1371/journal.pbio.1001745. http://journals.plos.org/plosbiology/article?id=10.1371/journal.pbio.1001745
2. Editorial (2012) Must try harder. Nature 483(509). doi:10.1038/483509a. http://www.nature.com/nature/journal/v483/n7391/full/483509a.html
3. Misset B, Nakache D, Vesin A, Darmon M, Garrouste-Orgeas M, Mourvillier B et al (2008) Reliability of diagnostic coding in intensive care patients. Crit Care 12(4):R95. http://www.ncbi.nlm.nih.gov/pmc/articles/PMC2575581/
4. Wickham H (2014) Tidy data. J Stat Softw 59(10):1–23. doi:10.18637/jss.v059.i10. https://www.jstatsoft.org/article/view/v059i10
5. Sustainability of Digital Formats Planning for Library of Congress Collections. Accessed: 24 Feb 2016. CSV, Comma Separated Values (RFC 4180). http://www.digitalpreservation.gov/formats/fdd/fdd000323.shtml
6. Editorial (2013) Unreliable research: trouble at the Lab. Economist. http://www.economist.com/news/briefing/21588057-scientists-think-science-self-correcting-alarming-degree-it-not-trouble
7. Goodman A, Pepe A, Blocker AW, Borgman CL, Cranmer K, Crosas M, et al (2014) Ten simple rules for the care and feeding of scientific data. PLoS Comput Biol 10(4):e1003542. doi:10.1371/journal.pcbi.1003542. http://journals.plos.org/ploscompbiol/article?id=10.1371/journal.pcbi.1003542
8. Karthik R (2013) Git can facilitate greater reproducibility and increased transparency in science. Source Code Biol Med 28; 8(1):7. doi:10.1186/1751-0473-8-7. http://scfbm.biomedcentral.com/articles/10.1186/1751-0473-8-7
9. GitHub. https://github.com. Accessed 24 Feb 2016
10. MIMIC website. http://mimic.physionet.org. Accessed 24 Feb 2016
11. MIMIC Code Repository. https://github.com/MIT-LCP/mimic-code. Accessed 24 Feb 2016

Chapter 12
Data Pre-processing

Brian Malley, Daniele Ramazzotti and Joy Tzung-yu Wu

Learning Objectives

- Understand the requirements for a "clean" database that is "tidy" and ready for use in statistical analysis.
- Understand the steps of cleaning raw data, integrating data, reducing and reshaping data.
- Be able to apply basic techniques for dealing with common problems with raw data including missing data inconsistent data, and data from multiple sources.

12.1 Introduction

Data pre-processing consists of a series of steps to transform raw data derived from data extraction (see Chap. 11) into a "clean" and "tidy" dataset prior to statistical analysis. Research using electronic health records (EHR) often involves the secondary analysis of health records that were collected for clinical and billing (non-study) purposes and placed in a study database via automated processes. Therefore, these databases can have many quality control issues. Pre-processing aims at assessing and improving the quality of data to allow for reliable statistical analysis.

Several distinct steps are involved in pre-processing data. Here are the general steps taken to pre-process data [1]:

- Data "cleaning"—This step deals with missing data, noise, outliers, and duplicate or incorrect records while minimizing introduction of bias into the database. These methods are explored in detail in Chaps. 13 and 14.
- "Data integration"—Extracted raw data can come from heterogeneous sources or be in separate datasets. This step reorganizes the various raw datasets into a single dataset that contain all the information required for the desired statistical analyses.

- "Data transformation"—This step translates and/or scales variables stored in a variety of formats or units in the raw data into formats or units that are more useful for the statistical methods that the researcher wants to use.
- "Data reduction"—After the dataset has been integrated and transformed, this step removes redundant records and variables, as well as reorganizes the data in an efficient and "tidy" manner for analysis.

Pre-processing is sometimes iterative and may involve repeating this series of steps until the data are satisfactorily organized for the purpose of statistical analysis. During pre-processing, one needs to take care not to accidentally introduce bias by modifying the dataset in ways that will impact the outcome of statistical analyses. Similarly, we must avoid reaching statistically significant results through "trial and error" analyses on differently pre-processed versions of a dataset.

12.2 Part 1—Theoretical Concepts

12.2.1 Data Cleaning

Real world data are usually "messy" in the sense that they can be incomplete (e.g. missing data), they can be noisy (e.g. random error or outlier values that deviate from the expected baseline), and they can be inconsistent (e.g. patient age 21 and admission service is neonatal intensive care unit).

The reasons for this are multiple. Missing data can be due to random technical issues with biomonitors, reliance on human data entry, or because some clinical variables are not consistently collected since EHR data were collected for non-study purposes. Similarly, noisy data can be due to faults or technological limitations of instruments during data gathering (e.g. dampening of blood pressure values measured through an arterial line), or because of human error in entry. All the above can also lead to inconsistencies in the data. Bottom line, all of these reasons create the need for meticulous data cleaning steps prior to analysis.

Missing Data
A more detailed discussion regarding missing data will be presented in Chap. 13. Here, we describe three possible ways to deal with missing data [1]:

- Ignore the record. This method is not very effective, unless the record (observation/row) contains several variables with missing values. This approach is especially problematic when the percentage of missing values per variable varies considerably or when there is a pattern of missing data related to an unrecognized underlying cause such as patient condition on admission.

- Determine and fill in the missing value manually. In general, this approach is the most accurate but it is also time-consuming and often is not feasible in a large dataset with many missing values.
- Use an expected value. The missing values can be filled in with predicted values (e.g. using the mean of the available data or some prediction method). It must be underlined that this approach may introduce bias in the data, as the inserted values may be wrong. This method is also useful for comparing and checking the validity of results obtained by ignoring missing records.

Noisy Data

We term noise a random error or variance in an observed variable—a common problem for secondary analyses of EHR data. For example, it is not uncommon for hospitalized patients to have a vital sign or laboratory value far outside of normal parameters due to inadequate (hemolyzed) blood samples, or monitoring leads disconnected by patient movement. Clinicians are often aware of the source of error and can repeat the measurement then ignore the known incorrect outlier value when planning care. However, clinicians cannot remove the erroneous measurement from the medical record in many cases, so it will be captured in the database. A detailed discussion on how to deal with noisy data and outliers is provided in Chap. 14; for now we limit the discussion to some basic guidelines [1].

- Binning methods. Binning methods smooth a sorted data value by considering their 'neighborhood', or values around it. These kinds of approaches to reduce noise, which only consider the neighborhood values, are said to be performing local smoothing.
- Clustering. Outliers may be detected by clustering, that is by grouping a set of values in such a way that the ones in the same group (i.e., in the same cluster) are more similar to each other than to those in other groups.
- Machine learning. Data can be smoothed by means of various machine learning approaches. One of the classical methods is the regression analysis, where data are fitted to a specified (often linear) function.

Same as for missing data, human supervision during the process of noise smoothing or outliers detection can be effective but also time-consuming.

Inconsistent Data

There may be inconsistencies or duplications in the data. Some of them may be corrected manually using external references. This is the case, for instance, of errors made at data entry. Knowledge engineering tools may also be used to detect the violation of known data constraints. For example, known functional dependencies among attributes can be used to find values contradicting the functional constraints.

Inconsistencies in EHR result from information being entered into the database by thousands of individual clinicians and hospital staff members, as well as captured from a variety of automated interfaces between the EHR and everything from telemetry monitors to the hospital laboratory. The same information is often entered in different formats by these different sources.

Take, for example, the intravenous administration of 1 g of the antibiotic vancomycin contained in 250 mL of dextrose solution. This single event may be captured in the dataset in several different ways. For one patient this event may be captured from the medication order as the code number (ITEMID in MIMIC) from the formulary for the antibiotic vancomycin with a separate column capturing the dose stored as a numerical variable. However, on another patient the same event could be found in the fluid intake and output records under the code for the IV dextrose solution with an associated free text entered by the provider. This text would be captured in the EHR as, for example "vancomycin 1 g in 250 ml", saved as a text variable (string, array of characters, etc.) with the possibility of spelling errors or use of nonstandard abbreviations. Clinically these are the exact same event, but in the EHR and hence in the raw data, they are represented differently. This can lead to the same single clinical event not being captured in the study dataset, being captured incorrectly as a different event, or being captured multiple times for a single occurrence.

In order to produce an accurate dataset for analysis, the goal is for each patient to have the same event represented in the same manner for analysis. As such, dealing with inconsistency perfectly would usually have to happen at the data entry or data extraction level. However, as data extraction is imperfect, pre-processing becomes important. Often, correcting for these inconsistencies involves some understanding of how the data of interest would have been captured in the clinical setting and where the data would be stored in the EHR database.

12.2.2 Data Integration

Data integration is the process of combining data derived from various data sources (such as databases, flat files, etc.) into a consistent dataset. There are a number of issues to consider during data integration related mostly to possible different standards among data sources. For example, certain variables can be referred by means of different IDs in two or more sources.

In the MIMIC database this mainly becomes an issue when some information is entered into the EHR during a different phase in the patient's care pathway, such as before admission in the emergency department, or from outside records. For example, a patient may have laboratory values taken in the ER before they are admitted to the ICU. In order to have a complete dataset it will be necessary to integrate the patient's full set of lab values (including those not associated with the same MIMIC ICUSTAY identifier) with the record of that ICU admission without repeating or missing records. Using shared values between datasets (such as a hospital stay identifier or a timestamp in this example) can allow for this to be done accurately.

Once data cleaning and data integration are completed, we obtain one dataset where entries are reliable.

12.2.3 Data Transformation

There are many possible transformations one might wish to do to raw data values depending on the requirement of the specific statistical analysis planned for a study. The aim is to transform the data values into a format, scale or unit that is more suitable for analysis (e.g. log transform for linear regression modeling). Here are few common possible options:

Normalization
This generally means data for a numerical variable are scaled in order to range between a specified set of values, such as 0–1. For example, scaling each patient's severity of illness score to between 0 and 1 using the known range of that score in order to compare between patients in a multiple regression analysis.

Aggregation
Two or more values of the same attribute are aggregated into one value. A common example is the transformation of categorical variables where multiple categories can be aggregated into one. One example in MIMIC is to define all surgical patients by assigning a new binary variable to all patients with an ICU service noted to be "SICU" (surgical ICU) or "CSRU" (cardiac surgery ICU).

Generalization
Similar to aggregation, in this case low level attributes are transformed into higher level ones. For example, in the analysis of chronic kidney disease (CKD) patients, instead of using a continuous numerical variable like the patient's creatinine levels, one could use a variable for CKD stages as defined by accepted guidelines.

12.2.4 Data Reduction

Complex analysis on large datasets may take a very long time or even be infeasible. The final step of data pre-processing is data reduction, i.e., the process of reducing the input data by means of a more effective representation of the dataset without compromising the integrity of the original data. The objective of this step is to provide a version of the dataset on which the subsequent statistical analysis will be more effective. Data reduction may or may not be lossless. That is the end database may contain all the information of the original database in more efficient format (such as removing redundant records) or it may be that data integrity is maintained but some information is lost when data is transformed and then only represented in the new form (such as multiple values being represented as an average value).

One common MIMIC database example is collapsing the ICD9 codes into broad clinical categories or variables of interest and assigning patients to them. This reduces the dataset from having multiple entries of ICD9 codes, in text format, for a given patient, to having a single entry of a binary variable for an area of interest to the study, such as history of coronary artery disease. Another example would be in the case of using blood pressure as a variable in analysis. An ICU patient will generally have their systolic and diastolic blood pressure monitored continuously via an arterial line or recorded multiple times per hour by an automated blood pressure cuff. This results in hundreds of data points for each of possibly thousands of study patients. Depending on the study aims, it may be necessary to calculate a new variable such as average mean arterial pressure during the first day of ICU admission.

Lastly, as part of more effective organization of datasets, one would also aim to reshape the columns and rows of a dataset so that it conforms with the following 3 rules of a "tidy" dataset [2, 3]:

1. Each variable forms a column
2. Each observation forms a row
3. Each value has its own cell

"Tidy" datasets have the advantage of being more easily visualized and manipulated for later statistical analysis. Datasets exported from MIMIC usually are fairly "tidy" already; therefore, rule 2 is hardly ever broken. However, sometimes there may still be several categorical values within a column even for MIMIC datasets, which breaks rule 1. For example, multiple categories of marital status or ethnicity under the same column. For some analyses, it is useful to split each categorical values of a variable into their own columns. Fortunately though, we do not often have to worry about breaking rule 3 for MIMIC data as there are not often multiple values in a cell. These concepts will become clearer after the MIMIC examples in Sect. 12.3

12.3 PART 2—Examples of Data Pre-processing in R

There are many tools for doing data pre-processing available, such as R, STATA, SAS, and Python; each differs in the level of programming background required. R is a free tool that is supported by a range of statistical and data manipulation packages. In this section of the chapter, we will go through some examples demonstrating various steps of data pre-processing in R, using data from various MIMIC dataset (SQL extraction codes included). Due to the significant content involved with the data cleaning step of pre-processing, this step will be separately addressed in Chaps. 13 and 14. The examples in this section will deal with some R basics as well as data integration, transformation, and reduction.

12.3.1 R—The Basics

The most common data output from a MIMIC database query is in the form of 'comma separated values' files, with filenames ending in '.csv'. This output file format can be selected when exporting the SQL query results from MIMIC database. Besides '.csv' files, R is also able to read in other file formats, such as Excel, SAS, etc., but we will not go into the detail here.

Understanding 'Data Types' in R
For many who have used other data analysis software or who have a programming background, you will be familiar with the concept of 'data types'.

R strictly stores data in several different data types, called 'classes':

- `Numeric` – e.g. 3.1415, 1.618
- `Integer` – e.g. -1, 0, 1, 2, 3
- `Character` – e.g. "vancomycin", "metronidazole"
- `Logical` – TRUE, FALSE
- `Factors/categorical` – e.g. male or female under variable, gender

R also usually does not allow mixing of data types for a variable, except in a:

- `List` – as a one dimensional vector, e.g. c("vancomycin", 1.618, "red")
- `Data-frame` – as a two dimensional table with rows (observations) and columns (variables)

Lists and data-frames are treated as their own 'class' in R.

Query output from MIMIC commonly will be in the form of data tables with different data types in different columns. Therefore, R usually stores these tables as 'data-frames' when they are read into R.

Special Values in R

- NA – 'not available', usually a default placeholder for missing values.
- NAN – 'not a number', only applying to numeric vectors.
- NULL – 'empty' value or set. Often returned by expressions where the value is undefined.
- Inf – value for 'infinity' and only applies to numeric vectors.

Setting Working Directory

This step tells R where to read in the source files.

Command: setwd("directory_path")

Example: (If all data files are saved in directory "MIMIC_data_files" on the Desktop)

```
setwd("~/Desktop/MIMIC_data_files")

# List files in directory:
list.files()
## [1] "c_score_sicker.csv"      "comorbidity_scores.csv"
## [3] "demographics.csv"        "mean_arterial_pressure.csv"
## [5] "population.csv"
```

Reading in .csv Files from MIMIC Query Results

The data read into R is assigned a 'name' for reference later on.

Command: set_var_name <- read.csv("filename.csv")

Example:

```
demo <- read.csv("demographics.csv")
```

12.3 PART 2—Examples of Data Pre-processing in R

Viewing the Dataset
There are several commands in R that are very useful for getting a 'feel' of your datasets and see what they look like before you start manipulating them.

- View the first and last 2 rows. E.g.:

```
head(demo, 2)

##   subject_id hadm_id marital_status_descr ethnicity_descr
## 1          4   17296               SINGLE           WHITE
## 2          6   23467              MARRIED           WHITE

tail(demo, 2)

##       subject_id hadm_id marital_status_descr    ethnicity_descr
## 27624      32807   32736              MARRIED UNABLE TO OBTAIN
## 27625      32805   34884             DIVORCED             WHITE
```

- View summary statistics. E.g.:

```
summary(demo)

##    subject_id        hadm_id       marital_status_descr
##  Min.   :    3    Min.   :    1    MARRIED  :13447
##  1st Qu.: 8063    1st Qu.: 9204    SINGLE   : 6412
##  Median :16060    Median :18278    WIDOWED  : 4029
##  Mean   :16112    Mean   :18035    DIVORCED : 1623
##  3rd Qu.:24119    3rd Qu.:26762             : 1552
##  Max.   :32809    Max.   :36118    SEPARATED:  320
##                                    (Other)  :  242
##
##             ethnicity_descr
##  WHITE                :19360
##  UNKNOWN/NOT SPECIFIED : 3446
##  BLACK/AFRICAN AMERICAN: 2251
##  ...
```

- View structure of data set (obs = number of rows). E.g.:

```
str(demo)

## 'data.frame':    27625 obs. of  4 variables:
##  $ subject_id           : int  4 6 3 9 15 14 11 18 18 19 ...
##  $ hadm_id              : int  17296 23467 2075 8253 4819 23919 28128 24759 33481 25788 ...
##  $ marital_status_descr: Factor w/ 8 levels "","DIVORCED",..: 6 4 4 1 6 4 4 4 4 1 ...
##  $ ethnicity_descr      : Factor w/ 39 levels "AMERICAN INDIAN/ALASKA NATIVE",..: 35 35 35 34 12 35 35 35 35 35 ...
```

- Find out the 'class' of a variable or dataset. E.g.:

```
class(demo)

## [1] "data.frame"
```

- View number of rows and column, or alternatively, the dimension of the dataset. E.g.:

```
nrow(demo)

## [1] 27625

ncol(demo)

## [1] 4

dim(demo)

## [1] 27625     4
```

- Calculate length of a variable. E.g.:

```
x <- c(1:10); x

## [1]  1  2  3  4  5  6  7  8  9 10

class(x)

## [1] "integer"
```

12.3 PART 2—Examples of Data Pre-processing in R

Subsetting a Dataset and Adding New Variables/Columns

Aim: Sometimes, it may be useful to look at only some columns or some rows in a dataset/data-frame—this is called subsetting.

Let's create a simple data-frame to demonstrate basic subsetting and other command functions in R. One simple way to do this is to create each column of the data-frame separately then combine them into a dataframe later. Note the different kinds of data types for the columns/variables created, and beware that R is case-sensitive.

Examples: Note that comments appearing after the hash sign (#) will not be evaluated.

```
subject_id <- c(1:6)                                    #integer
gender <- as.factor(c("F", "F", "M", "F", "M", "M"))#factor/categorical
height <- c(1.52, 1.65, 1.75, 1.72, 1.85, 1.78)     #numeric
weight <- c(56.7, 99.6, 90.4, 85.3, 71.4, 130.5)    #numeric
data <- data.frame(subject_id, gender, height, weight)

head(data, 4)                         # View only the first 4 rows

##   subject_id gender height weight
## 1          1      F   1.52   56.7
## 2          2      F   1.65   99.6
## 3          3      M   1.75   90.4
## ...

str(data)                   # Note the class of each variable/column

## 'data.frame':   6 obs. of  4 variables:
##  $ subject_id: int  1 2 3 4 5 6
##  $ gender    : Factor w/ 2 levels "F","M": 1 1 2 1 2 2
##  $ height    : num  1.52 1.65 1.75 1.72 1.85 1.78
##  $ weight    : num  56.7 99.6 90.4 85.3 71.4 ...
```

To subset or extract only e.g., weight, we can use either the dollar sign ($) after the dataset, data, or use the square brackets, []. The $ selects column with the column name (without quotation mark in this case). The square brackets [] here selected the column weight by its column number:

```
w1 <- data$weight; w1

## [1]  56.7  99.6  90.4  85.3  71.4 130.5

w2 <- data[, 4]; w2

## [1]  56.7  99.6  90.4  85.3  71.4 130.5
```

Generally one can subset a dataset by specifying the rows and column desired like this: data[row number, column number]. For example:

```
dat_sub <- data[2:4, 1:3]; dat_sub

##   subject_id gender height
## 2          2      F   1.65
## 3          3      M   1.75
## 4          4      F   1.72
```

The square brackets are useful for subsetting multiple columns or rows. Note that it is important to 'concatenate', c(), if selecting multiple variables/columns and to use quotation marks when selecting with columns names.

```
h_w1 <- data[, c(3, 4)]; h_w1

##   height weight
## 1   1.52   56.7
## 2   1.65   99.6
## 3   1.75   90.4
## ...

h_w2 <- data[, c("height", "weight")]; h_w2

##   height weight
## 1   1.52   56.7
## 2   1.65   99.6
## 3   1.75   90.4
## ...
```

To calculate the BMI (weight/height^2) in a new column—there are different ways to do this but here is a simple method:

12.3 PART 2—Examples of Data Pre-processing in R

```
data$BMI <- data$weight/data$height^2
head(data, 4)

##   subject_id gender height weight     BMI
## 1          1      F   1.52   56.7 24.54120
## 2          2      F   1.65   99.6 36.58402
## 3          3      M   1.75   90.4 29.51837
## 4          4      F   1.72   85.3 28.83315
```

Let's create a new column, obese, for BMI > 30, as TRUE or FALSE. This also demonstrates the use of 'logicals' in R.

```
data$obese <- data$BMI > 30
head(data)

##   subject_id gender height weight     BMI obese
## 1          1      F   1.52   56.7 24.54120 FALSE
## 2          2      F   1.65   99.6 36.58402  TRUE
## 3          3      M   1.75   90.4 29.51837 FALSE
## ...
```

One can also use logical vectors to subset datasets in R. A logical vector, named "ob" here, is created and then we pass it through the square brackets [] to tell R to select only the rows where the condition BMI > 30 is TRUE:

```
ob <- data$BMI > 30
data_ob <- data[ob, ];data_ob

##   subject_id gender height weight      BMI obese
## 2          2      F   1.65   99.6  36.58402  TRUE
## 6          6      M   1.78  130.5  41.18798  TRUE
```

Combining Datasets (Called Data Frames in R)
Aim: Often different variables (columns) of interest in a research question may come from separate MIMIC tables and could have been exported as separate.csv files if they were not merged via SQL queries. For ease of analysis and visualization, it is often desirable to merge these separate data frames in R on their shared ID column(s).

Occasionally, one may also want to attach rows from one data frame after rows from another. In this case, the column names and the number of columns of the two different datasets must be the same.

Examples: In general, there are a couple ways of combining columns and rows from different datasets in R:

- merge()—This function merges columns on shared ID column(s) between the data frames so the associated rows match up correctly.

  Command: merging on one ID column, e.g.:

```
df_merged <- merge(df1, df2, by = "column_ID_name")
```

  Command: merging on two ID columns, e.g.:

```
df_merged <- merge(df1, df2, by = c("column1", "column2"))
```

- cbind()—This function simply 'add' together the columns from two data frames (must have equal number of rows). It does not match up the rows by any identifier.

  Command: joining columns. E.g.:

```
df_total <- cbind(df1, df2)
```

- rbind()—The function 'row binds' the two data frames vertically (must have the same column names).

  Command: joining rows. E.g.:

```
df_total <- rbind(df1, df2)
```

Using Packages in R

There are many packages that make life so much easier when manipulating data in R. They need to be installed on your computer and loaded at the start of your R script before you can call the functions in them. We will introduce examples of of a couple of useful packages later in this chapter.

12.3 PART 2—Examples of Data Pre-processing in R

For now, the command for installing packages is:

`install.packages("name_of_package_case_sensitive")`

The command for loading the package into the R working environment:

`library(name_of_package_case_sensitive)`

Note—there are no quotation marks when loading packages as compared to installing; you will get an error message otherwise.

Getting Help in R
There are various online tutorials and Q&A forums for getting help in R. Stackoverflow, Cran and Quick-R are some good examples. Within the R console, a question mark, ?, followed by the name of the function of interest will bring up the help menu for the function, e.g.

`?head`

12.3.2 Data Integration

Aim: This involves combining the separate output datasets exported from separate MIMIC queries into a consistent larger dataset table.

To ensure that the associated observations or rows from the two different datasets match up, the right column ID must be used. In MIMIC, the ID columns could be subject_id, hadm_id, icustay_id, itemid, etc. Hence, knowing the context of what each column ID is used to identify and how they are related to each other is important. For example, subject_id is used to identify each individual patient, so includes their date of birth (DOB), date of death (DOD) and various other clinical detail and laboratory values in MIMIC. Likewise, the hospital admission ID, hadm_id, is used to specifically identify various events and outcomes from an unique hospital admission; and is also in turn associated with the subject_id of the patient who was involved in that particular hospital admission. Tables pulled from MIMIC can have one or more ID columns. The different tables exported from MIMIC may share some ID columns, which allows us to 'merge' them together, matching up the rows correctly using the unique ID values in their shared ID columns.

Examples: To demonstrate this with MIMIC data, a simple SQL query is constructed to extract some data, saved as: "population.csv" and "demographics.csv".

We will these extracted files to show how to merge datasets in R.

1. **SQL query**:

```
WITH
population AS(
SELECT subject_id, hadm_id, gender, dob, icustay_admit_age,
icustay_intime, icustay_outtime, dod, expire_flg
FROM mimic2v26.icustay_detail
  WHERE subject_icustay_seq = 1
  AND icustay_age_group = 'adult'
  AND hadm_id IS NOT NULL
)
, demo AS(
SELECT subject_id, hadm_id, marital_status_descr, ethnicity_descr
FROM mimic2v26.demographic_detail
WHERE subject_id IN (SELECT subject_id FROM population)
)

--# Extract the the datasets with each one of the following line of codes in turn:
--SELECT * FROM population
--SELECT * FROM demo
```

Note: Remove the – in front of the SELECT command to run the query.

12.3 PART 2—Examples of Data Pre-processing in R

2. **R code: Demonstrating data integration**

   Set working directory and read data files into R::

```
setwd("~/Desktop/MIMIC_data_files")
demo <- read.csv("demographics.csv", sep = ",")
pop <- read.csv("population.csv", sep = ",")
head(demo)

##   subject_id hadm_id marital_status_descr     ethnicity_descr
## 1          4   17296               SINGLE               WHITE
## 2          6   23467              MARRIED               WHITE
## 3          3    2075              MARRIED               WHITE
## ...
head(pop)

##   subject_id hadm_id gender                 dob icustay_admit_age
## 1          4   17296      F 3351-05-30 00:00:00          47.84414
## 2          6   23467      F 3323-07-30 00:00:00          65.94048
## 3          3    2075      M 2606-02-28 00:00:00          76.52892
## ...

##         icustay_intime         icustay_outtime                 dod expire_flg
## 1 3399-04-03 00:29:00 3399-04-04 16:46:00                             N
## 2 3389-07-07 20:38:00 3389-07-11 12:47:00                             N
## 3 2682-09-07 18:12:00 2682-09-13 19:45:00 2683-05-02 00:00:00          Y
## ...
```

Merging pop and demo: Note to get the rows to match up correctly, we need to merge on both the subject_id and hadm_id in this case. This is because each subject/patient could have multiple hadm_id from different hospital admissions during the EHR course of MIMIC database.

```
demopop <- merge(pop, demo, by = c("subject_id", "hadm_id"))
head(demopop)

##   subject_id hadm_id gender                 dob icustay_admit_age
## 1        100     445      F 3048-09-22 00:00:00          71.94482
## 2       1000   15170      M 2442-05-11 00:00:00          69.70579
## 3      10000   10444      M 3149-12-07 00:00:00          49.67315
## ...

##         icustay_intime       icustay_outtime                 dod expire_flg
## 1 3120-09-01 11:19:00 3120-09-03 14:06:00                                 N
## 2 2512-01-25 13:16:00 2512-03-02 06:05:00 2512-03-02 00:00:00              Y
## 3 3199-08-09 09:53:00 3199-08-10 17:43:00                                 N
## ...

##   marital_status_descr        ethnicity_descr
## 1              WIDOWED    UNKNOWN/NOT SPECIFIED
## 2              MARRIED    UNKNOWN/NOT SPECIFIED
## 3                            HISPANIC OR LATINO
## 4              MARRIED  BLACK/AFRICAN AMERICAN
## 5              MARRIED                   WHITE
## 6            SEPARATED  BLACK/AFRICAN AMERICAN
```

As you can see, there are still multiple problems with this merged database, for example, the missing values for 'marital_status_descr' column. Dealing with missing data is explored in Chap. 13.

12.3.3 Data Transformation

Aim: To transform the presentation of data values in some ways so that the new format is more suitable for the subsequent statistical analysis. The main processes involved are normalization, aggregation and generalization (See part 1 for explanation).

Examples: To demonstrate this with a MIMIC database example, let us look at a table generated from the following simple SQL query, which we exported as "comorbidity_scores.csv".

The SQL query selects all the patient comorbidity information from the mimic2v26.comorbidity_scores table on the condition of (1) being an adult, (2) in

12.3 PART 2—Examples of Data Pre-processing in R

his/her first ICU admission, and (3) where the hadm_id is not missing according to the mimic2v26.icustay_detail table.

1. **SQL query:**

```sql
SELECT *
FROM mimic2v26.comorbidity_scores
WHERE subject_id IN (SELECT subject_id
        FROM mimic2v26.icustay_detail
        WHERE subject_icustay_seq = 1
            AND icustay_age_group = 'adult'
            AND hadm_id IS NOT null)
```

2. **R code: Demonstrating data transformation:**

```r
setwd("~/Desktop/MIMIC_data_files")
c_scores <- read.csv("comorbidity_scores.csv", sep = ",")
```

Note the 'class' or data type of each column/variable and the total number of rows (obs) and columns (variables) in c_scores:

```r
str(c_scores)

## 'data.frame':    27525 obs. of  33 variables:
##  $ subject_id               : int  2848 21370 2026 11890 27223 27520 17928 31252 32083 9545 ...
##  $ hadm_id                  : int  16272 17542 11351 12730 32530 32724 20353 30062 32216 10809 ...
##  $ category                 : Factor w/ 1 level "ELIXHAUSER": 1 1 1 1 1 1 1 1 1 1 ...
##  $ congestive_heart_failure : int  0 0 0 0 1 0 0 0 1 1 ...
##  $ cardiac_arrhythmias      : int  0 1 1 0 1 0 0 0 0 1 ...
##  $ valvular_disease         : int  0 0 0 0 1 0 0 0 0 1 ...
##  $ ...
```

Here we add a column in c_scores to save the overall ELIXHAUSER. The rep() function in this case repeats 0 for nrow(c_scores) times. Function, colnames(), rename the new or last column, [ncol(c_scores)], as "ELIXHAUSER_overall".

```
c_scores <- cbind(c_scores, rep(0, nrow(c_scores)))
colnames(c_scores)[ncol(c_scores)] <- "ELIXHAUSER_overall"
```

Take a look at the result. Note the new "ELIXHAUSER_overall" column added at the end:

```
str(c_scores)

## 'data.frame':    27525 obs. of  34 variables:
##  $ subject_id            : int  2848 21370 2026 11890 27223 27520
17928 31252 32083 9545 ...
##  $ hadm_id               : int  16272 17542 11351 12730 32530
32724 20353 30062 32216 10809 ...
##  $ category              : Factor w/ 1 level "ELIXHAUSER": 1 1 1
1 1 1 1 1 ...
##  $ congestive_heart_failure: int  0 0 0 0 1 0 0 0 1 1 ...
##  $ cardiac_arrhythmias   : int  0 1 1 0 1 0 0 0 0 1 ...
##  $ valvular_disease      : int  0 0 0 0 1 0 0 0 0 1 ...
##  $ ...
```

Aggregation Step

Aim: To sum up the values of all the ELIXHAUSER comorbidities across each row. Using a 'for loop', for each i-th row entry in column "ELIXHAUSER_overall", we sum up all the comorbidity scores in that row.

```
for (i in 1:nrow(c_scores)) {
  c_scores[i, "ELIXHAUSER_overall"] <- sum(c_scores[i,4:33])
}
```

Let's take a look at the head of the resulting first and last column:

```
head(c_scores[, c(1, 34)])

##   subject_id ELIXHAUSER_overall
## 1       2848                  1
## 2      21370                  3
## 3       2026                  3
## ...
```

12.3 PART 2—Examples of Data Pre-processing in R

Normalization Step
Aim: Scale values in column ELIXHAUSER_overall to between 0 and 1, i.e. in [0, 1]. Function, max(), finds out the maximum value in column ELIXHAUSER overall. We then re-assign each entry in column ELIXHAUSERoverall as a proportion of the max_score to normalize/scale the column.

```
max_score <- max(c_scores[,"ELIXHAUSER_overall"])
c_scores[,"ELIXHAUSER_overall"] <- c_scores[ ,
"ELIXHAUSER_overall"]/max_score
```

We subset and remove all the columns in c_score, except for "subject_id", "hadm_id", and "ELIXHAUSER_overall":

```
c_scores <- c_scores[, c("subject_id", "hadm_id",
"ELIXHAUSER_overall")]
head(c_scores)

##   subject_id hadm_id ELIXHAUSER_overall
## 1       2848   16272         0.09090909
## 2      21370   17542         0.27272727
## 3       2026   11351         0.27272727
## ...
```

Generalization Step
Aim: Consider only the patient sicker than the average Elixhauser score. The function, which(), return the row numbers (indices) of all the TRUE entries of the logical condition set on c_scores inside the round () brackets, where the condition being the column entry for ELIXHAUSER_overall ≥ 0.5. We store the row indices information in the vector, 'sicker'. Then we can use 'sicker' to subset c_scores to select only the rows/patients who are 'sicker' and store this information in 'c_score_sicker'.

```
sicker <- which(c_scores[,"ELIXHAUSER_overall"]>=0.5)
c_score_sicker <- c_scores[sicker, ]
head(c_score_sicker)

##    subject_id hadm_id ELIXHAUSER_overall
## 10       9545   10809          0.5454545
## 15      12049   27692          0.5454545
## 59      29801   33844          0.5454545
## ...
```

Saving the results to file: There are several functions that will do this, e.g. write.table() and write.csv(). We will give an example here:

```
write.table(c_score_sicker, file = "c_score_sicker.csv", sep = ";",
row.names = F, col.names = F)
```

If you check in your working directory/folder, you should see the new "c_score_sicker.csv" file.

12.3.4 Data Reduction

Aim: To reduce or reshape the input data by means of a more effective representation of the dataset without compromising the integrity of the original data. One element of data reduction is eliminating redundant records while preserving needed data, which we will demonstrate in Example Part 1. The other element involves reshaping the dataset into a "tidy" format, which we will demonstrate in below sections.

Examples Part 1: Eliminating Redundant Records
To demonstrate this with a MIMIC database example, we will look at multiple records of non-invasive mean arterial pressure (MAP) for each patient. We will use the records from the following SQL query, which we exported as "mean_arterial_pressure.csv".

The SQL query selects all the patient subject_id's and noninvasive mean arterial pressure (MAP) measurements from the mimic2v26.chartevents table on the condition of (1) being an adult, (2) in his/her first ICU admission, and (3) where the hadm_id is not missing according to the mimic2v26.icustay_detail table.

12.3 PART 2—Examples of Data Pre-processing in R

1. **SQL query**:

```
SELECT subject_id, value1num
FROM mimic2v26.chartevents
WHERE subject_id IN (
SELECT subject_id
    FROM mimic2v26.icustay_detail
            WHERE subject_icustay_seq = 1
            AND icustay_age_group = 'adult'
            AND hadm_id IS NOT null)
AND itemid=456
AND value1num is not null

-- Export and save the query result as "mean_arterial_pressure.csv"
```

2. **R code**:

There are a variety of methods that can be chosen to aggregate records. In this case we will look at averaging multiple MAP records into a single average MAP for each patient. Other options which may be chosen include using the first recorded value, a minimum or maximum value, etc.

For a basic example, the following code demonstrates data reduction by averaging all of the multiple records of MAP into a single record per patient. The code uses the aggregate() function:

```
setwd("~/Desktop/MIMIC_data_files")
all_maps <- read.csv("mean_arterial_pressure.csv", sep = ",")

str(all_maps)

## 'data.frame':    790174 obs. of  2 variables:
##  $ subject_id: int  4 4 4 4 4 4 4 4 3 4 ...
##  $ value1num : num  80.7 71.7 74.3 69 75 ...
```

This step averages the MAP values for each distinct subject_id:

```
avg_maps <- aggregate(all_maps, by=list(all_maps[,1]), FUN=mean,
na.rm=TRUE)

head(avg_maps)

##   Group.1 subject_id value1num
## 1       3          3  75.10417
## 2       4          4  88.64102
## 3       6          6  91.37357
## ...
```

Examples Part 2: Reshaping Dataset

Aim: Ideally, we want a "tidy" dataset reorganized in such a way so it follows these 3 rules [2, 3]:

1. Each variable forms a column
2. Each observation forms a row
3. Each value has its own cell

Datasets exported from MIMIC usually are fairly "tidy" already. Therefore, we will construct our own data frame here for ease of demonstration for rule 3. We will also demonstrate how to use some common data tidying packages.

R code: To mirror our own MIMIC dataframe, we construct a dataset with a column of subject_id and a column with a list of diagnoses for the admission.

```
diag <- data.frame(subject_id = 1:6,  diagnosis = c("PNA, CHF", "DKA",
"DKA, UTI", "AF, CHF", "AF", "CHF"))
diag
##   subject_id diagnosis
## 1          1  PNA, CHF
## 2          2       DKA
## 3          3  DKA, UTI
## ...
```

Note that the dataset above is not "tidy". There are multiple categorical variables in column "diagnosis"—breaks "tidy" data rule 1. There are multiple values in column "diagnosis"—breaks "tidy" data rule 3.

There are many ways to "tidy" and reshape this dataset. We will show one way to do this by making use of R packages "splitstackshape" [5] and "tidyr" [4] to make reshaping the dataset easier.

R package example 1—"splitstackshape":
Installing and loading the package into R console.

```
install.packages("splitstackshape")
library(splitstackshape)
```

The function, cSplit(), can split the multiple categorical values in each cell of column "diagnosis" into different columns, "diagnosis_1" and "diagnosis_2". If the argument, direction, for cSplit() is not specified, then the function splits the original dataset "wide".

12.3 PART 2—Examples of Data Pre-processing in R

```
diag2 <- cSplit(diag, "diagnosis", ",")
diag2

##    subject_id diagnosis_1 diagnosis_2
## 1:          1         PNA         CHF
## 2:          2         DKA          NA
## 3:          3         DKA         UTI
## ...
```

One could possibly keep it as this if one is interested in primary and secondary diagnoses (though it is not strictly "tidy" yet).

Alternatively, if the direction argument is specified as "long", then cSplit split the function "long" like so:

```
diag3 <- cSplit(diag, "diagnosis", ",", direction = "long")
diag3
##    subject_id diagnosis
## 1:          1       PNA
## 2:          1       CHF
## 3:          2       DKA
## ...
```

Note diag3 is still not "tidy" as there are still multiple categorical variables under column diagnosis—but we no longer have multiple values per cell.

R package example 2—"tidyr":

To further "tidy" the dataset, package "tidyr" is pretty useful.

```
install.packages("tidyr")
library(tidyr)
```

The aim is to split each categorical variable under column, diagnosis, into their own columns with 1 = having the diagnosis and 0 = not having the diagnosis. To do this we first construct a third column, "yes", that hold all the 1 values initially (because the function we are going use require a value column that correspond with the multiple categories column we want to 'spread' out).

```
diag3$yes <- rep(1, nrow(diag3))
diag3

##     subject_id diagnosis yes
## 1:           1       PNA   1
## 2:           1       CHF   1
## 3:           2       DKA   1
## ...
```

Then we can use the spread function to split each categorical variables into their own columns. The argument, fill = 0, replaces the missing values.

```
diag4 <- spread(diag3, diagnosis, yes, fill = 0)
diag4

##     subject_id AF CHF DKA PNA UTI
## 1:           1  0   1   0   1   0
## 2:           2  0   0   1   0   0
## 3:           3  0   0   1   0   1
## ...
```

One can see that this dataset is now "tidy", as it follows all three "tidy" data rules.

12.4 Conclusion

A variety of quality control issues are common when using raw clinical data collected for non-study purposes. Data pre-processing is an important step in preparing raw data for statistical analysis. Several distinct steps are involved in pre-processing raw data as described in this chapter: cleaning, integration, transformation, and reduction. Throughout the process it is important to understand the choices made in pre-processing steps and how different methods can impact the validity and applicability of study results. In the case of EHR data, such as that in the MIMIC database, pre-processing often requires some understanding of the clinical context under which data were entered in order to guide these pre-processing choices. The objective of all the steps is to arrive at a "clean" and "tidy" dataset suitable for effective statistical analyses while avoiding inadvertent introduction of bias into the data.

12.4 Conclusion

Take Home Messages

- Raw data for secondary analysis is frequently "messy" meaning it is not in a form suitable for statistical analysis; data must be "cleaned" into a valid, complete, and effectively organized "tidy" database that can be analyzed.
- There are a variety of techniques that can be used to prepare data for analysis, and depending on the methods use, this pre-processing step can introduce bias into a study.
- The goal of pre-processing data is to prepare the available raw data for analysis without introducing bias by changing the information contained in the data or otherwise influencing end results.

Open Access This chapter is distributed under the terms of the Creative Commons Attribution-NonCommercial 4.0 International License (http://creativecommons.org/licenses/by-nc/4.0/), which permits any noncommercial use, duplication, adaptation, distribution and reproduction in any medium or format, as long as you give appropriate credit to the original author(s) and the source, a link is provided to the Creative Commons license and any changes made are indicated.

The images or other third party material in this chapter are included in the work's Creative Commons license, unless indicated otherwise in the credit line; if such material is not included in the work's Creative Commons license and the respective action is not permitted by statutory regulation, users will need to obtain permission from the license holder to duplicate, adapt or reproduce the material.

References

1. Son NH (2006) Data mining course—data cleaning and data preprocessing. Warsaw University. Available at URL http://www.mimuw.edu.pl/∼son/datamining/DM/4-preprocess.pdf
2. Grolemund G (2016) R for data science—data tidying. O'Reilly Media. Available at URL http://garrettgman.github.io/tidying/
3. Wickham H (2014) J Stat Softw 59(10). Tidy Data. Available at URL http://vita.had.co.nz/papers/tidy-data.pdf
4. Wickham H (2016) Package 'tidyr'—easily tidy data with spread() and gather() functions. CRAN. Available at URL https://cran.r-project.org/web/packages/tidyr/tidyr.pdf
5. Mahto A (2014) Package 'splitstackshape'—stack and reshape datasets after splitting concatenated values. CRAN. Available at URL https://cran.r-project.org/web/packages/splitstackshape/splitstackshape.pdf

Chapter 13
Missing Data

Cátia M. Salgado, Carlos Azevedo, Hugo Proença
and Susana M. Vieira

Learning Objectives

- What are the different types of missing data, and the sources for missingness.
- What options are available for dealing with missing data.
- What techniques exist to help choose the most appropriate technique for a specific dataset.

13.1 Introduction

Missing data is a problem affecting most databases and electronic medical records (EHR) are no exception. Because most statistical models operate only on complete observations of exposure and outcome variables, it is necessary to deal with missing data, either by deleting incomplete observations or by replacing any missing values with an estimated value based on the other information available, a process called imputation. Both methods can significantly effect the conclusions that can be drawn from the data.

Identifying the source of "missingness" is important, as it influences the choice of the imputation technique. Schematically, several cases are possible: (i) the value is missing because it was forgotten or lost; (ii) the value is missing because it was not applicable to the instance; (iii) the value is missing because it is of no interest to the instance. If we were to put this in a medical context: (i) the variable is measured but for some unidentifiable reason the values are not electronically recorded, e.g. disconnection of sensors, errors in communicating with the database server, accidental human omission, electricity failures, and others; (ii) the variable is not measured during a certain period of time due to an identifiable reason, for instance the patient is disconnected from the ventilator because of a medical decision;

Electronic supplementary material The online version of this chapter (doi:10.1007/978-3-319-43742-2_13) contains supplementary material, which is available to authorized users.

© The Author(s) 2016
MIT Critical Data, *Secondary Analysis of Electronic Health Records*,
DOI 10.1007/978-3-319-43742-2_13

(iii) the variable is not measured because it is unrelated with the patient condition and provides no clinical useful information to the physician [1].

An important distinction must be made between data missing for identifiable or unidentified reasons. In the first case, imputing values can be inadequate and add bias to the dataset, so the data is said to be non-recoverable. On the other hand, when data is missing for unidentifiable reasons it is assumed that values are missing because of random and unintended causes. This type of missing data is classified as recoverable.

The first section of this chapter focuses on describing the theory of some commonly used methods to handle missing data. In order to demonstrate the advantages and disadvantages of the methods, their application is demonstrated in the second part of the chapter on actual datasets that were created to study the relation between mortality and insertion of indwelling arterial catheters (IAC) in the intensive care unit (ICU).

13.2 Part 1—Theoretical Concepts

In knowledge discovery in databases, data preparation is the most crucial and time consuming task, that strongly influences the success of the research. Variable selection consists in identifying a useful subset of potential predictors from a large set of candidates (please refer to Chap. 5—Data Analysis for further information on feature selection). Rejecting variables with an excessive number of missing values (e.g. >50 %) is usually a good rule of thumb, however it is not a risk-free procedure. Rejecting a variable may lead to a loss of predictive power and ability to detect statistically significant differences and it can be a source of bias, affecting the representativeness of the results. For these reasons, variable selection needs to be tailored to the missing data mechanism. Imputation can be done before and/or after variable selection.

The general steps that should be followed for handling missing data are:

- Identify patterns and reasons for missing data;
- Analyse the proportion of missing data;
- Choose the best imputation method.

13.2.1 Types of Missingness

The mechanisms by which the data is missing will affect some assumptions supporting our data imputation methods. Three major mechanisms of missingness of the data can be described, depending on the relation between observed (available) and unobserved (missing) data.

For the sake of simplicity, lets consider missingness in the univariate case. To define missingness in mathematical terms, a dataset X can be divided in two parts:

13.2 Part 1—Theoretical Concepts

$$X = \{X_o, X_m\} \tag{1}$$

where X_o corresponds to the observed data, and X_m to the missing data, in the dataset.

For each observation we define a binary response whether or not that observation is missing:

$$R = \begin{cases} 1 & \text{if } X \text{ observed} \\ 0 & \text{if } X \text{ missing} \end{cases} \tag{2}$$

The missing value mechanism can be understood in terms of the probability that an observation is missing $\Pr(R)$ given the observed and missing observations, in the form:

$$\Pr(R|x_o, x_m) \tag{3}$$

The three mechanisms are subject to whether the probability of response R depends or not on the observed and/or missing values:

- **Missing Completely at Random (MCAR)**—When the missing observations are dependent on the observed and unobserved measurements. In this case the probability of an observation being missing depends only on itself, and reduces to $\Pr(R|x_o, x_m) = \Pr(R)$. As an example, imagine that a doctor forgets to record the gender of every six patients that enter the ICU. There is no hidden mechanism related to any variable and it does not depend on any characteristic of the patients.
- **Missing at Random (MAR)**—In this case the probability of a value being missing is related only to the observable data, i.e., the observed data is statistically related with the missing variables and it is possible to estimate the missing values from the observed data. This case is not completely 'random', but it is the most general case where we can ignore the missing mechanism, as we control the information upon which the missingness depends, the observed data. Said otherwise, the probability that some data is missing for a particular variable does not depend on the values of that variable, after adjusting for observed values. Mathematically the probability of missing reduces to $\Pr(R|x_o, x_m) = \Pr(R|x_o)$. Imagine that if elderly people are less likely to inform the doctor that they had had a pneumonia before, the response rate of the variable pneumonia will depend on the variable age.
- **Missing Not at Random (MNAR)**—This refers to the case when neither MCAR nor MAR hold. The missing data depends on both missing and observed values. Determining the missing mechanism is usually impossible, as it depends on unseen data. From that derives the importance of performing sensitivity analyses and test how the inferences hold under different assumptions. For example, we can imagine that patients with low blood pressure are more likely to have their blood pressure measured less frequently (the missing data for the variable "blood pressure" partially depends on the values of the blood pressure).

13.2.2 Proportion of Missing Data

The percentage of missing data for each variable (between patients) and each patient (between variables) must be computed, to help decide which variables and/or patients should be considered candidates for removal or data imputation. A crude example is shown in Table 13.1, where we might want to consider removing patient 1 and the variable "AST" from the analysis, considering that most of their values are missing.

13.2.3 Dealing with Missing Data

Overview of Methods for Handling Missing Data
The methods should be tailored to the dataset of interest, the reasons for missingness and the proportion of missing data. In general, a method is chosen for its simplicity and its ability to introduces as little bias as possible in the dataset.

When data are MCAR or MAR a researcher can ignore the reasons for missing data, which simplifies the choice of the methods to apply. In this case, any method can be applied. Nevertheless it is difficult to obtain empirical evidence about whether or not the data are MCAR or MAR. A valid strategy is to examine the sensitivity of results to the MCAR and MAR assumptions by comparing several analyses, where the differences in results across several analyses may provide some information about what assumptions may be the most relevant.

A significant body of evidence has focused on comparing the performance of missing data handling methods, both in general [2–4] and in context of specific factors such as proportion of missing data and sample size [5–7]. More detailed technical aspects, and application of these methods in various fields can also be found in the works of Jones and Little [8, 9].

In summary, the most widely used methods fall into three main categories, which are described in more detail below.

1. Deletion methods (listwise deletion, i.e. complete-case analysis, pairwise deletion, i.e. available-case analysis)
2. Single Imputation Methods (mean/mode substitution, linear interpolation, Hot deck and cold deck)
3. Model-Based Methods (regression, multiple imputation, k-nearest neighbors)

Table 13.1 Examples of missing data in EHR

	Gender	Glucose	AST	Age
Patient 1	?	120	?	?
Patient 2	M	105	?	68
Patient 3	F	203	45	63
Patient 4	M	145	?	42
Patient 5	M	89	?	80

13.2 Part 1—Theoretical Concepts

Deletion Methods

The simplest way to deal with missing data is to discard the cases or observations that have missing values. In general, case deletion methods lead to valid inferences only for MCAR [10]. There are three ways of doing this: complete-case analysis; available-case analysis; and weighting methods.

Complete-Case Analysis (Listwise Deletion)

In complete case analysis, all the observations with at least one missing variable are discarded (Fig. 13.1).

The principal assumption is that the remaining subsample is representative of the population, and will thus not bias the analysis towards a subgroup. This assumption is rather restrictive and assumes a MCAR mechanism. Listwise deletion often produces unbiased regression slope estimates, as long as missingness is not a function of the outcome variable. The biggest advantage of this method is its simplicity, it is always reasonable to use it when the number of discarded observations is relatively small when compared to the total. Its main drawbacks are the reduced statistical power (because it reduces the number of samples n, the estimates will have larger standard errors), waste of information, and possible bias of the analysis specially if data is not MCAR.

Fig. 13.1 Example of complete-case deletion. Cases highlighted in *red* are discarded

Gender	GLUCOSE	Age
M	?	65
F	120	71
F	99	?
F	140	52
M	88	?
F	85	63
M	170	68
?	153	80
M	115	59
F	103	?

Available-Case Analysis

The available-case method discards data only in the variables that are needed for a specific analysis. For example, if only 4 out of 20 variables are needed for a study, this method would only discard the missing observations of the 4 variables of interest. In Fig. 13.2, imagine that each one of the three represented variables would be used for a different analysis. The analysis is performed using all cases in which the variables of interest are present. Even though this method has the ability to preserve more information, the populations of each analysis would be different and possibly non-comparable.

Weighting-Case Analysis

Weighting is a way of weighting the complete-cases by modelling the missingness in order to reduce the bias introduced in the available-case.

Single-Value Imputation
In single imputation, missing values are filled by some type of "predicted" values [9, 11]. Single imputation ignores uncertainty and almost always underestimates the variance. Multiple imputation overcomes this problem, by taking into account both within—and between—imputation uncertainty.

Fig. 13.2 Example of available-case deletion. If each variable is used for separate analyses, only the cases in which the variable of interest is missing are discarded

Case Study		
S1	S2	S3
Gender	GLUCOSE	Age
M	?	65
F	120	71
F	99	?
F	140	52
M	88	?
F	85	63
M	170	68
?	153	80
M	115	59
F	103	?

13.2 Part 1—Theoretical Concepts

Mean and Median

The simplest imputation method is to substitute missing values by the mean or the median of that variable. Using the median is more robust in the presence of outliers in the observed data. The main disadvantages are that (1) it reduces variability, thereby lowering the estimate errors compared to deletion approaches, and (2) it disregards the relationship between variables, decreasing therefore their correlation. While this method diminishes the bias of using a non-representative sample, it introduces other bias.

Linear Interpolation

This method is particularly suitable for time-series. In linear interpolation, a missing value is computed by interpolating the values of the previous and next available measurements for the patient. For example, if the natremia changes from 132 to 136 mEq/L in 8 h, one can reasonably assume that its value was close to 134 mEq/L at midpoint.

Hot Deck and Cold Deck

In the hot deck method, a missing attribute value is replaced with a value from an estimated distribution of the current data. It is especially used in survey research [9]. Hot deck is typically implemented in two stages. First, the data is partitioned into clusters, and then each instance with missing data is associated with one cluster. The complete cases in a cluster are used to fill in the missing values. This can be done by calculating the mean or mode of the attribute within a cluster. Cold deck imputation is similar to hot deck, except that the data source is different from the current dataset. Hot-deck imputation replaces the missing data by realistic values that preserve the variable distribution. However it underestimates the standard errors and the variability [12].

Last Observation Carried Forward

Sometimes called "sample-and-hold" method [13]. The last value carried forward method is specific to longitudinal designs. This technique imputes the missing value with the last available observation of the individual. This method makes the assumption that the observation of the individual has not changed at all since the last measured observation, which is often unrealistic [14].

Model-Based Imputation

In model-based imputation, a predictive model is created to estimate values that will substitute the missing data. In this case, the dataset is divided into two subsets: one with no missing values for the variable under evaluation (used for training the model) and one containing missing values, that we want to estimate. Several modeling methods can be used such as: regression, logistic regression, neural networks and other parametric and non-parametric modeling techniques. There are two main drawbacks in this approach: the model estimates values are usually more well-behaved than the true values, and the models perform poorly if the observed and missing variables are independent.

Linear Regression

In this model, all the available variables are used to create a linear regression model using the available observations of the variable of interest as output. The advantages of this method is that it takes into account the relationship between variables, unlike the mean/median imputation. The disadvantages are that it overestimates the model fit and the correlation between the variables, as it does not take into account the uncertainty in the missing data and underestimates variances and covariances. A method that was created to introduce uncertainty is the stochastic linear regression (see below).

The case of multivariate imputation is more complex as missing values exist for several variables, which do not follow the same pattern of missingness through the observations. The method used is a multivariate extension of the linear model and relies on an iterative process carried until convergence.

Stochastic Regression

Stochastic regression imputation aims to reduce the bias by an extra step of augmenting each predicted score with a residual term. This residual term is normally distributed with a mean of zero and a variance equal to the residual variance from the regression of the predictor on the target. This method allows to preserve the variability in the data and unbiased parameter estimates with MAR data. However, the standard error tends to be underestimated, because the uncertainty about the imputed values is not included, which increases the risk of type I error [15].

Multiple-Value Imputation

Multiple Imputation (MI) is a powerful statistical technique developed by Rubin in the 1970s for analysing datasets containing missing values [7, 16]. It is a Monte Carlo technique that requires 3 steps (Fig. 13.3).

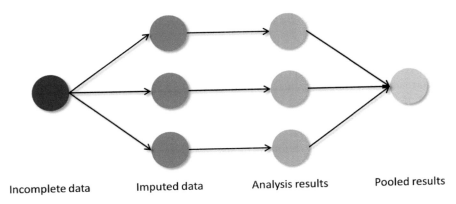

Fig. 13.3 The concept of multiple imputation, with $M = 3$

- Imputation, where the missing values are filled in using any method of choice, leading to $M \geq 2$ completed datasets (5–10 is generally sufficient) [10]. In these M multiply-imputed datasets, all the observed values are the same, but the imputed values are different, reflecting the uncertainty about imputation [10].
- Analysis: each of the M completed datasets is analysed (e.g. a logistic regression classifier for mortality prediction is built), which gives M analyses.
- Pooling: the M analyses are integrated into a final result, for example by computing the mean (and 95 % CI) of the M analyses.

K-Nearest Neighbors

K-nearest neighbors (kNN) can be used for handling missing values. Here, they will be filled with the mean of the k values coming from the k most similar complete observations. The similarity of two observations is determined, after normalization of the dataset, using a distance function which can be Euclidean, Manhattan, Mahalanobis, Pearson, etc. The main advantage of the kNN algorithm is that given enough data it can predict with a reasonable accuracy the conditional probability distribution around a point and thus make well informed estimations. It can predict qualitative and quantitative (discrete and continuous) attributes. Another advantage of this method is that the correlation structure of the data is taken into consideration. The choice of the k-value is very critical. A higher value of k would include attributes which are significantly different from our target observation, while lower value of k implies missing out of significant attributes.

13.2.4 Choice of the Best Imputation Method

Different imputation methods are expected to perform differently on various datasets. We describe here a generic and simple method that can be used to evaluate the performance of various imputation methods on your own dataset, in order to help selecting the most appropriate method. Of note, this simple approach does not test the effect of deletion methods. A more complex approach is described in the case study below, in which the performance of a predictive model is tested on the dataset completed by various imputation methods.

Here is how to proceed:

1. Use a sample of your own dataset that does not contain any missing data (will serve as ground truth).
2. Introduce increasing proportions of missing data at random (e.g. 5–50 % in 5 % increments).
3. Reconstruct the missing data using the various methods.
4. Compute the sum of squared errors between the reconstructed and the original data, for each method and each proportion of missing data.
5. Repeat steps 1–4 a number of times (10 times for example) and compute the average performance of each method (average SSE).
6. Plot the average SSE versus proportion of missing data (1 plot per imputation method), similarly to the example shown in Fig. 13.4.

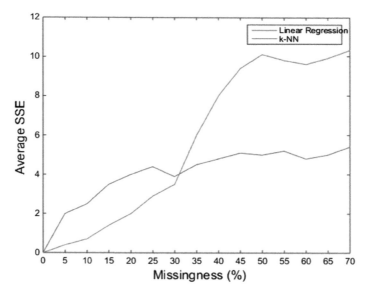

Fig. 13.4 Average SSE between original and reconstructed data, for various levels of missingness and 2 imputation methods (data only for illustrative purposes)

13.2 Part 1—Theoretical Concepts

7. Choose the method that performs best <u>at the level of missing data</u> in your dataset. E.g. if your data had 10 % of missing data, you would want to pick k-NN; at 40 % linear regression performs better (made-up data, for illustrative purpose only).

13.3 Part 2—Case Study

In this section, various imputation methods will be applied to two "real world" clinical datasets used in a study that investigated the effect of inserting an indwelling arterial catheter (IAC) in patients with respiratory failure. Two datasets are used, and include patients that received an IAC (IAC group) and patients that did not (non-IAC). Each dataset is subdivided into 2 classes, with class 1 corresponding to patients that died within 28 days and class 0 to survivors. The proportion of missing data and potential reasons for missingness are discussed first. The following analyses were then carried out:

1. Various proportions of missing data at random were inserted into the variable "age", then imputed using the various methods described above. The distribution of the imputed observations was compared to the original distribution for all the methods.
2. The performance of imputed datasets with different degrees of missingness was tested on a predictive model (logistic regression to predict mortality), first for univariate missing data (the variable age), then for all the variables (multivariate).

The code used to generate the analyses and the figures is provided in the in the accompanying R functions document.

13.3.1 Proportion of Missing Data and Possible Reasons for Missingness

Table 13.2 shows the proportion of missing data in some of the variables of the datasets. 26 variables represent the subset that was considered for testing the different imputation methods, and were selected based on the assumption that missing data occurring in these variables is recoverable.

Since IAC are mainly used for continuous hemodynamic monitoring and for arterial blood sampling for blood gas analysis, we can expect a higher percentage of missing data in blood gas-related variables in the non-IAC group. We can also expect that patient diagnoses are often able to provide an explanation for the lack of specific laboratory results: if a certain test is not ordered because it will most likely provide no clinical insight, a missing value will occur; it is fair to estimate that such

Table 13.2 Missing data in some of the variables of the IAC and non-IAC datasets

	IAC		Non-IAC	
	# points	%	# points	%
Arterial line time day	0	0	792	100
Hospital length of stay	0	0	0	0
Age	0	0	0	0
Gender	0	0	0	0
Weight first	39	3.96	71	8.96
SOFA first	2	0.20	4	0.51
Hemoglobin first	2	0.20	5	0.63
Bilirubin first	418	42.48	365	46.09
...				

value lies within a normal range. In both cases, the fact that data is missing contains information about the response, thus it is MNAR. Body mass index (BMI) has a relatively high percentage of missing data. Assuming that this variable is calculated automatically from the weight and height of patients, we can conclude that this data is MAR: because the height and/or weight are missing, BMI cannot be calculated. If the weight is missing because someone forgot to introduce it into the system then it is MCAR. Besides the missing data mechanism, it is also important to consider the sample distribution in each variable, as some imputation methods assume specific data distributions, usually the normal distribution.

13.3.2 Univariate Missingness Analysis

In this section, the specific influence of each imputation method will be explored for the variable age, using all the other variables. Two different levels of missingness (20 and 40 %) were artifically introduced in the datasets. The original dataset represents the ground truth, to which the imputed datasets were compared using frequency histograms.

Complete-Case Analysis
The complete-case analysis method discards all the incomplete observations with at least one missing value. The distribution of the "imputed" dataset is going to be equal to the original dataset minus the observations that have a missing value in variable age. Figure 13.5 shows an example of the distribution of the variable age in the IAC group.

13.3 Part 2—Case Study

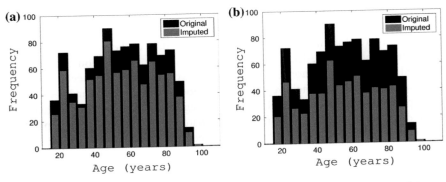

Fig. 13.5 Histogram of variable age in the IAC group before and after univariate complete case method

This method is only exploitable when there is a small percentage of missing data. This method does not require any assumption in the distribution of the missing data, besides that the complete cases should be representative of the original population, which is difficult to prove.

Single Value Imputation
Mean and Median Imputation
Mean and median methods are very crude imputation techniques, which ignore the relationship between age and the other variables and introduce a heavy bias towards the mean/median values. These simple methods allow us to better understand the biasing effect, something that is obvious in the examples Fig. 13.6.

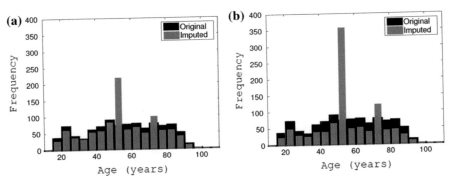

Fig. 13.6 Histogram of variable age in the IAC group before (original) and after (imputed) mean for univariate imputation

Linear Regression Imputation

The linear regression method imputes most of the data at the center of the distribution (example in Fig. 13.7). The extremities of the distribution are not well modeled and are easily ignored. This is due to two features of this technique: first, the assumption that the linear regression is a good fit to the data, and second, the assumption that the missing data lays over the regression line, bending the reality to fit the deterministic nature of the model. Compared to the mean/median imputation, the linear regression assumes a relation between the variables, however it overestimates this relation by assuming that the missing points are over the regression line. The model assumes that the percentage of variance explained is 100 %, thus it underestimates variability.

Stochastic Linear Regression Imputation

The stochastic linear regression is an attempt to loosen the deterministic assumption of the linear regression. In this case, the distribution of the imputed data fits better the original data than previous methods (Fig. 13.8). This method can introduce impossible values, such as negative age. It is a first step to model the uncertainty present in the dataset that represents a trade-off between the precision of the values and the uncertainty introduced by the missing data.

K-Nearest Neighbors
We limit the demonstration to the case where $k = 1$. In the extreme case where all neighbors are used without weights, this method converges to the mean imputation.

Figure 13.9 demonstrates that this method introduces in our particular dataset a huge bias towards the central value. The reason for this arises from the fact that

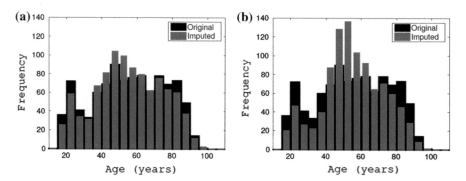

Fig. 13.7 Histogram of the variable age in the IAC group before (original) and after (imputed) linear for univariate imputation

13.3 Part 2—Case Study

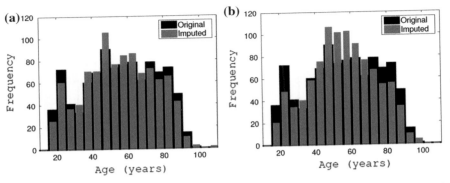

Fig. 13.8 Histogram of variable age in the IAC group before (original) and after (imputed) stochastic linear for univariate imputation

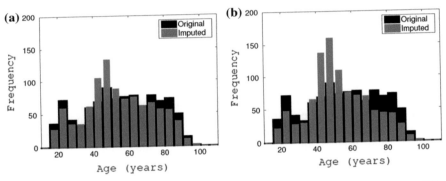

Fig. 13.9 Histogram of variable age in the IAC group before (original) and after (imputed) KNN for univariate imputation

almost half of the variables are binary, which end up having a much higher weight on the distances than continuous variables (which are always less than 1, due to the unitary normalization performed in data pre-processing). Computations with kNN increase in quality with the number of observations in the dataset, and indeed this method is very powerful given the right conditions.

Multiple Imputation
Multiple imputation with linear regression and multivariate normal regression are extensions of the single imputation methods of the same name and use sampling to create multiple different datasets, that represent different possibilities of what might be the original dataset. These methods allow a better modeling of the uncertainty present in the missing values and are, usually, more solid in terms of statistical

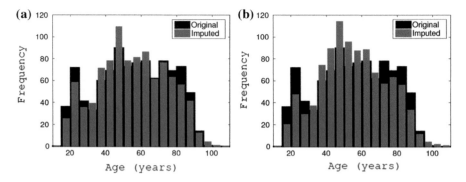

Fig. 13.10 Histogram of variable age in the IAC group before (original) and after (imputed) multiple imputation multivariate normal regression for univariate imputation

properties and results. We chose to work with 10 datasets, which were averaged so that the graphical representation would look similar to the previous methods.

Multivariate normal regression

Multiple imputation multivariate normal distribution gave more importance to the values of the center of the distribution (Fig. 13.10). The main assumption of this method is that the data follows a multivariate normal distribution, something that is not completely true for this dataset, which contains numerous binary variables. Nonetheless, even in the presence of categorical variables and distributions that are not strictly normal, it should perform reasonably well [10, 19]. The multiple imputation method enhances the modeling of uncertainty by adding a bootstrap sampling to the expectation maximization algorithm, giving raise to better predictions of the possible missing data by considering multiple possibilities of the original data. Obviously, when averaging the data for histogram representation, some of that richness is lost. Nonetheless, the quality of the regression is obvious when compared to the previous methods.

Linear regression

The multiple imputation linear regression method uses all the variables except the target variable (age) to estimate the missing data of this last variable. The data is modelled using linear regression and Gibbs sampling. Figure 13.11 demonstrates that this represents by far the most accurate imputation method in this particular dataset.

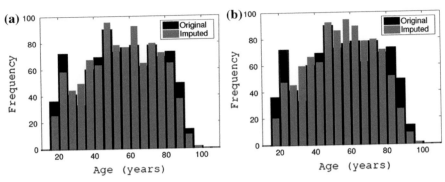

Fig. 13.11 Histogram of variable age in the IAC group before (original) and after (imputed) multiple imputation generalized regression for univariate imputation

13.3.3 Evaluating the Performance of Imputation Methods on Mortality Prediction

This test aims to assess the generalization capabilities of the models constructed using imputed data, and check their performance by comparing them to the original data. All the methods described previously were used to reconstruct a sample of both IAC and non-IAC datasets, with increasing proportions of missing data at random, first only on the variable age (univariate), then on all the variables in the dataset (multivariate). A logistic regression model was built on the reconstructed data and tested on a sample of the original data (that does not contain imputations or missing data).

The performance of the models is evaluated in terms of area under the receiver operating characteristic curve (AUC), accuracy (correct classification rate), sensitivity (true positive classification rate—TPR, also known as recall), specificity (true negative classification rate—TNR) and Cohen's kappa. All the methods were compared against a reference logistic regression that was fitted with the original data without missingness. The results were averaged over a 10-fold cross validation and the AUC results are presented graphically.

The influence of one variable has a limited effect, even if age is the variable most correlated with mortality (Fig. 13.12). At most, the AUC decreased from 0.84 to 0.81 for IAC and from 0.90 to 0.87 for the non-IAC case, if we exclude the complete-case analysis method that performs poorly from the beginning. For lower values of missingness (less than 50 %), all the other models perform similarly. Among univariate techniques, the methods that performed the best on both datasets are the two multiple imputation methods, namely the linear regression and the multivariate normal distribution, and the one-nearest neighbors algorithm. In the case of univariate missingness, the nearest neighbors reveals to be a good estimator if several complete observations exist, as it is the case. With increasing of the

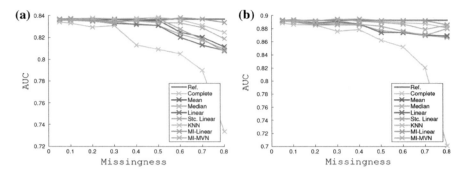

Fig. 13.12 Mean AUC performance of the logistic regression models modelled with different imputation methods for different degrees of univariate missingness of the Age variable

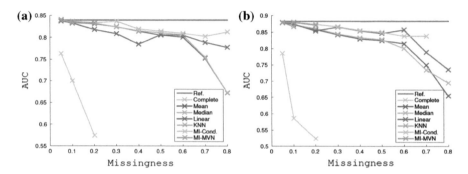

Fig. 13.13 Mean AUC of the logistic regression models for different degrees of multivariate missingness

missingness, the simpler methods introduced more bias in the modeling of the datasets.

The quality of the imputation methods was also evaluated in the presence of multivariate missingness with an uniform probability in all variables (Fig. 13.13). It has to be noted that obtaining results for more than 40 % of missingness in all the variables is quite infeasible in most cases, and there are no assurances of good performances with any of the methods. Some methods were not able to perform complete imputations over a certain degree of missingness (e.g. the complete-case analysis stopped having enough observations after 20 % of missingness).

Overall, and quite surprisingly, the methods had a reasonable performance even for 80 % of missingness in every variable. The reason behind this is that almost half of the variables are binary, and because of their relation with the output, reconstructing them from frequent values in each class is usually the best guess. The decrease in AUC was due to a decrease in the sensitivity, as the specificity values remained more or less unchanged with the increase in missingness. The method that performed the best overall in terms of AUC was the multiple imputation linear regression. In IAC it achieved a minimum value of AUC of 0.81 at 70 % of missingness, corresponding to a reference AUC of 0.84 and in non-IAC it achieved an AUC of 0.85 at 70 % of missingness, close to the reference AUC of 0.89.

13.4 Conclusion

Missing data is a widespread problem in EHR due to the nature of medical information itself, the massive amounts of data collected, the heterogeneity of data standards and recording devices, data transfers and conversions, and finally Human errors and omissions. When dealing with the problem of missing data, just like in many other domains of data mining, there is no one-size-fits-all approach, and the data scientist should ultimately rely on robust evaluation tools when choosing an imputation method to handle missing values in a particular dataset.

Take-Home Messages

- Always evaluate the reasons for missingness: is it MCAR/MAR/MNAR?
- What is the proportion of missing data per variable and per record?
- Multiple imputation approaches generally perform better than other methods.
- Evaluation tools must be used to tailor the imputation methods to a particular dataset.

Open Access This chapter is distributed under the terms of the Creative Commons Attribution-NonCommercial 4.0 International License (http://creativecommons.org/licenses/by-nc/4.0/), which permits any noncommercial use, duplication, adaptation, distribution and reproduction in any medium or format, as long as you give appropriate credit to the original author(s) and the source, a link is provided to the Creative Commons license and any changes made are indicated.

The images or other third party material in this chapter are included in the work's Creative Commons license, unless indicated otherwise in the credit line; if such material is not included in the work's Creative Commons license and the respective action is not permitted by statutory regulation, users will need to obtain permission from the license holder to duplicate, adapt or reproduce the material.

References

1. Cismondi F, Fialho AS, Vieira SM, Reti SR, Sousa JMC, Finkelstein SN (2013) Missing data in medical databases: impute, delete or classify? Artif Intell Med 58(1):63–72
2. Peng CY, Harwell MR, Liou SM, Ehman LH (2006) Advances in missing data methods and implications for educational research
3. Peugh JL, Enders CK (2004) Missing data in educational research: a review of reporting practices and suggestions for improvement. Rev Educ Res 74(4):525–556
4. Young W, Weckman G, Holland W (2011) A survey of methodologies for the treatment of missing values within datasets: limitations and benefits. Theor Issues Ergon Sci 12(1):15–43

5. Alosh M (2009) The impact of missing data in a generalized integer-valued autoregression model for count data. J Biopharm Stat 19(6):1039–1054
6. Knol MJ, Janssen KJM, Donders ART, Egberts ACG, Heerdink ER, Grobbee DE, Moons KGM, Geerlings MI (2010) Unpredictable bias when using the missing indicator method or complete case analysis for missing confounder values: an empirical example. J Clin Epidemiol 63(7):728–736
7. Little RJA, Rubin DB (2002) Missing data in experiments. In: Statistical analysis with missing data. Wiley, pp 24–40
8. Jones MP (1996) Indicator and stratification methods for missing explanatory variables in multiple linear regression. J Am Stat Assoc 91(433):222–230
9. Little RJA (2016) Statistical analysis with missing data. Wiley, New York
10. Schafer JL (1999) Multiple imputation: a primer. Stat Methods Med Res 8(1):3–15
11. de Waal T, Pannekoek J, Scholtus S (2011) Handbook of statistical data editing and imputation. Wiley, New York
12. Roth PL (1994) Missing data: a conceptual review for applied psychologists. Pers Psychol 47 (3):537–560
13. Hug CW (2009) Detecting hazardous intensive care patient episodes using real-time mortality models. Thesis, Massachusetts Institute of Technology
14. Wood AM, White IR, Thompson SG (2004) Are missing outcome data adequately handled? A review of published randomized controlled trials in major medical journals. Clin Trials 1 (4):368–376
15. Enders CK (2010) Applied missing data analysis, 1st edn. The Guilford Press, New York
16. Rubin DB (1988) An overview of multiple imputation. In: Proceedings of the survey research section, American Statistical Association, pp 79–84
17. Saeed M, Villarroel M, Reisner AT, Clifford G, Lehman L-W, Moody G, Heldt T, Kyaw TH, Moody B, Mark RG (2011) Multiparameter intelligent monitoring in intensive care II (MIMIC-II): a public-access intensive care unit database. Crit Care Med 39(5):952–960
18. Scott DJ, Lee J, Silva I, Park S, Moody GB, Celi LA, Mark RG (2013) Accessing the public MIMIC-II intensive care relational database for clinical research. BMC Med Inform Decis Mak 13(1):9
19. Schafer JL, Olsen MK (1998) Multiple imputation for multivariate missing-data problems: a data analyst's perspective. Multivar Behav Res 33(4):545–571

Chapter 14
Noise Versus Outliers

Cátia M. Salgado, Carlos Azevedo, Hugo Proença
and Susana M. Vieira

Learning Objectives

- What common methods for outlier detection are available.
- How to choose the most appropriate methods.
- How to assess the performance of an outlier detection method and how to compare different methods.

14.1 Introduction

An outlier is a data point which is different from the remaining data [1]. Outliers are also referred to as *abnormalities*, *discordants*, *deviants* and *anomalies* [2]. Whereas noise can be defined as mislabeled examples (class noise) or errors in the values of attributes (attribute noise), outlier is a broader concept that includes not only errors but also discordant data that may arise from the natural variation within the population or process. As such, outliers often contain interesting and useful information about the underlying system. These particularities have been exploited in fraud control, intrusion detection systems, web robot detection, weather forecasting, law enforcement and medical diagnosis [1], using in general methods of supervised outlier detection (see below).

Within the medical domain in general, the main sources of outliers are equipment malfunctions, human errors, anomalies arising from patient specific behaviors and natural variation within patients. Consider for instance an anomalous blood test result. Several reasons can explain the presence of outliers: severe pathological states, intake of drugs, food or alcohol, recent physical activity, stress, menstrual cycle, poor blood sample collection and/or handling. While some reasons may point to the existence of patient-specific characteristics discordant with the "average"

Electronic supplementary material The online version of this chapter (doi:10.1007/978-3-319-43742-2_14) contains supplementary material, which is available to authorized users.

patient, in which case the observation being an outlier provides useful information, other reasons may point to human errors, and hence the observation should be considered for removal or correction. Therefore, it is crucial to consider the causes that may be responsible for outliers in a given dataset before proceeding to any type of action.

The consequences of not screening the data for outliers can be catastrophic. The negative effects of outliers can be summarized in: (1) increase in error variance and reduction in statistical power; (2) decrease in normality for the cases where outliers are non-randomly distributed; (3) model bias by corrupting the true relationship between exposure and outcome [3].

A good understanding of the data itself is required before choosing a model to detect outliers, and several factors influence the choice of an outlier identification method, including the type of data, its size and distribution, the availability of ground truth about the data, and the need for interpretability in a model [2]. For example, regression-based models are better suited for finding outliers in linearly correlated data, while clustering methods are advisable when the data is not linearly distributed along correlation planes. While this chapter provides a description of some of the most common methods for outlier detection, many others exist.

Evaluating the effectiveness of an outlier detection algorithm and comparing the different approaches is complex. Moreover, the ground-truth about outliers is often unavailable, as in the case of unsupervised scenarios, hampering the use of quantitative methods to assess the effectiveness of the algorithms in a rigorous way. The analyst is left with the alternative of qualitative and intuitive evaluation of results [2]. To overcome this difficulty, we will use in this chapter logistic regression models to investigate the performance of different outlier identification techniques in the medically relevant case study.

14.2 Part 1—Theoretical Concepts

Outlier identification methods can be classified into supervised and unsupervised methods, depending on whether prior information about the abnormalities in the data is available or not. The techniques can be further divided into univariable and multivariable methods, conditional on the number of variables considered in the dataset of interest.

The simplest form of outlier detection is extreme value analysis of unidimensional data. In this case, the core principle of discovering outliers is to determine the statistical tails of the underlying distribution and assume that either too large or too small values are outliers. In order to apply this type of technique to a multidimensional dataset, the analysis is performed one dimension at a time. In such a multivariable analysis, outliers are samples which have unusual combinations with other samples in the multidimensional space. It is possible to have outliers with reasonable marginal values (i.e. the value appears normal when confining oneself to one dimension), but due to linear or non-linear combinations of multiple attributes

14.2 PART 1—Theoretical Concepts

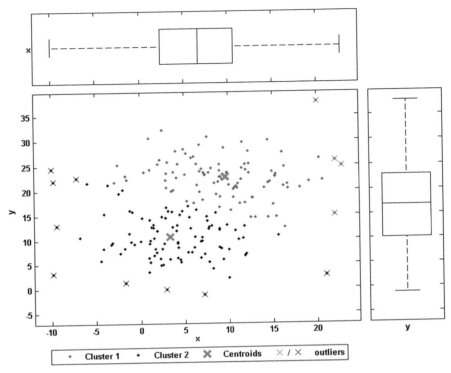

Fig. 14.1 Univariable (*boxplots*) versus multivariable (*scatter plot*) outlier investigation

these observations unveil unusual patterns in regards to the rest of the population under study.

To better understand this, the Fig. 14.1 provides a graphical example of a scenario where outliers are only visible in a 2-dimensional space. An inspection of the boxplots will reveal no outliers (no data point above and below 1.5 IQR (the interquartile range, refer to Chap. 15—Exploratory Data Analysis), a widely utilized outlier identification method), whereas a close observation of the natural clusters present in data will uncover irregular patterns. Outliers can be identified by visual inspection, highlighting data points that seem to be relatively out of the inherent 2-D data groups.

14.3 Statistical Methods

In the field of statistics, the data is assumed to follow a distribution model (e.g., normal distribution) and an instance is considered an outlier if it deviates significantly from the model [2, 4]. The use of normal distributions simplifies the analysis, as most of the existing statistical tests, such as the Z-score, can be directly interpreted in terms of probabilities of significance. However, in many real world datasets the underlying distribution of the data is unknown or complex. Statistical tests still provide a good approximation of outlier scores, but results of the tests need to be interpreted carefully and cannot be expressed statistically [2]. The next sections describe some of the most widely used statistical tests for outliers identification.

14.3.1 Tukey's Method

Quartiles are the values that divide an array of numbers into quarters. The (IQR) is the distance between the lower (Q1) and upper (Q3) quartiles in the boxplot, that is $IQR = Q3 - Q1$. It can be used as a measure of how spread out the values are. Inner "fences" are located at a distance of 1.5 IQR below Q1 and above Q3, and outer fences at a distance of 3 IQR below Q1 and above Q3 [5]. A value between the inner and outer fences is a possible outlier, whereas a value falling outside the outer fences is a probable outlier. The removal of all possible and probable outliers is referred to as the Interquartile (IQ) method, while in Tukey's method only the probable outliers are discarded.

14.3.2 Z-Score

The Z-value test computes the number of standard deviations by which the data varies from the mean. It presents a reasonable criterion for the identification of outliers when the data is normally distributed. It is defined as:

$$z_i = \frac{x_i - \bar{x}}{s} \tag{14.1}$$

where $\bar{x}$ and s denote the sample mean and standard deviation, respectively. In cases where mean and standard deviation of the distribution can be accurately estimated (or are available from domain knowledge), a good "rule of thumb" is to consider values with $|z_i| \geq 3$ as outliers. Of note, this method is of limited value for small datasets, since the maximum z-score is at most $n - 1/\sqrt{n}$ [6].

14.3.3 Modified Z-Score

The estimators used in the z-Score, the sample mean and sample standard deviation, can be affected by the extreme values present in the data. To avoid this problem, the

14.3 Statistical Methods

modified z-score uses the median $\widetilde{x}$ and the median absolute deviation (MAD) instead of the mean and standard deviation of the sample [7]:

$$M_i = \frac{0.6745(x_i - \widetilde{x})}{MAD} \tag{14.2}$$

where

$$MAD = median\{|x_i - \widetilde{x}|\} \tag{14.3}$$

The authors recommend using modified z-scores with $|M_i| \geq 3.5$ as potential outliers. The assumption of normality of the data still holds.

14.3.4 Interquartile Range with Log-Normal Distribution

The statistical tests discussed previously are specifically based on the assumption that the data is fairly normally distributed. In the health care domain it is common to find skewed data, for instance in surgical procedure times or pulse oxymetry [8]. Refer to Chap. 15-Exploratory Data Analysis for a formal definition of skewness. If a variable follows a log-normal distribution then the logarithms of the observations follow a normal distribution. A reasonable approach then is to apply the *ln* to the original data and they apply the tests intended to the "normalized" distributions. We refer to this method as the log-IQ.

14.3.5 Ordinary and Studentized Residuals

In a linear regression model, ordinary residuals are defined as the difference between the observed and predicted values. Data points with large residuals differ from the general regression trend and may represent outliers. The problem is that their magnitudes depend on their units of measurement, making it difficult to, for example, define a threshold at which a point is considered an outlier. Studentized residuals eliminate the units of measurement by dividing the residuals by an estimate of their standard deviation. One limitation of this approach is it assumes the regression model is correctly specified.

14.3.6 Cook's Distance

In a linear regression model, Cook's distance is used to estimate the influence of a data point on the regression. The principle of Cook's distance is to measure the effect of deleting a given observation. Data points with a large distance may represent outliers. For the ith point in the sample, Cook's distance is defined as:

$$D_i = \frac{\sum_{j=1}^{n}(\hat{y}_j \hat{y}_{j(i)})^2}{(k+1)s^2} \quad (14.4)$$

Where $\hat{y}_{j(i)}$ is the prediction of y_j by the revised regression model when the ith point is removed from the sample, and s is the estimated root mean square error. Instinctively, D_i is a normalized measure of the influence of the point i on all predicted mean values $\hat{y}_j$ with $j = 1, \ldots, n$. Different cut-off values can be used for flagging highly influential points. Cook has suggested that a distance >1 represents a simple operational guideline [9]. Others have suggested a threshold of $4/n$, with n representing the number of observations.

14.3.7 Mahalanobis Distance

This test is based on Wilks method designed to detect a single outlier from a normal multivariable sample. It approaches the maximum squared Mahalanobis Distance (MD) to an F-distribution function formulation, which is often more appropriate than a χ^2 distribution [10]. For a p-dimensional multivariate sample x_i ($i = 1,\ldots,n$), the Mahalanobis distance of the ith case is defined as:

$$MD_i = \sqrt{(x_i - t)^T C^{-1} (x_i - t)} \quad (14.5)$$

where t is the estimated multivariate location, which is usually the arithmetic mean, and C is the estimated covariance matrix, usually the sample covariance matrix.

Multivariate outliers can be simply defined as observations having a large squared Mahalanobis distance. In this work, the squared Mahalanobis distance is compared with quantiles of the F-distribution with p and $p - 1$ degrees of freedom. Critical values are calculated using Bonferroni bounds.

14.4 Proximity Based Models

Proximity-based techniques are simple to implement and unlike statistical models they make no prior assumptions about the data distribution model. They are suitable for both supervised and unsupervised multivariable outlier detection [4].

Clustering is a type of proximity-based technique that starts by partitioning a N–dimensional dataset into c subgroups of samples (clusters) based on their similarity. Then, some measure of the fit of the data points to the different clusters is used in order to determine if the data points are outliers [2]. One challenge associated with

14.4 Proximity Based Models

this type of technique is that it assumes specific shapes of clusters depending on the distance function used within the clustering algorithm. For example, in a 3-dimensional space, the Euclidean distance would consider spheres as equidistant, whereas the Mahalanobis distance would consider ellipsoids as equidistant (where the length of the ellipsoids in one axis is proportional to the variance of the data in that direction).

14.4.1 k-Means

The k-means algorithm is widely used in data mining due to its simplicity and scalability [11]. The difficulty associated with this algorithm is the need to determine k, the number of clusters, in advance. The algorithm minimizes the within-cluster sum of squares, the sum of distances between each point in a cluster and the cluster centroid. In k-means, the center of a group is the mean of measurements in the group. Metrics such as the Akaike Information Criterion or the Bayesian Information Criterion, which add a factor proportional to k to the cost function used during clustering, can help determine k. A k value which is too high will increase the cost function even if it reduces the within-cluster sum of squares [12, 13].

14.4.2 k-Medoids

Similarly to k-means, the k-medoids clustering algorithm partitions the dataset into groups so that it minimizes the sum of distances between a data point and its center. In contrast to the k-means algorithm, in k-medoids the cluster centers are members of the group. Consequently, if there is a region of outliers outside the area with higher density of points, the cluster center will not be pushed towards the outliers region, as in k-means. Thus, k-medoids is more robust towards outliers than k-means.

14.4.3 Criteria for Outlier Detection

After determining the position of the cluster center with either k-means or k-medoids, the criteria to classify an item as an outlier must be specified, and different options exist:

Criterion 1: The first criterion proposed to detect outliers is based on the Euclidean distance to the cluster centers C, such that points more distant to their center than the minimum interclusters distance are considered outliers:

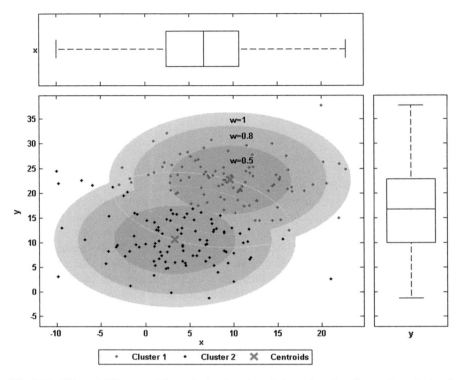

Fig. 14.2 Effect of different weights w in the detection of cluster-based outliers, using criterion 1

$$x \in C_k \text{ is outlier if } d(x, C_k) > \min_{k \neq j}\{\delta(C_k, C_j)\} \times w \quad (14.6)$$

where $d(x, C_k)$ is the Euclidean distance between point x and C_k center, $\delta(C_k, C_j)$ is the distance between C_k and C_j centers and $w = \{0.5, 0.7, 1, 1.2, 1.5, \ldots\}$ is a weighting parameter that determines how aggressively the method will remove outliers.

Figure 14.2 provides a graphical example of the effect of varying values of w in the creation of boundaries for outlier detection. While small values of w aggressively remove outliers, as w increases the harder it is to identify them.

Criterion 2: In this criterion, we calculate the distance of each data point to its centroid (case of k-means) or medoid (case of k-medoids) [14]. If the ratio of the distance of the nearest point to the cluster center and these calculated distances are smaller than a certain threshold, than the point is considered an outlier. The threshold is defined by the user and should depend on the number of clusters selected, since the higher the number of clusters the closer are the points inside the cluster, i.e., the threshold should decrease with increasing c.

14.5 Supervised Outlier Detection

In many scenarios, previous knowledge about outliers may be available and can be used to label the data accordingly and to identify outliers of interest. The methods relying on previous examples of data outliers are referred to as supervised outlier detection methods, and involve training classification models which can later be used to identify outliers in the data. Supervised methods are often devised for anomaly detection in application domains where anomalies are considered occurrences of interest. Examples include fraud control, intrusion detection systems, web robot detection or medical diagnosis [1]. Hence, the labels represent what an analyst might be specifically looking for rather than what one might want to remove [2]. The key difference comparing to many other classification problems is the inherent unbalanced nature of data, since instances labeled as "abnormal" are present much less frequently than "normal" labeled instances. Interested readers can find further information about this topic in the textbook by Aggarwal, for instance [2].

14.6 Outlier Analysis Using Expert Knowledge

In univariate analyses, expert knowledge can be used to define thresholds of values that are normal, critical (life-threatening) or impossible because they fall outside permissible ranges or have no physical meaning [15]. Negative measurements of heart rate or body temperatures are examples of impossible values. It is very important to check the dataset for these types of outliers, as they originated undoubtedly from human error or equipment malfunction, and should be deleted or corrected.

14.7 Case Study: Identification of Outliers in the Indwelling Arterial Catheter (IAC) Study

In this section, various methods will be applied to identify outliers in two "real world" clinical datasets used in a study that investigated the effect of inserting an indwelling arterial catheter (IAC) in patients with respiratory failure. Two datasets are used, and include patients that received an IAC (IAC group) and patients that did not (non-IAC). The code used to generate the analyses and the figures is available in the GitHub repository for this book.

Table 14.1 Normal, critical and impossible ranges for the selected variables, and maximum and minimum values present in the datasets

Variable	Reference value			Analyzed data		Units
	Normal range	Critical	Impossible	IAC	Non-IAC	
Age	–	–	<17 (adults)	15.2–99.1	15.2–97.5	Years
SOFA	–	–	<0 and >24	1–17	0–14	No units
WBC	3 9–10.7	≥ 100	<0	0.3–86.0	0 2–109.8	$\times 10^9$ cells/L
Hemoglobin	Male: 13.5–17.5	≤ 6 and ≥ 20	<0	Male: 3 2–19.0	4.9–18.6	g/dL
	Female: 12–16			Female: 2.0–18.1	4.2–18.1	
Platelets	150–400	≤ 40 and ≥ 1000	<0	7.0–680.0	9.0–988.0	$\times 10^9$/L
Sodium	136–145	≤ 120 and ≥ 160	<0	105 0–165.0	111.0–154.0	mmol/L
Potassium	3.5–5	≤ 2.5 and ≥ 6	<0	1 9–9.8	1.9–8.3	mmol/L
TCO$_2$	22–28	≤ 10 and ≥ 40 [4]	<0	2.0–62.0	5.0–52.0	mmol/L
Chloride [29]	95–105	≤ 70 and ≥ 120	<0 and ≥ 160	81.0–133.0	78.0–127.0	mmol/L
BUN	7–18	≥ 100 [1]	<0	2.0–139.0	2.0–126.0	mg/dL
Creatinine	0.6–1.2	≥ 10	<0	0.2–12 5	0.0–18.3	mg/dL
PO$_2$	75–105	≤ 40	<0	25 0–594.0	22.0–634.0	mmHg
PCO$_2$	33–45	≤ 20 and ≥ 70	<0	8.0–141.0	14.0–158.0	mmHg

14.8 Expert Knowledge Analysis

Table 14.1 provides maximum and minimum values for defining normal, critical and permissible ranges in some of the variables analyzed in the study, as well as maximum and minimum values present in the dataset.

14.9 Univariate Analysis

In this section, univariate outliers are identified for each variable within pre-defined classes (survivors and non-survivors), using the statistical methods described above.

Table 14.2 summarizes the number and percentage of outliers identified by each method in the Indwelling Arterial Catheter (IAC) and non-IAC groups. Overall, Tukey's and log-IQ are the most conservative methods, i.e., they identify the

14.9 Univariate Analysis

Table 14.2 Number and percentage of outliers identified by each method

IAC

	Class 0 (811 patients)					Class 1 (163 patients)				
	IQ	Tukey's	log–IQ	Z-score	Mod z-score	IQ	Tukey's	Log–IQ	Z-score	Mod z-score
Age	0 (0.0 %)	0 (0.0 %)	1 (0.1 %)	0 (0.0 %)	0 (0.0 %)	5 (0.6 %)	0 (0.0 %)	8 (1.0 %)	4 (0.5 %)	5 (0.6 %)
SOFA	13 (1.6 %)	0 (0.0 %)	6 (0.7 %)	2 (0.2 %)	20 (2.5 %)	**16 (2.0 %)**	3 (0.4 %)	8 (1.0 %)	1 (0.1 %)	5 (0.6 %)
WBC	20 (2.5 %)	3 (0.4 %)	21 (2.6 %)	5 (0.6 %)	10 (1.2 %)	6 (0.7 %)	1 (0.1 %)	5 (0.6 %)	1 (0.1 %)	3 (0.4 %)
Hemoglobin	8 (1.0 %)	1 (0.1 %)	13 (1.6 %)	5 (0.6 %)	4 (0.5 %)	0 (0.0 %)	0 (0.0 %)	0 (0.0 %)	0 (0.0 %)	0 (0.0 %)
Platelets	17 (2.1 %)	1 (0.1 %)	36 (4.4 %)	7 (0.9 %)	7 (0.9 %)	4 (0.5 %)	0 (0.0 %)	2 (0.2 %)	2 (0.2 %)	1 (0.1 %)
Sodium	30 (3.7 %)	8 (1.0 %)	30 (3.7 %)	10 (1.2 %)	26 (3.2 %)	8 (1.0 %)	1 (0.1 %)	8 (1.0 %)	2 (0.2 %)	2 (0.2 %)
Potassium	39 (4.8 %)	10 (1.2 %)	35 (4.3 %)	14 (1.7 %)	26 (3.2 %)	9 (1.1 %)	1 (0.1 %)	7 (0.9 %)	2 (0.2 %)	8 (1.0 %)
TCO$_2$	24 (3.0 %)	4 (0.5 %)	31 (3.8 %)	13 (1.6 %)	13 (1.6 %)	9 (1.1 %)	2 (0.2 %)	6 (0.7 %)	2 (0.2 %)	2 (0.2 %)
Chloride	21 (2.6 %)	3 (0.4 %)	24 (3.0 %)	13 (1.6 %)	18 (2.2 %)	4 (0.5 %)	0 (0.0 %)	3 (0.4 %)	1 (0.1 %)	1 (0.1 %)
BUN	**72 (8.9 %)**	**37 (4.6 %)**	**48 (5.9 %)**	**20 (2.5 %)**	**60 (7.4 %)**	13 (1.6 %)	**9 (1.1 %)**	7 (0.9 %)	**5 (0.6 %)**	**13 (1.6 %)**
Creatinine	50 (6.2 %)	31 (3.8 %)	43 (5.3 %)	18 (2.2 %)	40 (4.9 %)	11 (1.4 %)	2 (0.2 %)	2 (0.2 %)	2 (0.2 %)	8 (1.0 %)
PO$_2$	0 (0.0 %)	0 (0.0 %)	2 (0.2 %)	0 (0.0 %)	0 (0.0 %)	0 (0.0 %)	0 (0.0 %)	0 (0.0 %)	0 (0.0 %)	0 (0.0 %)
PCO$_2$	53 (6.5 %)	22 (2.7 %)	**48 (5.9 %)**	19 (2.3 %)	37 (4.6 %)	11 (1.4 %)	4 (0.5 %)	**13 (1.6 %)**	4 (0.5 %)	9 (1.1 %)
Total patients	**220 (27.1 %)**	86(10.6 %)	210 (25.9 %)	91 (11.2 %)	165 (20.3 %)	**63 (7.8 %)**	20 (2.5 %)	47 (5.8 %)	23 (2.8 %)	43 (5.3 %)

Non-IAC

	Class 0 (524 patients)					Class 1 (83 patients)				
	IQ	Tukey's	log–IQ	Z-score	Mod z-score	IQ	Tukey's	Log–IQ	Z-score	Mod z-score
Age	0 (0.0 %)	0 (0.0 %)	0 (0.0 %)	0 (0.0 %)	0 (0.0 %)	1 (0.2 %)	0 (0.0 %)	3 (0.6 %)	1 (0.2 %)	1 (0.2 %)
SOFA	**51 (9.7 %)**	2 (0.4 %)	**48 (9.2 %)**	2 (0.4 %)	7 (1.3 %)	**9 (1.7 %)**	1 (0.2 %)	8 (1.5 %)	1 (0.2 %)	3 (0.6 %)
WBC	21 (4.0 %)	4 (0.8 %)	10 (1.9 %)	4 (0.11 %)	11 (2.1 %)	4 (0.8 %)	1 (0.2 %)	4 (0.8 %)	1 (0.2 %)	3 (0.6 %)
Hemoglobin	1 (0.4 %)	0 (0.0 %)	6 (1.1 %)	2 (0.4 %)	2 (0.4 %)	0 (0.0 %)	0 (0.0 %)	2 (0.4 %)	0 (0.0 %)	0 (0.0 %)

(continued)

Table 14.2 (continued)

	Non-IAC					Class 1 (83 patients)				
	Class 0 (524 patients)									
	IQ	Tukey's	log–IQ	Z-score	Mod z-score	IQ	Tukey's	Log–IQ	Z-score	Mod z-score
Platelets	15 (2.9 %)	5 (1.0 %)	21 (4.0 %)	5 (1.0 %)	6 (1.1 %)	4 (0.8 %)	1 (0.2 %)	5 (1.0 %)	**2 (0.4 %)**	2 (0.4 %)
Sodium	25 (4.8 %)	9 (1.7 %)	25 (4.11 %)	9 (1.7 %)	20 (3.11 %)	5 (1.0 %)	1 (0.2 %)	5 (1.0 %)	1 (0.2 %)	1 (0.2 %)
Potassium	22 (4.2 %)	2 (0.4 %)	14 (2.7 %)	6 (1.1 %)	14 (2.7 %)	1 (0.2 %)	0 (0.0 %)	0 (0.0 %)	0 (0.0 %)	0 (0.0 %)
TCO$_2$	27 (5.2 %)	4 (0.8 %)	31 (5.9 %)	8 (1.5 %)	5 (1.0 %)	4 (0.8 %)	1 (0.2 %)	4 (0.8 %)	**2 (0.4 %)**	3 (0.6 %)
Chloride	21 (4.0 %)	4 (0.8 %)	20 (3.11 %)	9 (1.7 %)	11 (2.1 %)	**9 (1.7 %)**	1 (0.2 %)	**9 (1.7 %)**	1 (0.2 %)	4 (0.8 %)
BUN	**35 (6.7 %)**	**20 (3.8 %)**	27 (5.2 %)	**13 (2.5 %)**	**34 (6.5 %)**	6 (1.1 %)	2 (0.4 %)	2 (0.4 %)	**2 (0.4 %)**	6 (1.1 %)
Creatinine	29 (5.5 %)	17 (3.2 %)	25 (4.8 %)	8 (1.5 %)	22 (4.2 %)	7 (1.3 %)	2 (0.4 %)	3 (0.6 %)	**2 (0.4 %)**	5 (1.0 %)
PO$_2$	0 (0.0 %)	0 (0.0 %)	0 (0.0 %)	0 (0.0 %)	0 (0.0 %)	1 (0.2 %)	0 (0.0 %)	0 (0.0 %)	0 (0.0 %)	3 (0.6 %)
PCO$_2$	34 (6.5 %)	11 (2.1 %)	33 (6.3 %)	10 (1.9 %)	28 (5.3 %)	8 (1.5 %)	**4 (0.8 %)**	6 (1.1 %)	**2 (0.4 %)**	**8 (1.5 %)**
Total patients	**176 (33.6 %)**	59 (11.3 %)	172 (32.8 %)	56 (10.7 %)	111 (21.2 %)	**37 (7.1 %)**	11 (2.1 %)	29 (5.5 %)	11 (2.1 %)	28 (5.3 %)

"Total patients" represents the number of patients identified when considering all variables together. The results in bold highlight the variable with the most outliers in each method, and also the method that removes more patients in total, in each class. Class 0: represents survivors, Class 1: non-survivors

14.9 Univariate Analysis

smallest number of points as outliers, whereas IQ identifies more outliers than any other method. With a few exceptions, the modified z-score identifies more outliers than the z-score.

A preliminary investigation of results showed that values falling within reference normal ranges (see Table 14.1) are never identified as outliers, whatever the method. On the other hand, critical values are often identified as such. Additional remarks can be made as in general (1) more outliers are identified in the variable BUN than in any other and (2) the ratio of number of outliers and total number of patients is smaller in the class 1 cohorts (non-survivors). As expected, for variables that approximate more to lognormal distribution than to a normal distribution, such as potassium, BUN and PCO2, the IQ method applied to the logarithmic transformation of data (log-IQ method) identifies less outliers than the IQ applied to the real data. Consider for instance the variable BUN, which follows approximately a lognormal distribution. Figure 14.3 shows a scatter of all data points and the identified outliers in the IAC group.

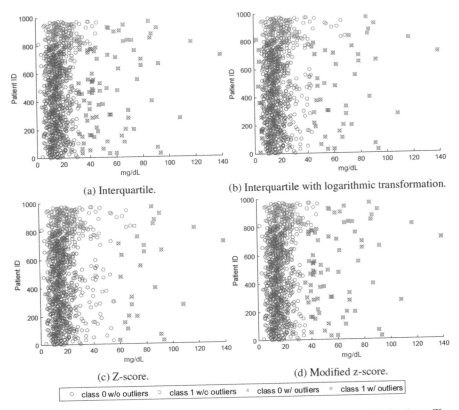

Fig. 14.3 Outliers identified by statistical analysis for the variable BUN, in the IAC cohort. Class 0: survivors; Class 1: non survivors

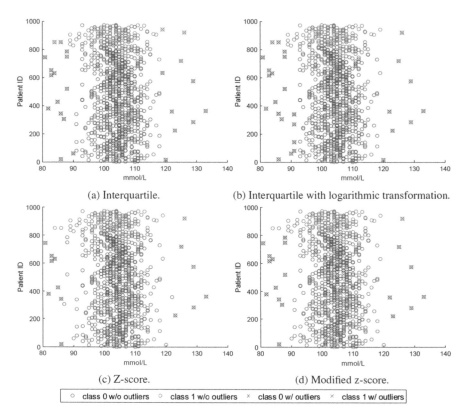

Fig. 14.4 Outliers identified by statistical analysis for the variable chloride, in the IAC cohort. Class 0: survivors; Class 1: non survivors

On the other hand, when the values follow approximately a normal distribution, as in the case of chloride (see Fig. 14.4), the IQ method identifies less outliers than log-IQ. Of note, the range of values considered outliers differs between classes, i.e., what is considered an outlier in class 0 is not necessarily an outlier in class 1. An example of this is values smaller than 90 mmol/L in the modified z-score.

Since this is a univariate analysis, the investigation of extreme values using expert knowledge is of interest. For chloride, normal values are in the range of 95–105 mmol/L, whereas values <70 or >120 mmol/L are considered critical, and concentrations above 160 mmol/L are physiologically impossible [15]. Figure 14.4 confirms that normal values are always kept, whatever the method. Importantly, some critical values are not identified in both z-score and modified z-score (especially in class 1). Thus, it seems that the methods identify outliers that should not be eliminated, as they likely represent actual values in extremely sick patients.

14.10 Multivariable Analysis

Using model based approaches, unusual combination of values for a number of variables can be identified. In this analysis we will be concerned with multivariable outliers for the complete set of variables in the datasets, including those that are binary. In order to investigate multivariable outliers in IAC and non-IAC patients, the Mahalanobis distance and cluster based approaches are tested within pre-defined classes. Table 14.3 shows the average results in terms of number of clusters c determined by the silhouette index, and the percentage of patients identified as

Table 14.3 Multivariable outliers identified by k-means, k-medoids and Mahalanobis distance

	Criterion	Weight	c		% of outliers Class 0	
			Class 0	Class 1	Class 0	Class 1
IAC						
K-means, silhouette index	1	1.2	4 ± 3.1	2 ± 0.0	25.2 ± 7.4	20.9 ± 11.0
	1	1.5	3 ± 2.9	2 ± 0.0	7.9 ± 4.6	3.3 ± 5.9
	1	1.7	3 ± 2.6	2 ± 0.0	3.6 ± 2.5	0.4 ± 2.2
	1	2.0	4 ± 3.1	2 ± 0.0	1.0 ± 1.1	0.1 ± 0.3
K-means, $c = 2$	2	0.05	2 ± 0.0	2 ± 0.0	28.5 ± 4.8	21.4 ± 11.9
	2	0.06	2 ± 0.0	2 ± 0.0	9.3 ± 4.2	2.9 ± 5.2
K-medoids, silhouette index	1	1.2	4 ± 3.0	2 ± 0.0	4.1 ± 2.2	0.8 ± 3.1
	1	1.5	3 ± 2.6	2 ± 0.0	1.1 ± 1.0	0.1 ± 0.3
	1	1.7	3 ± 2.9	2 ± 0.0	0.2 ± 0.2	0.0 ± 0.0
	1	2.0	4 ± 3.0	2 ± 0.0	0.7 ± 0.4	0.0 ± 0.0
K-medoids, $c = 2$	2	0.01	2 ± 0.0	2 ± 0.0	34.6 ± 8.6	2.5 ± 0.0
	2	0.02	2 ± 0.0	2 ± 0.0	20.8 ± 6.1	0.0 ± 0.0
Mahalanobis	–	–	–	–	16.7 ± 5.5	0.0 ± 0.0
Non-IAC						
K-means, silhouette index	1	1.2	9 ± 1.8	7 ± 2.4	12.8 ± 4.1	13.0 ± 9.5
	1	1.5	9 ± 1.7	7 ± 2.5	2.8 ± 1.8	1.0 ± 1.7
	1	1.7	9 ± 1.8	7 ± 2.5	0.9 ± 1.2	0.0 ± 0.2
	1	2.0	9 ± 2.4	7 ± 2.5	0.2 ± 0.7	0.0 ± 0.0
K-means, $c = 2$	2	0.05	2 ± 0.0	2 ± 0.0	25.5 ± 4.5	41.0 ± 11.9
	2	0.06	2 ± 0.0	2 ± 0.0	10.6 ± 2.6	4.8 ± 7.2
K-medoids, silhouette index	1	1.2	9 ± 1.5	7 ± 2.5	3.8 ± 1.6	1.4 ± 1.6
	1	1.5	9 ± 2.0	7 ± 2.4	0.9 ± 1.9	0.0 ± 0.0
	1	1.7	9 ± 2.0	7 ± 2.4	0.3 ± 0.6	0.0 ± 0.0
	1	2.0	9 ± 1.3	7 ± 2.5	0.4 ± 0.9	0.0 ± 0.0
K-medoids, $c = 2$	2	0.01	2 ± 0.0	2 ± 0.0	19.7 ± 4.0	2.7 ± 8.8
	2	0.02	2 ± 0.0	2 ± 0.0	11.0 ± 2.8	1.0 ± 5.0
Mahalanobis	–	–	–	–	6.8 ± 2.6	0.8 ± 4.0

Results are presented as mean ± standard deviation

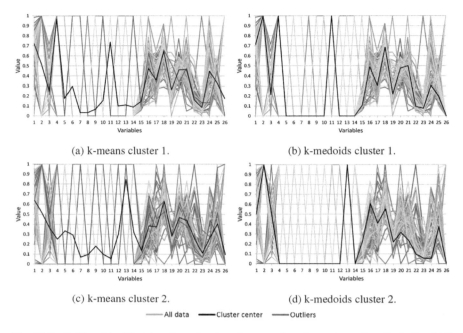

Fig. 14.5 Outliers identified by clustering based approaches for patients that died after IAC. Criterion 1, based on interclusters distance, with $c = 2$ and $w = 1.5$ was used. K-medoids does not identify outliers, whereas k-means identifies 1 outlier in cluster 1 and 2 outliers in cluster 2

outliers. In order to account for variability, the tests were performed 100 times. The data was normalized for testing the cluster based approaches only.

Considering the scenario where two clusters are created for the complete IAC dataset separated by classes, we investigate outliers by looking at multivariable observations around cluster centers. Figure 14.5 shows an example of the outliers detected using k-means and k-medoids with the criterion 1 and weight equal to 1.5. For illustrative purposes, we present only the graphical results of patients that died in the IAC group (class 1). The x-axis represents each of the selected features (see Table 14.1) and the y-axis represents the corresponding values normalized between 0 and 1. K-medoids does not identify any outlier, whereas k-means identifies 1 outlier in the first cluster and 2 outliers in the second cluster. This difference can be attributed to the fact that the intercluster distance is smaller in k-medoids than in k-means.

The detection of outliers seems to be more influenced by binary features than by continuous features: red lines are, with some exceptions, fairly close to black lines for the continuous variables (1 to 2 and 15 to 25) and distant in the binary variables. A possible explanation is that clustering was essentially designed for multivariable continuous data; binary variables produce a maximum separation, since only two values exist, 0 and 1, with nothing between them.

14.11 Classification of Mortality in IAC and Non-IAC Patients

Logistic regression models were created to assess the effect of removing outliers using the different methods in the classification of mortality in IAC and non-IAC patients, following the same rationale as in Chap. 13-Missing Data. A 10-fold cross validation approach was used to assess the validity and robustness of the models. In each round, every outlier identification method was applied separately for each class of the training set, and the results were averaged over the rounds. Before cross-validation, the values were normalized between 0 and 1 using the min-max procedure. For the log-IQ method, the data was log-transformed before normalization, except for variables containing null values (binary variables in Table 14.1, SOFA and creatinine). We also investigate the scenario where only the 10 % worst examples detected by each statistical method within each class are considered, and the case where no outliers were removed (all data is used). In the clustering based approaches, the number of clusters c was chosen between 2 and 10 using the silhouette index method. We also show the case where c is fixed as 2. The weight of the clustering based approaches was adjusted according to the particularities of the method. Since a cluster center in k-medoids is a data point belonging to the dataset, the distance to its nearest neighbor is smaller than in the case of k-means, especially because a lot of binary variables are considered. For this reason, we chose higher values of w for k-means criterion 2.

The performance of the models is evaluated in terms of area under the receiver operating characteristic curve (AUC), accuracy (ACC, correct classification rate), sensitivity (true positive classification rate), and specificity (true negative classification rate). A specific test suggested by DeLong and DeLong can then test whether the results differ significantly [16].

The performance results for the IAC group are shown in Table 14.4, and the percentage of patients removed using each method in Table 14.5. For conciseness, the results for the non-IAC group are not shown. The best performance for IAC is AUC = 0.83 and ACC = 0.78 (highlighted in bold). The maximum sensitivity is 87 % and maximum specificity is 79 %, however these two do not occur simultaneously. Overall, the best AUC is obtained when all the data is used and when only a few outliers are removed. The worst performances are obtained using the z-score without trimming the results and k-means and k-medoids using $c = 2$, criterion 1 and weight 1.2. As for non-IAC, the best performance corresponds to AUC = 0.88, ACC = 0.84, sensitivity = 0.85 and specificity = 0.85. Again, the best performance is achieved when all the data is used and in the cases where less outliers are removed. The worst performance by far is obtained when all outliers identified by the z-score are removed. Similarly to IAC, for k-means and k-medoids criterion 1, increasing values of weight provide better results.

Table 14.4 IAC logistic regression results using 10-fold cross validation, after removal of outliers and using the original dataset

Statistical	Cutoff	AUC	ACC	Sensitivity	Specificity
IQ	–	0.81 ± 0.05	0.76 ± 0.05	0.71 ± 0.14	0.76 ± 0.06
	10	0.82 ± 0.06	0.77 ± 0.06	0.76 ± 0.11	0.77 ± 0.07
Tukey's	–	0.82 ± 0.05	0.75 ± 0.06	0.76 ± 0.09	0.75 ± 0.06
	10	**0.83 ± 0.06**	0 78 ± 0.05	0.75 ± 0 10	0.78 ± 0.06
Log-IQ	–	0.82 ± 0.06	0.76 ± 0.05	0.74 ± 0 14	0.76 ± 0.06
	10	**0.83 ± 0.06**	**0.78 ± 0.04**	0.73 ± 0 10	0.79 ± 0.05
Z-score	–	0.78 ± 0.03	0.67 ± 0.06	0.85 ± 0 09	0.64 ± 0.08
	10	0.81 ± 0.07	0.75 ± 0.06	0.74 ± 013	0.75 ± 0.07
Modified z-score	–	0.82 ± 0.05	0.76 ± 0.05	0.77 ± 0 14	0.76 ± 0.05
	10	0.82 ± 0.06	0.77 ± 0.06	0.75 ± 0 10	0.77 ± 0.06
Mahalanobis	–	0.81 ± 0.08	0.75 ± 0.06	0.73 ± 0 10	0.76 ± 0.07
Cluster based	Weight	AUC	ACC	Sensitivity	Specificity
K-means silhouette criterion 1	1.2	0.81 ± 0.08	0.72 ± 0.05	0.80 ± 0.12	0.70 ± 0.06
	1.5	0.82 ± 0.05	0.76 ± 0.06	0.76 ± 011	0.76 ± 0.06
	1.7	**0.83 ± 0.06**	**0.78 ± 0.05**	0.77 ± 0 10	0.78 ± 0.06
	2	**0.83 ± 0.06**	**0.78 ± 0.05**	0.74 ± 0.09	0.78 ± 0.06
K-means $c = 2$ criterion 1	1.2	0.79 ± 0.08	0.66 ± 0.05	0.84 ± 0 10	0.63 ± 0.06
	1.5	0.82 ± 0.06	0.73 ± 0.06	0.79 ± 0 09	0.72 ± 0.07
	1.7	0.82 ± 0.06	0.75 ± 0.06	0.78 ± 0.08	0.75 ± 0.08
	2	**0.83 ± 0.07**	**0.78 ± 0.06**	0.76 ± 0 09	0.78 ± 0.06
K-means criterion 2	0 05	**0.83 ± 0.07**	0.77 ± 0.05	0.74 ± 0.09	0.78 ± 0.06
	0.06	**0.83 ± 0.06**	0.77 ± 0.06	0.75 ± 0 10	0.78 ± 0.06
K-medoids silhouette criterion 1	1.2	0.81 ± 0.04	0.68 ± 0.04	0.85 ± 0 09	0.64 ± 0.05
	1.5	**0.83 ± 0.05**	0.74 ± 0.04	0.80 ± 0 10	0.73 ± 0.06
	1.7	**0.83 ± 0.05**	0.75 ± 0.06	0.78 ± 0 10	0.74 ± 0.07
	2	**0.83 ± 0.06**	0.77 ± 0.05	0.77 ± 0 09	0.77 ± 0.06
K-medoids $c = 2$ criterion 1	1.2	0.78 ± 0.06	0.62 ± 0.07	0.87 ± 0 08	0.57 ± 0.07
	1.5	0.81 ± 0.06	0.70 ± 0.06	0.83 ± 0 10	0.68 ± 0.08
	1.7	0.82 ± 0.06	0.72 ± 0.06	0.80 ± 0 10	0.71 ± 0.08
	2	**0.83 ± 0.07**	0.76 ± 0.06	0.77 ± 0 10	0.75 ± 0.07
K-medoids criterion 2	0.01	**0.83 ± 0.07**	0.74 ± 0.07	0.77 ± 0 10	0.74 ± 0.08
	0 02	0.81 ± 0.06	0.67 ± 0.06	0.85 ± 0 09	0.63 ± 0.08
All data	–	**0.83 ± 0.06**	**0.78 ± 0.05**	0.76 ± 0.11	0.79 ± 0.06

Results are presented as mean ± standard deviation

14.12 Conclusions and Summary

Table 14.5 Percentage of IAC patients removed by each method in the train set, during cross-validation

Statistical	Cutoff	Class 0	Class 1	Total
IQ	–	23.1 ± 1.4	33.3 ± 1.9	24.8 ± 1.4
	10	3.3 ± 0.2	5.2 ± 0.3	3.6 ± 0.2
Tukey's	–	8.7 ± 0.05	10.1 ± 1.1	9.0 ± 0.5
	10	1.2 ± 0.1	1.3 ± 0.2	1.3 ± 0 1
Log-IQ	–	22.8 ± 1.1	25.4 ± 2.0	23.2 ± 1.1
	10	3.1 ± 0.2	3.7 ± 0.5	3.2 ± 0 1
Z-score	–	35.0 ± 1.6	0.67 ± 0.06	32.6 ± 1.4
	10	5.3 ± 0.2	2.9 ± 1.3	4.9 ± 0.3
Modified z-score	–	18.3 ± 0.05	24.5 ± 1.3	19.4 ± 0.5
	10	2.4 ± 0.1	3.5 ± 0.4	2.6 ± 0.1
Mahalanobis	–	19.6 ± 9.6	17.4 ± 3.0	19.2 ± 8.1

Cluster based	Weight	Class 0	Class 1	Total
K-means silhouette criterion 1	1.2	19.6 ± 9.6	17.4 ± 3.0	19.2 ± 8.1
	1.5	6.1 ± 5.1	1.9 ± 0.5	5.4 ± 4.2
	1.7	2.5 ± 2.6	0.3 ± 0.3	2.2 ± 2.2
	2	0.7 ± 0.9	0.0 ± 0.0	0.6 ± 0.8
K-means $c = 2$ criterion 1	1.2	29.7 ± 3.5	17.4 ± 3.0	27.6 ± 2.9
	1.5	11.9 ± 3.0	1.9 ± 0.5	10.2 ± 2.5
	1.7	5.5 ± 2.0	0.3 ± 0.3	4.7 ± 1.6
	2	1.7 ± 0.8	0.0 ± 0.0	1.4 ± 0 7
K-means criterion 2	0 05	0.3 ± 0.2	0.0 ± 0.0	0.3 ± 0.2
	0.06	1.1 ± 0.5	0.0 ± 0.0	0.9 ± 0 4
K-medoids silhouette criterion 1	1.2	25.0 ± 10.7	3.8 ± 2.0	21.5 ± 8.8
	1.5	12.9 ± 7.4	0.0 ± 0.0	10.8 ± 6.2
	1.7	9.5 ± 6.1	0.0 ± 0.0	7.9 ± 5.1
	2	3.1 ± 2.3	0.0 ± 0.0	2.5 ± 1.9
K-medoids $c = 2$ criterion 1	1.2	34.7 ± 0.7	3.8 ± 2.0	29.5 ± 0.7
	1.5	19.6 ± 0.6	0.0 ± 0.0	16.3 ± 0 5
	1.7	14.9 ± 1.1	0.0 ± 0.0	12.4 ± 0 9
	2	5.1 ± 0.4	0.0 ± 0.0	4.2 ± 0 4
K-medoids criterion 2	0.01	8.3 ± 2.1	0.0 ± 0.0	6.9 ± 1.7
	0 02	28.9 ± 3.9	1.8 ± 3.8	24.4 ± 3.6

Results are presented as mean ± standard deviation

14.12 Conclusions and Summary

The univariable outlier analysis provided in the case study showed that a large number of outliers were identified for each variable within the predefined classes, meaning that the removal of all the identified outliers would cause a large portion of data to be excluded. For this reason, ranking the univariate outliers according to score values and discarding only those with highest scores provided better classification results.

Overall, none of the outlier removal techniques was able to improve the performance of a classification model. As it had been cleaned these results suggest that the dataset did not contain impossible values, extreme values are probably due to biological variation rather than experimental mistakes. Hence, the "outliers" in this study appear to contain useful information in their extreme values, and automatically excluding resulted in a loss of this information.

Some modeling methods already accommodate for outliers so they have minimal impact in the model, and can be tuned to be more or less sensitive to them. Thus, rather than excluding outliers from the dataset before the modeling step, an alternative strategy would be to use models that are robust to outliers, such as robust regression.

Take Home Messages

1. Distinguishing outliers as useful or uninformative is not clear cut.
2. In certain contexts, outliers may represent extremely valuable information that must not be discarded.
3. Various methods exist and will identify possible or likely outliers, but the expert eye must prevail before deleting or correcting outliers.

Open Access This chapter is distributed under the terms of the Creative Commons Attribution-NonCommercial 4.0 International License (http://creativecommons.org/licenses/by-nc/4.0/), which permits any noncommercial use, duplication, adaptation, distribution and reproduction in any medium or format, as long as you give appropriate credit to the original author(s) and the source, a link is provided to the Creative Commons license and any changes made are indicated.

The images or other third party material in this chapter are included in the work's Creative Commons license, unless indicated otherwise in the credit line; if such material is not included in the work's Creative Commons license and the respective action is not permitted by statutory regulation, users will need to obtain permission from the license holder to duplicate, adapt or reproduce the material.

Code Appendix

The code used in this chapter is available in the GitHub repository for this book: https://github.com/MIT-LCP/critical-data-book. Further information on the code is available from this website.

References

1. Barnett V, Lewis T (1994) Outliers in statistical data, 3rd edn. Wiley, Chichester
2. Aggarwal CC (2013) Outlier analysis. Springer, New York
3. Osborne JW, Overbay A (2004) The power of outliers (and why researchers should always check for them). Pract Assess Res Eval 9(6):1–12
4. Hodge VJ, Austin J (2004) A survey of outlier detection methodologies. Artif Intell Rev 22(2):85–126
5. Tukey J (1977) Exploratory data analysis. Pearson
6. Shiffler RE (1988) Maximum Z scores and outliers. Am Stat 42(1):79–80
7. Iglewicz B, Hoaglin DC (1993) How to detect and handle outliers. ASQC Quality Press
8. Seo S (2006) A review and comparison of methods for detecting outliers in univariate data sets. 09 Aug 2006 [Online]. Available: http://d-scholarship.pitt.edu/7948/. Accessed 07-Feb-2016
9. Cook RD, Weisberg S (1982) Residuals and influence in regression. Chapman and Hall, New York
10. Penny KI (1996) Appropriate critical values when testing for a single multivariate outlier by using the Mahalanobis distance. Appl Stat 45(1):73–81
11. Macqueen J (1967) Some methods for classification and analysis of multivariate observations. Presented at the proceedings of 5th Berkeley symposium on mathematical statistics and probability, pp 281–297
12. Hu X, Xu L (2003) A comparative study of several cluster number selection criteria. In: Liu J, Cheung Y, Yin H (eds) Intelligent data engineering and automated learning. Springer, Berlin, pp 195–202
13. Jones RH (2011) Bayesian information criterion for longitudinal and clustered data. Stat Med 30(25):3050–3056
14. Cherednichenko S (2005) Outlier detection in clustering
15. Provan D (2010) Oxford handbook of clinical and laboratory investigation. OUP Oxford
16. DeLong ER, DeLong DM, Clarke-Pearson DL (1988) Comparing the areas under two or more correlated receiver operating characteristic curves: a nonparametric approach. Biometrics 44(3):837–845

Chapter 15
Exploratory Data Analysis

Matthieu Komorowski, Dominic C. Marshall, Justin D. Salciccioli and Yves Crutain

Learning Objectives

- Why is EDA important during the initial exploration of a dataset?
- What are the most essential tools of graphical and non-graphical EDA?

15.1 Introduction

Exploratory data analysis (EDA) is an essential step in any research analysis. The primary aim with exploratory analysis is to examine the data for distribution, outliers and anomalies to direct specific testing of your hypothesis. It also provides tools for hypothesis generation by visualizing and understanding the data usually through graphical representation [1]. EDA aims to assist the natural patterns recognition of the analyst. Finally, feature selection techniques often fall into EDA. Since the seminal work of Tukey in 1977, EDA has gained a large following as the gold standard methodology to analyze a data set [2, 3]. According to Howard Seltman (Carnegie Mellon University), "loosely speaking, any method of looking at data that does not include formal statistical modeling and inference falls under the term exploratory data analysis" [4].

EDA is a fundamental early step after data collection (see Chap. 11) and pre-processing (see Chap. 12), where the data is simply visualized, plotted, manipulated, without any assumptions, in order to help assessing the quality of the data and building models. "Most EDA techniques are graphical in nature with a few quantitative techniques. The reason for the heavy reliance on graphics is that by its very nature the main role of EDA is to explore, and graphics gives the analysts unparalleled power to do so, while being ready to gain insight into the data. There are many ways to categorize the many EDA techniques" [5].

Electronic supplementary material The online version of this chapter (doi:10.1007/978-3-319-43742-2_15) contains supplementary material, which is available to authorized users.

© The Author(s) 2016
MIT Critical Data, *Secondary Analysis of Electronic Health Records*,
DOI 10.1007/978-3-319-43742-2_15

The interested reader will find further information in the textbooks of Hill and Lewicki [6] or the NIST/SEMATECH e-Handbook [1]. Relevant R packages are available on the CRAN website [7].

The objectives of EDA can be summarized as follows:

1. Maximize insight into the database/understand the database structure;
2. Visualize potential relationships (direction and magnitude) between exposure and outcome variables;
3. Detect outliers and anomalies (values that are significantly different from the other observations);
4. Develop parsimonious models (a predictive or explanatory model that performs with as few exposure variables as possible) or preliminary selection of appropriate models;
5. Extract and create clinically relevant variables.

EDA methods can be cross-classified as:

- Graphical or non-graphical methods
- Univariate (only one variable, exposure or outcome) or multivariate (several exposure variables alone or with an outcome variable) methods.

15.2 Part 1—Theoretical Concepts

15.2.1 Suggested EDA Techniques

Tables 15.1 and 15.2 suggest a few EDA techniques depending on the type of data and the objective of the analysis.

Table 15.1 Suggested EDA techniques depending on the type of data

Type of data	Suggested EDA techniques
Categorical	Descriptive statistics
Univariate continuous	Line plot, Histograms
Bivariate continuous	2D scatter plots
2D arrays	Heatmap
Multivariate: trivariate	3D scatter plot or 2D scatter plot with a 3rd variable represented in different color, shape or size
Multiple groups	Side-by-side boxplot

15.2 Part 1—Theoretical Concepts

Table 15.2 Most useful EDA techniques depending on the objective

Objective	Suggested EDA techniques
Getting an idea of the distribution of a variable	Histogram
Finding outliers	Histogram, scatterplots, box-and-whisker plots
Quantify the relationship between two variables (one exposure and one outcome)	2D scatter plot +/curve fitting Covariance and correlation
Visualize the relationship between two exposure variables and one outcome variable	Heatmap
Visualization of high-dimensional data	t-SNE or PCA + 2D/3D scatterplot

t-SNE t-distributed stochastic neighbor embedding, *PCA* Principal component analysis

Table 15.3 Example of tabulation table

	Group count	Frequency (%)
Green ball	15	75
Red ball	5	25
Total	20	100

15.2.2 Non-graphical EDA

These non-graphical methods will provide insight into the characteristics and the distribution of the variable(s) of interest.

Univariate Non-graphical EDA

Tabulation of Categorical Data (Tabulation of the Frequency of Each Category)

A simple univariate non-graphical EDA method for categorical variables is to build a table containing the count and the fraction (or frequency) of data of each category. An example of tabulation is shown in the case study (Table 15.3).

Characteristics of Quantitative Data: Central Tendency, Spread, Shape of the Distribution (Skewness, Kurtosis)

Sample statistics express the characteristics of a sample using a limited set of parameters. They are generally seen as estimates of the corresponding population parameters from which the sample comes from. These characteristics can express the central tendency of the data (arithmetic mean, median, mode), its spread (variance, standard deviation, interquartile range, maximum and minimum value) or some features of its distribution (skewness, kurtosis). Many of those characteristics can easily be seen qualitatively on a histogram (see below). Note that these characteristics can only be used for quantitative variables (not categorical).

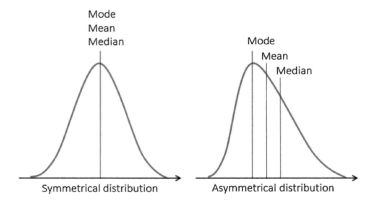

Fig. 15.1 Symmetrical versus asymmetrical (skewed) distribution, showing mode, mean and median

Central tendency parameters

The arithmetic mean, or simply called the mean is the sum of all data divided by the number of values. The median is the middle value in a list containing all the values sorted. Because the median is affected little by extreme values and outliers, it is said to be more "robust" than the mean (Fig. 15.1).

Variance

When calculated on the entirety of the data of a population (which rarely occurs), the variance σ^2 is obtained by dividing the sum of squares by n, the size of the population.

The sample formula for the variance of observed data conventionally has n-1 in the denominator instead of n to achieve the property of "unbiasedness", which roughly means that when calculated for many different random samples from the same population, the average should match the corresponding population quantity (here σ^2). s^2 is an unbiased estimator of the population variance σ^2.

$$s^2 = \frac{\sum_{i=1}^{n}(x_i - \underline{x})^2}{(n-1)} \qquad (15.1)$$

The standard deviation is simply the square root of the variance. Therefore it has the same units as the original data, which helps make it more interpretable.

The sample standard deviation is usually represented by the symbol s. For a theoretical Gaussian distribution, mean plus or minus 1, 2 or 3 standard deviations holds 68.3, 95.4 and 99.7 % of the probability density, respectively.

15.2 Part 1—Theoretical Concepts

Interquartile range (IQR)

The IQR is calculated using the boundaries of data situated between the 1st and the 3rd quartiles. Please refer to the Chap. 13 "Noise versus Outliers" for further detail about the IQR.

$$IQR = Q_3 - Q_1 \tag{15.2}$$

In the same way that the median is more robust than the mean, the IQR is a more robust measure of spread than variance and standard deviation and should therefore be preferred for small or asymmetrical distributions.

Important rule:

- **Symmetrical distribution** (not necessarily normal) **and N > 30**: express results as mean ± standard deviation.
- **Asymmetrical distribution** or N < 30 or evidence for outliers: use median ± IQR, which are more robust.

Skewness/kurtosis

Skewness is a measure of a distribution's asymmetry. Kurtosis is a summary statistic communicating information about the tails (the smallest and largest values) of the distribution. Both quantities can be used as a means to communicate information about the distribution of the data when graphical methods cannot be used. More information about these quantities can be found in [9]).

Summary

We provide as a reference some of the common functions in R language for generating summary statistics relating to measures of central tendency (Table 15.4).

Testing the Distribution

Several non-graphical methods exist to assess the normality of a data set (whether it was sampled from a normal distribution), like the Shapiro-Wilk test for example. Please refer to the function called "Distribution" in the GitHub repository for this book (see code appendix at the end of this Chapter).

Table 15.4 Main R functions for basic measure of central tendencies and variability

Function	Description
summary(x)	General description of a vector
max(x)	Maximum value
mean(x)	Average or mean value
median(x)	Median value
min(x)	Smallest value
sd(x)	Standard deviation
var(x)	Variance, measure the spread or dispersion of the values
IQR(x)	Interquartile range

Finding Outliers

Several statistical methods for outlier detection fall into EDA techniques, like Tukey's method, Z-score, studentized residuals, etc [8]. Please refer to the Chap. 14 "Noise versus Outliers" for more detail about this topic.

Multivariate Non-graphical EDA

Cross-Tabulation

Cross-tabulation represents the basic bivariate non-graphical EDA technique. It is an extension of tabulation that works for categorical data and quantitative data with only a few variables. For two variables, build a two-way table with column headings matching the levels of one variable and row headings matching the levels of the other variable, then fill in the counts of all subjects that share a pair of levels. The two variables may be both exposure, both outcome variables, or one of each.

Covariance and Correlation

Covariance and correlation measure the degree of the relationship between two random variables and express how much they change together (Fig. 15.2).

The covariance is computed as follows:

$$cov(x,y) = \frac{\sum_{i=1}^{n}(x_i - \bar{x})(y_i - \bar{y})}{n-1} \qquad (15.3)$$

where x and y are the variables, n the number of data points in the sample, $\bar{x}$ the mean of the variable x and $\bar{y}$ the mean of the variable y.

A positive covariance means the variables are positively related (they move together in the same direction), while a negative covariance means the variables are inversely related. A problem with covariance is that its value depends on the scale of the values of the random variables. The larger the values of x and y, the larger the

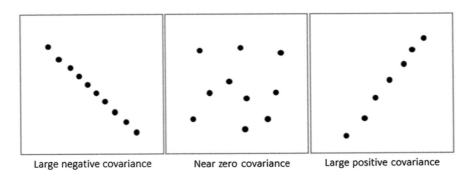

Fig. 15.2 Examples of covariance for three different data sets

15.2 Part 1—Theoretical Concepts

covariance. It makes it impossible for example to compare covariances from data sets with different scales (e.g. pounds and inches). This issue can be fixed by dividing the covariance by the product of the standard deviation of each random variable, which gives Pearson's correlation coefficient.

Correlation is therefore a scaled version of covariance, used to assess the linear relationship between two variables and is calculated using the formula below.

$$Cor(x, y) = \frac{Cov(x, y)}{s_x s_y} \qquad (15.4)$$

where $Cov(x, y)$ is the covariance between x and y and s_x, s_y are the sample standard deviations of x and y.

The significance of the correlation coefficient between two normally distributed variables can be evaluated using Fisher's z transformation (see the cor.test function in R for more details). Other tests exist for measuring the non-parametric relationship between two variables, such as Spearman's rho or Kendall's tau.

15.2.3 Graphical EDA

Univariate Graphical EDA

Histograms

Histograms are among the most useful EDA techniques, and allow you to gain insight into your data, including distribution, central tendency, spread, modality and outliers.

Histograms are bar plots of counts versus subgroups of an exposure variable. Each bar represents the frequency (count) or proportion (count divided by total count) of cases for a range of values. The range of data for each bar is called a bin. Histograms give an immediate impression of the shape of the distribution (symmetrical, uni/multimodal, skewed, outliers…). The number of bins heavily influences the final aspect of the histogram; a good practice is to try different values, generally from 10 to 50. Some examples of histograms are shown below as well as in the case studies. Please refer to the function called "Density" in the GitHub repository for this book (see code appendix at the end of this Chapter) (Figs. 15.3 and 15.4).

Histograms enable to confirm that an operation on data was successful. For example, if you need to log-transform a data set, it is interesting to plot the histogram of the distribution of the data before and after the operation (Fig. 15.5).

Histograms are interesting for finding outliers. For example, pulse oximetry can be expressed in fractions (range between 0 and 1) or percentage, in medical records. Figure 15.6 is an example of a histogram showing the distribution of pulse oximetry, clearly showing the presence of outliers expressed in a fraction rather than as a percentage.

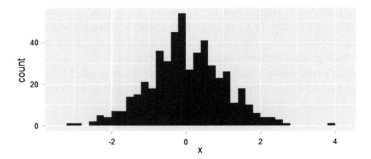

Fig. 15.3 Example of histogram

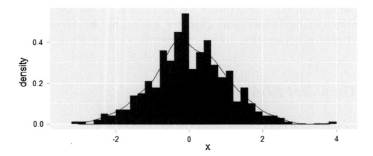

Fig. 15.4 Example of histogram with density estimate

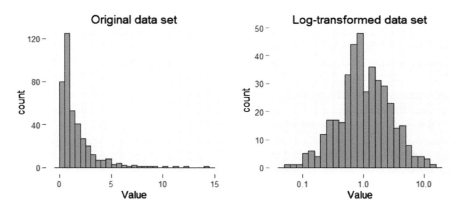

Fig. 15.5 Example of the effect of a log transformation on the distribution of the dataset

Stem Plots

Stem and leaf plots (also called stem plots) are a simple substitution for histograms. They show all data values and the shape of the distribution. For an example, Please refer to the function called "Stem Plot" in the GitHub repository for this book (see code appendix at the end of this Chapter) (Fig. 15.7).

15.2 Part 1—Theoretical Concepts

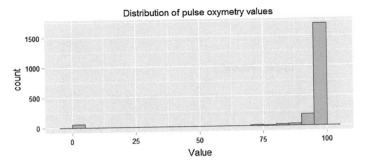

Fig. 15.6 Distribution of pulse oximetry

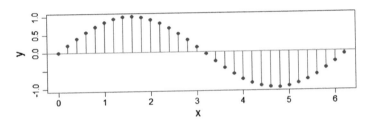

Fig. 15.7 Example of stem plot

Boxplots

Boxplots are interesting for representing information about the central tendency, symmetry, skew and outliers, but they can hide some aspects of the data such as multimodality. Boxplots are an excellent EDA technique because they rely on robust statistics like median and IQR.

Figure 15.8 shows an annotated boxplot which explains how it is constructed. The central rectangle is limited by Q1 and Q3, with the middle line representing the median of the data. The whiskers are drawn, in each direction, to the most extreme point that is less than 1.5 IQR beyond the corresponding hinge. Values beyond 1.5 IQR are considered outliers.

The "outliers" identified by a boxplot, which could be called "boxplot outliers" are defined as any points more than 1.5 IQRs above Q3 or more than 1.5 IQRs below Q1. This does not by itself indicate a problem with those data points. Boxplots are an exploratory technique, and you should consider designation as a boxplot outlier as just a suggestion that the points might be mistakes or otherwise unusual. Also, points not designated as boxplot outliers may also be mistakes. It is also important to realize that the number of boxplot outliers depends strongly on the size of the sample. In fact, for data that is perfectly normally distributed, we expect 0.70 % (about 1 in 140 cases) to be "boxplot outliers", with approximately half in either direction.

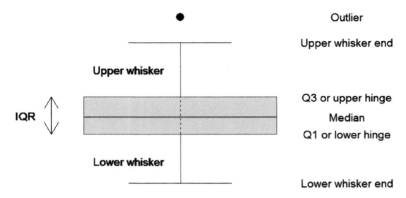

Fig. 15.8 Example of boxplot with annotations

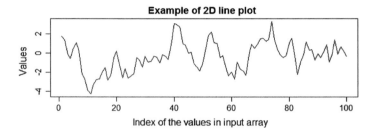

Fig. 15.9 Example of 2D line plot

2D Line Plot

2D line plots represent graphically the values of an array on the y-axis, at regular intervals on the x-axis (Fig. 15.9).

Probability Plots (Quantile-Normal Plot/QN Plot, Quantile-Quantile Plot/QQ Plot)

Probability plots are a graphical test for assessing if some data follows a particular distribution. They are most often used for testing the normality of a data set, as many statistical tests have the assumption that the exposure variables are approximately normally distributed. These plots are also used to examine residuals in models that rely on the assumption of normality of the residuals (ANOVA or regression analysis for example).

The interpretation of a QN plot is visual (Fig. 15.10): either the points fall randomly around the line (data set normally distributed) or they follow a curved pattern instead of following the line (non-normality). QN plots are also useful to identify skewness, kurtosis, fat tails, outliers, bimodality etc.

15.2 Part 1—Theoretical Concepts

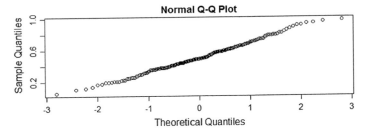

Fig. 15.10 Example of QQ plot

Besides the probability plots, there are many quantitative statistical tests (not graphical) for testing for normality, such as Pearson Chi^2, Shapiro-Wilk, and Kolmogorov-Smirnov.

Deviation of the observed distribution from normal makes many powerful statistical tools useless. Note that some data sets can be transformed to a more normal distribution, in particular with log-transformation and square-root transformations. If a data set is severely skewed, another option is to discretize its values into a finite set.

Multivariate Graphical EDA

Side-by-Side Boxplots

Representing several boxplots side by side allows easy comparison of the characteristics of several groups of data (example Fig. 15.11). An example of such boxplot is shown in the case study.

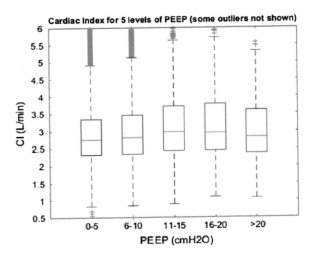

Fig. 15.11 Side-by-side boxplot showing the cardiac index for five levels of Positive end-expiratory pressure (PEEP)

Scatterplots

Scatterplots are built using two continuous, ordinal or discrete quantitative variables (Fig. 15.12). Each data point's coordinate corresponds to a variable. They can be complexified to up to five dimensions using other variables by differentiating the data points' size, shape or color.

Scatterplots can also be used to represent high-dimensional data in 2 or 3D (Fig. 15.13), using T-distributed stochastic neighbor embedding (t-SNE) or principal component analysis (PCA). t-SNE and PCA are dimension reduction features used to reduce complex data set in two (t-SNE) or more (PCA) dimensions.

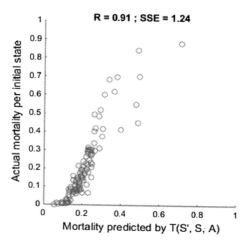

Fig. 15.12 Scatterpolot showing an example of actual mortality per rate of predicted mortality

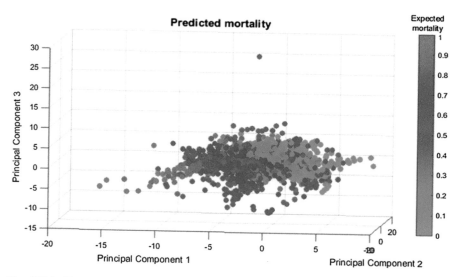

Fig. 15.13 3D representation of the first three dimension of a PCA

15.2 Part 1—Theoretical Concepts

For binary variables (e.g. 28-day mortality vs. SOFA score), 2D scatterplots are not very helpful (Fig. 15.14, left). By dividing the data set in groups (in our example: one group per SOFA point), and plotting the average value of the outcome in each group, scatterplots become a very powerful tool, capable for example to identify a relationship between a variable and an outcome (Fig. 15.14, right).

Curve Fitting

Curve fitting is one way to quantify the relationship between two variables or the change in values over time (Fig. 15.15). The most common method for curve fitting relies on minimizing the sum of squared errors (SSE) between the data and the

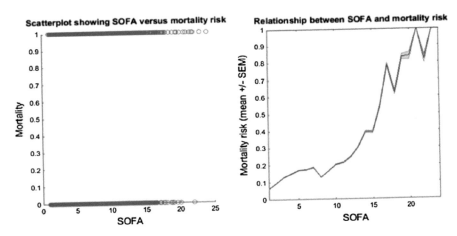

Fig. 15.14 Graphs of SOFA versus mortality risk

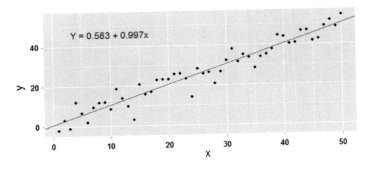

Fig. 15.15 Example of linear regression

fitted function. Please refer to the "Linear Fit" function to create linear regression slopes in R.

More Complicated Relationships

Many real life phenomena are not adequately explained by a straight-line relationship. An always increasing set of methods and algorithms exist to deal with that issue. Among the most common:

- Adding transformed explanatory variables, for example, adding x^2 or x^3 to the model.
- Using other algorithms to handle more complex relationships between variables (e.g., generalized additive models, spline regression, support vector machines, etc.).

Heat Maps and 3D Surface Plots

Heat maps are simply a 2D grid built from a 2D array, whose color depends on the value of each cell. The data set must correspond to a 2D array whose cells contain the values of the outcome variable. This technique is useful when you want to represent the change of an outcome variable (e.g. length of stay) as a function of two other variables (e.g. age and SOFA score).

The color mapping can be customized (e.g. rainbow or grayscale). Interestingly, the Matlab function *imagesc* scales the data to the full colormap range. Their 3D equivalent is mesh plots or surface plots (Fig. 15.16).

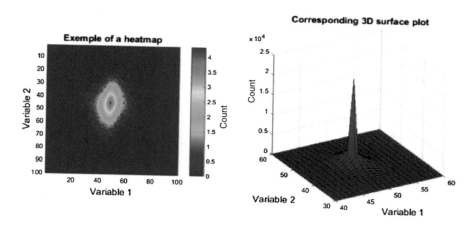

Fig. 15.16 Heat map (*left*) and surface plot (*right*)

15.3 Part 2—Case Study

This case study refers to the research that evaluated the effect of the placement of indwelling arterial catheters (IACs) in hemodynamically stable patients with respiratory failure in intensive care, from the MIMIC-II database.

For this case study, several aspects of EDA were used:

- The categorical data was first tabulated.
- Summary statistics were then generated to describe the variables of interest.
- Graphical EDA was used to generate histograms to visualize the data of interest.

15.3.1 Non-graphical EDA

Tabulation

To analyze, visualize and test for association or independence of categorical variables, they must first be tabulated. When generating tables, any missing data will be counted in a separate "NA" ("Not Available") category. Please refer to the Chap. 13 "Missing Data" for approaches in managing this problem. There are several methods for creating frequency or contingency tables in R, such as for example, tabulating outcome variables for mortality, as demonstrated in the case study. Refer to the "Tabulate" function found in the GitHub repository for this book (see code appendix at the end of this Chapter) for details on how to compute frequencies of outcomes for different variables.

Statistical Tests

Multiple statistical tests are available in R and we refer the reader to the Chap. 16 "Data Analysis" for additional information on use of relevant tests in R. For examples of a simple Chi-square…" as "For examples of a simple Chi-squared test, please refer to the "Chi-squared" function found in the GitHub repository for this book (see code appendix at the end of this Chapter). In our example, the hypothesis of independence between expiration in ICU and IAC is accepted ($p > 0.05$). On the contrary, the dependence link between day-28 mortality and IAC is rejected.

Summary statistics

Summary statistics as described above include, frequency, mean, median, mode, range, interquartile range, maximum and minimum values. An extract of summary statistics of patient demographics, vital signs, laboratory results and comorbidities, is shown in Table 6. Please refer to the function called "EDA Summary" in the

Table 15.5 Comparison between the two study cohorts (subsample of variables only)

Variables	Entire Cohort (N = 1776)		
	Non-IAC	IAC	p-value
Size	984 (55.4 %)	792 (44.6 %)	NA
Age (year)	51 (35–72)	56 (40–73)	0.009
Gender (female)	344 (43.5 %)	406 (41.3 %)	0.4
Weight (kg)	76 (65–90)	78 (67–90)	0.08
SOFA score	5 (4–6)	6 (5–8)	<0.0001
Co-morbidities			
CHF	97 (12.5 %)	116 (11.8 %)	0.7
...	...	...	...
Lab tests			
WBC	10.6 (7.8–14.3)	11.8 (8.5–15.9)	<0.0001
Hemoglobin (g/dL)	13 (11.3–14.4)	12.6 (11–14.1)	0.003
...	...	...	...

GitHub repository for this book (see code appendix at the end of this Chapter) (Table 15.5).

When separate cohorts are generated based on a common variable, in this case the presence of an indwelling arterial catheter, summary statistics are presented for each cohort.

It is important to identify any differences in subject baseline characteristics. The benefits of this are two-fold: first it is useful to identify potentially confounding variables that contribute to an outcome in addition to the predictor (exposure) variable. For example, if mortality is the outcome variable then differences in severity of illness between cohorts may wholly or partially account for any variance in mortality. Identifying these variables is important as it is possible to attempt to control for these using adjustment methods such as multivariable logistic regression. Secondly, it may allow the identification of variables that are associated with the predictor variable enriching our understanding of the phenomenon we are observing.

The analytical extension of identifying any differences using medians, means and data visualization is to test for statistically significant differences in any given subject characteristic using for example Wilcoxon-Rank sum test. Refer to Chap. 16 for further details in hypothesis testing.

15.3.2 Graphical EDA

Graphical representation of the dataset of interest is the principle feature of exploratory analysis.

15.3 Part 2—Case Study

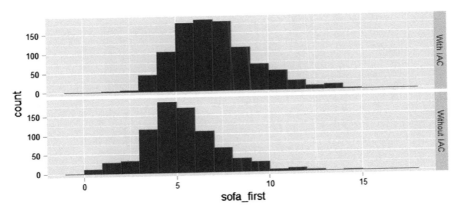

Fig. 15.17 histograms of SOFA scores by intra-arterial catheter status

Histograms

Histograms are considered the backbone of EDA for continuous data. They can be used to help the researcher understand continuous variables and provide key information such as their distribution. Outlined in *noise and outliers,* the histogram allows the researcher to visualize where the bulk of the data points are placed between the maximum and minimum values. Histograms can also allow a visual comparison of a variable between cohorts. For example, to compare severity of illness between patient cohorts, histograms of SOFA score can be plotted side by side (Fig. 15.17). An example of this is given in the code for this chapter using the "side-by-side histogram" function (see code appendix at the end of this Chapter).

Boxplot and ANOVA

Outside of the scope of this case study, the user may be interested in analysis of variance. When performing EDA and effective way to visualize this is through the use of boxplot. For example, to explore differences in blood pressure based on severity of illness subjects could be categorized by severity of illness with blood pressure values at baseline plotted (Fig. 15.18). Please refer to the function called "Box Plot" in the GitHub repository for this book (see code appendix at the end of this Chapter).

The box plot shows a few outliers which may be interesting to explore individually, and that people with a high SOFA score (>10) tend to have a lower blood pressure than people with a lower SOFA score.

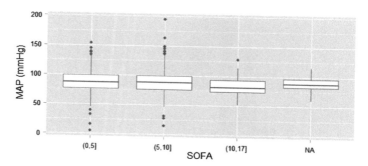

Fig. 15.18 Side-by-side boxplot of MAP for different levels of severity at admission

15.4 Conclusion

In summary, EDA is an essential step in many types of research but is of particular use when analyzing electronic health care records. The tools described in this chapter should allow the researcher to better understand the features of a dataset and also to generate novel hypotheses.

Take Home Messages

1. Always start by exploring a dataset with an open mind for discovery.
2. EDA allows to better apprehend the features and possible issues of a dataset.
3. EDA is a key step in generating research hypothesis.

Open Access This chapter is distributed under the terms of the Creative Commons Attribution-NonCommercial 4.0 International License (http://creativecommons.org/licenses/by-nc/4.0/), which permits any noncommercial use, duplication, adaptation, distribution and reproduction in any medium or format, as long as you give appropriate credit to the original author(s) and the source, a link is provided to the Creative Commons license and any changes made are indicated.

The images or other third party material in this chapter are included in the work's Creative Commons license, unless indicated otherwise in the credit line; if such material is not included in the work's Creative Commons license and the respective action is not permitted by statutory regulation, users will need to obtain permission from the license holder to duplicate, adapt or reproduce the material.

Code Appendix

The code used in this chapter is available in the GitHub repository for this book: https://github.com/MIT-LCP/critical-data-book. Further information on the code is available from this website.

References

1. Natrella M (2010) NIST/SEMATECH e-Handbook of Statistical Methods. NIST/SEMATECH
2. Mosteller F, Tukey JW (1977) Data analysis and regression. Addison-Wesley Pub. Co., Boston
3. Tukey J (1977) Exploratory data analysis. Pearson, London
4. Seltman HJ (2012) Experimental design and analysis. Online http://www.stat.cmu.edu/~hseltman/309/Book/Book.pdf
5. Kaski, Samuel (1997) "Data exploration using self-organizing maps." *Acta polytechnica scandinavica: Mathematics, computing and management in engineering series no. 82. 1997.*
6. Hill T, Lewicki P (2006) Statistics: methods and applications: a comprehensive reference for science, industry, and data mining. StatSoft, Inc., Tulsa
7. CRAN (2016) The Comprehensive R archive network—packages. Contributed Packages, 10 Jan 2016 [Online]. Available: https://cran.r-project.org/web/packages/. Accessed: 10 Jan 2016
8. Grubbs F (1969) Procedures for detecting outlying observations in samples. Technometrics 11(1)
9. Joanes DN, Gill CA (1998) Comparing measures of sample skewness and kurtosis. The Statistician 47:183–189.

Chapter 16
Data Analysis

Jesse D. Raffa, Marzyeh Ghassemi, Tristan Naumann,
Mengling Feng and Douglas Hsu

Learning Objectives

- Understand how the study objective and data types determine the type of data analysis.
- Understand the basics of the three most common analysis techniques used in the studies involving health data.
- Execute a case study to fulfil the study objective, and interpret the results.

16.1 Introduction to Data Analysis

16.1.1 Introduction

This chapter presents an overview of data analysis for health data. We give a brief introduction to some of the most common methods for data analysis of health care data, focusing on choosing appropriate methodology for different types of study objectives, and on presentation and the interpretation of data analysis generated from health data. We will provide an overview of three very powerful analysis methods: linear regression, logistic regression and Cox proportional hazards models, which provide the foundation for most data analysis conducted in clinical studies.

Chapter Goals
By the time you complete this chapter you should be able to:

1. Understand how different study objectives will influence the type of data analysis (Sect. 16.1).
2. Be able to carry out three different types of data analysis that are common for health data (Sects. 16.2–16.4).
3. Present and interpret the results of these analyses types (Sects. 16.2–16.4).

4. Understand the limitations and assumptions underlying the different types of analyses (Sects. 16.2–16.4).
5. Replicate an analysis from a case study using some of the methods learned in the chapter (Sect. 16.5)

Outline

This chapter is composed of five sections. First, in this section we will cover identifying data types and study objectives. These topics will enable us to pick an appropriate analysis method among linear (Sect. 16.2) or logistic (Sect. 16.3) regression, and survival analysis (Sect. 16.4), which comprise the next three sections. Following that, we will use what we learned on a case study using real data from Medical Information Mart for Intensive Care II (MIMIC-II), briefly discuss model building and finally, summarize what we have learned (Sect. 16.5)

16.1.2 Identifying Data Types and Study Objectives

In this section we will examine how different study objectives and data types affect the approaches one takes for data analysis. Understanding the data structure and study objective is likely the most important aspect to choosing an appropriate analysis technique.

Study Objectives

Identifying the study objective is an extremely important aspect of planning data analysis for health data. A vague or poorly described objective often leads to a poorly executed analysis. The study objective should clearly identify the study population, the outcome of interest, the covariate(s) of interest, the relevant time points of the study, and what you would like to do with these items. Investing time to make the objective very specific and clear often will save time in the long run.

An example of a clearly stated study objective would be:

> To estimate the reduction in 28 day mortality associated with vasopressor use during the first three days from admission to the MICU in MIMIC II.

An example of a vague and difficult to execute study objective may be:

> To predict mortality in ICU patients.

While both may be trying to accomplish the same goal, the first gives a much clearer path for the data scientist to perform the necessary analysis, as it identifies the study population (those admitted to the MICU in MIMIC II), outcome (28 day mortality), covariate of interest (vasopressor use in the first three days of the MICU admission), relevant time points (28 days for the outcome, within the first three days for the covariate). The objective does not need to be overly complicated, and it's often convenient to specify primary and secondary objectives, rather than an overly complex single objective.

Data Types

After specifying a clear study objective, the next step is to determine the types of data one is dealing with. The first distinction is between outcomes and covariates. Outcomes are what the study aims to investigate, improve or affect. In the above example of a clearly stated objective, our outcome is 28 day mortality. Outcomes are also sometimes referred to as response or dependent variables. Covariates are the variables you would like to study for their effect on the outcome, or believe may have some nuisance effect on the outcome you would like to control for. Covariates also go by several different names, including: features, predictors, independent variables and explanatory variables. In our example objective, the primary covariate of interest is vasopressor use, but other covariates may also be important in affecting 28 day mortality, including age, gender, and so on.

Once you have identified the study outcomes and covariates, determining the data types of the outcomes will often be critical in choosing an appropriate analysis technique. Data types can generally be identified as either continuous or discrete. Continuous variables are those which can plausibly take on any numeric (real number) value, although this requirement is often not explicitly met. This contrasts with discrete data, which usually takes on only a few values. For instance, gender can take on two values: male or female. This is a *binary* variable as it takes on two values. More discussion on data types can be found in Chap. 11.

There is a special type of data which can be considered simultaneously as continuous and discrete types, as it has two components. This frequently occurs in time to event data for outcomes like mortality, where both the occurrence of death and the length of survival are of interest. In this case, the discrete component is if the event (e.g., death) occurred during the observation period, and the continuous component is the time at which death occurred. The time at which the death occurred is not always available: in this case the time of the last observation is used, and the data is partially *censored*. We discuss censoring in more detail later in Sect. 16.4.

Figure 16.1 outlines the typical process by which you can identify outcomes from covariates, and determine which type of data type your outcome is. For each of the types of outcomes we highlighted—continuous, binary and survival, there are a set of analysis methods that are most common for use in health data—linear regression, logistic regression and Cox proportional hazards models, respectively.

Other Important Considerations

The discussion thus far has given a basic outline of how to choose an analysis method for a given study objective. Some caution is merited as this discussion has been rather brief and while it covers some of the most frequently used methods for analyzing health data, it is certainly not exhaustive. There are many situations where this framework and subsequent discussion will break down and other methods will be necessary. In particular, we highlight the following situations:

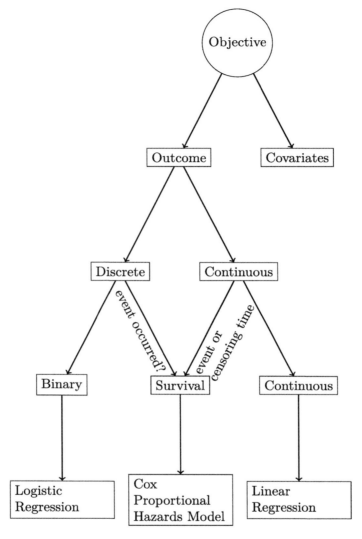

Fig. 16.1 Flow diagram of simplified process for choosing an analysis method based on the study objective and outcome data types

1. When the data is not patient level data, such as aggregated data (totals) instead of individual level data.
2. When patients contribute more than one observation (i.e., outcome) to the dataset.

   In these cases, other techniques should be used.

16.1.3 Case Study Data

We will be using a case study [1] to explore data analysis approaches in health data. The case study data originates from a study examining the effect of indwelling arterial catheters (IAC) on 28 day mortality in the intensive care unit (ICU) in patients who were mechanically ventilated during the first day of ICU admission. The data comes from MIMIC II v2.6. At this point you are ready to do data analysis (the data extraction and cleaning has already been completed) and we will be using a comma separated (.csv) file generated after this process, which you can load directly off of PhysioNet [2, 3]:

```
url <- "http://physionet.org/physiobank/database/mimic2-iaccd/full_cohort_data.csv";
dat <- read.csv(url)
# Or download the csv file from:
# http://physionet.org/physiobank/database/mimic2-iaccd/full_cohort_data.csv
# Type: dat <- read.csv(file.choose())
# And navigate to the file you downloaded (likely in your download directory)
```

The header of this file with the variable names can be accessed using the names function in R.

```
names(dat)
##  [1] "aline_flg"         "icu_los_day"      "hospital_los_day"
##  [4] "age"               "gender_num"       "weight_first"
##  [7] "bmi"               "sapsi_first"      "sofa_first"
## [10] "service_unit"      "service_num"      "day_icu_intime"
## [13] "day_icu_intime_num" "hour_icu_intime" "hosp_exp_flg"
## [16] "icu_exp_flg"       "day_28_flg"       "mort_day_censored"
## [19] "censor_flg"        "sepsis_flg"       "chf_flg"
## [22] "afib_flg"          "renal_flg"        "liver_flg"
## [25] "copd_flg"          "cad_flg"          "stroke_flg"
## [28] "mal_flg"           "resp_flg"         "map_1st"
## [31] "hr_1st"            "temp_1st"         "spo2_1st"
## [34] "abg_count"         "wbc_first"        "hgb_first"
## [37] "platelet_first"    "sodium_first"     "potassium_first"
## [40] "tco2_first"        "chloride_first"   "bun_first"
## [43] "creatinine_first"  "po2_first"        "pco2_first"
## [46] "iv_day_1"
```

There are 46 variables listed. The primary focus of the study was on the effect that IAC placement (aline_flg) has on 28 day mortality (day_28_flg). After we have covered the basics, we will identify a research objective and an appropriate analysis technique, and execute an abbreviated analysis to illustrate how to use these techniques to address real scientific questions. Before we do this, we need to cover the basic techniques, and we will introduce three powerful data analysis methods frequently used in the analysis of health data. We will use examples from the case study dataset to introduce these concepts, and will return to the the question of the effect of IAC has on mortality towards the end of thischapter.

16.2 Linear Regression

16.2.1 Section Goals

In this section, the reader will learn the fundamentals of linear regression, and how to present and interpret such an analysis.

16.2.2 Introduction

Linear regression provides the foundation for many types of analyses we perform on health data. In the simplest scenario, we try to relate one continuous outcome, y, to a single continuous covariate, x, by trying to find values for β_0 and β_1 so that the following equation:

$$y = \beta_0 + \beta_1 \times x$$

fits the data 'optimally'.[1] We call these optimal values: $\hat{\beta}_0$ and $\hat{\beta}_1$ to distinguish them from the true values of β_0 and β_1 which are often unknowable. In Fig. 16.2, we see a scatter plot of TCO2 (y: outcome) levels versus PCO2 (x: covariate) levels. We can clearly see that as PCO2 levels increase, the TCO2 levels also increase. This would suggest that we may be able to fit a linear regression model which predicts TCO2 from PCO2.

It is always a good idea to visualize the data when you can, which allows one to assess if the subsequent analysis corresponds to what you could see with your eyes. In this case, a scatter plot can be produced using the `plot` function:

```
plot(dat$pco2_first,dat$tco2_first,xlab="PCO2",ylab="TCO2",pch=19,xlim=c(0,175))
```

which produces the scattered points in Fig. 16.2.

Finding the best fit line for the scatter plot in Fig. 16.2 in R is relatively straightforward:

---

[1]Exactly what optimally means is beyond the scope of this chapter, but for those who are interested, we are trying to find values of β_0 and β_1 which minimize the squared distance between the fitted line and the observed data point, summed over all data points. This quantity is known as sum of squares error, or when divided by the number of observations is known as the mean squared error.

16.2 Linear Regression

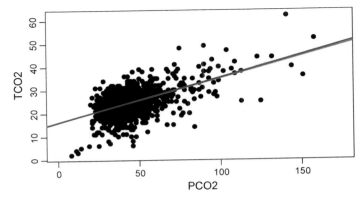

Fig. 16.2 Scatterplot of PCO2 (x-axis) and TCO2 (y-axis) along with linear regression estimates from the quadratic model (`co2.quad.lm`) and linear only model (`co2.lm`)

```
co2.lm <- lm(tco2_first ~ pco2_first,data=dat)
```

Dissecting this command from left to right. The `co2.lm <-` part assigns the right part of the command to a new variable or object called `co2.lm` which contains information relevant to our linear regression model. The right side of this command runs the `lm` function in R. `lm` is a powerful function in R that fits linear models. As with any command in R, you can find additional help information by running `?lm` from the R command prompt. The basic `lm` command has two parts. The first is the formula which has the general syntax outcome ~ covariates. Here, our outcome variable is called `tco2_first` and we are just fitting one covariate, `pco2_first`, so our formula is `tco2_first ~ pco2_first`. The second argument is separated by a comma and is specifying the data frame to use. In our case, the data frame is called `dat`, so we pass `data = dat`, noting that both `tco2_first` and `pco2_first` are columns in the dataframe `dat`. The overall procedure of specifying a model formula (`tco2_first ~ pco2_first`), a data frame (`data = dat`) and passing it an appropriate R function (`lm`) will be used throughout this chapter, and is the foundation for many types of statistical modeling in R.

We would like to see some information about the model we just fit, and often a good way of doing this is to run the `summary` command on the object we created:

```
summary(co2.lm)

##
## Call:
## lm(formula = tco2_first ~ pco2_first, data = dat)
##
## Residuals:
##      Min       1Q   Median       3Q      Max
## -18.8852  -2.5080   0.1891   2.8077  19.2005
##
## Coefficients:
##              Estimate Std. Error t value Pr(>|t|)
## (Intercept) 16.210859   0.359676   45.07   <2e-16 ***
## pco2_first   0.188572   0.007886   23.91   <2e-16 ***
## ---
## Signif. codes:  0 '***' 0.001 '**' 0.01 '*' 0.05 '.' 0.1 ' ' 1
##
## Residual standard error: 4.395 on 1588 degrees of freedom
##   (186 observations deleted due to missingness)
## Multiple R-squared:  0.2647, Adjusted R-squared:  0.2643
## F-statistic: 571.8 on 1 and 1588 DF,  p-value: < 2.2e-16
```

This outputs information about the `lm` object we created in the previous step. The first part recalls the model we fit, which is useful when we have fit many models, and are trying to compare them. The second part lists some summary information about what are called residuals—an important topic for validating modeling assumptions covered in [8]. Next lists the coefficient estimates—these are the $\hat{\beta}_0$, (`Intercept`), and $\hat{\beta}_1$, `pco2_first`, parameters in the best fit line we are trying to estimate. This output is telling us that the best fit equation for the data is:

$$\texttt{tco2\_first} = 16.21 + 0.189 \times \texttt{pco2\_first}.$$

These two quantities have important interpretations. The estimated intercept ($\hat{\beta}_0$) tells us what TCO2 level we would predict for an individual with a PCO2 level of 0. This is the mathematical interpretation, and often this quantity has limited practical use. The estimated slope ($\hat{\beta}_1$) on the other hand can be interpreted as how quickly the predicted value of TCO2 goes up for every unit increase in PCO2. In this case, we estimate that TCO2 goes up about 0.189 mmol/L for every 1 mm Hg increase in PCO2. Each coefficient estimate has a corresponding `Std. Error` (standard error). This is a measure of how certain we are about the estimate. If the standard error is large relative to the coefficient then we are less certain about our estimate. Many things can affect the standard error, including the study sample size. The next column in this table is the `t value`, which is simply the coefficient estimate divided by the standard error. This is followed by `Pr(>|t|)` which is also known as the *p*-value. The last two quantities are relevant to an area of statistics called hypothesis testing which we will cover briefly now.

16.2 Linear Regression

Hypothesis Testing

Hypothesis testing in statistics is fundamentally about evaluating two competing hypotheses. One hypothesis, called the *null hypothesis* is setup as a straw man (a sham argument set up to be defeated), and is the hypothesis you would like to provide evidence *against*. In the analysis methods we will discuss in this chapter, this is almost always $\beta_k = 0$, and it is often written as $H_0 : \beta_k = 0$. The alternative (second) hypothesis is commonly assumed to be $\beta_k \neq 0$, and will often be written as $H_A : \beta_k \neq 0$. A statistical significance level, α, should be established before any analysis is performed. This value is known as the Type I error, and is the probability of rejecting the null hypothesis when the null hypothesis is true, i.e. of incorrectly concluding that the null hypothesis is false. In our case, it is the probability that we falsely conclude that the coefficient is non-zero, when the coefficient is actually zero. It is common to set the Type I error at 0.05.

After specifying the null and alternative hypotheses, along with the significance level, hypotheses can be tested by computing a *p*-value. The actual computation of *p*-values is beyond the scope of this chapter, but we will cover the interpretation and provide some intuition. *P*-values are the probability of observing data as extreme or more extreme than what was seen, assuming the null hypothesis is *true*. The null hypothesis is $\beta_k = 0$, so when would this be unlikely? It is probably unlikely when we estimate β_k to be rather large. However, how large is large enough? This would likely depend on how certain we are about the estimate of β_k. If we were very certain, $\hat{\beta}_k$ likely would not have to be very large, but if we are less certain, then we might not think it to be unlikely for even very large values of $\hat{\beta}_k$. A *p*-value balances both of these aspects, and computes a single number. We reject the null hypothesis when the *p*-value is smaller than the significance level, α.

Returning to our fit model, we see that the *p*-value for both coefficients are tiny (`<2e-16`), and we would reject both null hypotheses, concluding that neither coefficient is likely zero. What do these two hypotheses mean at a practical level? The intercept being zero, $\beta_0 = 0$ would imply the best fit line goes through the origin [the (x, y) point (0, 0)], and we would reject this hypothesis. The slope being zero would mean that the best fit line would be a flat horizontal line, and did not increase as PCO2 increases. Clearly there is a relationship between TCO2 and PCO2, so we would also reject this hypothesis. In summary, we would conclude that we need both an intercept and a slope in the model. A next obvious question would be, could the relationship be more complicated than a straight line? We will examine this next.

16.2.3 Model Selection

Model selection are techniques related to selecting the best model from a list (perhaps rather large list) of candidate models. We will cover some basics here, as more complicated techniques will be covered in a later chapter. In the simplest case, we have two models, and we want to know which one we should use.

We will begin by examining if the relationship between TCO2 and PCO2 is more complicated than the model we fit in the previous section. If you recall, we fit a model where we considered a linear pco2_first term: tco2_first = $\beta_0 + \beta_1 \times$ pco2_first. One may wonder if including a quadratic term would fit the data better, i.e. whether:

$$\text{tco2\_first} = \beta_0 + \beta_1 \times \text{pco2\_first} + \beta_2 \times \text{pco2\_first}^2,$$

is a better model. One way to evaluate this is by testing the null hypothesis: $\beta_2 = 0$. We do this by fitting the above model, and looking at the output. Adding a quadratic term (or any other function) is quite easy using the lm function. It is best practice to enclose any of these functions in the I() function to make sure they get evaluated as you intended. The I() forces the formula to evaluate what is passed to it as is, as the ^ operator has a different use in formulas in R (see ?formula for further details). Fitting this model, and running the summary function for the model:

```
co2.quad.lm <- lm(tco2_first ~ pco2_first + I(pco2_first^2),data=dat)
summary(co2.quad.lm)$coef
```

```
##                      Estimate    Std. Error    t value     Pr(>|t|)
## (Intercept)      16.0916260327 0.7713394026 20.8619266 1.309513e-85
## pco2_first        0.1930281243 0.0266927962  7.2314689 7.401248e-13
## I(pco2_first^2)  -0.0000356873 0.0002042135 -0.1747548 8.612946e-01
```

You will note that we have abbreviated the output from the summary function by appending $coef to the summary function: this tells R we would like information about the coefficients only. Looking first at the estimates, we see the best fit line is estimated as:

$$\text{tco2\_first} = 160.09 + 0.19 \times \text{pco2\_first} + 0.00004 \times \text{pco2\_first}^2.$$

We can add both best fit lines to Fig. 16.2 using the abline function:

```
abline(co2.lm,col='red')
abline(co2.quad.lm,col='blue')
```

and one can see that the red (linear term only) and blue (linear and quadratic terms) fits are nearly identical. This corresponds with the relatively small coefficient estimate for the I(pco2_first^2) term. The *p*-value for this coefficient is about 0.86, and at the 0.05 significance level we would likely conclude that a quadratic

16.2 Linear Regression

term is not necessary in our model to fit the data, as the linear term only model fits the data nearly as well.

Statistical Interactions and Testing Nested Models

We have concluded that a linear (straight line) model fit the data quite well, but thus far we have restricted our exploration to just one variable at a time. When we include other variables, we may wonder if the same straight line is true for all patients. For example, could the relationship between PCO2 and TCO2 be different among men and women? We could subset the data into a data frame for men and a data frame for women, and then fit separate regressions for each gender. Another more efficient way to accomplish this is by fitting both genders in a single model, and including gender as a covariate. For example, we may fit:

$$\texttt{tco2\_first} = \beta_0 + \beta_1 \times \texttt{pco2\_first} + \beta_2 \times \texttt{gender\_num}.$$

The variable `gender_num` takes on values 0 for women and 1 for men, and for men the model is:

$$\texttt{tco2\_first} = \underbrace{(\beta_0 + \beta_2)}_{\text{intercept}} + \beta_1 \times \texttt{pco2\_first},$$

and in women:

$$\texttt{tco2\_first} = \beta_0 + \beta_1 \times \texttt{pco2\_first}.$$

As one can see these models have the same slope, but different intercepts (the distance between the slopes is β_2). In other words, the lines fit for men and women will be parallel and be separated by a distance of β_2 for all values of `pco2_first`. This isn't exactly what we would like, as the slopes may also be different. To allow for this, we need to discuss the idea of an interaction between two variables. An interaction is essentially the product of two covariates. In this case, which we will call the interaction model, we would be fitting:

$$\texttt{tco2\_first} = \beta_0 + \beta_1 \times \texttt{pco2\_first} + \beta_2 \times \texttt{gender\_num} + \beta_3 \\ \times \underbrace{\texttt{gender\_num} \times \texttt{pco2\_first}}_{\text{interaction term}}.$$

Again, separating the cases for men:

$$\texttt{tco2\_first} = \underbrace{(\beta_0 + \beta_2)}_{\text{intercept}} + \underbrace{(\beta_1 + \beta_3)}_{\text{slope}} \times \texttt{pco2\_first},$$

and women:

$$\texttt{tco2\_first} = \underbrace{(\beta_0)}_{\text{intercept}} + \underbrace{(\beta_1)}_{\text{slope}} \times \texttt{pco2\_first}.$$

Now men and women have different intercepts *and* slopes.

Fitting these models in R is relatively straightforward. Although not absolutely required in this particular circumstance, it is wise to make sure that R handles data types in the correct way by ensuring our variables are of the right class. In this particular case, men are coded as 1 and women as 0 (a discrete binary covariate) but R thinks this is numeric (continuous) data:

```
class(dat$gender_num)
```

```
## [1] "integer"
```

Leaving this unaltered, will not affect the analysis in this instance, but it can be problematic when dealing with other types of data such as categorical data with several categories (e.g., ethnicity). Also, by setting the data to the right type, the output R generates can also be more informative. We can set the gender_num variable to the class factor by using the as.factor function.

```
dat$gender_num <- as.factor(dat$gender_num)
```

Here we have just overwritten the old variable in the dat data frame with a new copy which is of class

```
factor:
```
```
class(dat$gender_num)
```

```
## [1] "factor"
```

Now that we have the gender variable correctly encoded, we can fit the models we discussed above. First the model with gender as a covariate, but no interaction. We can do this by simply adding the variable gender_num to the previous formula for our co2.lm model fit.

16.2 Linear Regression

```
co2.gender.lm <- lm(tco2_first ~ pco2_first + gender_num,data=dat)
summary(co2.gender.lm)$coef
```

```
##                  Estimate  Std. Error    t value      Pr(>|t|)
## (Intercept)   16.3043942 0.377712532 43.1661457  6.337240e-270
## pco2_first     0.1888542 0.007894741 23.9215128  3.015777e-108
## gender_num1   -0.1816540 0.223738366 -0.8119036  4.169687e-01
```

This output is very similar to what we had before, but now there's a gender_num term as well. The 1 is present in the first column after gender_num, and it tells us who this coefficient is relevant to (subjects with 1 for the gender_num — men). This is always relative to the baseline group, and in this case this is women.

The estimate is negative, meaning that the line fit for males will be below the line for females. Plotting this fit curve in Fig. 16.3:

```
plot(dat$pco2_first, dat$tco2_first, col = dat$gender_num, xlab = "PCO2", ylab = "TCO2",
    xlim = c(0, 40), type = "n", ylim = c(15, 25))
abline(a = c(coef(co2.gender.lm)[1]), b = coef(co2.gender.lm)[2])
abline(a = coef(co2.gender.lm)[1] + coef(co2.gender.lm)[3], b = coef(co2.gender.lm)[2],
    col = "red")
```

we see that the lines are parallel, but almost indistinguishable. In fact, this plot has been cropped in order to see any difference at all. From the estimate from the summary output above, the difference between the two lines is -0.182 mmol/L, which is quite small, so perhaps this isn't too surprising. We can also see in the above summary output that the *p*-value is about 0.42, and we would likely *not* reject the null hypothesis that the true value of the gender_num coefficient is zero.

And now moving on to the model with an interaction between pco2_first and gender_num. To add an interaction between two variables use the * operator within a model formula. By default, R will add all of the main effects (variables contained in the interaction) to the model as well, so simply adding pco2_first*gender_num will add effects for pco2_first and gender_num in addition to the interaction between them to the model fit.

```
co2.gender.interaction.lm <- lm(tco2_first ~ pco2_first*gender_num,data=dat)
summary(co2.gender.interaction.lm)$coef
```

```
##                              Estimate  Std. Error    t value      Pr(>|t|)
## (Intercept)               15.85443226 0.48869107 32.442648  1.591490e-177
## pco2_first                 0.19939518 0.01072876 18.585105   6.559901e-70
## gender_num1                0.81437833 0.72225677  1.127547   2.596819e-01
## pco2_first:gender_num1    -0.02297002 0.01583758 -1.450348   1.471591e-01
```

The estimated coefficients are $\hat{\beta}_0, \hat{\beta}_1, \hat{\beta}_2$ and $\hat{\beta}_3$, respectively, and we can determine the best fit lines for men:

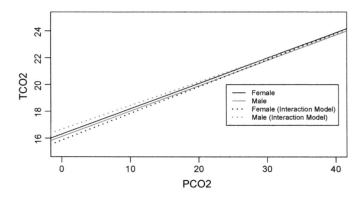

Fig. 16.3 Regression fits of PCO2 on TCO2 with gender (*black* female; *red* male; *solid* no interaction; *dotted* with interaction). *Note* Both axes are cropped for illustration purposes

$$\text{tco2\_first} = (15.85 + 0.81) + (0.20 - 0.023) \times \text{pco2\_first}$$
$$= 16.67 + 0.18 \times \text{pco2\_first},$$

and for women:

$$\text{tco2\_first} = 15.85 + 0.20 \times \text{pco2\_first}.$$

Based on this, the men's intercept should be higher, but their slope should be not as steep, relative to the women. Let's check this and add the new model fits as dotted lines and add a legend to Fig. 16.3.

```
abline(a = coef(co2.gender.interaction.lm)[1], b = coef(co2.gender.interaction.lm)[2],
    lty = 3, lwd = 2)
abline(a = coef(co2.gender.interaction.lm)[1] + coef(co2.gender.interaction.lm)[3],
    b = coef(co2.gender.interaction.lm)[2] + coef(co2.gender.interaction.lm)[4],
    col = "red", lty = 3, lwd = 2)
legend(24, 20, lty = c(1, 1, 3, 3), lwd = c(1, 1, 2, 2), col = c("black", "red",
    "black", "red"), c("Female", "Male", "Female (Interaction Model)", "Male (Interaction Model)"))
```

We can see that the fits generated from this plot are a little different than the one generated for a model without the interaction. The biggest difference is that the dotted lines are no longer parallel. This has some serious implications, particularly when it comes to interpreting our result. First note that the estimated coefficient for the gender_num variable is now positive. This means that at pco2_first = 0, men (red) have higher tco2_first levels than women (black). If you recall in the previous model fit, women had higher levels of tco2_first at all levels of pco2_first. At some point around pco2_first = 35 this changes and women (black) have higher tco2_first levels than men (red). This means that the effect of gender_num *may* vary as you change the level of pco2_first, and is why interactions are often referred to as effect modification in the epidemiological

16.2 Linear Regression

literature. The effect need not change signs (i.e., the lines do not need to cross) over the observed range of values for an interaction to be present.

The question remains, is the variable `gender_num` important? We looked at this briefly when we examined the `t value` column in the no interaction model which included `gender_num`. What if we wanted to test (simultaneously) the null hypothesis: β_2 and $\beta_3 = 0$. There is a useful test known as the F-test which can help us in this exact scenario where we want to look at if we should use a larger model (more covariates) or use a smaller model (fewer covariates). The F-test applies only to *nested models*—the larger model *must* contain each covariate that is used in the smaller model, and the smaller model *cannot* contain covariates which are not in the larger model. The interaction model and the model with gender are nested models since all the covariates in the model with gender are also in the larger interaction model. An example of a non-nested model would be the quadratic model and the interaction model: the smaller (quadratic) model has a term (`pco2_first`^{2}) which is not in the larger (interaction) model. An F-test would not be appropriate for this latter case.

To perform an F-test, first fit the two models you wish to consider, and then run the `anova` command passing the two model objects.

```
anova(co2.lm,co2.gender.interaction.lm)

## Analysis of Variance Table
##
## Model 1: tco2_first ~ pco2_first
## Model 2: tco2_first ~ pco2_first * gender_num
##   Res.Df   RSS Df Sum of Sq      F Pr(>F)
## 1   1588 30674
## 2   1586 30621  2    53.349 1.3816 0.2515
```

As you can see, the `anova` command first lists the models it is considering. Much of the rest of the information is beyond the scope of this chapter, but we will highlight the reported F-test *p*-value (`Pr(>F)`), which in this case is 0.2515. In nested models, the null hypothesis is that all coefficients in the larger model and not in the smaller model are zero. In the case we are testing, our null hypothesis is β_2 and $\beta_3 = 0$. Since the *p*-value exceeds the typically used significance level ($\alpha = 0.05$), we would not reject the null hypothesis, and likely say the smaller model explains the data just as well as the larger model. If these were the only models we were considering, we would use the smaller model as our final model and report the final model in our results. We will now discuss what exactly you should report and how you can interpret the results.

16.2.4　Reporting and Interpreting Linear Regression

We will briefly discuss how to communicate a linear regression analysis. In general, before you present the results, some discussion of how you got the results should be done. It is a good idea to report: whether you transformed the outcome or any covariates in anyway (e.g., by taking the logarithm), what covariates you considered and how you chose the covariates which were in the model you reported. In our above example, we did not transform the outcome (TCO2), we considered PCO2 both as a linear and quadratic term, and we considered gender on its own and as an interaction term with PCO2. We first evaluated whether a quadratic term should be included in the model by using a t-test, after which we considered a model with gender and a gender-PCO2 interaction, and performed model selection with an F-test. Our final model involved only a linear PCO2 term and an intercept.

When reporting your results, it's a good idea to report three aspects for each covariate. Firstly, you should always report the coefficient estimate. The coefficient estimate allows the reader to assess the magnitude of the effect. There are many circumstances where a result may be statistically significant, but practically meaningless. Secondly, alongside your estimate you should always report some measure of uncertainty or precision. For linear regression, the standard error (Std. Error column in the R output) can be reported. We will cover another method called a confidence interval later on in this section. Lastly, reporting a p-value for each of the coefficients is also a good idea. An example of appropriate presentation of our final model would be something similar to: TCO2 increased 0.18 (SE: 0.008, p-value <0.001) units per unit increase of PCO2. You will note we reported p-value <0.001, when in fact it is smaller than this. It is common to report very small p-values as <0.001 or <0.0001 instead of using a large number of decimal places. While sometimes it's simply reported whether $p < 0.05$ or not (i.e., if the result is statistically significant or not), this practice should be avoided.

Often it's a good idea to also discuss how well the overall model fit. There are several ways to accomplish this, but reporting a unitless quantity known as R^2 (pronounced r-squared) is often done. Looking back to the output R provided for our chosen final model, we can find the value of R^2 for this model under Multiple R-squared: 0.2647. This quantity is a proportion (a number between 0 and 1), and describes how much of the total variability in the data is explained by the model. An R^2 of 1 indicates a perfect fit, where 0 explains no variability in the data. What exactly constitutes a 'good' R^2 depends on subject matter and how it will be used. Another way to describe the fit in your model is through the residual standard error. This is also in the lm output when using the summary function. This roughly estimates square-root of the average squared distance between the model fit and the data. While it is in the same units as the outcome, it is in general more difficult to interpret than R^2. It should be noted that for evaluating prediction error, these values are likely too optimistic when applied to new data, and a better estimate of the error should be evaluated by other methods (e.g., cross-validation), which will be covered in another chapter and elsewhere [4, 5].

16.2 Linear Regression

Interpreting the Results

Interpreting the results is an important component to any data analysis. We have already covered interpreting the intercept, which is the prediction for the outcome when all covariates are set at zero. This quantity is not of direct interest in most studies. If one does want to interpret it, subtracting the mean from each of the model's covariates will make it more interpretable—the expected value of the outcome when all covariates are set to the study's averages.

The coefficient estimates for the covariates are in general the quantities most of scientific interest. When the covariate is binary (e.g., gender_num), the coefficient represents the difference between one level of the covariate (1) relative to the other level (0), while holding any other covariates in the model constant. Although we won't cover it until the next section, extending discrete covariates to the case when they have more than two levels (e.g., ethnicity or service_unit) is quite similar, with the noted exception that it's important to reference the baseline group (i.e., what is the effect relative to). We will return to this topic later on in the chapter. Lastly, when the covariate is continuous the interpretation is the expected change in the outcome as a result of increasing the covariate in question by one unit, while holding all other covariates fixed. This interpretation is actually universal for any non-intercept coefficient, including for binary and other discrete data, but relies more heavily on understanding how R is coding these covariates with dummy variables.

We examined statistical interactions briefly, and this topic can be very difficult to interpret. It is often advisable, when possible, to represent the interaction graphically, as we did in Fig. 16.3.

Confidence and Prediction Intervals

As mentioned above, one method to quantify the uncertainty around coefficient estimates is by reporting the standard error. Another commonly used method is to report a confidence interval, most commonly a 95 % confidence interval. A 95 % confidence interval for β is an interval for which if the data were collected repeatedly, about 95 % of the *intervals* would contain the *true value* of the parameter, β, assuming the modeling assumptions are correct.

To get 95 % confidence intervals of coefficients, R has a confint function, which you pass an lm object to. It will then output 2.5 and 97.5 % confidence interval limits for each coefficient.

```
confint(co2.lm)

##                  2.5 %      97.5 %
## (Intercept) 15.5053693  16.9163494
## pco2_first   0.1731033   0.2040403
```

The 95 % confidence interval for pco2_first is about 0.17–0.20, which may be slightly more informative than reporting the standard error. Often people will look at if the confidence interval includes zero (no effect). Since it does not, and in fact since the interval is quite narrow and not very close to zero, this provides some additional evidence of its importance. There is a well known link between hypothesis testing and confidence intervals which we will not get into detail here.

When plotting the data with the model fit, similar to Fig. 16.2, it is a good idea to include some sort of assessment of uncertainty as well. To do this in R, we will first create a data frame with PCO2 levels which we would like to predict. In this case, we would like to predict the outcome (TCO2) over the range of observed covariate (PCO2) values. We do this by creating a data frame, where the variable names in the data frame must match the covariates used in the model. In our case, we have only one covariate (pco2_first), and we predict the outcome over the range of covariate values we observed determined by the min and max functions.

```
grid.pred <- data.frame(pco2_first=seq.int(from=min(dat$pco2_first,na.rm=T),
                                           to=max(dat$pco2_first,na.rm=T)));
```

Then, by using the predict function, we can predict TCO2 levels at these PCO2 values. The predict function has three arguments: the model we have constructed (in this case, using lm), newdata, and interval. The newdata argument allows you to pass any data frame with the same covariates as the model fit, which is why we created grid.pred above. Lastly, the interval argument is optional, and allows for the inclusion of any confidence or prediction intervals. We want to illustrate a prediction interval which incorporates both uncertainty about the model coefficients, in addition to the uncertainty generated by the data generating process, so we will pass interval = "prediction".

```
preds <- predict(co2.lm,newdata=grid.pred,interval = "prediction")
preds[1:2,]

##        fit      lwr      upr
## 1 17.71943 9.078647 26.36022
## 2 17.90801 9.268186 26.54783
```

We have printed out the first two rows of our predictions, preds, which are the model's predictions for PCO2 at 8 and 9. We can see that our predictions (fit) are about 0.18 apart, which make sense given our estimate of the slope (0.18). We also see that our 95 % prediction intervals are very wide, spanning about 9 (lwr) to 26 (upr). This indicates that, despite coming up with a model which is very statistically significant, we still have a lot of uncertainty about the predictions generated from such a model. It is a good idea to capture this quality when plotting how well your model fits by adding the interval lines as dotted lines. Let's plot our final model fit, co2.lm, along with the scatterplot and prediction interval in Fig. 16.4.

16.2 Linear Regression

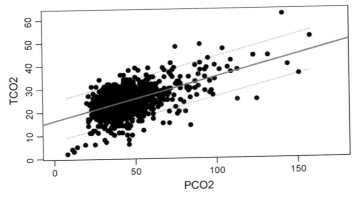

Fig. 16.4 Scatterplot of PCO2 (x-axis) and TCO2 (y-axis) along with linear regression estimates from the linear only model (co2.lm). The *dotted line* represents 95 % prediction intervals for the model

```
plot(dat$pco2_first,dat$tco2_first,xlab="PCO2",ylab="TCO2",pch=19,xlim=c(0,175))
co2.lm <- lm(tco2_first ~ pco2_first,data=dat)
abline(co2.lm,col='red',lwd=2)
lines(grid.pred$pco2_first,preds[,2],lty=3)
lines(grid.pred$pco2_first,preds[,3],lty=3)
```

16.2.5 Caveats and Conclusions

Linear regression is an extremely powerful tool for doing data analysis on continuous outcomes. Despite this, there are several aspects to be aware of when performing this type of analysis.

1. Hypothesis testing and the interval generation are reliant on modelling assumptions. Doing diagnostic plots is a critical component when conducting data analysis. There is subsequent discussion on this elsewhere in the book, and we will refer you to [6–8] for more information about this important topic.
2. Outliers can be problematic when fitting models. When there are outliers in the covariates, it's often easiest to turn a numeric variable into a categorical one (2 or more groups cut along values of the covariate). Removing outliers should be avoided when possible, as they often tell you a lot of information about the data generating process. In other cases, they may identify problems for the extraction process. For instance, a subset of the data may use different units for the same covariate (e.g., inches and centimeters for height), and thus the data needs to be converted to common units. Methods robust to outliers are available in R, a brief introduction of how to get started with some of the functions in R is available [7].

3. Be concerned about missing data. R reports information about missing data in the `summary` output. For our model fit `co2.lm`, we had 186 observations with missing `pco2_first` observations. R will leave these observations out of the analysis, and fit on the remaining non-missing observations. Always check the output to ensure you have as many observations as you think that you are supposed to. When many observations have missing data and you try to build a model with a large number of coefficients, you may be fitting the model on only a handful of observations.
4. Assess potential multi-colinearity. Co-linearity can occur when two or more covariates are highly correlated. For instance, if blood pressure on the left and right arms were simultaneously measured, and both used as covariates in the model. In this case, consider taking the sum, average or difference (whichever is most useful in the particular case) to craft a single covariate. Co-linearity can also occur when a categorical variable has been improperly generated. For instance, defining groups along the PCO2 covariate of 0–25, 5–26, 26–50, >50 may cause linear regression to encounter some difficulties as the first and second groups are nearly identical (usually these types of situations are programming errors). Identifying covariates which may be colinear is a key part of the exploratory analysis stage, where they can often (but not always) be seen by plotting the data.
5. Check to see if outcomes are dependent. This most commonly occurs when one patient contributes multiple observations (outcomes). There are alternative methods for dealing with this situation [9], but it is beyond the scope of this chapter.

These concerns should not discourage you from using linear regression. It is extremely powerful and reasonably robust to some of the problems discussed above, depending on the situation. Frequently a continuous outcome is converted to a binary outcome, and often there is no compelling reason this is done. By discretizing the outcome you may be losing information about which patients may benefit or be harmed most by a therapy, since a binary outcome may treat patients who had very different outcomes on the continuous scale as the same. The overall framework we took in linear regression will closely mirror the way in which we approach the other analysis techniques we discuss later in this chapter.

16.3 Logistic Regression

16.3.1 Section Goals

In this section, the reader will learn the fundamentals of logistic regression, and how to present and interpret such an analysis.

16.3.2 Introduction

In Sect. 16.2 we covered a very useful methodology for modeling quantitative or continuous outcomes. We of course know though that health outcomes come in all different kinds of data types. In fact, the health outcomes we often care about most —cured/not cured, alive/dead, are discrete binary outcomes. It would be ideal if we could extend the same general framework for continuous outcomes to these binary outcomes. Logistic regression allows us to incorporate much of what we learned in the previous section and apply the same principles to binary outcomes.

When dealing with binary data, we would like to be able to model the probability of a type of outcome given one or more covariates. One might ask, why not just simply use linear regression? There are several reasons why this is generally a bad idea. Probabilities need to be somewhere between zero and one, and there is nothing in linear regression to constrain the estimated probabilities to this interval. This would mean that you could have an estimated probability 2, or even a negative probability! This is one unattractive property of such a method (there are others), and although it is sometimes used, the availability of good software such as R allows us to perform better analyses easily and efficiently. Before introducing such software, we should introduce the analysis of small contingency tables.

16.3.3 2 × 2 Tables

Contingency tables are the best way to start to think about binary data. A contingency table cross-tabulates the outcome across two or more levels of a covariate. Let's begin by creating a new variable (age.cat) which dichotomizes age into two age categories: ≤ 55 and > 55. Note, because we are making age a discrete variable, we also change the data type to a factor. This is similar to what we did for the gender_num variable when discussing linear regression in the previous section. We can get a breakdown of the new variable using the table function.

```
dat$age.cat <- as.factor(ifelse(dat$age<=55, "<=55",">55"))
table(dat$age.cat)
```

```
##
## <=55  >55
##  923  853
```

We would like to see how 28 day mortality is distributed among the age categories. We can do so by constructing a contingency table, or in this case what is commonly referred to as a 2 × 2 table.

```
table(dat$age.cat,dat$day_28_flg)
```

```
##       
##         0   1
##   <=55 883  40
##   >55  610 243
```

From the above table, you can see that 40 patients in the young group (≤ 55) died within 28 days, while 243 in the older group died. These correspond to $P(\text{die}|\text{age} \leq 55) = 0.043$) or 4.3 % and $P(\text{die}|\text{age} > 55) = 0.284$ or 28.4 %, where the "|" can be interpreted as "given" or "for those who have." This difference is quite marked, and we know that age is an important factor in mortality, so this is not surprising.

The odds of an event happening is a positive number and can be calculated from the probability of an event, p, by the following formula

$$\text{Odds} = \frac{p}{1-p}.$$

An event with an odds of zero never happens, and an event with a very large odds (>100) is very likely to happen. Here, the odds of dying within 28 days in the young group is $0.043/(1 - 0.043) = 0.045$, and in the older group is $0.284/(1 - 0.284) = 0.40$. It is convenient to represent these two figures as a ratio, and the choice of what goes in the numerator and the denominator is somewhat arbitrary. In this case, we will choose to put the older group's odds on the numerator and the younger in the denominator, and it's important to make it clear which group is in the numerator and denominator in general. In this case the *Odds ratio* is $0.40/0.045 = 8.79$, which indicates a very strong association between age and death, and means that the odds of dying in the older group is nearly 9 fold higher than when compared to the younger group. There is a convenient shortcut for doing odds ratio calculation by making an X on a 2 × 2 table and multiplying top left by bottom right, then dividing it by the product of bottom left and top right. In this case $\frac{883 \times 243}{610 \times 40} = 8.79$.

Now let us look at a slightly different case—when the covariate takes on more than two values. Such a variable is the `service_unit`. Let's see how the deaths are distributed among the different units:

```
deathbyservice <- table(dat$service_unit,dat$day_28_flg)
deathbyservice
```

```
##       
##          0   1
##   FICU  59   3
##   MICU 605 127
##   SICU 829 153
```

16.3 Logistic Regression

we can get frequencies of these service units by applying the `prop.table` function to our cross-tabulated table.

```
dbys.proptable <- prop.table(deathbyservice,1)
dbys.proptable
```

```
##
##                0         1
##   FICU 0.9516129 0.0483871
##   MICU 0.8265027 0.1734973
##   SICU 0.8441955 0.1558045
```

It appears as though the `FICU` may have a lower rate of death than either the `MICU` or `SICU`. To compute an odds ratios, first compute the odds:

```
dbys.proptable[,"1"]/dbys.proptable[,"0"]
```

```
##       FICU       MICU       SICU
## 0.05084746 0.20991736 0.18455971
```

and then we need to pick which of `FICU`, `MICU` or `SICU` will serve as the reference or baseline group. This is the group which the other two groups will be compared to. Again the choice is arbitrary, but should be dictated by the study objective. If this were a clinical trial with two drug arms and a placebo arm, it would be foolish to use one of the treatments as the reference group, particularly if you wanted to compare the efficacy of the treatments. In this particular case, there is no clear reference group, but since the FICU is so much smaller than the other two units, we will use it as the reference group. Computing the odds ratio for MICU and SICU we get 4.13 and 3.63, respectively. These are also very strong associations, meaning that the odds of dying in the SICU and MICU are around 4 times higher than in the FICU, but relatively similar.

Contingency tables and 2×2 tables in particular are the building blocks of working with binary data, and it's often a good way to begin looking at the data.

16.3.4 Introducing Logistic Regression

While contingency tables are a fundamental way of looking at binary data, they are somewhat limited. What happens when the covariate of interest is continuous? We could of course create categories from the covariate by establishing cut points, but we may still miss some important aspect of the relationship between the covariate and the outcome by not choosing the right cut points. Also, what happens when we know that a nuisance covariate is related to both the outcome and the covariate of interest. This type of nuisance variable is called a confounder and occurs frequently in observational data, and although there are ways of accounting for confounding in contingency tables, they become more difficult to use when there are more than one present.

Logistic regression is a way of addressing both of these issues, among many others. If you recall, using linear regression is problematic because it is prone to estimating probabilities outside of the [0, 1] range. Logistic regression has no such problem per se, because it uses a link function known as the logit function which maps probabilities in the interval [0, 1] to a real number $(-\infty, \infty)$. This is important for many practical and technical reasons. The logit of p_x (i.e. the probability of an event for certain covariate values x) is related to the covariates in the following way

$$\text{logit}(p_x) = \log(Odds_x) = \log\left(\frac{p_x}{1-p_x}\right) = \beta_0 + \beta_1 \times x.$$

It is worth pointing out here that log here, and in most places in statistics is referring to the natural logarithm, sometimes denoted *ln*.

The first covariate we were considering, age.cat was also a binary variable, where it takes on values 1 when the age > 55 and 0 when age ≤ 55. So plugging these values in, first for the young group ($x = 0$):

$$\text{logit}(p_{x=0}) = \log(Odds_{x=0}) = \log\left(\frac{p_{x=0}}{1-p_{x=0}}\right) = \beta_0 + \beta_1 \times 0 = \beta_0,$$

and then for the older group ($x = 1$):

$$\text{logit}(p_{x=1}) = \log(Odds_{x=1}) = \log\left(\frac{p_{x=1}}{1-p_{x=1}}\right) = \beta_0 + \beta_1 \times 1 = \beta_0 + \beta_1.$$

If we subtract the two cases $\text{logit}(p_{x=1}) - \text{logit}(p_{x=0}) = \log(Odds_{x=1}) - \log(Odds_{x=0})$, and we notice that this quantity is equal to β_1. If you recall the properties of logarithms, that the difference of two logs is the log of their ratio, so $\log(Odds_{x=1}) - \log(Odds_{x=0}) = \log(Odds_{x=1}/Odds_{x=0})$, which may be looking familiar. This is the log ratio of the odds or the *log odds ratio* in the $x = 1$ group relative to the $x = 0$ group. Hence, we can estimate odds ratios using logistic regression by exponentiating the coefficients of the model (the intercept notwithstanding, which we will get to in a moment).

Let's fit this model, and see how this works using a real example. We fit logistic regression very similarly to how we fit linear regression models, with a few exceptions. First, we will use a new function called glm, which is a very powerful function in R which allow one to fit a class of models known as generalized linear models or GLMs [10]. The glm function works in much the same way the lm function does. We need to specify a formula of the form: outcome ~ co-variates, specify what dataset to use (in our case the dat data frame), and then specify the family. For logistic regression family = 'binomial' will be our choice. You can run the summary function, just like you did for lm and it produces output very similar to what lm did.

16.3 Logistic Regression

```
age.glm <- glm(day_28_flg ~ age.cat,data=dat,family="binomial")
summary(age.glm)
```

```
## 
## Call:
## glm(formula = day_28_flg ~ age.cat, family = "binomial", data = dat)
## 
## Deviance Residuals:
##     Min       1Q   Median       3Q      Max
## -0.8189  -0.8189  -0.2977  -0.2977   2.5055
## 
## Coefficients:
##             Estimate Std. Error z value Pr(>|z|)
## (Intercept)  -3.0944     0.1616  -19.14   <2e-16 ***
## age.cat>55    2.1740     0.1785   12.18   <2e-16 ***
## ---
## Signif. codes:  0 '***' 0.001 '**' 0.01 '*' 0.05 '.' 0.1 ' ' 1
## 
## (Dispersion parameter for binomial family taken to be 1)
## 
##     Null deviance: 1557.9  on 1775  degrees of freedom
## Residual deviance: 1348.7  on 1774  degrees of freedom
## AIC: 1352.7
## 
## Number of Fisher Scoring iterations: 5
```

As you can see, we get a coefficients table that is similar to the lm table we used earlier. Instead of a t value, we get a z value, but this can be interpreted similarly. The rightmost column is a *p*-value, for testing the null hypothesis $\beta = 0$. If you recall, the non-intercept coefficients are log-odds ratios, so testing if they are zero is equivalent to testing if the odds ratios are one. If an odds ratio is one the odds are equal in the numerator group and denominator group, indicating the probabilities of the outcome are equal in each group. So, assessing if the coefficients are zero will be an important aspect of doing this type of analysis.

Looking more closely at the coefficients. The intercept is -3.09 and the age.cat coefficient is 2.17. The coefficient for age.cat is the log odds ratio for the 2 × 2 table we previously did the analysis on. When we exponentiate 2.17, we get exp(2.17) = 8.79. This corresponds with the estimate using the 2 × 2 table. For completeness, let's look at the other coefficient, the intercept. If you recall, $\log(Odds_{x=0}) = \beta_0$, so β_0 is the log odds of the outcome in the younger group. Exponentiating again, exp(-3.09) = 0.045, and this corresponds with the previous analysis we did. Similarly, $\log(Odds_{x=1}) = \beta_0 + \beta_1$, and the estimated odds of 28 day death in the older group is exp($-3.09 + 2.17$) = 0.4, as was found above. Converting estimated odds into a probability can be done directly using the plogis function, but we will cover a more powerful and easier way of doing this later on in the section.

Beyond a Single Binary Covariate

While the above analysis is useful for illustration, it does not readily demonstrate anything we could not do with our 2 × 2 table example above. Logistic regression allows us to extend the basic idea to at least two very relevant areas. The first is the case where we have more than one covariate of interest. Perhaps we have a confounder, we are concerned about, and want to adjust for it. Alternatively, maybe there are two covariates of interest. Secondly, it allows use to use covariates as continuous quantities, instead of discretizing them into categories. For example, instead of dividing age up into exhaustive strata (as we did very simply by just dividing the patients into two groups, ≤ 55 and > 55), we could instead use age as a continuous covariate.

First, having more than one covariate is simple. For example, if we wanted to add `service_unit` to our previous model, we could just add it as we did when using the `lm` function for linear regression. Here we specify ~`day_28_flg` `age.cat` + `service_unit` and run the `summary` function.

```
ageunit.glm <- glm(day_28_flg ~ age.cat + service_unit,data=dat,family="binomial")
summary(ageunit.glm)$coef
```

```
##                   Estimate Std. Error   z value     Pr(>|z|)
## (Intercept)      -4.209013  0.6222758 -6.763903 1.343230e-11
## age.cat>55        2.161142  0.1787575 12.089800 1.195779e-33
## service_unitMICU  1.178865  0.6151757  1.916307 5.532607e-02
## service_unitSICU  1.123442  0.6135095  1.831173 6.707466e-02
```

A coefficient table is produced, and now we have four estimated coefficients. The same two, (`Intercept`) and `age.cat` which were estimated in the unadjusted model, but also we have `service_unitMICU` and `service_unitSICU` which correspond to the log odds ratios for the MICU and SICU relative to the FICU. Taking the exponential of these will result in an odds ratio for each variable, adjusted for the other variables in the model. In this case the adjusted odds ratios for Age > 55, MICU and SICU are 8.68, 3.25, and 3.08, respectively. We would conclude that there is an almost 9-fold increase in the odds of 28 day mortality for those in the >55 year age group relative to the younger ≤ 55 group while holding service unit constant. This adjustment becomes important in many scenarios where groups of patients may be more or less likely to receive treatment, but also more or less likely to have better outcomes, where one effect is confounded by possibly many others. Such is almost always the case with observational data, and this is why logistic regression is such a powerful data analysis tool in this setting.

Another case we would like to be able to deal with is when we have a continuous covariate we would like to include in the model. One can always break the continuous covariate into mutually exclusive categories by selecting break or cut points, but selecting the number and location of these points can be arbitrary, and in many cases unnecessary or inefficient. Recall that in logistic regression we are fitting a model:

16.3 Logistic Regression

$$\text{logit}(p_x) = \log(Odds_x) = \log(\frac{p_x}{1-p_x}) = \beta_0 + \beta_1 \times x,$$

but now assume x is continuous. Imagine a hypothetical scenario where you know β_0 and β_1 and have a group of 50 year olds, and a group of 51 year olds. The difference in the log Odds between the two groups is:

$$\log(Odds_{51}) - \log(Odds_{50}) = (\beta_0 + \beta_1 \times 51) - (\beta_0 + \beta_1 \times 50) = \beta_1(51-50)$$
$$= \beta_1.$$

Hence, the odds ratio for 51 year olds versus 50 year olds is $\exp(\beta_1)$. This is actually true for any group of patients which are 1 year apart, and this gives a useful way to interpret and use these estimated coefficients for continuous covariates. Let's work with an example. Again fitting the 28 day mortality outcome as a function of age, but treating age as it was originally recorded in the dataset, a continuous variable called age.

```
agects.glm <- glm(day_28_flg ~ age,data=dat,family="binomial")
summary(agects.glm)$coef
```

```
##                 Estimate  Std. Error    z value      Pr(>|z|)
## (Intercept) -5.77800634 0.320774776 -18.01266 1.550034e-72
## age          0.06523274 0.004469569  14.59486 3.028256e-48
```

We see the estimated coefficient is 0.07 and still very statistically significant. Exponentiating the log odds ratio for age, we get an estimated odds ratio of 1.07, which is per 1 year increase in age. What if the age difference of interest is ten years instead of one year? There are at least two ways of doing this. One is to replace age with I(age/10), which uses a new covariate which is age divided by ten. The second is to use the agects.glm estimated log odds ratio, and multiple by ten prior to exponentiating. They will yield equivalent estimates of 1.92, but it is now per 10 year increases in age. This is useful when the estimated odds ratios (or log odds ratios) are close to one (or zero). When this is done, one unit of the covariate is 10 years, so the generic interpretation of the coefficients remains the same, but the units (per 10 years instead of per 1 year) changes.

This of course assumes that the form of our equation relating the log odds of the outcome to the covariate is correct. In cases where odds of the outcome decreases and increases as a function of the covariate, it is possible to estimate a relatively small effect of the linear covariate, when the outcome may be strongly affected by the covariate, but not in the way the model is specified. Assessing the linearity of the log odds of the outcome and some discretized form of the covariate can be done graphically. For instance, we can break age into 5 groups, and estimate the log odds of 28 day mortality in each group. Plotting these quantities in Fig. 16.5 (left), we can see in this particular case, age is indeed strongly related to the odds of the outcome. Further, expressing age linearly appears like it would be a good approximation. If on the other hand, 28 day mortality has more of a "U"-shaped curve, we may falsely conclude that no relationship between age and mortality exists, when the relationship may be rather strong. Such may be the case when looking at the the log odds of mortality by the first temperature (temp_1st) in Fig. 16.5 (right).

16.3.5 Hypothesis Testing and Model Selection

Just as in the case for linear regression, there is a way to test hypotheses for logistic regression. It follows much of the same framework, with the null hypothesis being $\beta = 0$. If you recall, this is the log odds ratio, and testing if it is zero is equivalent to a test for the odds ratio being equal to one. In this chapter, we focus on how to conduct such a test in R.

As was the case when using lm, we first fit the two competing models, a larger (alternative model), and a smaller (null model). Provided that the models are nested, we can again use the anova function, passing the smaller model, then the larger model. Here our larger model is the one which contained service_unit and age.cat, and the smaller only contains age.cat, so they are nested. We are then testing if the log odds ratios for the two coefficients associated with service_unit are zero. Let's call these coefficients β_{MICU} and β_{SICU}. To test if β_{MICU} and $\beta_{SICU} = 0$, we can use the anova function, where this time we will specify the type of test, in this case set the test parameter to "Chisq".

```
anova(age.glm,ageunit.glm,test="Chisq")

## Analysis of Deviance Table
##
## Model 1: day_28_flg ~ age.cat
## Model 2: day_28_flg ~ age.cat + service_unit
##   Resid. Df Resid. Dev Df Deviance Pr(>Chi)
## 1      1774     1348.7
## 2      1772     1343.8  2   4.9315   0.08495 .
## ---
## Signif. codes:  0 '***' 0.001 '**' 0.01 '*' 0.05 '.' 0.1 ' ' 1
```

Here the output of the anova function when applied to glm objects looks similar to the output generated when used on lm objects. A couple good practices to get in a habit are to first make sure the two competing models are correctly specified. He we are are testing ~ age.cat versus age.cat + service_unit. Next, the difference between the residual degrees of freedom (Resid. Df) in the two models tell us how many more parameters the larger model has when compared

16.3 Logistic Regression

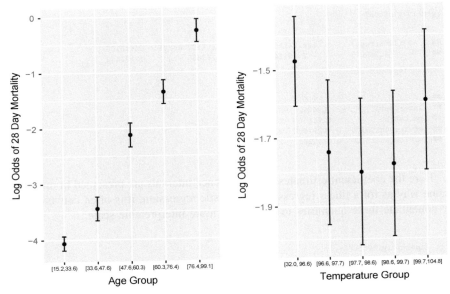

Fig. 16.5 Plot of log-odds of mortality for each of the five age and temperature groups. *Error bars* represent 95 % confidence intervals for the log odds

to the smaller model. Here we see $1774 - 1772 = 2$ which means that there are two more coefficients estimated in the larger model than the smaller one, which corresponds with the output from the `summary` table above. Next looking at the *p*-value (`Pr(>Chi)`), we see a test for β_{MICU} and $\beta_{SICU} = 0$ has a *p*-value of around 0.08. At the typical 0.05 significance level, we would not reject the null, and use the simpler model without the service unit. In logistic regression, this is a common way of testing whether a categorical covariate should be retained in the model, as it can be difficult to assess using the `z value` in the `summary` table, particularly when one is very statistically significant, and one is not.

16.3.6 Confidence Intervals

Generating confidence intervals for either the log-odds ratios or the odds ratios are relatively straightforward. To get the log-odds ratios and respective confidence intervals for the `ageunit.glm` model which includes both age and service unit,

```
ageunit.glm$coef
```

```
##   (Intercept)    age.cat>55 service_unitMICU service_unitSICU
##     -4.209013      2.161142         1.178865         1.123442
```

```
confint(ageunit.glm)
```

```
##                       2.5 %    97.5 %
## (Intercept)      -5.66202924 -3.139732
## age.cat>55        1.82211403  2.524682
## service_unitMICU  0.12291680  2.620797
## service_unitSICU  0.07182767  2.563132
```

Here the coefficient estimates and confidence intervals are presented in much the same way as for a linear regression. In logistic regression, it is often convenient to exponentiate these quantities to get it on a more interpretable scale.

```
exp(ageunit.glm$coef[-1])
```

```
##       age.cat>55 service_unitMICU service_unitSICU
##         8.681049         3.250684         3.075423
```

```
exp(confint(ageunit.glm)[-1,])
```

```
##                      2.5 %   97.5 %
## age.cat>55        6.18492 12.48693
## service_unitMICU  1.13079 13.74668
## service_unitSICU  1.07447 12.97640
```

Similar to linear regression, we will look at if the confidence intervals for the log odds ratios include zero. This is equivalent to seeing if the intervals for the odds ratios include 1. Since the odds ratios are more directly interpretable it is often more convenient to report them instead of the coefficients on the log odds ratio scale.

16.3.7 Prediction

Once you have decided on your final model, you may want to generate predictions from your model. Such a task may occur when doing a propensity score analysis (Chap. 25) or creating tools for clinical decision support. In the logistic regression setting this involves attempting to estimate the probability of the outcome given the characteristics (covariates) of a patient. This quantity is often denoted $P(outcome|X)$. This is relatively easy to accomplish in R using the predict function. One must pass a dataset with all the variables contained in the model. Let's assume that we decided to include the service_unit in our final model, and want to generate predictions from this based on a new set of patients. Let's first

16.3 Logistic Regression

create a new data frame called `newdat` using the `expand.grid` function which computes all combinations of the values of variables passed to it.

```
newdat <- expand.grid(age.cat=c("<=55",">55"),service_unit=c("FICU","MICU","SICU"))
newdat$pred <- predict(ageunit.glm,newdata=newdat,type="response")
newdat
##   age.cat service_unit       pred
## 1    <=55         FICU 0.01464341
## 2     >55         FICU 0.11426771
## 3    <=55         MICU 0.04608233
## 4     >55         MICU 0.29546130
## 5    <=55         SICU 0.04370639
## 6     >55         SICU 0.28405645
```

We followed this by adding a `pred` column to our new data frame by using the `predict` function. The `predict` function for logistic regression works similar to when we used it for linear regression, but this time we also specify type = "response" which ensures the quantities computed are what we need, $P(outcome|X)$. Outputting this new object shows our predicted probability of 28 day mortality for six hypothetical patients. Two in each of the service units, where one is in the younger group and another in the older group. We see that our lowest prediction is for the youngest patients in the FICU, while the patients with highest risk of 28 day mortality are the older group in the MICU, but the predicted probability is not all that much higher than the same age patients in the SICU.

To do predictions on a different dataset, just replace the `newdata` argument with the other dataset. We could, for instance, pass newdata = dat and receive predictions for the dataset we built the model on. As was the case with linear regression, evaluating the predictive performance of our model on data used to build the model will generally be too optimistic as to how well it would perform *in the real world*. How to get a better sense of the accuracy of such models is covered in Chap. 17.

16.3.8 *Presenting and Interpreting Logistic Regression Analysis*

In general, presenting the results from a logistic regression model will follow quite closely to what was done in the linear regression setting. Results should always be put in context, including what variables were considered and which variables were in the final model. Reporting the results should always include some form of the coefficient estimate, a measure of uncertainty and likely a *p*-value. In medical and epidemiological journals, coefficients are usually exponentiated so that they are no longer on the log scale, and reported as odds ratios. Frequently, multivariable analyses (analysis with more than one covariate) is distinguished from univariate analyses (one covariate) by denoting the estimated odds ratios as adjusted odds ratios (AOR).

For the `age.glm` model, an example of what could be reported is:

> Mortality at 28 days was much higher in the older (> 55 years) group than the younger group (≤ 55 years), with rates of 28.5 and 4.3 %, respectively (OR = 8.79, 95 % CI: 6.27–12.64, p < 0.001).

When treating age as a continuous covariate in the `agects.glm` model we could report:

> Mortality at 28 days was associated with older age (OR = 1.07 per year increase, 95 % CI: 1.06–1.08, p < 0.001).

And for the case with more than one covariate, (`ageunit.glm`) an example of what could be reported is:

> Older age (> 55 versus ≤ 55 years) was independently associated with 28 day mortality (AOR = 8.68, 95 % CI: 6.18–12.49, p < 0.001) after adjusting for service unit.

16.3.9 Caveats and Conclusions

As was the case with linear regression, logistic regression is an extremely powerful tool for data analysis of health data. Although the study outcomes in each approach are different, the framework and way of thinking of the problem have similarities. Likewise, many of the problems encountered in linear regression are also of concern in logistic regression. Outliers, missing data, colinearity and dependent/correlated outcomes are all problems for logistic regression as well, and can be dealt with in a similar fashion. Modelling assumptions are as well, and we briefly touched on this when discussing whether it was appropriate to use age as a continuous covariate in our models. Although continuous covariates are frequently modeled in this way, it is important to ensure if the relationship between the log odds of the outcome is indeed linear with the covariate. In cases where the data has been divided into too many subgroups (or the study may be simply too small), you may encounter a level of a discrete variable where none (or very few) of one of the outcomes occurred. For example, if we had an additional `service_unit` with 50 patients, all of whom lived. In such a case, the estimated odds ratios and subsequent confidence intervals or hypothesis testing may not be appropriate to use. In such a case, collapsing the discrete covariate into fewer categories will often help return the analysis into a manageable form. For our hypothetical new service unit, creating a new group of it and FICU would be a possible solution. Sometimes a covariate is so strongly related to the outcome, and this is no longer possible, and the only solution may be to report this finding, and remove these patients.

Overall, logistic regression is a very valuable tool in modelling binary and categorical data. Although we did not cover this latter case, a similar framework is

16.3 Logistic Regression

available for discrete data which is ordered or has more than one category (see ?multinom in the nnet package in R for details about multinomial logistic regression). This and other topics such as assessing model fit, and using logistic regression in more complicated study designs are discussed in [11].

16.4 Survival Analysis

16.4.1 Section Goals

In this section, the reader will learn the fundamentals of survival analysis, and how to present and interpret such an analysis.

16.4.2 Introduction

As you will note that in the previous section on logistic regression, we specifically looked at the mortality outcome at 28 days. This was deliberate, and illustrates a limitation of using logistic regression for this type of outcome. For example, in the previous analysis, someone who died on day 29 was treated identically as someone who went on to live for 80+ years. You may wonder, why not just simply treat the survival time as a continuous variable, and perform linear regression analysis on this outcome? There are several reasons, but the primary reason is that you likely won't be able to wait around for the lifetime for each study participant. It is likely in your study only a fraction of your subjects will die before you're ready to publish your results.

While we often focus on mortality this can occur for many other outcomes, including times to patient relapse, re-hospitalization, reinfection, etc. In each of these types of outcomes, it is presumed the patients are at risk of the outcome until the event happens, or until they are *censored*. Censoring can happen for a variety of different reasons, but indicates the event was not observed during the observation time. In this sense, survival or more generally time-to-event data is a bivariate outcome incorporating the observation or study time in which the patient was observed and whether the event happened during the period of observation. The particular case we will be most interested is *right censoring* (subjects are observed only up to a point in time, and we don't know what happens beyond this point), but there is also *left censoring* (we only know the event happened before some time point) and *interval censoring* (events happen inside some time window). Right censoring is generally the most common type, but it is important to understand how the data was collected to make sure that it is indeed right censored.

Establishing a common time origin (i.e., a place to start counting time) is often easy to identify (e.g., admission to the ICU, enrollment in a study, administration of a drug, etc.), but in other scenarios it may not be (e.g., perhaps interest lies in survival time since disease onset, but patients are only followed from the time of disease diagnosis). For a good treatment on this topic and other issues, see Chap. 3 of [12].

With this additional complexity in the data (relative to logistic and linear regression), there are additional technical aspects and assumptions to the data analysis approaches. In general, each approach attempts to compare groups or identify covariates which modify the survival rates among the patients studied.

Overall survival analysis is a complex and fascinating area of study, and we will only touch briefly on two types of analysis here. We largely ignore the technical details of these approaches focusing on general principles and intuition instead. Before we begin doing any survival analysis, we need to load the survival package in R, which we can do by running:

```
library(survival);
```

Normally, you can skip the next step, but since this dataset was used to analyze the data in a slightly different way, we need to correct the observation times for a subset of the subjects in the dataset.

```
dat$mort_day_censored[dat$censor_flg==1] <- 731;
```

16.4.3 Kaplan-Meier Survival Curves

Now that we have the technical issues sorted out, we can begin by visualizing the data. Just as the 2 × 2 table is a fundamental step in the analysis of binary data, the fundamental step for survival data is often plotting what is known as a Kaplan-Meier survival function [13]. The *survival function* is a function of time, and is the probability of surviving at least that amount of time. For example, if there was 80 % survival at one year, the survival function at one year is 0.8. Survival functions normally start at time = 0, where the survivor function is 1 (or 100 % – everyone is alive), and can only stay the same or decrease. If it were to increase as time progressed, that would mean people were coming back to life! Kaplan-Meier plots are one of the most widely used plots in medical research.

Before plotting the Kaplan-Meier plot, we need to setup a survfit object. This object has a familiar form, but differs slightly from the previous methodologies we covered. Specifying a formula for survival outcomes is somewhat more complicated, since as we noted, survival data has two components. We do this by creating a Surv object in R. This will be our survival outcome for subsequent analysis.

16.4 Survival Analysis

```
datSurv <- Surv(dat$mort_day_censored,dat$censor_flg==0)
datSurv[101:105]
```

```
## [1] 236.08   731.00+ 731.00+ 731.00+   2.00
```

The first step setups a new kind of R object useful for survival data. The `Surv` function normally takes two arguments: a vector of times, and some kind of indicator for which patients had an event (death in our case). In our case, the vector of death and censoring times are the `mort_day_censored`, and deaths are coded with a zero in the `censor_flg` variable (hence we identify the events where `censor_flg == 0`). The last step prints out 5 entries of the new object (observations 101 to 105). We can see there are three entries of 731.00+. The + indicates that this observation is censored. The other entries are not censored, indicating deaths at those times.

Fitting a Kaplan-Meier curve is quite easy after doing this, but requires two steps. The first specifies a formula similar to how we accomplished this for linear and logistic regression, but now using the `survfit` function. We want to 'fit' by gender (`gender_num`), so the formula is, `datSurv ~ gender_num`. We can then `plot` the newly created object, but we pass some additional arguments to the plot function which include 95 % confidence intervals for the survival functions (`conf.int = TRUE`), and includes a x- and y- axis label (`xlab` and `ylab`). Lastly we add a legend, coding black for the women and red for the men. This plot is in Fig. 16.6.

```
gender.surv <- survfit(datSurv~gender_num,data=dat)
plot(gender.surv,col=1:2,conf.int = TRUE,xlab="Days",ylab="Proportion Who Survived")
legend(400,0.4,col=c("black","red"),lty=1,c("Women","Men"))
```

In Fig. 16.6, there appears to be a difference between the survival function between the two gender groups, with again the male group (red) dying at slightly slower rate than the female group (black). We have included 95 % point-wise confidence bands for the survival function estimate, which assesses how much certain we are about the estimated survivorship at each point in time. We can do the same for `service_unit`, but since it has three groups, we need to change the color argument and legend to ensure the plot is properly labelled. This plot is in Fig. 16.7.

```
unit.surv <- survfit(datSurv~service_unit,data=dat)
plot(unit.surv,col=1:3,conf.int = FALSE,xlab="Days",ylab="Proportion Who Survived")
legend(400,0.4,col=c("black","red","green"),lty=1,c("FICU","MICU","SICU"))
```

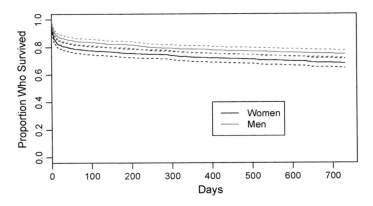

Fig. 16.6 Kaplan-Meier plot of the estimated survivor function stratified by gender

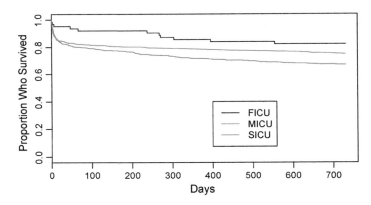

Fig. 16.7 Kaplan-Meier plot of the estimated survivor function stratified by service unit

16.4.4 Cox Proportional Hazards Models

Kaplan-Meier curves are a good first step in examining time to event data before proceeding with any more complex statistical model. Time to event outcomes are in general more complex than the other types of outcomes we have examined thus far. There are several different modelling approaches, each of which has some advantages and limitations. The most popular approach for health data is likely the Cox Proportional Hazards Model [14], which is also sometimes called the Cox model or Cox Regression. As the name implies this method models something called the hazard function. We will not dwell on the technical details, but attempt to provide some intuition. The hazard function is a function of time (hours, days, years) and is approximately the instantaneous probability of the event occurring (i.e., chance the event is happening in some very small time window) given the event has not

16.4 Survival Analysis

already happened. It is frequently used to study mortality, sometimes going by the name force of mortality or instantaneous death rate, and can be interpreted simply as the risk of death at a particular time, given that the person has survived up until that point. The "proportional" part of Cox's model assumes that the way covariates effect the hazard function for different types of patients is through a proportionality assumption relative to the baseline hazard function. For illustration, consider a simple case where two treatments are given, for treatment 0 (e.g., the placebo) we determine the hazard function is $h_0(t)$, and for treatment 1 we determine the hazard function is $h_1(t)$, where t is time. The proportional hazards assumption is that:

$$h_1(t) = HR \times h_0(t).$$

It's easy to see that $HR = h_1(t)/h_0(t)$. This quantity is often called the hazard ratio, and if for example it is two, this would mean that the risk of death in the treatment 1 group was twice as high as the risk of death in the treatment zero group. We will note, that HR is *not* a function of time, meaning that the risk of death is *always* twice as high in the first group when compared to the second group. This assumption means that if the proportional hazards assumption is valid we need only know the hazard function from group 0, and the hazard ratio to know the hazard function for group 1. Estimation of the hazard function under this model is often considered a nuisance, as the primary focus is on the hazard ratio, and this is key to being able to fit and interpret these models. For a more technical treatment of this topic, we refer you to [12, 15–17].

As was the case with logistic regression, we will model the log of the hazard ratio instead of the hazard ratio itself. This allows us to use the familiar framework we have used thus far for modeling other types of health data. Like logistic regression, when the $\log(HR)$ is zero, the HR is one, meaning the risk between the groups is the same. Furthermore, this extends to multiple covariate models or continuous covariates in the same manner as logistic regression.

Fitting Cox regression models in R will follow the familiar pattern we have seen in the previous cases of linear and logistic regressions. The `coxph` function (from the `survival` package) is the fitting function for Cox models, and it continues the general pattern of passing a model formula (`outcome ~ covariate`), and the dataset you would like to use. In our case, let's continue our example of using gender (`gender_num`) to model the `datSurv` outcome we created, and running the `summary` function to see what information is outputted.

```
gender.coxph <- coxph(datSurv ~ gender_num,data=dat)
summary(gender.coxph)
```

```
## Call:
## coxph(formula = datSurv ~ gender_num, data = dat)
##
## n= 1775, number of events= 497
##    (1 observation deleted due to missingness)
##
##                coef exp(coef) se(coef)     z Pr(>|z|)
## gender_num -0.29094   0.74756  0.08978 -3.24  0.00119 **
## ---
## Signif. codes:  0 '***' 0.001 '**' 0.01 '*' 0.05 '.' 0.1 ' ' 1
##
##            exp(coef) exp(-coef) lower .95 upper .95
## gender_num    0.7476      1.338    0.6269    0.8914
##
## Concordance= 0.537  (se = 0.011 )
## Rsquare= 0.006   (max possible= 0.983 )
## Likelihood ratio test= 10.43  on 1 df,   p=0.001243
## Wald test            = 10.5   on 1 df,   p=0.001193
## Score (logrank) test = 10.58  on 1 df,   p=0.001146
```

The coefficients table has the familiar format, which we've seen before. The coef for gender_num is about −0.29, and this is the estimate of our log-hazard ratio. As discussed, taking the exponential of this gives the hazard ratio (HR), which the summary output computes in the next column (exp(coef)). Here, the HR is estimated at 0.75, indicating that men have about a 25 % reduction in the hazards of death, under the proportional hazards assumption.

The next column in the coefficient table has the standard error for the log hazard ratio, followed by the z score and p-value (Pr(>|z|)), which is very similar to what we saw in the case of logistic regression. Here we see the p-value is quite small, and we would reject the null hypothesis that the hazard functions are the same between men and women. This is consistent with the exploratory figures we produced using Kaplan-Meier curves in the previous section. For coxph, the summary function also conveniently outputs the confidence interval of the HR a few lines down, and here our estimate of the HR is 0.75 (95 % CI: 0.63–0.89, p = 0.001). This is how the HR would typically be reported.

Using more than one covariate works the same as our other analysis techniques. Adding a co-morbidity to the model such as atrial fibrillation (afib_flg) can be done as you would do for logistic regression.

```
genderafib.coxph <- coxph(datSurv~gender_num + afib_flg,data=dat)
summary(genderafib.coxph)$coef
```

```
##                 coef exp(coef)  se(coef)        z     Pr(>|z|)
## gender_num -0.2591201 0.7717304 0.08997143 -2.883231 0.003936189
## afib_flg    1.3443975 3.8358747 0.10200099 13.180239 0.000000000
```

16.4 Survival Analysis

Here again male gender is associated with reduced time to death, while atrial fibrillation increases the hazard of death by almost four-fold. Both are statistically significant in the summary output, and we know from before that we can test a large number of other types of statistical hypotheses using the `anova` function. Again we pass `anova` the smaller (`gender_num only`) and larger (`gender_num and afib_flg`) nested models.

```
anova(gender.coxph,genderafib.coxph)

## Analysis of Deviance Table
##  Cox model: response is  datSurv
##  Model 1: ~ gender_num
##  Model 2: ~ gender_num + afib_flg
##     loglik  Chisq Df P(>|Chi|)
## 1 -3636.1
## 2 -3567.4 137.37  1 < 2.2e-16 ***
## ---
## Signif. codes:  0 '***' 0.001 '**' 0.01 '*' 0.05 '.' 0.1 ' ' 1
```

As expected, atrial fibrillation is very statistically significant, and therefore we would like to keep it in the model.

Cox regression also allows one to use covariates which change over time. This would allow one to incorporate changes in treatment, disease severity, etc. within the same patient without need for any different methodology. The major challenge to do this is mainly in the construction of the dataset, which is discussed in some of the references at the end of this chapter. Some care is required when the time dependent covariate is only measure periodically, as the method requires that it be known at every event time for the entire cohort of patients, and not just those relevant to the patient in question. This is more practical for changes in treatment which may be recorded with some precision, particularly in a database like MIMIC II, and less so for laboratory results which may be measured at the resolution of hours, days or weeks. Interpolating between lab values or carrying the last observation forward has been shown to introduce several types of problems.

16.4.5 Caveats and Conclusions

We will conclude this brief overview of survival analysis, but acknowledge we have only scratched the surface. There are many topics we have not covered or we have only briefly touched on.

Survival analysis is distinguished from other forms of analyses covered in this Chapter, as it allows the data to be censored. As was the case for the other approaches we considered, there are modeling assumptions. For instance, it is important that the censoring is not informative of the survival time. For example, if censoring occurs when treatment is withdrawn *because* the patient is too sick to continue therapy, this would be an example of informative censoring. The validity of all methods discussed in this section are then invalid. Care should be taken to make sure you understand the censoring mechanism as to avoid any false inferences drawn.

Assessment of the proportional hazards assumption is an important part of any Cox regression analysis. We refer you to the references (particularly [17] and see ?cox.zph) at the end of this chapter for strategies and alternatives for when the proportional hazards assumption breaks down. In some circumstances, the proportional hazards assumption is not valid, and alternative approaches can be used. As is always the case, when outcomes are dependent (e.g., one patient may contribute more than one observation), the methods discussed in this section should not be used directly. Generally the standard error estimates will be too small, and p-values will be incorrect. The concerns in logistic regression regarding outliers, co-linearity, missing data, and covariates with sparse outcomes apply here as well, as do the concerns about model misspecification for continuous covariates.

Survival analysis is a powerful analysis technique which is extremely relevant for health studies. We have only given a brief overview of the subject, and would encourage you to further explore these methods.

16.5 Case Study and Summary

16.5.1 Section Goals

In this section, we will work through a case study, and discuss the data analysis components which should be included in an original research article suitable for a clinical journal. We will also discuss some approaches for model and feature selection.

16.5.2 Introduction

We will now use what we learned in the previous sections to examine if indwelling arterial catheters (IAC) have any effect on patient mortality. As reiterated throughout, clearly identifying a study objective is important for a smooth data analysis. In our case, we'd like to estimate the effect of IAC on mortality, but acknowledge a few potential problem areas. First, the groups who receive IAC and and those who don't are likely different in many respects, and many of these differences likely also have some effect on mortality. Second, we would like to be able to limit ourselves on mortality events which occur in close proximity to the ICU admission. The dataset includes 28 day mortality, so that would seem to be in close proximity to the ICU admission. As for the first issue, we also have many

16.5 Case Study and Summary

covariates which capture some of the features we may be concerned with, including severity of illness (`sapsi_first` and `sofa_first`), age (`age`), patient gender (`gender_num`) and co-morbidities (`chf_flg`, `afib_flg`, `renal_flg`, etc.).

With all these in mind, we should have a good start on determining our study objective. In our case, it might be,

> To estimate the effect that administration of IAC during an ICU admission has on 28 day mortality in patients within the MIMIC II study who received mechanical ventilation, while adjusting for age, gender, severity of illness and comorbidities.

For now, this describes our outcome and covariates quite well. One of the first things that is often done is to describe our population by computing summary statistics of all or a subset of variables collected in the study. This description allows the reader to understand how well the study would generalize to other populations. We have made available an R package on GitHub that will allow one to construct preliminary forms of such a table quite quickly. To install the R package, first install and load the `devtools` package:

```
install.package("devtools")
library(devtools)
```

and then install and load our package by using the `install_github` function.

```
install_github("jraffa/MIMICbook")
library(MIMICbook);
```

Before we do any in depth analysis, let's make sure we are using the original dataset, first by removing and then reloading the `dat` data frame. In order to ensure our research is reproducible, it's a good idea to make sure the entire process of doing the analysis is documented. By starting from the original copy of the dataset, we are able to present precisely what methods we used in an analysis.

```
rm(dat)
dat <- read.csv(url)
```

As mentioned before, recoding binary encoded variables (ones which are 0s and 1s) to the R data class `factor` can sometimes make interpreting the R output easier. The following piece of code cycles through all the columns in `dat` and converts any binary variables to a `factor`.

```
# Identify which columns are binary coded
bincols <- colMeans((dat == 1 | dat == 0), na.rm = T) == 1
for (i in 1:length(bincols)) {
    # Turn the binary columns into a factor
    if (bincols[i]) {
        dat[[i]] <- as.factor(dat[[i]])
    }
}
```

We are now ready to generate a summary of the patient characteristics in our study. The MIMICbook package has a produce.table1 function. This generates a summary table of the data frame you pass to it, using an appropriate summary for continuous variables (average and standard deviation) and categorical variables (number and percentages) for each variable. In its most simple form, produce.table1 can be passed a data frame as an argument, which we do (passing it the dat data frame). This output is not very nice, and we can make it look nicer by using a powerful R package called knitr, which provides many tools to assist in performing reproducible research. You can find out more about knitr (which can be installed using install.packages ('knitr')), by running ?knitr on the R console after loading it. We will be using the kable command, which will take our tab1 variable—a summary table we generated using the produce.table1 function, and make it look a little nicer.

```
tab1 <- produce.table1(dat);
library(knitr);
kable(tab1,caption = "Overall patient characteristics")
```

The row descriptors are not very informative, and what we have produced would not be usable for final publication, but it suits our purposes for now. knitr allows one to output such tables in HTML, LaTeX or even a Word document, which you can edit and make the table more informative. The results are contained in Table 16.1.

A couple things we may notice from the baseline characteristics are:

1. Some variables have a lot of missing observations (e.g., bmi, po2_first, iv_day_1).
2. None of the patients have sepsis.

Both of these points are important, and illustrates why it is always a good idea to perform basic descriptive analyses before beginning any modeling. The missing data is primarily related to weight/BMI, or lab values. For the purpose of this chapter, we are going to ignore both of these classes of variables. While we would likely want to adjust for some of these covariates in a final version of the paper, and Chap. 11 gives some useful techniques for dealing with such a situation, we are going to focus on the set of covariates we had identified in our study objective, which do not include these variables. The issue related to sepsis is also of note.

16.5 Case Study and Summary

Table 16.1 Overall patient characteristics

	Average (SD), or N (%)
aline_flg==1	984 (55.4 %)
icu_los_day	3.3 (3.4)
hospital_los_day	8.1 (8.2)
age	54.4 (21.1)
gender_num==1	1025 (57.7 %) [Missing: 1]
weight_first	80.1 (22.5) [Missing: 110]
bmi	27.8 (8.2) [Missing: 466]
sapsi_first	14.1 (4.1) [Missing: 85]
sofa_first	5.8 (2.3) [Missing: 6]
service_unit==SICU	982 (55.3 %)
service_num==1	982 (55.3 %)
day_icu_intime==Saturday	278 (15.7 %)
day_icu_intime_num	4.1 (2)
hour_icu_intime	10.6 (7.9)
hosp_exp_flg==0	1532 (86.3 %)
icu_exp_flg==0	1606 (90.4 %)
day_28_flg ==0	1493 (84.1 %)
mort_day_censored	614.3 (403.1)
censor_flg==1	1279 (72 %)
sepsis_flg==0	1776 (100 %)
chf_flg==0	1563 (88 %)
afib_flg==0	1569 (88.3 %)
renal_flg==0	1716 (96.6 %)
liver_flg==0	1677 (94.4 %)
copd_flg==0	1619 (91.2 %)
cad_flg==0	1653 (93.1 %)
stroke_flg==0	1554 (87.5 %)
mal_flg==0	1520 (85.6 %)
resp_flg==0	1211 (68.2 %)
map_1st	88.2 (17.6)
hr_1st	87.9 (18.8)
temp_1st	97.8 (4.5) [Missing: 3]
spo2_1st	98.4 (5.5)
abg_count	6 (8.7)
wbc_first	12.3 (6.6) [Missing: 8]
hgb_first	12.6 (2.2) [Missing: 8]
platelet_first	246.1 (99.9) [Missing: 8]
sodium_first	139.6 (4.7) [Missing: 5]
potassium_first	4.1 (0.8) [Missing: 5]
tco2_first	24.4 (5) [Missing: 5]
chloride_first	103.8 (5.7) [Missing: 5]

(continued)

Table 16.1 (continued)

	Average (SD), or N (%)
aline_flg==1	984 (55.4 %)
bun_first	19.3 (14.4) [Missing: 5]
creatinine_first	1.1 (1.1) [Missing: 6]
po2_first	227.6 (144.9) [Missing: 186]
pco2_first	43.4 (14) [Missing: 186]
iv_day_1	1622.9 (1677.1) [Missing: 143]

Sepsis certainly would contribute to higher rates of mortality when compared to patients without sepsis, but since we do not have any patients with sepsis, we cannot and do not need to adjust for this covariate per se. What we do need to do is acknowledge this fact by revising our study objective. We originally identified our population as patients within MIMIC, but because this is a subset of MIMIC—those without sepsis, we should revise the study objective to:

> To estimate the effect that administration of IAC during an ICU admission has on 28 day mortality in patients without sepsis who received mechanical ventilation within MIMIC II, while adjusting for age, gender, severity of illness and comorbidities.

We will also *not* want to include the sepsis_flg variable as a covariate in any of our models, as there are no patients with sepsis within this study to estimate the effect of sepsis. Now that we have examined the basic overall characteristics of the patients, we can begin the next steps in the analysis.

The next steps will vary slightly, but it is often useful to put yourself in the shoes of a peer reviewer. What problems will a reviewer likely find with your study and how can you address them? Usually, the reviewer will want to see how the population differs for different values of the covariate of interest. In our case study, if the treated group (IAC) differed substantially from the untreated group (no IAC), then this may account for any effect we demonstrate. We can do this by summarizing the two groups in a similar fashion as was done for Table 16.1. We can reuse the produce.table1 function, but we pass it the two groups separately by splitting the dat data frame into two using the split function (by the aline_flg variable), later combining them into one table using cbind to yield Table 16.2. It's important to ensure that the same reference groups are used across the two study groups, and that's what the labels argument is used for (see ?produce.table1 for more details).

```
datby.aline <- split(dat, dat$aline_flg)
reftable <- produce.table1(datby.aline[[1]])
tab2 <- cbind(produce.table1(datby.aline[[1]], labels = attr(reftable, "labels")),
    produce.table1(datby.aline[[2]], labels = attr(reftable, "labels")))
colnames(tab2) <- paste0("Average (SD), or N (%)", c(", No-IAC", ", IAC"))
kable(tab2, caption = "Patient characteristics stratified by IAC administration")
```

16.5 Case Study and Summary

Table 16.2 Patient characteristics stratified by IAC administration

	Average (SD), or N (%), No-IAC	Average (SD), or N (%), IAC
aline_flg==0	792 (100 %)	0 (0 %)
icu_los_day	2.1 (1.9)	4.3 (3.9)
hospital_los_day	5.4 (5.4)	10.3 (9.3)
age	53 (21.7)	55.5 (20.5)
gender_num==1	447 (56.5 %) [Missing: 1]	578 (58.7 %)
weight_first	79.2 (22.6) [Missing: 71]	80.7 (22.4) [Missing: 39]
bmi	28 (9.1) [Missing: 220]	27.7 (7.5) [Missing: 246]
sapsi_first	12.7 (3.8) [Missing: 70]	15.2 (4) [Missing: 15]
sofa_first	4.8 (2.1) [Missing: 4]	6.6 (2.2) [Missing: 2]
service_unit==MICU	480 (60.6 %)	252 (25.6 %)
service_num==0	504 (63.6 %)	290 (29.5 %)
day_icu_intime==Saturday	138 (17.4 %)	140 (14.2 %)
day_icu_intime_num	4 (2)	4.1 (2)
hour_icu_intime	9.9 (7.7)	11.2 (8.1)
hosp_exp_flg==0	702 (88.6 %)	830 (84.3 %)
icu_exp_flg==0	734 (92.7 %)	872 (88.6 %)
day_28_flg==0	679 (85.7 %)	814 (82.7 %)
mort_day_censored	619.1 (388.3)	610.5 (414.8)
censor_flg==1	579 (73.1 %)	700 (71.1 %)
sepsis_flg==0	792 (100 %)	984 (100 %)
chf_flg==0	695 (87.8 %)	868 (88.2 %)
afib_flg==0	710 (89.6 %)	859 (87.3 %)
renal_flg==0	764 (96.5 %)	952 (96.7 %)
liver_flg==0	754 (95.2 %)	923 (93.8 %)
copd_flg==0	711 (89.8 %)	908 (92.3 %)
cad_flg==0	741 (93.6 %)	912 (92.7 %)
stroke_flg==0	722 (91.2 %)	832 (84.6 %)
mal_flg==0	700 (88.4 %)	820 (83.3 %)
resp_flg==0	514 (64.9 %)	697 (70.8 %)
map_1st	87.5 (15.9)	88.9 (18.8)
hr_st	88.4 (18.8)	87.5 (18.7)
temp_1st	97.9 (3.8) [Missing: 3]	97.7 (5.1)
spo2_1st	98.4 (5.7)	98.5 (5.4)
abg_count	1.4 (1.6)	9.7 (10.2)
wbc_first	11.7 (6.5) [Missing: 6]	12.8 (6.6) [Missing: 2]
hgb_first	12.7 (2.2) [Missing: 6]	12.4 (2.2) [Missing: 2]
platelet_first	254.3 (104.5) [Missing: 6]	239.5 (95.6) [Missing: 2]
sodium_first	139.8 (4.8) [Missing: 3]	139.4 (4.7) [Missing: 2]
potassium_first	4.1 (0.8) [Missing: 3]	4.1 (0.8) [Missing: 2]

(continued)

Table 16.2 (continued)

	Average (SD), or N (%), No-IAC	Average (SD), or N (%), IAC
tco2_first	24.7 (4.9) [Missing: 3]	24.2 (5.1) [Missing: 2]
chloride_first	103.3 (5.4) [Missing: 3]	104.3 (5.9) [Missing: 2]
bun_first	18.9 (14.5) [Missing: 3]	19.6 (14.3) [Missing: 2]
creatinine_first	1.1 (1.2) [Missing: 4]	1.1 (1) [Missing: 2]
po2_first	223.8 (152.9) [Missing: 178]	230.1 (139.6) [Missing: 8]
pco2_first	44.9 (15.9) [Missing: 178]	42.5 (12.5) [Missing: 8]
iv_day_1	[1364.2 (1406.8) Missing: 110]	1808.4 (1825) [Missing: 33]

As you can see in Table 16.2, the IAC group differs in many respects to the non-IAC group. Patients who were given IAC tended to have higher severity of illness at baseline (`sapsi_first` and `sofa_first`), slightly older, less likely to be from the MICU, and have slightly different co-morbidity profiles when compared to the non-IAC group.

Next, we can see how the covariates are distributed among the different outcomes (death within 28 days versus alive at 28 days). This will give us an idea of which covariates may be important for affecting the outcome. The code to generate this is nearly identical to that used to produce Table 16.2, but instead, we replace `aline_flg` with `day_28_flg` (the outcome) to get Table 16.3.

```
datby.28daymort <- split(dat, dat$day_28_flg)
reftablemort <- produce.table1(datby.28daymort[[1]])
tab3 <- cbind(produce.table1(datby.28daymort[[1]], labels = attr(reftablemort,
    "labels")), produce.table1(datby.28daymort[[2]], labels = attr(reftablemort,
    "labels")))
colnames(tab3) <- paste0("Average (SD), or N (%)", c(",Alive", ",Dead"))
kable(tab3, caption = "Patient characteristics stratified by 28 day mortality")
```

As can be seen in Table 16.3, those patients who died within 28 days differ in many ways with those who did not. Those who died had higher SAPS and SOFA scores, were on average older, and had different co-morbidity profiles.

16.5.3 Logistic Regression Analysis

In Table 16.3, we see that of the 984 subjects receiving IAC, 170 (17.2 %) died within 28 days, whereas 113 of 792 (14.2 %) died in the no-IAC group. In a univariate analysis we can assess if the lower rate of mortality is statistically significant, by fitting a single covariate `aline_flg` logistic regression.

16.5 Case Study and Summary

Table 16.3 Patient characteristics stratified by 28 day mortality

	Average (SD), or N (%), alive	Average (SD), or N (%), dead
aline_flg==1	814 (54.5 %)	170 (60.1 %)
icu_los_day	3.2 (3.2)	4 (4)
hospital_los_day	8.4 (8.4)	6.4 (6.4)
age	50.8 (20.1)	73.3 (15.3)
gender_num==1	886 (59.4 %) [Missing: 1]	139 (49.1 %)
weight_first	81.4 (22.7) [Missing: 77]	72.4 (19.9) [Missing: 33]
bmi	28.2 (8.3) [Missing: 392]	26 (7.2) [Missing: 74]
sapsi_first	13.6 (3.9) [Missing: 51]	17.3 (3.8) [Missing: 34]
sofa_first	5.7 (2.3) [Missing: 3]	6.6 (2.4) [Missing: 3]
service_unit==SICU	829 (55.5 %)	153 (54.1 %)
service_num==1	829 (55.5 %)	153 (54.1 %)
day_icu_intime==Saturday	235 (15.7 %)	43 (15.2 %)
day_icu_intime_num	4 (2)	4.1 (2)
hour_icu_intime	10.5 (7.9)	11 (8)
hosp_exp_flg==0	1490 (99.8 %)	42 (14.8 %)
icu_exp_flg==0	1493 (100 %)	113 (39.9 %)
day_28_flg==0	1493 (100 %)	0 (0 %)
mort_day_censored	729.6 (331.4)	6.1 (6.4)
censor_flg==1	1279 (85.7 %)	0 (0 %)
sepsis_flg==0	1493 (100 %)	283 (100 %)
chf_flg==0	1348 (90.3 %)	215 (76 %)
afib_flg==0	1372 (91.9 %)	197 (69.6 %)
renal_flg==0	1447 (96.9 %)	269 (95.1 %)
liver_flg==0	1413 (94.6 %)	264 (93.3 %)
copd_flg==0	1377 (92.2 %)	242 (85.5 %)
cad_flg==0	1403 (94 %)	250 (88.3 %)
stroke_flg==0	1386 (92.8 %)	168 (59.4 %)
mal_flg==0	1294 (86.7 %)	226 (79.9 %)
resp_flg==0	1056 (70.7 %)	155 (54.8 %)
map_1st	88.2 (17.5)	88.3 (17.9)
hr_1st	88.3 (18.4)	85.8 (20.6)
temp_1st	97.8 (4.6) [Missing: 1]	97.7 (4.5) [Missing: 2]
spo2_1st	98.6 (5)	97.8 (7.6)
abg_count	5.7 (7.7)	7.5 (12.5)
wbc_first	12.2 (6.4) [Missing: 6]	12.7 (7.5) [Missing: 2]
hgb_first	12.7 (2.2) [Missing: 6]	11.9 (2.1) [Missing: 2]

(continued)

Table 16.3 (continued)

	Average (SD), or N (%), alive	Average (SD), or N (%), dead
platelet_first	246.8 (97.3) [Missing: 6]	242.1 (112.6) [Missing: 2]
sodium_first	139.6 (4.6) [Missing: 4]	139.1 (5.4) [Missing: 1]
potassium_first	4.1 (0.8) [Missing: 4]	4.2 (0.9) [Missing: 1]
tco2_first	24.3 (4.8) [Missing: 4]	25 (5.8) [Missing: 1]
chloride_first	104.1 (5.6) [Missing: 4]	102.6 (6.4) [Missing: 1]
bun_first	18 (12.9) [Missing: 4]	26.2 (19) [Missing: 1]
creatinine_first	1.1 (1.1) [Missing: 5]	1.2 (0.9) [Missing: 1]
po2_first	231.3 (146.3) [Missing: 153]	207.9 (135.8) [Missing: 33]
pco2_first	43.3 (12.9) [Missing: 153]	43.8 (18.6) [Missing: 33]
iv_day_1	1694.2 (1709.5) [Missing: 127]	1258 (1449.4) [Missing: 16]

```
uvr.glm <- glm(day_28_flg ~ aline_flg,data=dat,family="binomial")
exp(uvr.glm$coef[-1])

## aline_flg1
##   1.254919

exp(confint(uvr.glm)[-1,]);

##     2.5 %    97.5 %
## 0.9701035 1.6285165
```

Those who received IAC had over a 25 % increase in odds of 28 day mortality when compared to those who did not receive IAC. The confidence interval includes one, so we would expect the p-value would be >0.05. Running the summary function, we see that this is the case.

```
##              Estimate Std. Error   z value  Pr(>|z|)
## (Intercept) -1.7932333  0.1015988 -17.650149 1.014880e-69
## aline_flg1   0.2270714  0.1320347   1.719786 8.547142e-02
```

Indeed, the p-value for aline_flg is about 0.09. As we saw in Table 16.2, there are likely several important covariates that differed among those who received IAC and those who did not. These may serve as confounders, and the possible association we observed in the univariate analysis may be stronger, non-existent or in the opposite direction (i.e., IAC having lower rates of mortality) depending on the situation. Our next step would be to adjust for these confounders. This is an

16.5 Case Study and Summary

exercise in what is known as model building, and there are several ways people do this in the literature. A common approach is to fit all univariate models (one covariate at a time, as we did with `aline_flg`, but separately for each covariate and without `aline_flg`), and perform a hypothesis test on each model. Any variables which had statistical significance under the univariate models would then be included in a multivariable model. Another approach begins with the model we just fit (`uvr.glm` which only has `aline_flg` as a covariate), and then sequentially adds variables one at a time. This approach is often called *step-wise forward selection*. We will make a choice to do *step-wise backwards selection*, which is as it sounds—the opposite direction of step-wise forward selection. Model selection is a challenging task in data analysis, and there are many other methods [18] we couldn't possibly describe in full detail here. As an overall philosophy, it is important to outline and describe the process by which you will do model selection before you actually do it and stick with the process.

In our stepwise backwards elimination procedure, we are going to fit a model containing IAC (`aline_flg`), age (`age`), gender, (`gender_num`), disease severity (`sapsi_first` and `sofa_first`), service type (`service_unit`), and comorbidities (`chf_flg`, `afib_flg`, `renal_flg`, `liver_flg`, `copd_flg`, `cad_flg`, `stroke_flg`, `mal_flg` and `resp_flg`). This is often called the *full model*, and is fit below (`mva.full.glm`). From the full model, we will proceed by eliminating one variable at a time, until we are left with a model with only statistically significant covariates. Because `aline_flg` is the covariate of interest, it will remain in the model regardless of its statistical significance. At each step we need to come up with a criteria to choose which variable we will eliminate. There are several ways of doing this, but one way we can make this decision is performing a hypothesis test for each covariate, and choosing to eliminate the covariate with the largest p-value, unless all p-values are <0.05 or the largest p-value is `aline_flg`, in which case we would stop or eliminate the next largest p-value, respectively.

Most of the covariates are binary or categorical in nature, and we've already converted them to factors. The disease severity scores (SAPS and SOFA) are continuous. We could add them as we did age, but this assumes a linear trend in the odds of death as these scores change. This may or may not be appropriate (see Fig. 16.8). Indeed, when we plot the log odds of 28 day death by SOFA score, we note that while the log odds of death generally increase as the SOFA score increases the relationship may not be linear (Fig. 16.8).

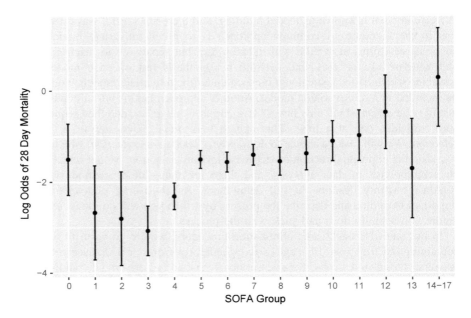

Fig. 16.8 Plot of log-odds of mortality for each of the SOFA groups. *Error bars* represent 95 % confidence intervals for the log odds

What can be done in this situation is to turn a continuous covariate into a discrete one. A quick way of doing this is using the `cut2` function in the `Hmisc` package.[2] Applying `cut2(sofa_first, g = 5)` turns the `sofa_first` variable into five approximately equal sized groups by SOFA score. For illustration, SOFA breaks down into the following sized groups by SOFA scores:

```
library(Hmisc)
table(cut2(dat$sofa_first,g=5))

## 
## [0, 5)     5     6 [7, 9) [9,17]
##    523   346   294    391    216
```

with not quite equal groups, due to the already discretized nature of SOFA to begin with. We will treat both SAPS and SOFA in this way in order to avoid any model misspecification that may occur as a result of assuming a linear relationship.

Returning to fitting the full model, we use these new disease severity scores, along with the other covariates we identified to include in the full model.

---

[2]You may need to install `Hmisc`, which can be done by running `install.packages` ('Hmisc') from the R command prompt.

16.5 Case Study and Summary

```
mva.full.glm <- glm(day_28_flg ~ aline_flg + age + gender_num + cut2(sapsi_first,
    g = 5) + cut2(sofa_first, g = 5) + service_unit + chf_flg + afib_flg + renal_flg +
    liver_flg + copd_flg + cad_flg + stroke_flg + mal_flg + resp_flg, data = dat,
    family = "binomial")
summary(mva.full.glm)
```

```
## 
## Call:
## glm(formula = day_28_flg ~ aline_flg + age + gender_num + cut2(sapsi_first,
##     g = 5) + cut2(sofa_first, g = 5) + service_unit + chf_flg +
##     afib_flg + renal_flg + liver_flg + copd_flg + cad_flg + stroke_flg +
##     mal_flg + resp_flg, family = "binomial", data = dat)
## 
## Deviance Residuals:
##     Min       1Q   Median       3Q      Max
## -2.2912  -0.4710  -0.2330  -0.1104   2.9640
## 
## Coefficients:
##                                 Estimate Std. Error z value Pr(>|z|)
## (Intercept)                     -7.61471    0.86262  -8.827  < 2e-16 ***
## aline_flg1                       0.01085    0.20443   0.053 0.957679
## age                              0.04020    0.00627   6.412 1.44e-10 ***
## gender_num1                      0.16214    0.17296   0.937 0.348527
## cut2(sapsi_first, g = 5)[12,14)  0.36961    0.40348   0.916 0.359637
## cut2(sapsi_first, g = 5)[14,16)  1.01794    0.36214   2.811 0.004940 **
## cut2(sapsi_first, g = 5)[16,19)  0.92803    0.36794   2.522 0.011662 *
## cut2(sapsi_first, g = 5)[19,32]  1.77615    0.37446   4.743 2.10e-06 ***
## cut2(sofa_first, g = 5)5         0.49761    0.30267   1.644 0.100159
## cut2(sofa_first, g = 5)6         0.58530    0.30300   1.932 0.053396 .
## cut2(sofa_first, g = 5)[7, 9)    0.68011    0.29439   2.310 0.020876 *
## cut2(sofa_first, g = 5)[9,17]    0.75134    0.34062   2.206 0.027397 *
## service_unitMICU                 1.08086    0.67839   1.593 0.111100
## service_unitSICU                 0.64257    0.67144   0.957 0.338562
## chf_flg1                         0.23350    0.23381   0.999 0.317962
## afib_flg1                        0.52408    0.21122   2.481 0.013092 *
## renal_flg1                      -0.76796    0.40904  -1.877 0.060452 .
## liver_flg1                       0.47238    0.34032   1.388 0.165125
## copd_flg1                        0.23440    0.24631   0.952 0.341287
## cad_flg1                        -0.25674    0.28823  -0.891 0.373065
## stroke_flg1                      2.04301    0.21966   9.301  < 2e-16 ***
## mal_flg1                         0.49319    0.20897   2.360 0.018274 *
## resp_flg1                        0.69330    0.19166   3.617 0.000298 ***
## ---
## Signif. codes:  0 '***' 0.001 '**' 0.01 '*' 0.05 '.' 0.1 ' ' 1
## 
## (Dispersion parameter for binomial family taken to be 1)
## 
##     Null deviance: 1400.58  on 1683  degrees of freedom
## Residual deviance:  954.39  on 1661  degrees of freedom
##   (92 observations deleted due to missingness)
## AIC: 1000.4
## 
## Number of Fisher Scoring iterations: 6
```

The `summary` output show that some of the covariates are very statistically significant, while others may be expendable. Ideally, we would like as simple of a model as possible that can explain as much of the variation in the outcome as possible. We will attempt to remove our first covariate by the procedure we outlined above. For each of the variables we consider removing, we could fit a logistic regression model without that covariate, and then test it against the current model. R has a useful function that automates this process for us, called `drop1`. We pass to `drop1` our logistic regression object (`mva.full.glm`) and the type of test you would like to do. If you recall from the logistic regression section, we used `test = "Chisq"`, and this is what we will pass the `drop1` function as well.

```
drop1(mva.full.glm,test="Chisq")
```

```
## Single term deletions
## 
## Model:
## day_28_flg ~ aline_flg + age + gender_num + cut2(sapsi_first,
##     g = 5) + cut2(sofa_first, g = 5) + service_unit + chf_flg +
##     afib_flg + renal_flg + liver_flg + copd_flg + cad_flg + stroke_flg +
##     mal_flg + resp_flg
##                         Df Deviance    AIC     LRT  Pr(>Chi)
## <none>                        954.39 1000.39
## aline_flg                1   954.39  998.39   0.003 0.9576771
## age                      1  1000.60 1044.60  46.210 1.063e-11 ***
## gender_num               1   955.27  999.27   0.883 0.3475044
## cut2(sapsi_first, g = 5) 4   989.69 1027.69  35.304 4.023e-07 ***
## cut2(sofa_first, g = 5)  4   960.95  998.95   6.558 0.1611514
## service_unit             2   960.11 1002.11   5.716 0.0573820 .
## chf_flg                  1   955.38  999.38   0.990 0.3196816
## afib_flg                 1   960.47 1004.47   6.080 0.0136708 *
## renal_flg                1   958.20 1002.20   3.814 0.0508182 .
## liver_flg                1   956.23 1000.23   1.839 0.1750410
## copd_flg                 1   955.28  999.28   0.893 0.3445691
## cad_flg                  1   955.20  999.20   0.811 0.3678829
## stroke_flg               1  1045.22 1089.22  90.831 < 2.2e-16 ***
## mal_flg                  1   959.80 1003.80   5.410 0.0200201 *
## resp_flg                 1   967.57 1011.57  13.177 0.0002834 ***
## ---
## Signif. codes:  0 '***' 0.001 '**' 0.01 '*' 0.05 '.' 0.1 ' ' 1
```

As you see from the output, each covariate is listed, along with a *p*-value (`Pr(>Chi)`). Each row represents a hypothesis test with the bigger (alternative model) being the full model (`mva.full.glm`), and each null being the full model without the row's covariate. The *p*-values here should match those output if you were to do this exact test with `anova`. As we can see from the listed *p*-values, `aline_flg` has the largest *p*-value, but we stipulated in our model selection plan that we would retain this covariate as it's our covariate of interest. We will then go to the next largest *p*-value which is the `cad_flg` variable (coronary artery disease). We will update our model, and repeat the backwards elimination step on the updated model. We could just cut and paste the `mva.full.glm` command and remove + `cad_flg`, but an easier way less prone to errors is to use the `update`

16.5 Case Study and Summary

command. The `update` function can take a `glm` or `lm` object, and alter one of the covariates. To do a backwards elimination, the second argument is `. ~ . - variable`. The `. ~ .` part indicates keep the outcome and the rest of the variables the same, and the `- variable` indicates to fit the model without the variable called `variable`. Hence, to fit a new model from the full model, but without the `cad_flg` variable, we would run:

```
mva.tmp.glm <- update(mva.full.glm, .~. - cad_flg)
```

We then repeat the `drop1` step:

```
drop1(mva.tmp.glm,test="Chisq")
```

```
## Single term deletions
##
## Model:
## day_28_flg ~ aline_flg + age + gender_num + cut2(sapsi_first,
##     g = 5) + cut2(sofa_first, g = 5) + service_unit + chf_flg +
##     afib_flg + renal_flg + liver_flg + copd_flg + stroke_flg +
##     mal_flg + resp_flg
##                     Df Deviance     AIC     LRT  Pr(>Chi)
## <none>                   955.20  999.20
## aline_flg            1   955.20  997.20   0.002 0.9674503
## age                  1  1000.92 1042.92  45.715 1.368e-11 ***
## gender_num           1   955.98  997.98   0.784 0.3760520
## cut2(sapsi_first, g = 5)  4  990.38 1026.38  35.180 4.266e-07 ***
## cut2(sofa_first, g = 5)   4  961.75  997.75   6.552 0.1615399
## service_unit         2   960.98 1000.98   5.782 0.0555160 .
## chf_flg              1   955.92  997.92   0.719 0.3965762
## afib_flg             1   961.32 1003.32   6.115 0.0134006 *
## renal_flg            1   959.97 1001.97   4.774 0.0288966 *
## liver_flg            1   957.06  999.06   1.862 0.1723427
## copd_flg             1   956.02  998.02   0.824 0.3640764
## stroke_flg           1  1045.73 1087.73  90.526 < 2.2e-16 ***
## mal_flg              1   960.64 1002.64   5.435 0.0197326 *
## resp_flg             1   968.84 1010.84  13.638 0.0002217 ***
## ---
## Signif. codes:  0 '***' 0.001 '**' 0.01 '*' 0.05 '.' 0.1 ' ' 1
```

and see that `aline_flg` still has the largest *p*-value, but `chf_flag` has the second largest, so we'll choose to remove it next. To update the new model, and run another elimination step, we would run:

```
mva.tmp.glm2 <- update(mva.tmp.glm, .~. - chf_flg)
drop1(mva.tmp.glm2,test="Chisq")
```

```
## Single term deletions
##
## Model:
## day_28_flg ~ aline_flg + age + gender_num + cut2(sapsi_first,
##     g = 5) + cut2(sofa_first, g = 5) + service_unit + afib_flg +
##     renal_flg + liver_flg + copd_flg + stroke_flg + mal_flg +
##     resp_flg
##                          Df Deviance    AIC     LRT  Pr(>Chi)
## <none>                       955.92  997.92
## aline_flg                 1   955.93  995.93   0.016 0.9003547
## age                       1  1005.90 1045.90  49.976 1.556e-12 ***
## gender_num                1   956.65  996.65   0.734 0.3916088
## cut2(sapsi_first, g = 5)  4   991.04 1025.04  35.121 4.387e-07 ***
## cut2(sofa_first, g = 5)   4   962.39  996.39   6.467 0.1669071
## service_unit              2   962.45 1000.45   6.529 0.0382253 *
## afib_flg                  1   963.01 1003.01   7.090 0.0077512 **
## renal_flg                 1   960.24 1000.24   4.321 0.0376445 *
## liver_flg                 1   957.70  997.70   1.780 0.1821692
## copd_flg                  1   956.95  996.95   1.035 0.3088774
## stroke_flg                1  1045.73 1085.73  89.808 < 2.2e-16 ***
## mal_flg                   1   961.15 1001.15   5.231 0.0221921 *
## resp_flg                  1   970.13 1010.13  14.214 0.0001632 ***
## ---
## Signif. codes:  0 '***' 0.001 '**' 0.01 '*' 0.05 '.' 0.1 ' ' 1
```

where again `aline_flg` has the largest *p*-value, and `gender_num` has the second largest. We continue, eliminating `gender_num`, `copd_flg`, `liver_flg`, `cut2(sofa_first, g = 5)`, `renal_flg`, and `service_unit`, in that order (results omitted). The table produced by `drop1` from our final model is as follows:

```
drop1(mva.tmp.glm8,test="Chisq")
```

```
## Single term deletions
##
## Model:
## day_28_flg ~ aline_flg + age + cut2(sapsi_first, g = 5) + afib_flg +
##     stroke_flg + mal_flg + resp_flg
##                          Df Deviance    AIC     LRT  Pr(>Chi)
## <none>                       989.10 1011.1
## aline_flg                 1   989.10 1009.1   0.001 0.977380
## age                       1  1037.65 1057.7  48.556 3.209e-12 ***
## cut2(sapsi_first, g = 5)  4  1037.88 1051.9  48.788 6.465e-10 ***
## afib_flg                  1   995.60 1015.6   6.502 0.010777 *
## stroke_flg                1  1078.58 1098.6  89.485 < 2.2e-16 ***
## mal_flg                   1   997.37 1017.4   8.274 0.004021 **
## resp_flg                  1  1022.30 1042.3  33.200 8.317e-09 ***
## ---
## Signif. codes:  0 '***' 0.001 '**' 0.01 '*' 0.05 '.' 0.1 ' ' 1
```

All variables are statistically significant at the 0.05 significance level. Looking at the `summary` output, we see that `aline_flg` is not statistically significant (p = 0.98), but all other terms are statistically significant, with the exception of the `cut2(sapsi_first, g = 5)[12,14)`, which suggest that the second to

16.5 Case Study and Summary

lowest SAPS group may not be statistically significantly different than the baseline (lowest SAPS group).

```
mva.final.glm <- mva.tmp.glm8;
summary(mva.final.glm)

## 
## Call:
## glm(formula = day_28_flg ~ aline_flg + age + cut2(sapsi_first,
##     g = 5) + afib_flg + stroke_flg + mal_flg + resp_flg, family = "binomial",
##     data = dat)
## 
## Deviance Residuals:
##     Min       1Q   Median       3Q      Max
## -2.3025  -0.4928  -0.2433  -0.1289   3.1103
## 
## Coefficients:
##                             Estimate Std. Error z value Pr(>|z|)
## (Intercept)                 -6.081944   0.445625 -13.648  < 2e-16 ***
## aline_flg1                   0.005078   0.179090   0.028  0.97738
## age                          0.037205   0.005644   6.592 4.33e-11 ***
## cut2(sapsi_first, g = 5)[12,14)  0.302084   0.391502   0.772  0.44035
## cut2(sapsi_first, g = 5)[14,16)  1.127302   0.344670   3.271  0.00107 **
## cut2(sapsi_first, g = 5)[16,19)  1.030901   0.347842   2.964  0.00304 **
## cut2(sapsi_first, g = 5)[19,32]  1.883738   0.347311   5.424 5.84e-08 ***
## afib_flg1                    0.522664   0.203485   2.569  0.01021 *
## stroke_flg1                  1.870553   0.199980   9.354  < 2e-16 ***
## mal_flg1                     0.592458   0.202297   2.929  0.00340 **
## resp_flg1                    0.976808   0.171629   5.691 1.26e-08 ***
## ---
## Signif. codes:  0 '***' 0.001 '**' 0.01 '*' 0.05 '.' 0.1 ' ' 1
## 
## (Dispersion parameter for binomial family taken to be 1)
## 
##     Null deviance: 1413.4  on 1690  degrees of freedom
## Residual deviance:  989.1  on 1680  degrees of freedom
##   (85 observations deleted due to missingness)
## AIC: 1011.1
## 
## Number of Fisher Scoring iterations: 6
```

We would call this model our final model, and would present it in a table similar to Table 16.4. Since the effect of IAC was of particular focus, we will highlight it by saying that it is not associated with 28 day mortality with an estimated adjusted odds ratio of 1.01 (95 % CI: 0.71–1.43, p = 0.98). We may conclude that after adjusting for the other potential confounders found in Table 16.4, we do not find any statistically significant impact of using IAC on mortality.

16.5.4 Conclusion and Summary

This brief overview of the modeling techniques for health data has provided you with the foundation to perform the most common types of analyses in health studies. We have cited how important having a clear study objective before

Table 16.4 Multivariable logistic regression analysis for mortality at 28 days outcome (final model)

Covariate	AOR	Lower 95 % CI	Upper 95 % CI	p-value
IAC	1.01	0.71	1.43	0.977
Age (per year increase)	1.04	1.03	1.05	<0.001
SAPSI [12–14]* (relative to SAPSI <2)	1.35	0.63	2.97	0.440
SAPSI [14–16]*	3.09	1.61	6.28	0.001
SAPSI [16–19]*	2.80	1.45	5.74	0.003
SAPSI [19–32]*	6.58	3.42	13.46	<0.001
Atrial fibrillation	1.69	1.13	2.51	0.010
Stroke	6.49	4.40	9.64	<0.001
Malignancy	1.81	1.21	2.68	0.003
Non-COPD respiratory disease	2.66	1.90	3.73	<0.001

conducting data analysis is, as it identifies all the important aspects you need to plan and execute your analysis. In particular by identifying the outcome, you should be able to determine what analysis methodology would be most appropriate. Often you will find that you will be using multiple analysis techniques for different study objectives within the same study. Table 16.5 summarizes some of the important aspects of each analysis approach.

Fortunately, R's framework for conducting these analyses is very similar across the different types of techniques, and this framework will often extend more generally to other more complex models (including machine learning algorithms) and data structures (including dependent/correlated data such as longitudinal data).

Table 16.5 Summary of different methods

	Linear regression	Logistic regression	Cox proportional hazards model
Outcome data type	Continuous	Binary	Time to an event (possibly censored)
Useful preliminary analysis	Scatterplot	Contingency and 2 × 2 tables	Kaplan-Meier survivor function estimate
Presentation Output	Coefficient	Odds Ratio	Hazard ratio
R output	Coefficient	Log Odds ratio	Log hazard ratio
Presentation Interpretation	An estimate of the expected change in the outcome per one unit increase in the covariate, while keeping all other covariates constant	An estimate of the fold change in the odds of the outcome per unit increase in the covariate, while keeping all other covariates constant	An estimate of the fold change in the hazards of the outcome per unit increase in the covariate, while keeping all other covariates constant

16.5 Case Study and Summary

We have highlighted some areas of concern that careful attention should be paid to including missing data, colinearity, model misspecification, and outliers. Some of these items will be looked at more closely in Chap. 17.

Open Access This chapter is distributed under the terms of the Creative Commons Attribution-NonCommercial 4.0 International License (http://creativecommons.org/licenses/by-nc/4.0/), which permits any noncommercial use, duplication, adaptation, distribution and reproduction in any medium or format, as long as you give appropriate credit to the original author(s) and the source, a link is provided to the Creative Commons license and any changes made are indicated.

The images or other third party material in this chapter are included in the work's Creative Commons license, unless indicated otherwise in the credit line; if such material is not included in the work's Creative Commons license and the respective action is not permitted by statutory regulation, users will need to obtain permission from the license holder to duplicate, adapt or reproduce the material.

References

1. Hsu DJ, Feng M, Kothari R, Zhou H, Chen KP, Celi LA (2015) The association between indwelling arterial catheters and mortality in hemodynamically stable patients with respiratory failure: a propensity score analysis. CHEST J 148(6):1470–1476
2. Goldberger AL, Amaral LA, Glass L, Hausdorff JM, Ivanov PC, Mark RG, Mietus JE, Moody GB, Peng C-K, Stanley HE (2000) Physiobank, physiotoolkit, and physionet components of a new research resource for complex physiologic signals. Circulation 101(23):e215–e220
3. Indwelling arterial catheter clinical data from the MIMIC II database (2016) Available http://physionet.org/physiobank/database/mimic2-iaccd/. Accessed: 02 Jun 2016
4. Friedman J, Hastie T, Tibshirani R (2009) The elements of statistical learning: data mining, inference, and prediction. Springer series in statistics
5. James G, Witten D, Hastie T, Tibshirani R (2013) An introduction to statistical learning, vol 112. Springer, Berlin
6. Harrell F (2015) Regression modeling strategies: with applications to linear models, logistic and ordinal regression, and survival analysis. Springer, Berlin
7. Venables WN, Ripley BD (2013) Modern applied statistics with S-plus. Springer Science & Business Media
8. Weisberg S (2005) Applied linear regression, vol 528. Wiley, New York
9. Diggle P, Heagerty P, Liang KY, Zeger S (2013) Analysis of longitudinal data. OUP Oxford
10. McCullagh P, Nelder JA (1989) Generalized linear models, vol 37. CRC press, Boca Raton
11. Hosmer DW, Lemeshow S (2004) Applied logistic regression. Wiley, New York
12. Kleinbaum DG, Klein M (2006) Survival analysis: a self-learning text. Springer Science & Business Media
13. Kaplan EL, Meier P (1958) Nonparametric estimation from incomplete observations. J Am Stat Assoc 53(282):457–481
14. Cox DR (1972) Regression models and life-tables. J R Stat Soc Ser B (Methodol) 34(2):187–220
15. Collett D (2015) Modelling survival data in medical research. CRC press, Boca Raton
16. Kalbfleisch JD, Prentice RL (2011) The statistical analysis of failure time data, vol 360. Wiley, New York
17. Therneau TM, Grambsch PM (2000) Modeling survival data: extending the Cox model. Springer Science & Business Media
18. Dash M, Liu H (1997) Feature selection for classification. Intel Data Anal 1(3):131–156

Chapter 17
Sensitivity Analysis and Model Validation

Justin D. Salciccioli, Yves Crutain, Matthieu Komorowski
and Dominic C. Marshall

Learning Objectives

- Appreciate that all models possess inherent limitations for generalizability.
- Understand the assumptions for making causal inferences from available data.
- Check model fit and performance.

17.1 Introduction

Imagine that you have now finished the primary analyses of your current research and have been able to reject the null hypothesis. Even after your chosen methods have been applied and robust models generated, some doubts may remain. *"How confident are you in the results? How much will the results change if your basic data is slightly wrong? Will that have a minor impact on your results? Or will it give a completely different outcome?"* Causal inference is often limited by the assumptions made in study design and analysis and this is particularly pronounced when working with observational health data. An important approach for any investigator is to avoid relying on any single analytical approach to assess the hypothesis and as such, a critical next step is to test the assumptions made in the analysis.

Sensitivity Analysis and Model Validation are linked in that they are both attempts to assess the appropriateness of a particular model specification and to appreciate the strength of the conclusions being drawn from such a model. Whereas model validation is useful for assessing the model fit within a specific research dataset, sensitivity analysis is particularly useful in gaining confidence in the results of the primary analysis and is important in situations where a model is likely to be used in a future research investigation or in clinical practice. Herein, we discuss concepts relating to the assessment of model fit and outline broadly the steps relating to cross and external validation with direct application to the arterial line project. We will discuss briefly a few of the common reasons why models fail validity testing and the potential implications of such failure.

17.2 Part 1—Theoretical Concepts

17.2.1 Bias and Variance

In statistics and machine learning, the bias–variance trade-off (or dilemma) is the problem of simultaneously minimizing two sources of error that prevent supervised learning algorithms from generalizing beyond their training set. A model with high bias fails to accurately estimate the data. For example, a linear regression model would have high bias when trying to model a quadratic relationship—no matter how the parameters are set (as shown in Fig. 17.1). Variance, on the other hand, relates to the stability of your model in response to new training examples. An algorithm that fits the training data very well but generalizes poorly to new examples (showing over-fitting) is said to have high variance.

Some common strategies for dealing with bias and variance are outlined below.

- High bias:
  - Adding features (predictors) tends to decrease bias, at the expense of introducing additional variance.
  - Adding training examples will not fix high bias, because the underlying model will still not be able to approximate the correct function.
- High variance:
  - Reducing model complexity can help decrease variance. Dimensionality reduction and feature selection are two examples of methods to decrease model parameters and thus reduce variance (parameter selection is discussed below).
  - A larger training set tends to decrease variance.

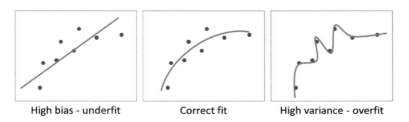

Fig. 17.1 Comparison between bias and variance in model development

17.2.2 Common Evaluation Tools

A variety of statistical techniques exist to quantitatively assess the performance of statistical models. These techniques are important, but generally beyond the scope of this textbook. We will, however, briefly mention two of the most common techniques: the R^2 value used for regressions and the Receiver Operating Characteristic (ROC) curve used for binary classifier (dichotomous outcome).

The R^2 value is a summary statistic representing the proportion of total variance in the outcome variable that is captured by the model. The R^2 has a range from 0 to 1 where values close to 0 reflect situations where the model does not appreciably summarise variation in the outcome of interest and values close to 1 indicate that the model captures nearly all of the variation in the outcome of interest. High R^2 values means that a high proportion of the variance is explained by the regression model. In R programming, the R^2 is computed when the linear regression function is used. For an example of R-code to produce the R^2 value please refer to the "R^2" function.

The R^2 value is an overall measure of strength of association between the model and the outcome and does not reflect the contribution of any single independent predictor variable. Further, while we may expect intuitively that there is a proportional relationship between the number of predictor variables and the overall model R^2, in practice, adding predictors does not necessarily increase R^2 in new data. It is possible for an individual predictor to decrease the R^2 depending on how this variable interacts with the other parameters in the model.

For the purpose of this discussion we expect the reader to be familiar with the computation and utility of the values of sensitivity and specificity. In situations such as developing a new diagnostic test, investigators may define a single threshold value to classify a test result as positive. When dealing with a dichotomous outcome, the Receiver Operating Characteristic (ROC) curve is a more complete description of a model's ability to classify outcomes. The ROC curve is a common method to show the relationship between the sensitivity of a classification model and its false positive rate (1 - specificity). The resultant Area Under the Curve of the ROC reflects the prediction estimate of the model, can take values from 0.5 to 1 with values of 0.5 implying near random chance in outcomes and values nearer to 1 reflecting greater prediction. For an example of ROC curves in R, please refer to the "ROC" function in the accompanying code. For further reading on the ROC curve, see for example the article by Fawcett [1] (Fig. 17.2).

17.2.3 Sensitivity Analysis

Sensitivity analysis involves a series of methods to quantify how the uncertainty in the output of a model is related to the uncertainty in its inputs. In other words, sensitivity analysis assesses how "sensitive" the model is to fluctuations in the parameters and data on which it is built. The results of sensitivity analysis can have

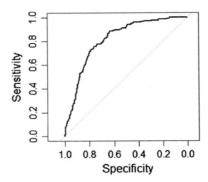

Fig. 17.2 Example of receiver operator characteristic (ROC) curve which may be used to assess the ability of a model to discriminate between dichotomous outcomes

important implications at many stages of the modeling process, including for identifying errors in the model itself, informing the calibration of model parameters, and exploring more broadly the relationship between the inputs and outputs of the model.

The principles of a sensitivity analysis are: (a) to allow the investigator to quantify the uncertainty in a model, (b) to test the model of interest using a secondary experimental design, and (c) using the results of the secondary experimental design to calculate the overall sensitivity of the model of interest. The justification for sensitivity analysis is that a model will always perform better (i.e. over-perform) when tested on the dataset from which it was derived. Sub-group analysis is a common variation of sensitivity analysis [2].

17.2.4 Validation

As discussed in Chap. 16—Data Analysis validation is used to confirm that the model of interest will perform similarly under modified testing conditions. As such, it is the primary responsibility of the investigator to assess the suitability of model fit to the data. This may be accomplished with a variety of methodological approaches and for a more detailed discussion of model fit diagnostics the reader is referred to other sources [3]. Although it is beyond the scope of this textbook to discuss validation in detail, the general theory is to select a model based on two principles: model parsimony and clinical relevance. A number of pre-defined model selection algorithm-based approaches including Forward selection, Backward, and Stepwise selection, but also lasso and genetic algorithms, available in common statistical packages. Please refer to Chap. 16 for further information about model selection.

Cross validation is a technique used to assess the predictive ability of a regression model. The approach has been discussed in detail previously [4]. The concept of cross-validation relies on the principle that a large enough dataset can split into two or more (not necessarily equally sized) sub-groups, the first being used to derive the model and the additional data set(s) reserved for model testing and validation. To avoid losing information by training the model only on a subset of available data, a variant called k-fold cross validation exist (not discussed here).

External validation is defined as testing the model on a sample of subjects taken from a population different than the original cohort. External validation is usually a more robust approach for testing the derived model in that the maximum amount of information has been used from the initial dataset to derive a model and an entirely independent dataset is used subsequently to verify the suitability of the model of interest. Although external validation is the most rigorous and an essential validation method, finding a suitably similar albeit entirely independent cohort for external validation is challenging and is often unavailable for researchers. However, with the increasing amount of healthcare data being captured electronically it is likely that researchers will also have increasing capacity for external validation.

17.3 Case Study: Examples of Validation and Sensitivity Analysis

This case study used the dataset produced for the "IAC study", which evaluated the impact of inserting an arterial line in intensive care patients with respiratory failure. Three different sensitivity analyses were performed:

1. Test the effects of varying the inclusion criteria of time to mechanical ventilation and mortality;
2. Test the effects of changes in caliper level for propensity matching on association between arterial catheter insertion and the mortality;
3. Hosmer-Lemeshow Goodness-of-Fit test to assess the overall fit of the data to the model of interest.

A number of R packages from CRAN, were used to conduct these analyses: Multivariate and Propensity Score Matching [5], analysis of complex survey samples [6], ggplot2 for generating graphics [7], pROC for ROC curves [8] and Twang for weighting and analyzing non-equivalent groups [9].

17.3.1 Analysis 1: Varying the Inclusion Criteria of Time to Mechanical Ventilation

The first sensitivity analysis evaluates the effect of varying the inclusion criteria of time to mechanical ventilation and mortality. Mechanical ventilation is one of the more common invasive interventions performed in the ICU and the timing of intervention may serve as a surrogate for the severity of critical illness, as we might

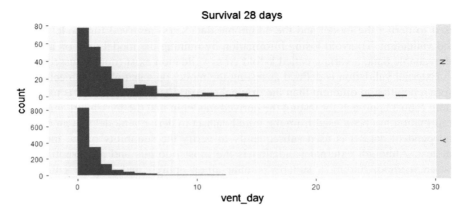

Fig. 17.3 Simple sensitivity analysis to compare outcomes between groups by varying the inclusion criteria. Modification of the inclusion criteria for subjects entered into the model is a common sensitivity analysis

expect patients with worse illness to require assisted ventilation earlier in the course of intensive care. As such, mechanical ventilation along with indwelling arterial catheter (IAC), another invasive intervention, may both be related to the outcome of interest, 28-day mortality. An example of R-code to inspect the distribution across groups of patients by ventilation status is provided in the "Cohort" function, in the accompanying R functions document (Fig. 17.3).

By modifying the time of first assisted mechanical ventilation we may also obtain important information about the effect of the primary exposure on the outcome. An example of R-code for this analysis is provided in the "Ventilation" function.

17.3.2 Analysis 2: Changing the Caliper Level for Propensity Matching

The second sensitivity analysis performed tests the impact of different caliper levels for propensity matching on the association between arterial catheter and the mortality. In this study, the propensity score matches a subject who did not received an arterial catheter with a subject who did. The matching algorithm creates a pair of two independent subjects whose propensity scores are the most similar. However, the investigator is responsible for setting a maximum reasonable difference in propensity score which would allow the matching algorithm to generate a suitable match; this maximum reasonable difference is also known as the propensity score 'caliper'. The choice of caliper for the propensity score match will directly influence the variance bias trade-off such that a wider caliper will result in matching of subjects which are more dissimilar with respect to likelihood of treatment. An

17.3 Case Study: Examples of Validation ...

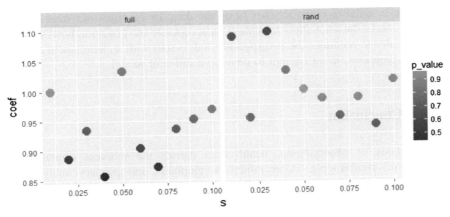

Fig. 17.4 A sensitivity analysis to assess the effect of modifying the propensity score caliper level

example of the R-code to produce a sensitivity analysis for varying the propensity score caliper level is provided in the accompanying R functions document as the "Caliper" function.

The Fig. 17.4 displays the effect of adjustments of the caliper level on the propensity score. The full model shows a lower coefficient due to the presence of additional variables.

17.3.3 Analysis 3: Hosmer-Lemeshow Test

The Hosmer-Lemeshow Goodness-of-Fit test may be used to assess the overall fit of the data to the model of interest [10]. For this test, the subjects are grouped according to a percentile of risk (usually deciles). A Pearson Chi square statistic is generated to compare observed subject grouping with the expected risk according to the model. An example of the R-code to conduct this test is provided in the accompanying R functions document as the "HL" function.

17.3.4 Implications for a 'Failing' Model

In the favorable situation of a robust model, each sensitivity analysis and validation technique supports the model as an appropriate summary of the data. However, in some situations, the chosen validation method or sensitivity analysis reveals an inadequate fit of the model for the data such that the model fails to accurately predict the outcome of interest. A 'failing' model may be the result of a number of different factors. Occasionally, it is possible to modify the model derivation procedure in order to claim a better fit on the data. In the situations where modifying the model does not allow to achieve an acceptable level of error, however, it is good practice to renounce the investigation and re-start with an assessment of the a priori assumptions, in an attempt to develop a different model.

17.4 Conclusion

The analysis of observational health data carries the inherent limitation of unmeasured confounding. After model development and primary analysis, an important step is to confirm a model's performance with a series of confirmatory tests to verify a valid model. While validation may be used to check that the model is an appropriate fit for the data and is likely to perform similarly in other cohorts, sensitivity analysis may be used to interrogate inherent assumptions of the primary analysis. When performed adequately these additional steps help improve the robustness of the overall analysis and aid the investigator in making meaningful inferences from observational health data.

Take Home Messages

1. Validation and sensitivity analyses test the robustness of the model assumptions and are a key step in the modeling process;
2. The key principle of these analyses is to vary the model assumptions and observe how the model responds;
3. Failing the validation and sensitivity analyses might require the researcher to start with a new model.

Open Access This chapter is distributed under the terms of the Creative Commons Attribution-NonCommercial 4.0 International License (http://creativecommons.org/licenses/by-nc/4.0/), which permits any noncommercial use, duplication, adaptation, distribution and reproduction in any medium or format, as long as you give appropriate credit to the original author(s) and the source, a link is provided to the Creative Commons license and any changes made are indicated.

The images or other third party material in this chapter are included in the work's Creative Commons license, unless indicated otherwise in the credit line; if such material is not included in the work's Creative Commons license and the respective action is not permitted by statutory regulation, users will need to obtain permission from the license holder to duplicate, adapt or reproduce the material.

Code Appendix

The code used in this chapter is available in the GitHub repository for this book: https://github.com/MIT-LCP/critical-data-book. Further information on the code is available from this website.

References

1. Fawcett T (2006) An introduction to ROC analysis. Pattern Recogn Lett 27(8):861–874
2. Brookes ST, Whitely E, Egger M, Smith GD, Mulheran PA, Peters TJ (2004) Subgroup analyses in randomized trials: risks of subgroup-specific analyses; power and sample size for the interaction test. J Clin Epidemiol 57(3):229–236
3. Pregibon D (1981) Logistic regression diagnostics. Ann Stat 9(4):705–724
4. Picard RR, Cook RD (1984) Cross-validation of regression models. J Am Stat Assoc 79(387):575–583
5. Sekhon JS (2011) Multivariate and propensity score matching software with automated balance optimization: the matching package for R. J Stat Softw 42(i07)
6. Lumley T (2004) Analysis of complex survey samples. J Stat Softw 09(i08)
7. Wickham H (2009) ggplot2. Springer, New York
8. Robin X, Turck N, Hainard A, Tiberti N, Lisacek F, Sanchez J-C, Müller M (2011) pROC: an open-source package for R and S + to analyze and compare ROC curves. BMC Bioinf 12:77
9. Ridgeway G, Mccaffrey D, Morral A, Burgette L, Griffin BA (2006) Twang: toolkit for weighting and analysis of nonequivalent groups. R package version 1.4-9.3. In: R Foundation for Statistical Computing, 2006. (http://www.cran.r-project.org). Accessed 2015
10. Hosmer DW, Lemesbow S (1980) Goodness of fit tests for the multiple logistic regression model. Commun Stat Theory Methods 9(10):1043–1069

Part III
Case Studies Using MIMIC

Introduction

This section presents twelve case studies of secondary analyses of electronic health records (EHRs). The case studies exhibit a wide range of research topics and methodologies, making them of interest to a wide range of researchers. They are written primarily for the beginner, although the experienced researcher will also benefit much from the detailed explanations offered by experts in the field. The case studies provide an opportunity to thoroughly engage with high-level research studies, since they are accompanied by both publicly available data and analytical code. This section should not be approached as a continuous narrative. Rather, each case study can be read independently. Indeed, it is advisable to begin with those which lie closest to your interests. An overview of the research areas and methodologies of the case studies is now provided.

The case studies are ordered according to their research areas. The first two case studies concern system-level analyses, beginning with an analysis of the trends in clinical practice with regard to mechanical ventilation (Chap. 18). This is followed by an investigation into the effect of caring for critically-ill patients in "non-target ICUs", otherwise known as boarding, on mortality (Chap. 19). The next three case studies focus on mortality prediction using a plethora of inputs such as demographics, vital signs and laboratory test results (Chaps. 20–22). Two case studies investigate the effectiveness of a clinical intervention, with assessments of clinical effectiveness (Chap. 23) and cost effectiveness (Chap. 24). A study of the relationship between blood pressure and the risk of Acute Kidney Injury is presented, illustrating the physiological insights that can be gained by analysis of EHRs (Chap. 25). Two case studies are then presented on monitoring techniques: an investigation into the estimation of respiratory rate, a key physiological parameter, from routinely acquired physiological signals (Chap. 26); and a detailed study of the potential for false alarm reduction using machine learning classification techniques (Chap. 27). Finally two studies consider particular aspects of research methodology, focusing on patient cohort identification (Chap. 28) and mathematical techniques for selection of hyperparameters (Chap. 29).

A plethora of methodologies are demonstrated in the case studies. The machine learning techniques used include: regression, support vector machines, decision trees (Chap. 21), random forest classification (Chap. 27), Markov models (Chap. 24), and a Super Learner algorithm to fuse multiple techniques (Chap. 20). Other analytical approaches include instrumental variable analysis (Chap. 19), propensity score matching (Chap. 23), case-control and case-crossover designs (Chap. 25), signal processing (Chaps. 26 and 27), and natural language processing (Chap. 28).

The aim of this section is to provide readers with examples of secondary EHR analyses to empower them in their own research. We hope that the clinical relevance of the investigations will inspire researchers to realize the full potential of EHRs for the benefit of the patients of tomorrow. The detailed descriptions of study methodologies are intended to provide an understanding of the nuances of EHR analyses. Finally, a range of tools are available to underpin novel investigations: both the data and the analytical code used in this Section are publicly available. Further details of these tools are provided in the accompanying GitHub repository: https://github.com/MIT-LCP/critical-data-book.

Chapter 18
Trend Analysis: Evolution of Tidal Volume Over Time for Patients Receiving Invasive Mechanical Ventilation

Anuj Mehta, Franck Dernoncourt and Allan Walkey

Learning Objectives

Learn the importance of trend analysis

- To understand epidemiological changes in health and delivery of healthcare.
- To assess the implementation of new evidence into clinical practice.
- Assess real world effectiveness of discoveries (interrupted time series design; difference in differences, regression discontinuity).

Learn methods of performing trend analysis

- Cochrane-Armitage test for trend.
- Differences Logistic/linear regression analysis with time as an independent variable.

Addressing changes in aspects of the study population over time with relation to the main dependent and independent variables

- Adjustment/confounding.
- Interaction of covariates with time and outcomes.

Refining the research question

- Addressing limitations in the data.

18.1 Introduction

Healthcare is a dynamic field that is constantly evolving in response to changes in disease epidemiology, population demographics, and new discoveries. Epidemiologic changes in disease prevalence and outcomes have important implications for determining healthcare resource allocation. For example, identifying trends that show increasing utilization of invasive mechanical ventilation may suggest local or societal needs for more intensive care unit beds, critical care nurses and physicians, and mechanical ventilators. Additionally, changes in healthcare outcomes over time can provide insight into the adoption of new scientific knowledge and identify targets for quality improvement where implementation of evidence has been slow or where results from tightly-controlled trials are not realized in the "real world". Trend analyses utilize statistical methods in an attempt to quantify changes to better understand the evolution of health and healthcare delivery.

To highlight the uses of trend analysis, we present a study evaluating how scientific evidence supporting treatment of one condition may be generalized by healthcare professionals to other conditions in which the treatment is untested. We investigated adoption of evidence supporting lower tidal volumes during mechanical ventilation for patients admitted to the medical intensive care unit (MICU) compared to the cardiac care unit (CCU).

Critically ill patients can develop severe difficulty breathing and may require the assistance of a breathing machine (ventilator) through a process called invasive mechanical ventilation. Patients may require invasive mechanical ventilation for a wide variety of conditions such as pneumonia, asthma, and heart failure. In some cases, the lungs fall victim to massive inflammation triggered by severe systemic diseases such as infection, trauma, or aspiration. The inflammation leads to leakage of fluid into the lungs (pulmonary edema) in a condition called the acute respiratory distress syndrome (ARDS). ARDS is defined by four criteria [1]:

1. Acute in nature
2. Bilateral infiltrates on chest x-ray
3. Not caused by heart failure (as heart failure can also cause pulmonary edema)
4. Severe hypoxia defined by the partial pressure of arterial oxygen to fraction of inspired oxygen (P/F) ratio

Regardless of the cause of respiratory failure, many patients receiving invasive mechanical ventilation develop ARDS.

Mechanical Ventilators are most often set to deliver one volume of air for each breath (i.e. tidal volume). Too much air delivered during each breath can cause over-stretch and injury to already impaired lungs, resulting in yet further damage by the systemic release of inflammatory chemicals. In the setting of ARDS, large tidal volumes cause already inflamed lungs to release more inflammatory chemicals that can cause further lung damage but also damage to other organs. Based on the theory that lower tidal volumes may act to protect the lungs and other organs by decreasing lung over-distention and release of inflammatory chemicals during invasive mechanical ventilation, a landmark study demonstrated that use of lower tidal volumes for patients receiving invasive mechanical ventilation with ARDS resulted in an absolute mortality reduction of 8.8 % [2]. Since then, several studies have demonstrated improvements in mortality over time for patients with ARDS [3–6] as well as a reduction in the tidal volumes used in all patients in MICUs [3, 7].

Because the definition of ARDS strictly excludes patients with heart failure, patients with heart failure have been excluded from studies evaluating effects and

18.1 Introduction

epidemiology of tidal volume reduction. In order to fill current knowledge gaps regarding tidal volume selection among patients with heart failure, we sought to use trend analysis to explore temporal changes in tidal volumes among patients with heart failure as compared to patients with ARDS. In order to address difficulties with identifying the indication for mechanical ventilation in electronic health records, we adjusted our analytic plan to focus on trends in tidal volume selection in CCUs (where heart failure is the most common cause of invasive mechanical ventilation) as compared to MICUs (where most patients with ARDS receive care).

18.2 Study Dataset

In this case study we used the Medical Information Mart for Intensive Care II (MIMIC-II) database version 3 [8], which contains de-identified, granular patient-level information for 48,018 patients across 57,995 ICU hospitalizations at a single academic center from 2002 to 2011. The MIMIC II Clinical Database is a relational database that contains individual values for a variety of patient variables such as lab results, vital signs, and billing codes.

18.3 Study Pre-processing

We identified patients in MIMIC-II who received invasive mechanical ventilation. We excluded patients <18 years of age; pediatric critical care practices and the physiology of pediatric patients differ from adult patients. While we initially sought to compare patients with ARDS to patients with heart failure, accurate identification of specific indications for mechanical ventilation in electronic health records was difficult and subject to misclassification. Thus, we selected patients admitted to the MICU as a surrogate for patients with ARDS [3, 7] and patients admitted to the CCU as a surrogate for patients with heart failure. We excluded patients whose initial ICU service was a surgical ICU as the majority of patients would likely have been receiving invasive mechanical ventilation for routine post-operative care. For patients who were admitted to multiple different intensive care units (ICU) during a single hospitalization, we based inclusion/exclusion criteria on the initial ICU admission. We further excluded patients who had missing data on tidal volume.

18.4 Study Methods

Our primary outcome was average tidal volume ordered by clinicians during assist-control ventilation. We used the Cochrane-Armitage test for trends to evaluate changes over time in the percentage of patients in each unit who required invasive mechanical ventilation. We calculated the average tidal volume for the entire period of assisted invasive mechanical ventilation for each patient and then calculated the average of tidal volumes for the MICU and CCU each year. In order to assess for a temporal trend in tidal volume, we performed multivariable linear regression (see Sect. 5.2 in Chap. 5 on Data Analysis for details) stratified by ICU type. Analyses for trends in tidal volume change over time included a dependent (outcome) variable of tidal volume and independent variable (exposure) of time (year of intensive care admission). Year of admission is a common time variable chosen for trend analysis. Smaller sample sizes can result in large amounts of noise and fluctuations when analyzing shorter time frames such as 'month'. We chose multivariable linear regression because tidal volume is a continuous variable and because regression techniques allowed for adjustment of effect estimates for possible confounders of the relationship between time and tidal volume. We adjusted for patient age and gender as both could affect tidal volume selection. To determine differences in tidal volume trends between the MICU and CCU, we included an interaction term between time and patient location in regression models. In order to determine if variability in average tidal volumes had changed over time, we compared the coefficient of variation (standard deviation normalized to the sample mean) at the beginning of the study to the end of the study, in each unit [9]. All testing was done at an alpha level = 0.05.

All studies were deemed exempt by the Institutional Review Boards of Boston Medical Center and Beth Israel Deaconess. All statistical testing was performed with SAS 9.4 (Cary, NC).

18.5 Study Analysis

We identified 7083 patients receiving invasive mechanical ventilation in the MICU and 3085 patients in the CCU from 2002 to 2011. The number of patients receiving invasive mechanical ventilation in the MICU fluctuated during the study period, but the net change was consistent with a 20.2 % increase in mechanical ventilation between 2002 and 2011. The percentage of MICU patients who received invasive mechanical ventilation decreased from 48.1 % in 2002 to 30.8 % in 2011 ($p < 0.0001$ for trend) (Fig. 18.1). Thus, the driver of increasing mechanical ventilation utilization was a rising MICU census rather than a greater likelihood of using mechanical ventilation among MICU patients. In contrast to trends in the MICU, mechanical ventilation in the CCU declined by 35.6 %, with trends driven by a lower CCU census and a reduction in the proportion of patients receiving invasive mechanical ventilation decreased (from 58.4 % in 2002 to 46.8 % in 2011) ($p < 0.0001$ for trend) (Fig. 18.2).

Average tidal volumes in the CCU decreased by 24.4 % over the study period, from 661 mL (SD = 132 mL) in 2002 to 500 mL (SD = 59) in 2011 ($p < 0.0001$).

18.5 Study Analysis

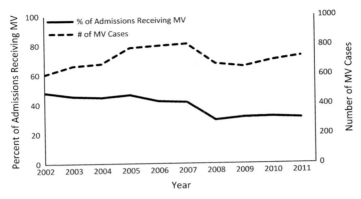

Fig. 18.1 Percent of all admissions (*left* y-axis) and number of cases (*right* y-axis) receiving invasive mechanical ventilation in the MICU. *MV*—invasive mechanical ventilation, *MICU*—medical intensive care unit

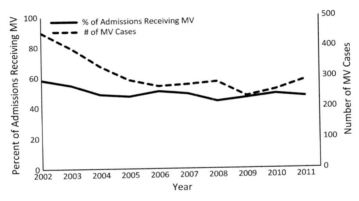

Fig. 18.2 Percent of all admissions (*left* y-axis) and number of cases (*right* y-axis) receiving invasive mechanical ventilation in the CCU. *MV*—invasive mechanical ventilation, *CCU*—cardiac care unit

Tidal volume in the MICU decreased by 17.6 %, from 568 mL (SD = 121 mL) in 2002 to 468 mL (SD = 65 mL) in 2011 ($p < 0.0001$) (Fig. 18.3). During each year of the study period, the CCU used higher tidal volumes than the MICU ($p < 0.0001$ for comparison between units for each year). After adjusting for age and gender, tidal volume in the CCU decreased by an average of 18 mL per year (95 % CI 16–19 mL, $p < 0.0001$) while tidal volumes in the MICU decreased by 11 mL per year (95 % CI 10–11, $p < 0.0001$). The decrease in tidal volume in the CCU was greater than the decrease in the MICU ($p_{interaction} < 0.0001$). Additionally, the coefficient of variation decreased in both units during the study period (MICU: 20.0 % in 2002 to 11.8 % in 2011, $p < 0.0001$; CCU: 21.3 % in 2002 to 13.9 % in 2011, $p < 0.0001$).

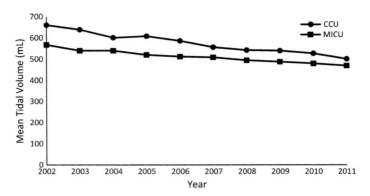

Fig. 18.3 Average tidal volume in the MICU and CCU per year. For each year, the average tidal volume was higher in the CCU, $p < 0.0001$ for comparison for each year. The decrease (slope) of the change in tidal volume was greater for the CCU, $p < 0.001$. *MICU*—medical intensive care unit. *CCU*—cardiac care unit

18.6 Study Conclusions

While there is strong evidence indicating survival benefits for lower tidal volumes in patients with non-cardiogenic pulmonary edema (ARDS) [2] there is little evidence for its use in patients with cardiogenic pulmonary edema (heart failure). Using the MIMIC-II database, we identified a decrease in rates of invasive mechanical ventilation in both the MICU and CCU, despite an increase in the actual number of invasive mechanical ventilation cases in the MICU. Tidal volumes decreased in both ICUs over the course of the study period. Interestingly, tidal volumes decreased at a faster rate in the CCU as compared to the MICU, with tidal volumes nearly equivalent in the MICU and CCU by 2011. The more rapid rate of tidal volume decline in the CCU occurred despite little evidence supporting use of low tidal volumes for patients with cardiogenic pulmonary edema or heart failure. In addition to declining tidal volumes, variability in tidal volume selection also declined over time, demonstrating an evolving tendency towards greater uniformity in tidal volume selection. Our findings demonstrate a generalization of the evidence for ARDS towards the treatment of patients previously excluded from studies investigating tidal volumes during mechanical ventilation.

18.7 Next Steps

Our analysis has several limitations. First, many factors affect tidal volume choice in ICUs including patient height, respiratory drive, and acid/base status. If these unmeasured factors were to have changed over time in our study population, they would be potential confounders of our observation that tidal volumes have been set

18.7 Next Steps

lower over time. Including covariates related to these factors in the regression analysis could reduce possible confounding. For the purposes of this case study, we limited our covariates to demographic characteristics, but others could be added to the model in future analyses. Second, our primary outcome variable is mean tidal volume. We did not look at changes in tidal volumes during a patient's hospitalization, an analysis that may also be performed in future studies. Third, tidal volumes are generally normalized to the ideal body weight, as normal lung size correlates with ideal body weight. We did not have ideal body weights available in MIMIC-II.

The next step from this study would be determine associations between changes in tidal volume and changes in clinical outcomes. Studies attempting to assess the association of changing tidal volumes with clinical outcomes would need to be vigilant to measure multiple potentially confounding variables that may have been co-linear secular trends along with decreasing tidal volumes. Additionally, we used patients admitted to the MICU as a surrogate for patients with ARDS and to the CCU as a surrogate for patients with heart failure. In future studies we would hope to refine our search algorithms within EHR databases to be able to identify patients with ARDS and heart failure with minimal risk of misclassification bias. The strengths of EHR databases such as MIMIC-II lie in their unique granularity, providing a wealth of opportunities to measure clinical details such as pharmacy data, laboratory results, physician notes (via natural language processing), etc., that allow a greater ability to attenuate confounding.

18.8 Connections

Trend analyses assess health care changes over time. In our case study we used linear regression techniques to determine the association of time on a continuous variable (tidal volume). Regression methods allow researchers to account for confounding variables that may have changed over time along with exposures and outcomes of interest. However linear regression techniques are limited to data that have a linear relationship. For non-linear data, transformation techniques (e.g. log-transformation) can be used to convert a nonlinear distribution to a more linear relationship, higher-order polynomial regression, or spline regression may be used; alternatively Poisson regression may be used for count data.

Other techniques should be used for categorical outcomes. The Cochrane-Armitage test for trends is a modified Pearson chi-squared test that allows for ordering of one of the variables (i.e. a time variable). Additionally multivariable logistic regression tools allow for trend analysis for categorical data with the potential for addition of possible confounders as covariates.

These analytic techniques can be applied broadly beyond our case study. The fundamental aspect of trend analyses stems from the fact that the main independent/exposure variable is time. With this concept, numerous conditions and treatments can be studied to see how their utilization changes over time such as subgroups of patients receiving invasive mechanical ventilation [10], patients with tracheostomy [11], etc. Trend analysis is important to evaluate how well clinical trial findings have penetrated usual care by assessing changes in trends with relationship to new research findings or new guidelines. Additionally, trend analyses are critical for quality assessment in determining if certain interventions or process have significantly changed outcomes. As with all statistics, one must understand the assumptions involved in the types of tests being performed and ensure that the data meet those criteria.

Open Access This chapter is distributed under the terms of the Creative Commons Attribution-NonCommercial 4.0 International License (http://creativecommons.org/licenses/by-nc/4.0/), which permits any noncommercial use, duplication, adaptation, distribution and reproduction in any medium or format, as long as you give appropriate credit to the original author(s) and the source, a link is provided to the Creative Commons license and any changes made are indicated.

The images or other third party material in this chapter are included in the work's Creative Commons license, unless indicated otherwise in the credit line; if such material is not included in the work's Creative Commons license and the respective action is not permitted by statutory regulation, users will need to obtain permission from the license holder to duplicate, adapt or reproduce the material.

Code Appendix

The code used in this case study is available from the GitHub repository accompanying this book: https://github.com/MIT-LCP/critical-data-book. Further information on the code is available from this website.

References

1. The ARDS Definition Task Force (2012) Acute respiratory distress syndrome: the Berlin definition. JAMA 307(23):2526–2533
2. Amato MB, Barbas CS, Medeiros DM, Laffey JG, Engelberts D, Kavanagh BP (2000) Ventilation with lower tidal volumes as compared with traditional tidal volumes for acute lung injury and the acute respiratory distress syndrome. The acute respiratory distress syndrome network. N Engl J Med 342(18):1301–1308
3. Esteban A, Frutos-VIvar F, Muriel A et al (2013) Evolution of mortality over time in patients receiving mechanical ventilation. Am J Respir Crit Car Med 188(2):220
4. Rubenfeld GD, Caldwell E, Peabody E et al (2005) Incidence and outcomes of acute lung injury. N Engl J Med 353(16):1685–1693
5. Erickson SE, Martin GS, Davis JL et al (2009) Recent trends in acute lung injury mortality: 1996–2005. Crit Care Med 37(5):1574–1579
6. Zambon M, Vincent JL (2008) Mortality rates for patients with acute lung injury/ARDS have decreased over time. Chest 133(5):1120–1127
7. Esteban A, Ferguson ND, Meade MO et al (2008) Evolution of mechanical ventilation in response to clinical research. Am J Respir Crit Care Med 177(2):170–177

References

8. Scott DJ, Lee J, Silva I et al (2013) Accessing the public MIMIC-II intensive care relational database for clinical research. BMC Med Inform Decis Mak 13:9. doi:10.1186/1472-6947-13-9
9. United States Forest Service (2015) A likelihood ratio test of the equality of the coefficients of variation of k normally distributed populations. http://www1.fpl.fs.fed.us/covtestk.html. 28 July 2015
10. Mehta AB, Syeda SN, Wiener RS et al (2015) Epidemiological trends in invasive mechanical ventilation in the United States: a population-based study. J Crit Care 30(6):1217–1221
11. Mehta AB, Syeda SN, Bajpayee L et al (2015) Trends in tracheostomy for mechanically ventilated patients in the United States, 1993–2012. Am J Respir Crit Care Med 192(4):446–454

Chapter 19
Instrumental Variable Analysis of Electronic Health Records

Nicolás Della Penna, Jennifer P. Stevens and Robert Stretch

Learning Objectives
In this case study we Illustrate how to

- Estimate causal effects of a potential intervention when there is an instrumental variable available.
- Identify appropriate model classes with which to estimate effects using instrumental variables.
- Examine potential sources of treatment effect heterogeneity.

19.1 Introduction

The goal of observational research is to identify the causal effects of exposures or treatments on clinical outcomes of interest. The availability of data derived from electronic health records (EHRs) has improved the feasibility of large-scale observational studies. However, both treatments and patient characteristics (co-variates) affect outcomes. Since in general the two are dependent, it is not accurate to simply compare the outcomes of those receiving different treatments to decide which treatment is more effective. While regression analysis can account for the variation in those covariates that can be observed, estimates remain biased if there are unobservable covariates that affect treatment propensity and outcomes.

Idealized randomized controlled experiments overcome the problem of unobserved covariates by virtue of them being randomly distributed in a balanced manner between the treatment and control groups as the sample size becomes large. In practice, however, such experiments are affected by participant non-compliance. Instrumental variable techniques, which use treatment assignment as the instrument and actual treatment taken as the endogenous variables (those that result from choices that may be affected by unobservables), are useful in this setting.

Instrumental variable analyses (IVAs) attempt to exploit "natural experiments"—sources of unintentional but effective randomization of subjects to

Fig. 19.1 Instrumental variable analyses employ instruments that affect the likelihood of the exposure but do not otherwise affect the outcome

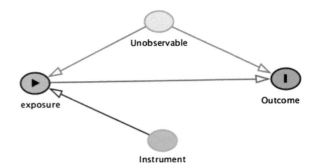

different treatments. To take advantage of such natural experiments, subjects must find themselves in a situation in which some observable characteristic makes them more likely to receive a specified treatment, but does not otherwise affect the outcome of interest, and is independent of unobservable covariates (see Fig. 19.1). The estimation then relies on using only the variation caused by this observable characteristic, called an *instrument* or *instrumental variable* (*IV*), to identify the effect.

There are three key considerations in the selection of appropriate controls and valid instruments:

1. **Control variables should be pre-treatment characteristics of the patients or providers**: One should not control for outcomes or decisions that occur after the treatment, even if they are not the outcome of interest, as this would bias results. Drawing the causal model and analyzing the paths provides a principled way of understanding the underlying assumptions that are being made. Web-based software [1] is available to facilitate this.
2. **The instrument must be correlated with the treatment and explain a substantial portion of the variation in the treatment**: The less variation in the treatment that the instrument explains (the "weaker" the instrument), the higher the variance of the estimates obtained. This higher variance may deny any benefits from bias reduction.
3. **The instrument must be *independent of* the outcome through any mechanism other than the treatment**: This remains one of the greatest challenges of employing IVAs accurately in medical data, as identifying instruments that have no relationship with any unobservable clinical variation beyond the treatment is difficult.

To illustrate these concepts we propose using an IVA to estimate the effect on intensive care unit (ICU) mortality of receiving care in a "non-target" ICU, defined as a unit that has a different specialty focus than the ICU to which patients would have been assigned in the absence of capacity constraints. For example, patients being cared for by a medical ICU team ideally care for their patients in a defined

19.1 Introduction

geographic area designated as the medical ICU (MICU), but when no beds are available in that unit a patient may instead be assigned to an unoccupied bed in a non-target ICU such as a surgical ICU (SICU). In this study, we define those patients assigned beds in non-target ICUs as *boarders*.

Although the physicians of the MICU team retain responsibility for the care of boarders, most other staff involved in the patient's care (e.g. nurses, respiratory therapists, physical therapists) will change as a result of boarding status. This is because these staff are assigned to a specific geographically-defined ICU such as the SICU. As a result, boarders are typically cared for by nurses and other staff who possess expertise more appropriate for managing surgical patients than medical patients. Additionally, since physicians and nurses who work in different ICUs may not be as familiar with each other's clinical practices, communication difficulties can arise. Lastly, there are also greater geographic distances between boarders and their physicians compared to non-boarders. This can contribute to delays in care and impairment of a physician's level of situational awareness. It therefore seems reasonable to hypothesize that boarding may negatively impact upon clinical outcomes, including survival.

19.2 Methods

19.2.1 *Dataset*

The Medical Information Mart for Intensive Care (MIMIC-III) database contains clinical and administrative data on over 60,000 ICU stays at Beth Israel Deaconess Medical Center (BIDMC) between 2001 and 2012. It includes operational-level data on bed assignments and service transfers, as well as ICD-9-CM diagnoses and several mortality measures (ICU stay mortality, hospital mortality, and survival duration up to one year).

19.2.2 *Methodology*

Cohort Selection
We included all adult subjects, aged 18 years or older, cared for by the MICU at any point during their admission. The study period was defined as June, 2002 through December, 2012. In order to ensure independence of observations only the last ICU admission for each subject was included in the analysis.

Exclusion criteria included subjects whose primary hospital team at any point during their admission was non-medical (i.e. surgical or cardiac), as this might imply a specific reason aside from capacity constraints for a patient to be a boarder in a non-medical ICU (for example, a postoperative subject in the surgical ICU being transferred from the surgical ICU team to the medical ICU team for persistent respiratory failure).

The final study population included 8442 subjects, of whom 1881 (22 %) were exposed to the effects of boarding.

Statistical Approach

A naive estimate of the effect of boarding on mortality would compare the outcomes of patients who were boarders to those who were not. However, the decision to board a patient is not random. It takes into account the level of severity of a given patient's condition, as well as how that compares with the severity levels of other incoming patients also in need of an ICU bed. It is likely that much of the information that informs this decision is unobservable. As a consequence, if we conducted this study as a simple regression analysis we would obtain biased estimates of the effect of boarding.

For example, assume that boarding *increases* mortality, but also that ICU staff preferentially select *less* severely ill patients to be boarders. In this hypothetical scenario, the *observed* association between boarding and mortality could appear protective if the negative effect of boarding on mortality is smaller than the positive effect on observed mortality of selecting healthier patients. While one may, and should, control for patients' severity of illness and pre-existing health levels, it is not usually possible to observe these with the same granularity and accuracy as the hospital staff who decide whether the patient will become a boarder. As a result, boarders may still be healthier than non-boarders even after conditioning on a measure of severity of illness.

An IVA is an attractive approach in this situation. In this study, we focus on MICU patients. We propose that the number of remaining available beds in the western campus MICU at time of patient intake (*west_initial_remaining_beds*) may serve as a valid instrument for boarding status. It is important to note that *west_initial_remaining_beds* does not include beds that are available outside of the MICU (i.e. beds to which boarders can be assigned). The boarder status of the patient is the *causal variable* and the *outcome* is death during ICU stay (Fig. 19.2).

The Oxford Acute Severity of Illness Score (OASIS) is employed to help account for residual differences between the health status of boarders and non-boarders at the time of their intake into the ICU. OASIS is an ICU scoring system that has been shown to have non-inferior performance characteristics relative to APACHE (Acute Physiology and Chronic Health Evaluation), MPM (Mortality Probability Model), and SAPS (Simplified Acute Physiology Score) [2]. We preferentially use OASIS for severity of illness adjustment because its scores can be more accurately reconstructed in MIMIC-III in a retrospective manner than the aforementioned alternatives.

At times when hospital load is high, the total number of patients being cared for by the ICU team (*west_initial_team_census*) is likely to be high, and

19.2 Methods

Fig. 19.2 Simplified causal diagram illustrating confounding of the relationship between boarding and mortality due to unobservable heterogeneity in patient risk, and potential conditional instrument *west_initial_remaining_beds*. The diagram can be manipulated at http://dagitty.net/dags.html?id=AVKMi0

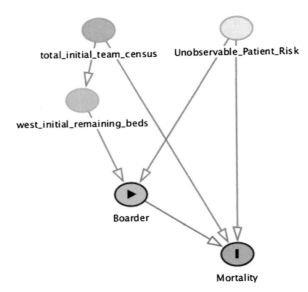

west_initial_remaining_beds is likely to be low. Furthermore, it is plausible that higher values of *west_initial_team_census* might affect mortality as a relatively fixed quantity of ICU resources (e.g. physicians) is stretched across a greater number of patients.

At first it may be unclear why there is imperfect correlation between *west_initial_team_census* and *west_initial_remaining_beds,* as one might anticipate that the number of remaining beds is simply inversely proportional to the total number of patients being cared for by the ICU team. The source of variation between these variables is two-fold. The primary driver is the stochastic pattern of ICU discharges. It is improbable that all boarders will be discharged prior to any of the non-boarders. Discharging a non-boarder while other patients remain as boarders creates a situation where the total team census may continue to be higher than the bed capacity of the MICU, yet the number of available beds in the MICU becomes non-zero. The second, smaller source of variation is occupancy of MICU beds by patients being cared for by other ICU teams (e.g a SICU patient boarding in the MICU).

Using *west_initial_remaining_beds* as an instrument is therefore valid, but we must control for *west_initial_team_census*. To check that *west_initial_remaining_beds* is correlated to the propensity of patients to board, we fit a generalized additive model with a logistic link function.

Once a natural experiment has been identified and the validity of the instrumental variable confirmed, an IVA can be conducted to estimate the causal effect of the treatment. The standard in the econometrics literature has been to use a two-step ordinary least squares (OLS) regression. There are two important limitations to this approach in biomedical settings. Firstly, it requires continuous treatment and outcome variables, both of which tend to be discrete or binary in medical applications.

Secondly, it requires knowledge of the functional form of the underlying relationships such that the data can be transformed to make the relationships linear in the parameters of the estimated model. This is often beyond what is known in the biomedical field.

Several approaches have been developed to address these limitations. Probit models are part of a family of generalized linear models (GLM) that is well suited to working with discrete data, thereby addressing the first aforementioned limitation. Furthermore, use of a basis expansion may allow the functional form to be approximated flexibly using penalized splines, substantially relaxing the second limitation related to knowledge of functional forms. At least one statistical package, *SemiParBIVProbit* for R, combines these two approaches in an accessible implementation.

In addition to the probit model, we used the *survival* package for R to estimate a non-instrumental Cox proportional hazards model as a robustness check. In order to minimize selection bias in this non-instrumental model, we used a subset of the dataset in which it is intuitive that selective pressures would be reduced or non-existent: *west_initial_remaining_beds* equal to zero (all patients must board irrespective of their severity of illness) or *west_initial_remaining_beds* greater than or equal to three (no imminent capacity constraint exerting pressure on physicians to board patients). The linear assumptions of the Cox models are strong and not justified *a priori*, therefore in order to test for potential nonlinearities in the instrumental model we used the *Vuong and Clarke* tests of the *SemiParBIVProbit* package.

All of our models included controls for patient age, gender, OASIS and Elixhauser comorbidity scores, length of hospital stay prior to ICU admission, and calendar year. In addition to controlling for the *west_initial_team_census*, we also controlled for the total number of boarders under the care of the MICU team.

19.2.3 Pre-processing

We used a software package called *Chatto-Transform* [3] that connects to a local PostgreSQL instance of MIMIC-III and simplifies the process of importing table data into an interactive *Jupyter* notebook [4]. Python 3 and the *Pandas* library [5] were used for data extraction and analysis (see code supplement).

The publicly available version of MIMIC-III applies random time-shifts to records to help prevent subjects from being identified. After institutional review board approval, we obtained the exact dates and bed assignments for each subject's ICU stay and used this to reconstruct the entire hospital ICU census.

The *services* table in MIMIC-III documents the specific service (e.g. medicine, general surgery, cardiology) responsible for a patient at a given moment in time. The service providing MICU care is classified as 'medicine'. Therefore general medicine patients who are initially admitted to a ward and later require a MICU bed will still only have one entry per admission in this table, provided that they are not transferred to the care of a different service. We consider a refined copy of the

19.2 Methods

services table ('*med_service_only*') that retains only those rows pertaining to patients cared for exclusively by the medicine service during their stay. The resulting table therefore has only one row per hospital admission.

The *transfers* table documents every change in a patient's location during their hospital admission, including exact bed assignments and timestamp data. A new table *df* can be created by performing a left join between *transfers* and *med_service_only*. In the resulting table, rows pertaining to the population of interest (i.e. medicine patients who incurred a MICU stay at some point during their admission) will have data corresponding to both the left (*transfers*) and right (*med_service_only*) tables. Rows pertaining to all other patients will only have data from the *transfers* table. We further subdivide this table into *inboarders* (which contains rows pertaining to non-MICU patients occupying beds in the MICU) and *df5* (which contains rows pertaining to our population of interest).

Looping through each row in *df5*, we identify rows in *inboarders* that represent a MICU bed occupied by a non-MICU patient at the time a MICU patient began their ICU stay. We also determine whether the new MICU patient was assigned a bed outside the geographic confines of the MICU, in which case they were classified as a boarder. Lastly, a count of the total number of patients being cared for by the MICU team is generated and added to each row of *df5*. These variables allow for calculation of the number of remaining MICU beds through the formula:

$$\text{Remaining Beds} = (\text{MICU Capacity} - \text{No. of Inboarders}) - (\text{Team Census} - \text{No. of Boarders})$$

Death during ICU stay was determined *a priori* to be our primary outcome of interest. We identified a number of instances in the dataset where death occurred within minutes or hours of discharge from the ICU. This was most likely due to combination of expected deaths (subjects transitioned to comfort-focused care who were transferred out of the ICU shortly prior to death), unexpected deaths, and minor time discrepancies inherent to large datasets that include administrative details. Prior to data analysis it was decided that our preferred definition of *death during ICU stay* would include those within 24 h of leaving the ICU.

19.3 Results

Looking at the fitted models, we observe an increase in mortality from boarding across the different specifications. In the semiparametric bivariate probit model, using the *west_initial_remaining_beds* as an instrument, the estimated causal [6] average risk ratio is 1.44 (95 % interval: 1.17, 1.79). In the non-instrumental Cox proportional hazards model we observe a similar estimate of 1.34 (1.06, 1.70).

Often treatments result in different effects of different patients, thus it is sensible to think of average treatment effects (ATE). Instrumental variable analyses, however, restrict the estimation to the variation in the data that is attributable to the instrument. That is, the effect they estimate is the *local* effect on those patients whose treatment is affected by the instrument. This is termed the Local Average Treatment Effect (LATE), and is what is estimated by an IVA when there is heterogeneity in treatment effects.

19.4 Next Steps

Much of the existing medical literature utilizing IVAs has addressed policy questions as opposed to the effect of medical treatments. This has been driven by the interest in such questions by health care economists, as well as the greater availability and suitability of administrative—rather than clinical—data within the medical field. In contrast, the growing adoption and increasing sophistication of EHRs now presents us with an opportunity to investigate the effects of medical treatments through their provision of a rich source of observable variables and potential instruments. Examples include measurable variation in the number and characteristics of hospital staff, as well as load levels that cause spillover between units and thus are exogenous to a particular patient in a given unit. There is also a large body of literature that has explored Mendelian randomization as a source of instruments, however these usually create limited variation therefore instrument weakness is a substantial concern.

Aside from serving as candidate instruments or controls, some variables easily extracted from EHRs may be useful for checking the plausibility of a proposed pseudo-randomization process: if an instrument is truly randomizing patients with respect to a treatment then we would expect a balanced distribution of a wide range of observable variables (e.g. patient demographics). This is akin to tables that compare the baseline characteristics between groups in the results of randomized controlled trial. Estimating causal effects from natural experiments is an important part of the econometrics literature. For an influential practitioners reference, see *Mostly Harmless Econometrics* [7]. A excellent counterpoint can be found in part III of Shalizi [8].

Instrumental variables are powerful tools in the identification of causal relationships, but it is critical to remain mindful of potential sources of confounding. Garabedian et al. reviewed the studies published in the medical literature using IVAs and found that the four most commonly used instrument categories—distance to facility, regional variation, facility variation, and physician variation—all suffered from "potential unadjusted instrument–outcome confounders ... including patient race, socioeconomic status, clinical risk factors, health status, and urban or rural residency; facility and procedure volume; and co-occurring treatments" [9].

19.5 Conclusions

This case study demonstrates the steps involved in the identification and validation of an instrumental variable. It also illustrates the process of conducting an IVA to estimate effect sizes and infer causal relationships from observational data.

The results of our study support the hypothesis that boarding of critically ill patients has deleterious effects on ICU survival. We recommend that institutions take steps to minimize boarding among ICU patients and that further studies be undertaken to more precisely characterize the effect size. Better understanding of the mediators through which boarding influences mortality is also important, and may help to identify groups of patients who are able to board without detrimental effects, and those for whom boarding should be particularly avoided.

Open Access This chapter is distributed under the terms of the Creative Commons Attribution-NonCommercial 4.0 International License (http://creativecommons.org/licenses/by-nc/4.0/), which permits any noncommercial use, duplication, adaptation, distribution and reproduction in any medium or format, as long as you give appropriate credit to the original author(s) and the source, a link is provided to the Creative Commons license and any changes made are indicated.

The images or other third party material in this chapter are included in the work's Creative Commons license, unless indicated otherwise in the credit line; if such material is not included in the work's Creative Commons license and the respective action is not permitted by statutory regulation, users will need to obtain permission from the license holder to duplicate, adapt or reproduce the material.

Code Appendix

The code used in this case study is available from the GitHub repository accompanying this book: https://github.com/MIT-LCP/critical-data-book. Further information on the code is available from this website.

References

1. Textor J, Hardt J, Knüppel S (2011) DAGitty: a graphical tool for analyzing causal diagrams. Epidemiology 22(5):745
2. Johnson AEW, Kramer AA, Clifford GD (2013) A new severity of illness scale using a subset of acute physiology and chronic health evaluation data elements shows comparable predictive accuracy. Crit Care Med 41(7):1711–1718
3. Spitz D, Spencer D (2015) Chatto-transform
4. Jupyter Team, "Project Jupyter."
5. PyData Development Team (2015) Pandas data analysis library
6. Marra G, Giampiero M, Rosalba R (2011) Estimation of a semiparametric recursive bivariate probit model in the presence of endogeneity. Can J Stat 39(2):259–279

7. Angrist JD, Pischke J-S (2008) Mostly harmless econometrics: an empiricist's companion. Princeton University Press, Princeton
8. Shalizi CR (2016) Advanced data analysis from an elementary point of view, 18 Jan 2016
9. Garabedian LF, Chu P, Toh S, Zaslavsky AM, Soumerai SB (2014) Potential bias of instrumental variable analyses for observational comparative effectiveness research. Ann Intern Med 161(2):131–138

Chapter 20
Mortality Prediction in the ICU Based on MIMIC-II Results from the Super ICU Learner Algorithm (SICULA) Project

Romain Pirracchio

Learning Objectives
In this chapter, we illustrate the use of MIMIC II clinical data, non-parametric prediction algorithm, ensemble machine learning, and the Super Learner algorithm.

20.1 Introduction

Predicting mortality in patients hospitalized in intensive care units (ICU) is crucial for assessing severity of illness and adjudicating the value of novel treatments, interventions and health care policies. Several severity scores have been developed with the objective of predicting hospital mortality from baseline patient characteristics, defined as measurements obtained within the first 24 h after ICU admission. The first scores proposed, APACHE [1] (Acute Physiology and Chronic Health Evaluation), APACHE II [2], and SAPS [3] (Simplified Acute Physiology Score), relied upon subjective methods for variable importance measure, namely by prompting a panel of experts to select and assign weights to variables according to perceived relevance for mortality prediction. Further scores, such as the SAPS II [4] were subsequently developed using statistical modeling techniques [4–7]. To this day, the SAPS II [4] and APACHE II [2] scores remain the most widely used in clinical practice. However, since first being published, they have been modified several times in order to improve their predictive performance [6–11]. Despite these extensions of SAPS, predicted hospital mortality remains generally overestimated [8, 9, 12–14]. As an illustration, Poole et al. [9] compared the SAPS II and the SAPS3 performance in a cohort of more than 28,000 admissions to 10 different Italian ICUs. They concluded that both scores provided unreliable predictions, but unexpectedly the newer SAPS 3 turned out to overpredict mortality more than the older SAPS II. Consistently, Nassar et al. [8] assessed the performance of the APACHE IV, the SAPS 3 and the Mortality Probability Model III [MPM(0)-III] in a population admitted at 3 medical-surgical Brazilian intensive care units and found that all models showed poor calibration, while discrimination was very good for all of them.

Most ICU severity scores rely on a logistic regression model. Such models impose stringent constraints on the relationship between explanatory variables and risk of death. For instance, main term logistic regression relies on the assumption of a linear and additive relationship between the outcome and its predictors. Given the complexity of the processes underlying death in ICU patients, this assumption might be unrealistic.

Given that the true relationship between risk of mortality in the ICU and explanatory variables is unknown, we expect that prediction can be improved by using an automated nonparametric algorithm to estimate risk of death without requiring any specification about the shape of the underlying relationship. Indeed, nonparametric algorithms offer the great advantage of not relying on any assumption about the underlying distribution, which make them more suited to fit such complex data. Some studies have evaluated the benefit of nonparametric approaches, namely based on neural networks or data-mining, to predict hospital mortality in ICU patients [15–20]. These studies unanimously concluded that nonparametric methods might perform at least as well as standard logistic regression in predicting ICU mortality.

Recently, the *Super Learner* was developed as a nonparametric technique for selecting an optimal regression algorithm among a given set of candidate algorithms provided by the user [21]. The *Super Learner* ranks the algorithms according to their prediction performance, and then builds an aggregate algorithm obtained as the optimal weighted combination of the candidate algorithms. Theoretical results have demonstrated that the *Super Learner* performs no worse than the optimal choice among the provided library of candidate algorithms, at least in large samples. It capitalizes on the richness of the library it builds upon and generally offers gains over any specific candidate algorithm in terms of flexibility to accurately fit the data.

The primary aim of this study was to develop a scoring procedure for ICU patients based on the *Super Learner* using data from the Medical Information Mart for Intensive Care II (MIMIC-II) study [22–24], and to determine whether it results in improved mortality prediction relative to the SAPS II, the APACHE II and the SOFA scores. Complete results of this study have been published in 2015 in the Lancet Respiratory Medicine [25]. We also wished to develop an easily-accessible user-friendly web implementation of our scoring procedure, even despite the complexity of our approach (http://webapps.biostat.berkeley.edu:8080/sicula/).

20.2 Dataset and Pre-preprocessing

20.2.1 Data Collection and Patients Characteristics

The MIMIC-II study [22–24] includes all patients admitted to an ICU at the Beth Israel Deaconess Medical Center (BIDMC) in Boston, MA since 2001. For the sake of the present study, only data from MIMIC-II version 26 (2001–2008) on adult ICU patients were included. Patients younger than 16 years were not included. For patients with multiple admission, we only considered the first ICU stay. A total of 24,508 patients were included in this study.

20.2.2 Patient Inclusion and Measures

Two categories of data were collected: clinical data, aggregated from ICU information systems and hospital archives, and high-resolution physiologic data (waveforms and time series of derived physiologic measurements), recorded on bedside monitors. Clinical data were obtained from the CareVue Clinical Information System (Philips Healthcare, Andover, Massachusetts) deployed in all study ICUs, and from hospital electronic archives. The data included time-stamped nurse-verified physiologic measurements (e.g., hourly documentation of heart rate, arterial blood pressure, pulmonary artery pressure), nurses' and respiratory therapists' progress notes, continuous intravenous (IV) drip medications, fluid balances, patient demographics, interpretations of imaging studies, physician orders, discharge summaries, and ICD-9 codes. Comprehensive diagnostic laboratory results (e.g., blood chemistry, complete blood counts, arterial blood gases, microbiology results) were obtained from the patient's entire hospital stay including periods outside the ICU. In the present study, we focused exclusively on outcome variables (specifically, ICU and hospital mortality) and variables included in the SAPS II [4] and SOFA scores [26].

We first took an inventory of all available recorded characteristics required to evaluate the different scores considered. Raw data from the MIMIC II database version 26 were then extracted. We decided to use only R functions (without any SQL routines) as most of our researchers only have R package knowledge. Each table within each patient datafile were checked for the different characteristics and extracted. Finally, we created a global CSV file including all data and easily manipulable with R.

Baseline variables and outcomes are summarized in Table 20.1.

Table 20.1 Baseline characteristics and outcome measures

	Overall population (n = 24,508)	Dead at hospital discharge (n = 3002)	Alive at hospital discharge (n = 21,506)
Age	65 [51–77]	74 [59–83]	64 [50–76]
Gender (female)	13,838 (56.5 %)	1607 (53.5 %)	12,231 (56.9 %)
First SAPS	13 [10–17]	18 [14–22]	13 [9–17]
First SAPS II	38 [27–51]	53 [43–64]	36 [27–49]
First SOFA	5 [2–8]	8 [5–12]	5 [2–8]
Origin			
Medical	2453 (10 %)	240 (8 %)	2213 (10.3 %)
Trauma	7703 (31.4 %)	1055 (35.1 %)	6648 (30.9 %)
Emergency surgery	10,803 (44.1 %)	1583 (52.7 %)	9220 (42.9 %)
Scheduled surgery	3549 (14.5 %)	124 (4.1 %)	3425 (15.9 %)
Site			
MICU	7488 (30.6 %)	1265 (42.1 %)	6223 (28.9 %)
MSICU	2686 (11 %)	347 (11.6 %)	2339 (10.9 %)
CCU	5285 (21.6 %)	633 (21.1 %)	4652 (21.6 %)
CSRU	8100 (33.1 %)	664 (22.1 %)	7436 (34.6 %)
TSICU	949 (3.9 %)	93 (3.1 %)	856 (4 %)
HR (bpm)	87 [75–100]	92 [78–109]	86 [75–99]
MAP (mmHg)	81 [70–94]	78 [65–94]	82 [71–94]
RR (cpm)	14 [12–20]	18 [14–23]	14 [12–18]
Na (mmol/l)	139 [136–141]	138 [135–141]	139 [136–141]
K (mmol/l)	4.2 [3.8–4.6]	4.2 [3.8–4.8]	4.2 [3.8–4.6]
HCO_3 (mmol/l)	26 [22–28]	24 [20–28]	26 [23–28]
WBC (10^3/mm^3)	10.3 [7.5–14.4]	11.6 [7.9–16.9]	10.2 [7.4–14.1]
P/F ratio	281 [130–447]	174 [90–352]	312 [145–461]
Ht (%)	34.7 [30.4–39]	33.8 [29.8–38]	34.8 [30.5–39.1]
Urea (mmol/l)	20 [14–31]	28 [18–46]	19 [13–29]
Bilirubine (mg/dl)	0.6 [0.4–1]	0.7 [0.4–1.5]	0.6 [0.4–0.9]
Hospital LOS (days)	8 [4–14]	9 [4–17]	8 [4–14]
ICU death (%)	1978 (8.1 %)	1978 (65.9 %)	–
Hospital death (%)	3002 (12.2 %)	–	–

Continuous variables are presented as median [InterQuartile Range]; binary or categorical variables as count (%)

20.3 Methods

20.3.1 Prediction Algorithms

The primary outcome measure was hospital mortality. A total of 1978 deaths occurred in ICU (estimated mortality rate: 8.1 %, 95 %CI: 7.7–8.4), and 1024 additional deaths were observed after ICU discharge, resulting in an estimated hospital mortality rate of 12.2 % (95 %CI: 11.8–12.7).

The data recorded within the first 24 h following ICU admission were used to compute two of the most widely used severity scores, namely the SAPS II [4] and SOFA [26] scores. Individual mortality prediction for the SAPS II score was calculated as defined by its authors [4]:

$$\log\left[\frac{\text{pr(death)}}{1 - \text{pr(death)}}\right] = -7.7631 + 0.0737 * \text{SAPSII} + 0.9971 * \log(1 + \text{SAPSII})$$

In addition, we developed a new version of the SAPS II score, by fitting to our data a main-term logistic regression model using the same explanatory variables as those used in the original SAPS II score [4]: age, heart rate, systolic blood pressure, body temperature Glasgow Coma Scale, mechanical ventilation, PaO_2, FiO_2, urine output, BUN (blood urea nitrogen), blood sodium, potassium, bicarbonates, bilirubin, white blood cells, chronic disease (AIDS, metastatic cancer, hematologic malignancy) and type of admission (elective surgery, medical, unscheduled surgery). The same procedure was used to build a new version of the APACHE II score [2]. Finally, because the SOFA score [26] is widely used in clinical practice as a proxy for outcome prediction, it was also computed for all subjects. Mortality prediction based on the SOFA score was obtained by regressing hospital mortality on the SOFA score using a main-term logistic regression. These two algorithms for mortality prediction were compared to our *Super Learner*-based proposal.

The *Super Learner* has been proposed as a method for selecting via cross-validation the optimal regression algorithm among all weighted combinations of a set of given candidate algorithms, henceforth referred to as the library [21, 27, 28] (Fig. 20.1). To implement the *Super Learner*, a user must provide a customized collection of various data-fitting algorithms. The *Super Learner* then estimates the risk associated to each algorithm in the provided collection using cross-validation. One round of cross-validation involves partitioning a sample of data into complementary subsets, performing the analysis on one subset (called the *training set*), and validating the analysis on the other subset (called the *validation set* or *testing set*). To reduce variability, multiple rounds of cross-validation are performed using different partitions, and the validation results are averaged over the rounds. From this estimation of the risk associated with each candidate algorithm, the *Super Learner* builds an aggregate algorithm obtained as the optimal weighted combination of the candidate algorithms. Theoretical results suggest that to optimize the performance of the

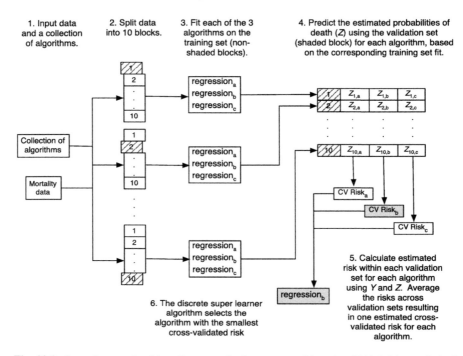

Fig. 20.1 Super learner algorithm. From van der Laan, targeted learning 2011 (with permission) [41]

resulting algorithm, the inputted library should include as many sensible algorithms as possible.

In this study, the library size was limited to 12 algorithms (list available in the Appendix) for computational reasons. Among these 12 algorithms, some were parametric such as logistic regression of affiliated methods classically used for ICU scoring systems, and some non-parametric i.e. methods that fit the data without any assumption concerning the underlying data distribution. In the present study, we chose the library to include most of parametric (including regression models with various combinations of main and interaction terms as well as splines, and fitted using maximum likelihood with or without penalization) and nonparametric algorithm, previously evaluated for the prediction of mortality in critically ill patients in the literature. The main term logistic regression is the parametric algorithm that has been used for constructing both the SAPS II and APACHE II scores. This algorithm was included in the SL library so that revised fits of the SAPS II score based on the current data also competed against other algorithms.

Comparison of the 12 algorithms relied on 10-fold cross-validation. The data are first split into 10 mutually exclusive and exhaustive blocks of approximately equal size. Each algorithm is fitted on a the 9 blocks corresponding to the training set and then this fit used to predict mortality for all patients in the remaining block used a validation set. The squared errors between predicted and observed outcomes are averaged. The performance of each algorithm is evaluated in this manner. This procedure is repeated exactly 10 times, with a different block used as validation set every time. Performance measures are aggregated over all 10 iterations, yielding a cross-validated estimate of the mean-squared error (CV-MSE) for each algorithm. A crucial aspect of this approach is that for each iteration not a single patient appears in both the training and validation sets. The potential for overfitting, wherein the fit of an algorithm is overly tailored to the available data at the expense of performance on future data, is thereby mitigated, as overfitting is more likely to occur when training and validation sets intersect.

Candidate algorithms were ranked according to their CV-MSE and the algorithm with least CV-MSE was identified. This algorithm was then refitted using all available data, leading to a prediction rule referred to as the *Discrete Super Learner*. Subsequently, the prediction rule consisting of the CV-MSE-minimizing weighted convex combination of all candidate algorithms was also computed and refitted on all data. This is what we refer to as the *Super Learner* combination algorithm [28].

The data used in fitting our prediction algorithm included the 17 variables used in the SAPS II score: 13 physiological variables (age, Glasgow coma scale, systolic blood pressure, heart rate, body temperature, PaO_2/FiO_2 ratio, urinary output, serum urea nitrogen level, white blood cells count, serum bicarbonate level, sodium level, potassium level and bilirubin level), type of admission (scheduled surgical, unscheduled surgical, or medical), and three underlying disease variables (acquired immunodeficiency syndrome, metastatic cancer, and hematologic malignancy derived from ICD-9 discharge codes). Two sets of predictions based on the *Super Learner* were produced: the first based on the 17 variables as they appear in the SAPS II score (SL1), and the second, on the original, untransformed variables (SL2).

20.3.2 Performance Metrics

A key objective of this study was to compare the predictive performance of scores based on the *Super Learner* to that of the SAPS II and SOFA scores. This comparison hinged on a variety of measures of predictive performance, described below.

1. A mortality prediction algorithm is said to have adequate discrimination if it tends to assign higher severity scores to patients that died in the hospital compared to those that did not. We evaluated discrimination using the cross-validated area under the receiver-operating characteristic curve (AUROC), reported with corresponding 95 % confidence interval (95 % CI). Discrimination can be graphically illustrated using the receiver-operating (ROC) curves. Additional tools for assessing discrimination include boxplots of predicted probabilities of death for survivors and non-survivors, and

corresponding discrimination slopes, defined as the difference between the mean predicted risks in survivors and non-survivors. All these are provided below.

2. A mortality prediction algorithm is said to be adequately calibrated if predicted and observed probabilities of death coincide rather well. We assessed calibration using the Cox calibration test [9, 29, 30]. Because of its numerous shortcoming, including poor performance in large samples, the more conventional Hosmer-Lemeshow statistic was avoided [31, 32]. Under perfect calibration, a prediction algorithm will satisfy the logistic regression equation 'observed log-odds of death = $\alpha + \beta*$ predicted log-odds of death' with $\alpha = 0$. To implement the Cox calibration test, a logistic regression is performed to estimate α and β; these estimates suggest the degree of deviation from ideal calibration. The null hypothesis $(\alpha, \beta) = (0, 1)$ is tested formally using a U-statistic [33].

3. Summary reclassification measures, including the Continuous Net Reclassification Index (cNRI) and the Integrated Discrimination Improvement (IDI), are relative metrics which have been devised to overcome the limitations of usual discrimination and calibration measures [34–36]. The cNRI comparing severity score A to score B is defined as twice the difference between the proportion of non-survivors and of survivors, respectively, deemed more severe according to score A rather than score B. The IDI comparing severity score A to score B is the average difference in score A between survivors and non-survivors minus the average difference in score B between survivors and non-survivors. Positive values of the cNRI and IDI indicate that score A has better discriminative ability than score B, whereas negative values indicate the opposite. We computed the reclassification tables and associated summary measures to compare each *Super Learner* proposal to the original SAPS II score and each of the revised fits of the SAPS II and APACHE II scores.

All analyses were performed using statistical software R version 2.15.2 for Mac OS X (The R Foundation for Statistical Computing, Vienna, Austria; specific packages: cvAUC, Super Learner and ROCR). Relevant R codes are provided in Appendix.

20.4 Analysis

20.4.1 *Discrimination*

The ROC curves for hospital mortality prediction are provided below (Fig. 20.2). The cross-validated AUROC was 0.71 (95 %CI: 0.70–0.72) for the SOFA score, and 0.78 (95 %CI: 0.77–0.78) for the SAPS II score. When refitting the SAPS II score on our data, the AUROC reached 0.83 (95 %CI: 0.82–0.83); this is similar to the results obtained with the revised fit of the APACHE II, which led to an AUROC of 0.82 (95 %CI: 0.81–0.83). The two *Super Learner* (SL1 and SL2) prediction models substantially outperformed the SAPS II and the SOFA score. The AUROC

20.4 Analysis

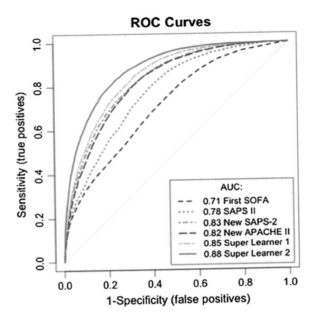

Fig. 20.2 Receiver-operating characteristics curves. Super learner 1: super learner with categorized variables; super learner 2: super learner with non-transformed variables

was 0.85 (95 %CI: 0.84–0.85) for SL1, and 0.88 (95 %CI: 0.87–0.89) for SL2, revealing a clear advantage of the Super Learner-based prediction algorithms over both the SOFA and SAPS II scores.

Discrimination was also evaluated by comparing differences between the predicted probabilities of death among the survivors and the non-survivors using each prediction algorithm. The discrimination slope equaled 0.09 for the SOFA score, 0.26 for the SAPS II score, 0.21 for SL1, and 0.26 for SL2.

20.4.2 Calibration

Calibration plots (Fig. 20.3) indicate a lack of fit for the SAPS II score. The estimated values of α and β were of -1.51 and 0.72 respectively (U statistic = 0.25, $p < 0.0001$). The calibration properties were markedly improved by refitting the SAPS II score: $\alpha < 0.0001$ and $\beta = 1$ (U < 0.0001, $p = 1.00$). The prediction based on the SOFA and the APACHE II scores exhibited excellent calibration properties, as reflected by $\alpha < 0.0001$ and $\beta = 1$ (U < 0.0001, $p = 1.00$). For the Super Learner-based predictions, despite U-statistics significantly different from zero, the estimates of α and β were close to the null values: SL1: 0.14 and 1.04, respectively (U = 0.0007, $p = 0.0001$); SL2: 0.24 and 1.25, respectively (U = 0.006, $p < 0.0001$).

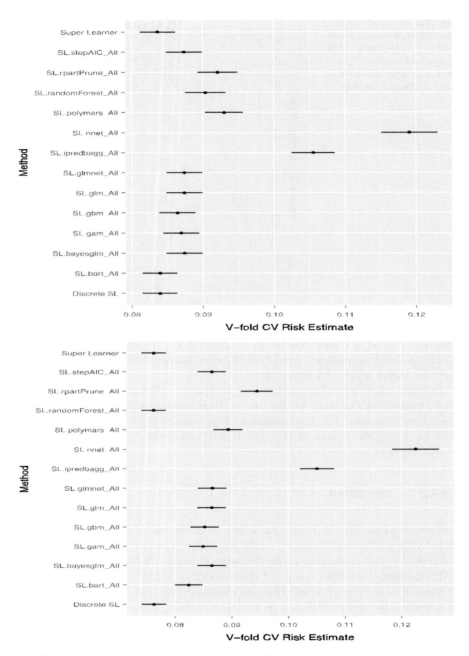

Fig. 20.3 Calibration and discrimination plots for SAPS 2 (*upper panel*) and SL1 (*lower panel*)

20.4.3 Super Learner Library

The performance of the 12 candidate algorithms, the Discrete *Super Learner* and the *Super Learner* combination algorithms, as evaluated by CV-MSE and CV-AUROC, are illustrated in Fig. 20.4.

As suggested by theory, when using either categorized variables (SL1) or untransformed variables (SL2), the *Super Learner* combination algorithm achieved the same performance as the best of all 12 candidates, with an average CV-MSE of 0.084 (SE = 0.001) and an average AUROC of 0.85 (95 %CI: 0.84–0.85) for SL1 [best single algorithm: Bayesian Additive Regression Trees, with CV-MSE = 0.084 and AUROC = 0.84 (95 %CI: 0.84, 0.85)]. For the SL2, the average CV-MSE was of 0.076 (SE = 0.001) and the average AUROC of 0.88 (95 %CI: 0.87–0.89) [best single algorithm: Random Forests, with CV-MSE = 0.076 and AUROC = 0.88 (95 %CI: 0.87–0.89)]. In both cases (SL1 and SL2), the *Super Learner* outperformed the main term logistic regression used to develop the SAPS II or the APACHE II score [main term logistic regression: CV-MSE = 0.087 (SE = 0.001) and AUROC = 0.83 (95 %CI: 0.82–0.83)].

20.4.4 Reclassification Tables

The reclassification *tables involving the SAPS* II score in its original and its actualized versions, the revised APACHE II score, and the SL1 and SL2 scores are provided in Table 20.2. When compared to the classification provided by the original SAPS II, the actualized SAPS II or the revised APACHE II score, the Super Learner-based scores resulted in a downgrade of a large majority of patients to a lower risk stratum. This was especially the case for patients with a predicted probability of death above 0.5.

We computed the cNRI and the IDI considering each Super Learner proposal (score A) as the updated model and the original SAPS II, the new SAPS II and the new APACHE II scores (score B) as the initial model. In this case, positive values of the cNRI and IDI would indicate that score A has better discriminative ability than score B, whereas negative values indicate the opposite. For SL1, both the cNRI (cNRI = 0.088 (95 %CI: 0.050, 0.126), $p < 0.0001$) and IDI (IDI = -0.048 (95 % CI: -0.055, -0.041), $p < 0.0001$) were significantly different from zero. For SL2, the cNRI was significantly different from zero (cNRI = 0.247 (95 %CI: 0.209, 0.285), $p < 0.0001$), while the IDI was close to zero (IDI = -0.001 (95 %CI: -0.010, -0.008), $p = 0.80$). When compared to the classification provided by the actualized SAPS II, the cNRI and IDI were significantly different from zero for both SL1 and SL2: cNRI = 0.295 (95 %CI: 0.257, 0.333), $p < 0.0001$ and IDI = 0.012 (95 %CI: 0.008, 0.017), $p < 0.0001$ for SL1; cNRI = 0.528 (95 %CI: 0.415, 0.565), $p < 0.0001$ and IDI = 0.060 (95 %CI: 0.054, 0.065), $p < 0.0001$ for SL2. When compared to the actualized APACHE II score, the cNRI and IDI were also

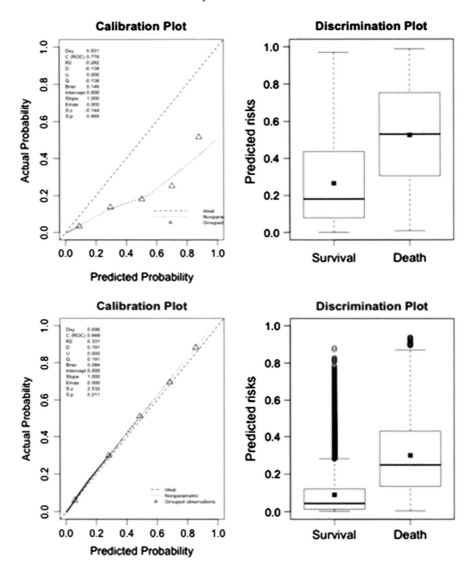

Fig. 20.4 Cross-validated mean-squared error for the super learner and the 12 candidate algorithms included in the library. Upper panel concerns the super learner with categorized variables (super learner 1): mean squared error (MSE) associated with each candidate algorithm (*top figure*)—receiver operating curves (ROC) for each candidate algorithm (*bottom figure*); lower panel concerns the super learner with non-transformed variables (super learner 2): mean squared error (MSE) associated with each candidate algorithm (*top figure*)—receiver operating curves (ROC) for each candidate algorithm (*bottom figure*)

20.4 Analysis

Table 20.2 Reclassification tables

	Updated model				
	0–0.25	0.25–0.5	0.5–0.75	0.75–1	% Reclassified
Super learner 1					
Initial model: original SAPS II					
0–0.25	13,341	134	3	0	1 %
0.25–0.5	4529	723	50	0	86 %
0.5–0.75	2703	1090	174	2	96 %
0.75–1	444	705	473	137	92 %
Super learner 2					
Initial model: original SAPS II					
0–0.25	12,932	490	55	1	4 %
0.25–0.5	4062	1087	142	11	79 %
0.5–0.75	2531	1165	258	15	93 %
0.75–1	485	775	448	51	97 %
Super learner 1					
Initial model: new SAPS II					
0–0.25	20,104	884	30	2	4 %
0.25–0.5	894	1426	238	9	44 %
0.5–0.75	18	328	361	62	53 %
0.75–1	1	14	71	66	57 %
Super learner 2					
Initial model: new SAPS II					
0–0.25	19,221	1667	124	8	9 %
0.25–0.5	765	1478	318	6	42 %
0.5–0.75	24	346	367	32	52 %
0.75–1	0	26	94	32	79 %
Super learner 1					
Initial model: new APACHE II					
0–0.25	19,659	1140	107	6	6 %
0.25–0.5	1262	1195	296	34	57 %
0.5–0.75	89	298	264	71	63 %
0.75–1	7	19	33	28	68 %
Super learner 2					
Initial model: new APACHE II					
0–0.25	18,930	1764	200	18	9 %
0.25–0.5	1028	1395	345	19	50 %

(continued)

Table 20.2 (continued)

	Updated model				
	0–0.25	0.25–0.5	0.5–0.75	0.75–1	% Reclassified
0.5–0.75	50	333	309	30	57 %
0.75–1	2	25	49	11	87 %

Super learner 1: super learner with categorized variables; super learner 2: super learner with non-transformed variables

significantly different from zero for both SL1 and SL2: cNRI = 0.336 (95 %CI: 0.298, 0.374), $p < 0.0001$ and IDI = 0.029 (95 %CI: 0.023, 0.035), $p < 0.0001$ for SL1; cNRI = 0.561 (95 %CI: 0.524, 0.598), $p < 0.0001$ and IDI = 0.076 (95 %CI: 0.069, 0.082) for SL2. When compared either to the new SAPS II or the new APACHE II score, both Super Learner proposals resulted in a large proportion of patients reclassified, especially from high predicted probability strata to lower ones.

20.5 Discussion

The new scores based on the *Super Learner* improve the prediction of hospital mortality in this sample, both in terms of discrimination and calibration, as compared to the SAPS II or the APACHE II scoring systems. The Super Learner severity score based on untransformed variables, also referred to as SL2 or SICULA, is available online through a web application. An ancillary important result is that the MIMIC-II database can easily and reliably serve to develop new severity score for ICU patients.

Our results illustrate the crucial advantage of the Super Learner that can include as many candidate algorithms as inputted by investigators, including algorithms reflecting available scientific knowledge, and in fact borrows strength from diversity in its library. Indeed, established theory indicates that in large samples the *Super Learner* performs at least as well as the (unknown) optimal choice among the library of candidate algorithms [28]. This is illustrated by comparing the CV-MSE associated with each algorithm included in the library: SL1 achieves similar performance as BART, which is the best candidate in the case, while SL2 achieves similar performance as random forest, which outperformed all other candidates in this case. Hence, the *Super Learner* offers a more flexible alternative to other nonparametric methods.

Given the similarity in calibration of the two Super Learner-based scores (SL1 and SL2), we recommend using the Super Learner with untransformed explanatory variables (SL2) in view of its greater discrimination. When considering risk reclassification, the two Super Learner prediction algorithms had similar cNRI, but SL2 clearly had a better IDI. It should be emphasized that, when considering the IDI, the SL1 seemed to perform worse that the SAPS II score. Nonetheless, the IDI must be used carefully since it suffers from similar drawbacks as the AUROC: it

20.5 Discussion

summarizes prediction characteristics uniformly over all possible classification thresholds even though many of these are unacceptable and would never be considered in practice [37].

20.6 What Are the Next Steps?

The SICULA should be compared to more recent severity scores. Nonetheless, such scores (e.g., SAPS 3 and APACHE III) have been reported to face the same drawbacks as SAPS II [9, 12, 38]. Moreover, those scores remain the most widely used scores in practice [39]. Despite the fact that MIMIC II encompasses data from multiple ICUs, the sample still comes from a single hospital and thus needs further external validation. However, the patients included in the MIMIC-II cohort seem representative of the overall ICU patient population, as reflected by a hospital mortality rate in the MIMIC-II cohort that is similar to the one reported for ICU patients during the same time period [40]. Consequently, our score can be reasonably expected to exhibit, in other samples, performance characteristics similar to those reported here, at least in samples drawn from similar patient populations. A large representation in our sample of CCU or CSRU patients, who often have lower severity scores than medical or surgical ICU patients, may have limited our score's applicability to more critically ill patients. Finally, a key assumption justifying this study was that the poor calibration associated with current severity scores derives from the use of insufficiently flexible statistical models rather than an inappropriate selection of variables included in the model. For this reason and for the sake of providing a fair comparison of our novel score with the SAPS II score, we included the same explanatory variables as used in SAPS II. Expanding the set of explanatory variables used could potentially result in a score with even better predictive performance. In the future, expending the number of explanatory variables will probably further improve the predictive performances of the score.

20.7 Conclusions

Thanks to a large collection of potential predictors and a sufficient sample size, MIMIC II dataset offers a unique opportunity to develop and validate new severity scores. In this population, the prediction of hospital mortality based on the Super Learner achieves significantly improved performance, both in terms of calibration and discrimination, as compared to conventional severity scores. The SICULA prediction algorithm is a promising alternative that could prove valuable in clinical practice and for research purposes. Externally validating results of this study in different populations (especially population outside the U.S.), providing regular update of the SICULA fit and assessing the potential benefit of including additional variables in the score remain important future challenges that are to be faced in the second stage of the SICULA project.

Open Access This chapter is distributed under the terms of the Creative Commons Attribution-NonCommercial 4.0 International License (http://creativecommons.org/licenses/by-nc/4.0/), which permits any noncommercial use, duplication, adaptation, distribution and reproduction in any medium or format, as long as you give appropriate credit to the original author(s) and the source, a link is provided to the Creative Commons license and any changes made are indicated.

The images or other third party material in this chapter are included in the work's Creative Commons license, unless indicated otherwise in the credit line; if such material is not included in the work's Creative Commons license and the respective action is not permitted by statutory regulation, users will need to obtain permission from the license holder to duplicate, adapt or reproduce the material.

Code Appendix

This case study used code from the Super Learner Library, implemented in R. Further details and code are available from the GitHub repository accompanying this book: https://github.com/MIT-LCP/critical-data-book. The following algorithms are included in the Super Learner Library.

Parametric algorithms:

- Logistic regression: standard logistic regression, including only main terms for each covariate and including interaction terms [42] (SL.glm),
- Stepwise regression: logistic regression using a variable selection procedure based on the Akaike Information Criteria [43] (SL.stepAIC),
- Generalized additive model [43] (SL.gam):,
- Generalized linear model with penalized maximum likelihood [44] (SL.glmnet),
- Multivariate adaptive polynomial spline regression [44] (SL.polymars),
- Bayesian generalized linear model [45] (SL.bayesglm).

Non parametric algorithms:

- Random Forest [46] (SL.randomForest),
- Neural Networks [47] (SL.nnet),
- Bagging classification trees [48] (SL.ipredbagg),
- Generalized boosted regression model [49] (SL.gbm),
- Pruned Recursive Partitioning and Regression Trees [50] (SL.rpartPrune),
- Bayesian Additive Regression Trees [51] (SL.bart).

References

1. Knaus WA, Zimmerman JE, Wagner DP, Draper EA, Lawrence DE (1981) APACHE-acute physiology and chronic health evaluation: a physiologically based classification system. Crit Care Med 9(8):591–597
2. Knaus WA, Draper EA, Wagner DP, Zimmerman JE (1985) APACHE II: a severity of disease classification system. Crit Care Med 13(10):818–829
3. Le Gall JR, Loirat P, Alperovitch A, Glaser P, Granthil C, Mathieu D, Mercier P, Thomas R, Villers D (1984) A simplified acute physiology score for ICU patients. Crit Care Med 12(11):975–977
4. Le Gall JR, Lemeshow S, Saulnier F (1993) A new simplified acute physiology score (SAPS II) based on a European/North American multicenter study. JAMA 270(24):2957–2963
5. Lemeshow S, Teres D, Klar J, Avrunin JS, Gehlbach SH, Rapoport J (1993) Mortality probability models (MPM II) based on an international cohort of intensive care unit patients. JAMA 270(20):2478–2486
6. Knaus WA, Wagner DP, Draper EA, Zimmerman JE, Bergner M, Bastos PG, Sirio CA, Murphy DJ, Lotring T, Damiano A (1991) The APACHE III prognostic system. Risk prediction of hospital mortality for critically ill hospitalized adults. Chest 100(6):1619–1636
7. Le Gall JR, Neumann A, Hemery F, Bleriot JP, Fulgencio JP, Garrigues B, Gouzes C, Lepage E, Moine P, Villers D (2005) Mortality prediction using SAPS II: an update for French intensive care units. Crit Care 9(6):R645–R652
8. Nassar AP, Jr, Mocelin AO, Nunes ALB, Giannini FP, Brauer L, Andrade FM, Dias CA (2012) Caution when using prognostic models: a prospective comparison of 3 recent prognostic models. J Crit Care 27(4), 423.e1–423.e7
9. Poole D, Rossi C, Latronico N, Rossi G, Finazzi S, Bertolini G (2012) Comparison between SAPS II and SAPS 3 in predicting hospital mortality in a cohort of 103 Italian ICUs. Is new always better? Intensive Care Med 38(8):1280–1288
10. Metnitz B, Schaden E, Moreno R, Le Gall J-R, Bauer P, Metnitz PGH (2009) Austrian validation and customization of the SAPS 3 admission score. Intensive Care Med 35(4):616–622
11. Moreno RP, Metnitz PGH, Almeida E, Jordan B, Bauer P, Campos RA, Iapichino G, Edbrooke D, Capuzzo M, Le Gall J-R (2005) SAPS 3–From evaluation of the patient to evaluation of the intensive care unit. Part 2: development of a prognostic model for hospital mortality at ICU admission. Intensive Care Med 31(10):1345–1355
12. Beck DH, Smith GB, Pappachan JV, Millar B (2003) External validation of the SAPS II, APACHE II and APACHE III prognostic models in South England: a multicentre study. Intensive Care Med 29(2):249–256
13. Aegerter P, Boumendil A, Retbi A, Minvielle E, Dervaux B, Guidet B (2005) SAPS II revisited. Intensive Care Med 31(3):416–423
14. Ledoux D, Canivet J-L, Preiser J-C, Lefrancq J, Damas P (2008) SAPS 3 admission score: an external validation in a general intensive care population. Intensive Care Med 34(10):1873–1877
15. Dybowski R, Weller P, Chang R, Gant V (1996) Prediction of outcome in critically ill patients using artificial neural network synthesised by genetic algorithm. Lancet 347(9009):1146–1150
16. Clermont G, Angus DC, DiRusso SM, Griffin M, Linde-Zwirble WT (2001) Predicting hospital mortality for patients in the intensive care unit: a comparison of artificial neural networks with logistic regression models. Crit Care Med 29(2):291–296
17. Ribas VJ, López JC, Ruiz-Sanmartin A, Ruiz-Rodríguez JC, Rello J, Wojdel A, Vellido A (2011) Severe sepsis mortality prediction with relevance vector machines. Conf Proc IEEE Eng Med Biol Soc 2011:100–103
18. Kim S, Kim W, Park RW (2011) A comparison of intensive care unit mortality prediction models through the use of data mining techniques. Health Inform Res 17(4):232–243

19. Foltran F, Berchialla P, Giunta F, Malacarne P, Merletti F, Gregori D (2010) Using VLAD scores to have a look insight ICU performance: towards a modelling of the errors. J Eval Clin Pract 16(5):968–975
20. Gortzis LG, Sakellaropoulos F, Ilias I, Stamoulis K, Dimopoulou I (2008) Predicting ICU survival: a meta-level approach. BMC Health Serv Res 8:157–164
21. Dudoit S, Van Der Laan MJ (2003) Asymptotics of cross-validated risk estimation in estimator selection and performance assessment. Statistical Methodology 2(2):131–154
22. Lee J, Scott DJ, Villarroel M, Clifford GD, Saeed M, Mark RG (2011) Open-access MIMIC-II database for intensive care research. Conf Proc IEEE Eng Med Biol Soc 2011:8315–8318
23. Saeed M, Villarroel M, Reisner AT, Clifford G, Lehman L-W, Moody G, Heldt T, Kyaw TH, Moody B, Mark RG (2011) Multiparameter intelligent monitoring in intensive care II: a public-access intensive care unit database. Crit Care Med 39(5):952–960
24. Goldberger AL, Amaral LA, Glass L, Hausdorff JM, Ivanov PC, Mark RG, Mietus JE, Moody GB, Peng CK, Stanley HE (2000) PhysioBank, PhysioToolkit, and PhysioNet: components of a new research resource for complex physiologic signals. Circulation 101(23): E215–E220
25. Pirracchio R, Petersen ML, Carone M, Rigon MR, Chevret S, van der Laan MJ (2015) Mortality prediction in intensive care units with the super ICU learner algorithm (SICULA): a population-based study. Lancet Respir Med 3(1)
26. Vincent JL, Moreno R, Takala J, Willatts S, De Mendonça A, Bruining H, Reinhart CK, Suter PM, Thijs LG (1996) The SOFA (Sepsis-related Organ Failure Assessment) score to describe organ dysfunction/failure. On behalf of the working group on sepsis-related problems of the European Society of Intensive Care Medicine. Intensive Care Med 22 (7):707–710
27. Van Der Laan MJ, Dudoit S (2003) Unified cross-validation methodology for selection among estimators and a general cross-validated adaptive epsilon-net estimator: finite sample oracle inequalities and examples. U.C. Berkeley Division of Biostatistics Working Paper Series, Working Paper, no 130, pp 1–103
28. van der Laan MJ, Polley EC, Hubbard AE (2007) Super learner. Stat Appl Genet Mol Biol 6:25
29. Cox DR (1958) Two further applications of a model for binary regression. Biometrika 45 (3/4):562–565
30. Harrison DA, Brady AR, Parry GJ, Carpenter JR, Rowan K (2006) Recalibration of risk prediction models in a large multicenter cohort of admissions to adult, general critical care units in the United Kingdom. Crit Care Med 34(5):1378–1388
31. Kramer AA, Zimmerman JE (2007) Assessing the calibration of mortality benchmarks in critical care: the Hosmer-Lemeshow test revisited. Crit Care Med 35(9):2052–2056
32. Bertolini G, D'Amico R, Nardi D, Tinazzi A, Apolone G (2000) One model, several results: the paradox of the Hosmer-Lemeshow goodness-of-fit test for the logistic regression model. J Epidemiol Biostat 5(4):251–253
33. Miller ME, Hui SL, Tierney WM (1991) Validation techniques for logistic regression models. Stat Med 10(8):1213–1226
34. Cook NR (2007) Use and misuse of the receiver operating characteristic curve in risk prediction. Circulation 115(7):928–935
35. Cook NR (2008) Statistical evaluation of prognostic versus diagnostic models: beyond the ROC curve. Clin Chem 54(1):17–23
36. Pencina MJ, D'Agostino RB, Sr, D'Agostino RB, Jr, Vasan RS (2008) Evaluating the added predictive ability of a new marker: from area under the ROC curve to reclassification and beyond. Stat Med 27(2):157–172; discussion 207–212, Jan 2008
37. Greenland S (2008) The need for reorientation toward cost-effective prediction: comments on 'Evaluating the added predictive ability of a new marker: From area under the ROC curve to reclassification and beyond' by M. J. Pencina et al., Statistics in Medicine 10.1002/sim.2929. Stat Med 27(2):199–206

References

38. Sakr Y, Krauss C, Amaral ACKB, Réa-Neto A, Specht M, Reinhart K, Marx G (2008) Comparison of the performance of SAPS II, SAPS 3, APACHE II, and their customized prognostic models in a surgical intensive care unit. Br J Anaesth 101(6):798–803
39. Rosenberg AL (2002) Recent innovations in intensive care unit risk-prediction models. Curr Opin Crit Care 8(4):321–330
40. Zimmerman JE, Kramer AA, Knaus WA (2013) Changes in hospital mortality for United States intensive care unit admissions from 1988 to 2012. Crit Care 17(2):R81
41. Van der Laan MJ, Rose S (2011) Targeted learning: causal inference for observational and experimental data. Springer, Berlin
42. McCullagh P, Nelder JA (1989) Generalized linear models, vol 37. Chapman & Hall/CRC
43. Venables WN, Ripley BD (2002) Modern applied statistics with S. Springer, Berlin
44. Friedman JH (1991) Multivariate adaptive regression splines. Ann Stat 1–67
45. Gelman A, Jakulin A, Pittau MG, Su YS (2008) A weakly informative default prior distribution for logistic and other regression models. Ann Appl Stat 1360–1383
46. Breiman L (2001) Random forests. Mach Learn 45(1):5–32
47. Ripley BD (2008) Pattern recognition and neural networks. Cambridge university press, Cambridge
48. Breiman L (1996) Bagging predictors. Mach Learn 24(2):123–140
49. Elith J, Leathwick JR, Hastie T (2008) A working guide to boosted regression trees. J Anim Ecol 77(4):802–813
50. Breiman L, Friedman J, Olshen R, Stone C (1984) Classification and regression trees. Chapman & Hall, New York
51. Chipman HA, George EI, McCulloch RE (2010) BART: Bayesian additive regression trees. Ann Appl Stat 4(1):266–298

Chapter 21
Mortality Prediction in the ICU

Joon Lee, Joel A. Dubin and David M. Maslove

Learning Objectives
Build and evaluate mortality prediction models.

1. Learn how to extract predictor variables from MIMIC-II.
2. Learn how to build logistic regression, support vector machine, and decision tree models for mortality prediction.
3. Learn how to utilize adaptive boosting to improve the predictive performance of a weak learner.
4. Learn how to train and evaluate predictive models using cross-validation.

21.1 Introduction

Patients admitted to the ICU suffer from critical illness or injury and are at high risk of dying. ICU mortality rates differ widely depending on the underlying disease process, with death rates as low as 1 in 20 for patients admitted following elective surgery, and as high as 1 in 4 for patients with respiratory diseases [1]. The risk of death can be approximated by evaluating the severity of a patient's illness as determined by important physiologic, clinical, and demographic determinants.

In clinical practice, estimates of mortality risk can be useful in triage and resource allocation, in determining appropriate levels of care, and even in discussions with patients and their families around expected outcomes. Estimates of mortality risk are, however, based on studying aggregate data from large, heterogeneous groups of patients, and as such their validity in the context of any single patient encounter cannot be assured. This shortcoming can be mitigated by personalized mortality risk estimation, which is well discussed in [2, 3], but is not a subject of the present study.

Perhaps even more noteworthy uses of mortality prediction in the ICU are in the areas of health research and administration, which often involve looking at cohorts of critically ill patients. Traditionally, such population-level studies have been more widely accepted as applications of mortality prediction given the cohort-based derivation of prediction models. In this context, mortality prediction is used to compare the average severity of illness between groups of critically ill patients (for example, between patients in different ICUs, hospitals, or health care systems) and between groups of patients enrolled in clinical trials. Predicted mortality can be compared with observed mortality rates for the purpose of benchmarking and performance evaluation of ICUs and health systems.

A number of severity of illness (SOI) scores have been introduced in the ICU to predict outcomes including death. These include the APACHE scores [4], the Simplified Acute Physiology Score (SAPS) [5], the Mortality Probability Model (MPM) [6], and the Sequential Organ Failure Assessment (SOFA) score [7]. These scoring systems perform well, with areas under the receiver operator characteristic (ROC) curves (AUROCs) typically between 0.8 and 0.9 [5, 6, 8]. Current research is exploring ways to leverage the enhanced completeness and expressivity of modern electronic medical records (EMRs) in order to improve prediction accuracy. In particular, the granular nature (i.e., a rich set of clinical variables recorded in high temporal resolution) of EMRs can lead to creating a personalized predictive model for a given patient by identifying and utilizing data from similar patients.

21.2 Study Dataset

This case study aimed to create mortality prediction models using the first ICU admissions from all adult patients in MIMIC-II version 2.6. In the *icustay_detail* table, adult patients in MIMIC-II can be identified by *icustay_age_group='adult'*, whereas the first ICU admission of each patient can be selected by *subject_icustay_seq=1*. In addition, all ICU stays with a null *icustay_id* were excluded, since *icustay_id* was used to find the data in other tables that correspond to the included ICU stays. A total of 24,581 ICU admissions in MIMIC-II met these inclusion criteria.

The following demographic/administrative variables were extracted to be used as predictors: age at ICU admission, gender, admission type (elective, urgent, emergency), and first ICU service type of the ICU admission. Furthermore, the first measurement in the ICU of the following vital signs and lab tests was each extracted as a predictor: heart rate, mean and systolic blood pressure (invasive and noninvasive measurements combined), body temperature, SpO_2, respiratory rate, creatinine, potassium, sodium, chloride, bicarbonate, hematocrit, white blood cell count, glucose, magnesium, calcium, phosphorus, and lactate. Although the very

21.2 Study Dataset

first measurements in the ICU were extracted, the exact measurement time with respect to the ICU admission time would have varied between patients. Also, this approach to variable-by-variable data extraction does not ensure concurrent measurements within patient. For the vast majority of the ICU admissions in MIMIC-II, however, measurements of these common clinical variables were obtained at the beginning of the ICU admission, or at most within the first 24 h.

As the patient outcome to be predicted, mortality at 30 days post-discharge from the hospital was extracted. In MIMIC-II, this binary outcome variable can be obtained by comparing the date of death (found in the *d_patients* table) and the hospital discharge date (found in the *icustay_detail* table). If our focus were on a greater time period to post-discharge death, we would have extracted mortality date in an attempt to predict survival time.

21.3 Pre-processing

Some of the extracted variables require further processing before they can be used for predictive modeling. In MIMIC-II, some ages are unrealistically large (~ 200 years), as they were intentionally inserted to mask the actual ages of those patients who were 90 years or older and still alive (according to the latest social security death index data), which is protected health information. For these patients, the median of such masked ages (namely, 91.4) was substituted. Furthermore, regarding ICU service type, FICU (Finard ICU; this is a term specific to Beth Israel Deaconess Medical Center where MIMIC-II data were collected) was converted to MICU (medical ICU) since there are only a small number of FICU admissions in MIMIC-II and FICU is nothing more than a special MICU.

There are abundant missing data in MIMIC-II. Although there are ways to make use of ICU admissions with incomplete data (e.g., imputation), this case study simply excluded cases with incomplete data since missing data is discussed in depth in [insert reference to Missing Data Chapter, Part 2]. After exclusion of cases with incomplete data, only 9269 ICU admissions remained. This still is a sufficient sample size to conduct the present case study, but approaches such as imputation and/or exclusion of variables with frequent missing data should be considered if a larger patient sample size is required.

With default settings in R, numeric variables are normally imported correctly with proper handling of missing data (flagged as NA), but special care may be needed for importing categorical variables. In order to avoid the empty field being imported as a category on its own, this case study (1) imported the categorical variables as strings, (2) converted all empty fields to NA, and then (3) converted the categorical variables to factors. This case study includes the following categorical variables: gender, admission type, ICU service type, and 30-day mortality.

21.4 Methods

The following predictive models were employed: logistic regression (LR), support vector machine (SVM), and decision tree (DT). These models were chosen due to their widespread use in machine learning. Although the reader should refer to appropriate chapters in Part 2 to learn more about these models, a brief description of each model is provided here.

LR is a model that can learn the mathematical relationship, within a restricted framework using a logistic function, between a set of covariates (i.e., predictor variables in this case study) and a binary outcome variable (i.e., mortality in this case study). Once this relationship is learned, the model can make a prediction for a new case given the predictor values from the new case. LR is very widely used in health research thanks to its easy interpretability.

SVMs are similar to LR in the sense that it can classify (or predict) a given case in terms of the outcome, but they do so by coming up with an optimal decision boundary in the data space where the dimensions are the covariates and all available data points are plotted. In other words, SVMs attempt to draw a decision boundary that puts as many negative (survived) cases as possible on one side of the boundary and as many positive (expired) cases as possible on the other side.

Lastly, DTs have a tree-like structure that consists of decision nodes in a hierarchy. Each decision node leads to two branches depending on the value of a particular covariate (e.g., age >65 or not). Each case follows appropriate branches until it reaches a terminal leaf node which is associated with a particular outcome. DT learning algorithms automatically learn an optimal decision tree structure given a set of data.

We also attempted to improve the predictive performance of the DT by applying adaptive boosting, i.e., AdaBoost [9]. AdaBoost can effectively improve a weak predictive model by building an ensemble of models that progressively focus more on the cases that are inaccurately predicted by the previous model. In other words, AdaBoost allowed us to build a series of DTs where the ones built later were experts on more challenging cases. In AdaBoost, the final prediction is the average of the predictions from the individual models.

In order to run the provided R code, the following R packages should be installed via *install.packages()*: *e1071*, *ada*, *rpart*, and *ROCR*. The training functions for LR, SVM, and DT are *glm()*, *svm()*, and *rpart()*, respectively. For all models, default parameter settings were used.

For training and testing, 10-fold cross-validation was utilized. Under such a scheme, the ICU admissions included in the case study were randomly partitioned into 10 similarly sized groups (a.k.a. folds). The procedure rotated through the 10 folds to train predictive models based on 9 folds (training data) and test them on the remaining fold (test data), until each fold is utilized as test data.

Predictive performance was measured using AUROC which is a widely used performance metric for binary classification. For each predictive model, the

21.4 Methods

AUROC was calculated for each fold of the cross-validation. In the provided R code, the *comp.auc()* function is called to calculate the AUROC given a set of predicted probabilities from a model and the corresponding actual mortality data.

21.5 Analysis

The following were the AUROCs of the predictive models (shown in mean [standard deviation]): LR—0.790 [0.015]; SVM—0.782 [0.014]; DT—0.616 [0.049]; AdaBoost—0.801 [0.013]. Hence, in terms of mean AUROC, AdaBoost resulted in the best performance, while DT was clearly the worst predictive model. DT was only moderately better than random guessing (which would correspond to an AUROC of 0.5) and as a result can be considered a weak learner. Note that AdaBoost was able to substantially improve DT, which is consistent with its known ability to effectively improve weak learners. Because of the random data partitioning of cross-validation, slightly different results will be produced every time the provided R code is run. Using *set.seed()* in R can seed the random number generation in *sample()* and make the results reproducible, but this was not used in this case study for a more robust evaluation of the results.

As a comparison, a previous study [2] reported mean AUROCs of 0.658 (95 % confidence interval (CI): [0.648,0.668]) and 0.633 (95 % CI: [0.624,0.642]) for SAPS I and SOFA, respectively, for predicting 30-day mortality for 17,152 adult ICU stays in MIMIC-II, despite that the analyzed patient cohort was a bit different from the one in this case study. More advanced SOI scores such as APACHE IV would have achieved a comparable or better performance than the predictive models investigated in this case study (only SAPS I and SOFA are available in MIMIC-II), but it should be noted that those advanced SOI scores tend to use a much more comprehensive set of predictors than the ones used in this case study.

21.6 Visualization

Figure 21.1 shows the performances of the predictive models in a boxplot. It is visually apparent that AdaBoost, LR, and SVM resulted in similar performance, while DT yielded not only the worst performance but also the largest variability in AUROC, which sheds light on its sensitivity to the random data partitioning in cross-validation.

Figure 21.2 is an interesting visualization of the prediction results, where each circle represents a patient and the color of the circle indicates the prediction result (correct or incorrect) of the patient. Random horizontal jitter was added to each point (this simply means that a small random shift was applied to the x-value of each point) to reduce overlap with other points. Prediction results from only one of the ten cross-validation folds are shown, with a threshold of 0.5 (arbitrarily selected;

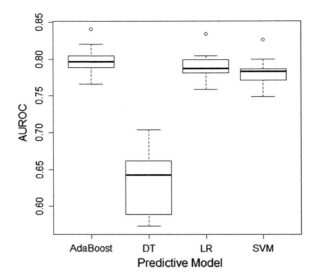

Fig. 21.1 A *box* and *whisker* plot showing mortality prediction performances of several predictive models from 10-fold cross-validation. *AUROC* Area under the receiver operating characteristic curve; *DT* Decision tree; *LR* Logistic regression; *SVM* Support vector machine

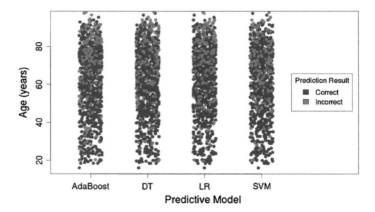

Fig. 21.2 Prediction results for individual patients as a function of age, stratified by predictive model. Results from only one of the ten cross-validation folds are plotted here

the reader may be interested in studying how this threshold affects this figure) applied to the estimated mortality risks from the predictive models (by calling the *th.pred()* function in the R code). Figure 21.2 shows the prediction results as a function of age, but the variable on the y-axis can easily be changed to some other variable of interest (e.g., heart rate, creatinine). One observation that is clear in Fig. 21.2 but not in Fig. 21.1 is that predictive accuracy is higher for younger

21.6 Visualization

patients (e.g., <40 years) than for older patients, across all predictive models. This is most likely due to the fact that mortality rate is much lower among younger patients than older patients, and predictive models can achieve a high accuracy by biasing towards predicting low mortality risks (however, this would lead to a low sensitivity). Hence, it is important to note that although Fig. 21.2 conveys a sense of overall accuracy, it does not reveal sensitivity, specificity, positive predictive value, or negative predictive value.

21.7 Conclusions

Using clinical and demographic data from the MIMIC II database, this case study used machine learning algorithms to classify patients as alive or dead at 30 days after hospital discharge. Results were comparable to those obtained by the most up to date SOI scores currently in use. Unlike these scores, however, the learning algorithms used did not have access to specific diagnoses and procedures, which can add considerable predictive power. An advantage of using only clinical and demographic data, however, is that they are more routinely available and as a result predictive models based on them can be used more widely. Moreover, our algorithms were applied to an undifferentiated population of critically ill patients, rather than tailored to specific groups such as those following cardiovascular surgery (i.e., cardiac surgery recovery unit (CSRU) patients), which has also been shown to enhance predictive performance [3]. The success of prediction seen in this case study likely reflects the power of the learning algorithms used, as well as the utility of both the size and granularity of the database studied.

One useful prospect that leverages the dynamic nature of EMR data is the potential to update training data and prediction models as the most recent clinical data become available. This would theoretically lead to equally dynamic scoring systems that generate more accurate predictions by reflecting current practices. A trade-off becomes apparent between the use of the most current data, which is likely to be the most representative, and the inclusion of older data as well, which may be less relevant but provides greater statistical power.

21.8 Next Steps

Although AUROCs near 0.8 represent good performance, the fact that LR, SVM, and AdaBoost resulted in similar performance may imply that performance could be limited by the predictor variables rather than model selection. A meaningful future study could further investigate predictor selection or different representations of the same variables (e.g., temporal patterns rather than measurements at a specific time point; see the Hyperparameter Selection chapter of Part 3).

Since the default parameter settings were used for the LR, SVM, DT, and AdaBoost, another reasonable next step is to investigate how changing the parameters affect predictive performance. Please refer to R Help or appropriate R package documentation to learn more about the model parameters.

To improve predictive performance, we have previously considered a personalized mortality prediction approach where only the data from patients that are similar to an index patient (for whom prediction is to be made) are used for training customized predictive models [2]. Using a particular cosine-similarity-based patient similarity metric and LR, the maximum AUROC this study reported was 0.83. In light of this promising result, the reader is invited to pursue similar personalized approaches with new patient similarity metrics.

Bayesian methods [10] offer another prediction paradigm that may be worth investigating. Bayesian methods strike a balance between subject-matter expertise (for mortality prediction in the ICU, this would correspond to clinical expertise regarding mortality risk) and empirical evidence in the clinical data. Since the machine learning models discussed in this chapter were purely empirical, the explicit addition of clinical expertise through the Bayesian paradigm can potentially improve predictive performance.

Aside from AUROC, there are other ways to evaluate predictive performance, including the scaled Brier score. Please see [11] for more information. Once a threshold is applied to predicted mortality risk, more conventional performance measures such as accuracy, sensitivity, specificity, etc. can also be calculated. Since each performance measure has pros and cons (e.g., while AUROC provides a more complete assessment than simple accuracy, it becomes biased for skewed datasets [12]), it may be best to calculate a variety of measures for a holistic assessment of predictive performance.

Lastly, data quality is often overlooked but plays an important role in determining what predictive performance is possible with a given set of data. This is a particularly critical issue with retrospective EMR data, the recording of which may have had minimal data quality checks. Implementation of more rigorous data quality checks (e.g., outliers, physiologic feasibility) prior to predictive model training is a meaningful next step.

21.9 Connections

While this chapter focused on mortality prediction, the data extraction and analytic techniques discussed here are widely applicable to prediction of other discrete (e.g., hospital re-admission) and continuous (e.g., length of stay) patient outcomes. In addition, the nuances related to MIMIC-II such as handling ages near 200 years and the service type FICU are important issues for any MIMIC-II study.

The machine learning models (LR, DT, SVM) and techniques (cross-validation, AdaBoost, AUROC) are widely used in a variety of prediction, detection, and data

21.9 Connections

mining applications, not only in but beyond medicine. Furthermore, given that R is one of the most popular programming languages in data science, being able to manipulate EMR data and apply machine learning in R is an invaluable skill to have.

Open Access This chapter is distributed under the terms of the Creative Commons Attribution-NonCommercial 4.0 International License (http://creativecommons.org/licenses/by-nc/4.0/), which permits any noncommercial use, duplication, adaptation, distribution and reproduction in any medium or format, as long as you give appropriate credit to the original author(s) and the source, a link is provided to the Creative Commons license and any changes made are indicated.

The images or other third party material in this chapter are included in the work's Creative Commons license, unless indicated otherwise in the credit line; if such material is not included in the work's Creative Commons license and the respective action is not permitted by statutory regulation, users will need to obtain permission from the license holder to duplicate, adapt or reproduce the material.

Code Appendix

The code used in this case study is available from the GitHub repository accompanying this book: https://github.com/MIT-LCP/critical-data-book. Further information on the code is available from this website. The reader can reproduce the present case study by running the following SQL and R codes verbatim:

- `query.sql`: used to extract data from the MIMIC II database.
- `analysis.R`: used to perform data processing.

References

1. Kuzniewicz MW, Vasilevskis EE, Lane R, Dean ML, Trivedi NG, Rennie DJ, Clay T, Kotler PL, Dudley RA (2008) Variation in ICU risk-adjusted mortality: impact of methods of assessment and potential confounders. Chest 133(6):1319–1327
2. Lee J, Maslove DM, Dubin JA (2015) Personalized mortality prediction driven by electronic medical data and a patient similarity metric. PLoS ONE 10(5):e0127428
3. Lee J, Maslove DM (2015) Customization of a severity of illness score using local electronic medical record data. J. Intensive Care Med, 0885066615585951
4. Knaus WA, Draper EA, Wagner DP, Zimmerman JE (1985) APACHE II: a severity of disease classification system. Crit Care Med 13(10):818–829
5. Legall JR, Lemeshow S, Saulnier F (1993) A new simplified acute physiology score (SAPS-II) based on a european north-american multicenter study. Jama-J Am Med Assoc 270:2957–2963
6. Lemeshow S, Teres D, Klar J, Avrunin JS, Gehlbach SH, Rapoport J (1993) Mortality Probability Models (MPM II) based on an international cohort of intensive care unit patients. JAMA 270(20):2478–2486

7. Vincent J, Moreno R, Takala J, Willatts S, De Mendonca A, Bruining H, Reinhart C, Suter P, Thijs L (1996) The SOFA (sepsis-related organ failure assessment) score to describe organ dysfunction/failure. Intensive Care Med 22(7):707–710
8. Gursel G, Demirtas S (2006) Value of APACHE II, SOFA and CPIS scores in predicting prognosis in patients with ventilator-associated pneumonia. Respiration. 73(4):503–508
9. Freund Y, Schapire R (1995) A desicion-theoretic generalization of on-line learning and an application to boosting. Comput Learn Theory 55(1):119–139
10. Gelman A, Carlin JB, Stern HS, Rubin DB (2014) Bayesian data analysis, vol 2. Taylor & Francis, UK
11. Wu YC, Lee WC (2014) Alternative performance measures for prediction models. PLoS One 9(3)
12. Davis J, Goadrich M (2006) The relationship between precision-recall and ROC curves. In: Proceedings of the 23rd international conference on Machine learning—ICML'06, pp 233–240

Chapter 22
Data Fusion Techniques for Early Warning of Clinical Deterioration

Peter H. Charlton, Marco Pimentel and Sharukh Lokhandwala

Learning Objectives
Design and evaluate early warning score (EWS) algorithms which fuse vital signs with additional physiological parameters commonly available in hospital electronic health records (EHRs).

1. Extract physiological, demographic and biochemical variables from the MIMIC II database.
2. Extract patient outcomes from the MIMIC II database.
3. Prepare EHR data for analysis in Matlab®.
4. Design data fusion algorithms in Matlab®.
5. Compare the performances of data fusion algorithms.

22.1 Introduction

Acutely-ill hospitalized patients are at risk of clinical deteriorations such as infection, congestive heart failure and cardiac arrest [1]. The early detection and management of such deteriorations can improve patient outcomes, and reduce healthcare resource utilization [2, 3]. Currently, early warning scores (EWSs) are used to assist in the identification of deteriorating patients. EWSs were designed for use at the bedside: they can be calculated by hand, and the required inputs (vital signs) can be easily measured at the bedside. Now that EHRs are becoming more widespread in acute hospital care there is scope to develop improved EWSs by using more complex algorithms calculated by computer, and by incorporating additional physiological data from the EHR.

Most methods for detection of deteriorations are based on the assumption that changes in physiology are manifested during the early stages of deteriorations. This assumption is well documented. Schein et al. published landmark results in 1990 that 84 % of patients "had documented observations of clinical deterioration or new complaints" in the eight hours preceding cardiac arrest [4]. This was further supported by a study by Franklin et al. [5]. Physiological abnormalities have also been observed prior to other deteriorations such as unplanned Intensive Care Unit (ICU) admissions [6] and preventable deaths [7]. Evidence of deterioration can be observed 8–12 h before major events [8, 9].

It was proposed that the incidence of deteriorations could be reduced by recognising and responding to early changes in physiology [10–12]. Subsequently, EWSs were developed to allow timely recognition of patients at risk of deterioration. EWSs are aggregate scores calculated from a set of routinely and frequently measured physiological parameters, known as vital signs. The higher the score, the more abnormal the patient's physiology, and the higher the risk of future deterioration. EWSs are now in widespread use in acute hospital wards [13].

Current EWSs correlate with important patient-centered endpoints such as levels of intervention [14], hospital mortality [14, 15], and length of stay [15], and have been shown to be a better predictor of cardiac arrest than individual parameters [16]. However, there is scope for improving their performance since most EWSs use simple formulae which can be calculated by hand at the bedside, and use only a limited set of vital signs as inputs [17]. Now that electronic health records (EHRs) are becoming widely used in acute hospital care, there is opportunity to use more complex, automated algorithms and a broader range of inputs. Consequently, algorithms have been proposed in the literature which improve performance by using data fusion techniques to combine vital signs with other parameters such as biochemistry and demographic data [18, 19].

The remainder of this chapter is designed to equip the reader with the necessary tools to develop and evaluate data fusion algorithms for prediction of clinical deteriorations.

22.2 Study Dataset

Data was extracted from the MIMIC II database (v. 2.26) [21], which is publicly available on PhysioNet [22]. This database was chosen because it contains routinely recorded EHR data for thousands of patients who, being critically-ill, are at high risk of deterioration. Data extraction was performed using the three SQL queries `cohort_labs.sql`, `cohort_vitals.sql`, and `cohort_selection.sql`. For ease of analysis data were extracted from only 500 patients. Only adult data were extracted since paediatrics have different normal physiological ranges to those of adults. The parameters extracted from the database, listed in Table 22.1, were chosen in line with those used previously in the literature [18, 19].

Traditionally the performance of EWSs has been assessed using three outcome measures with which rapid response systems have been assessed: mortality, cardiopulmonary arrest and ICU admission rates [20]. However, cardiopulmonary arrests are difficult to reliably identify in the MIMIC II dataset, and the dataset only

22.2 Study Dataset

Table 22.1 EHR Parameters extracted from the MIMIC II database records for input into data fusion algorithms

Biochemisty	Vital signs
Albumin	Respiratory rate
Anion gap	Heart rate
Arterial pCO$_2$	Blood pressure—systolic and diastolic
Arterial pH	Temperature
Aspartate aminotransferase (AST)	Oxygen saturation
Bicarbonate	Level of consciousness
Blood urea nitrogen (BUN)	**Demographics**
Calcium	Age
Creatinine	Gender
Glucose	
Hemoglobin	
Platelets	
Potassium	
Sodium	
Total bilirubin	
White blood cell count (WBC)	

contains data from patients already staying on the ICU. Therefore, mortality, which can be reliably and easily extracted from the dataset, was chosen as the outcome measure for this case study.

22.3 Pre-processing

Data analysis was conducted in Matlab®. The first pre-processing step was to import the *CSV* files generated by the *SQL* query into Matlab® (using `LoadData.m`). The purpose of this step was to create:

1. A design matrix of predictor variables (the parameters listed in Table 22.1): This MxN matrix contained values for each of the N parameters at each of M time points. This was performed using the methodology in [19]: the time-points were calculated as the end times of successive four-hour periods spanning each patient's ICU stay; parameter values at the time-points were set to the last measured value during that time period.
2. An Mx3 response matrix of the three easily acquired dependent variables, namely, binary variables of death in ICU and death in ICU within the next 24 h, and a continuous variable of time to ICU death.

The remaining pre-processing steps and analyses were conducted using only data from within these matrices.

Further pre-processing was required to prepare the data for analysis (`PreProcessing.m`). Firstly, it was observed that the temperature values exhibited a bimodal distribution centred on 37.1 and 98.8 °C, indicating that some had been measured in Celsius, and others in Fahrenheit. Those measured in

Fahrenheit were converted to Celcius. Secondly, the dataset contained blood pressures (BPs) acquired invasively and non-invasively. Invasive measurements were retained since they had been acquired more frequently. Non-invasive measurements were replaced with surrogate invasive values by correcting for the observed biases between the two measurement techniques when both had been used in the same four-hour periods (the median differences between invasive and non-invasive measurements were 2, 7 and 6 mmHg for systolic, diastolic and mean BPs respectively). Finally, the dataset contained missing values where parameters had not been measured within particular four-hour periods. These missing data had to be imputed since the analysis technique to be used, logistic regression, requires a complete data set. To do so, we followed the approach proposed previously of imputing the last measured value, unless no value had yet been measured in which case the population median value was imputed [19]. Note that this approach could be applied to a dataset in real-time.

22.4 Methods

Novel data fusion algorithms were created using `CreateDataFusionAlgs.m`. Generalized linear models were used to fuse both continuous and binary variables to provide an output indicative of the patient's risk of deterioration. A training dataset, containing 50 % of the data, was used to create the algorithms.

Logistic regression was used to estimate the probability of each of the binary response variables of "death in ICU", and "death in ICU within 24 h" being true. Logistic regression differs from ordinary linear regression in that it bounds the output to be between 0 and 1, thus making it suitable for estimation of the probability of a response variable being true. Logistic regression provides an estimate for

$$y = \ln\left[\frac{p(x)}{1 - p(x)}\right]$$

where $p(x)$ is the probability of the response variable being true and x is a vector of predictor variables. Notice that $p(x)$ is constrained to be between 0 and 1 for all real values of y.

When using logistic regression one must decide how to model the relationships between the n predictor variables contained within x, and the output, y. The simplest method is to assume that y is linearly related to the predictor variables as $y = \alpha + \sum_{i=1}^{n} \beta_i x_i$, where α is the intercept term, and β is a vector of coefficients. For variables such as diastolic blood pressure the assumption of a linear relationship is reasonable because they consistently change in one particular direction during a deterioration. However, other variables such as sodium level could change in either

22.4 Methods

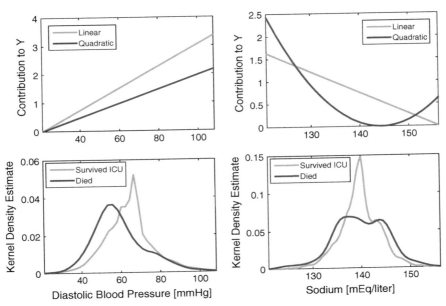

Fig. 22.1 A comparison of the contributions of input variables to the algorithm output, Y, under the assumptions of either a linear or a non-linear relationship between the input variables and Y. The choice of relationship had little impact on the contribution of Diastolic Blood Pressure (*above left*), since it tended to be reduced in those patients who died (*below left*). However, a quadratic relationship provided a very different contribution for Sodium Level (*above right*), since the Sodium Levels of those patients who died exhibited a biomodal distribution indicating either an increase or a decrease away from the normal range (*below right*)

direction away from normality. For these variables a non-linear relationship is more appropriate, such as the quadratic

$$y = \alpha + \sum_{i=1}^{n} \beta_i x_i + \sum_{i=1}^{n} \gamma_i x_i^2,$$

where γ is a vector of coefficients for the squares of the predictor variables. Note that this 'purely quadratic' relationship does not contain interaction terms such as $x_i x_j$. The importance of the choice of relationship between the predictor variables and the estimate is demonstrated in Fig. 22.1.

In this case study separate algorithms were created using linear and quadratic relationships. Firstly, only the parameters which are used in EWSs (vital signs) were included. Secondly, all the extracted EHR parameters were included. Thirdly, stepwise regression was used to avoid including terms which do not increase the performance of the model. This consisted of building a model by including terms until no further terms would increase the performance of the model, and then removing terms whose removal would not significantly decrease the performance of the model.

22.5 Analysis

EWS algorithms must trigger an effective clinical response in order to impact patient outcomes. Typically, a particular response is mandated when the algorithm's output is elevated above a threshold value. The response may include clinical review by ward staff or a centralised rapid response team. The following analysis is based on the assumption that the algorithms would be used to mandate responses such as this.

The performance of each algorithm was analysed using the latter 50 % of the data—the validation dataset. At all 4 h time points the model was used to estimate the probability of a patient dying during their ICU stay. Figure 22.2 shows exemplary plots of the output for four patients throughout their ICU stays. Throughout the analysis, each time point was classified as either positive or negative, indicating that the model predicted that the patient either subsequently died on ICU, or survived to ICU discharge. Hence, a true positive is identified at a particular time point when the model correctly predicts the death of a patient who died on ICU, whereas a false positive is identified when the model incorrectly predicts the death of a patient who survived to ICU discharge. True and false negatives were similarly identified.

Table 22.2 shows the performances of each algorithm assessed using the area under the receiver operating characteristic (ROC) curve (AUROC). The algorithm with the highest AUROC of 0.810 used stepwise inclusion of parameters and the quadratic relationship. The ROC curves for this algorithm and the corresponding algorithm using vital signs alone are shown in Fig. 22.3. Algorithms using all available parameters as inputs had higher AUROCs than those using vital signs

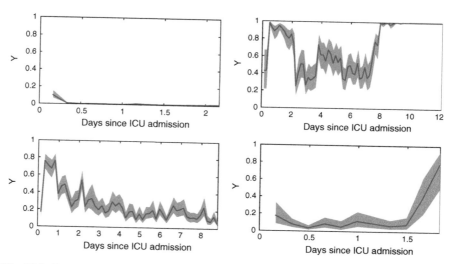

Fig. 22.2 Exemplary plots of the output of algorithm outputs (Y) over the duration of patients' ICU stays. The *left hand* plots show patients who survived their ICU stays, whereas the *right hand* plots show patients who died. The *upper plots* show examples in which the algorithm performed well, whereas the *lower plots* show examples in which the algorithm did not perform well

22.5 Analysis

Table 22.2 The performances of data fusion algorithms for prediction of death in ICU, given as the area under the receiver-operator curve (AUROC), and the maximum sensitivities when the algorithms were constrained to satisfy the clinical requirements of a PPV ≥ 0.33, and an alert rate of ≤ 17 %

Relationship between predictor variables and output	Candidate predictor variables	Number of predictor variables included	AUROC	Maximum Sensitivities [%]	
				PPV ≥ 0.33	Alert rate ≤ 17 %
Linear	Vital signs only	6	0.757	14.4	42.5
Linear	All	25	0.800	46.6	49.7
Linear	Stepwise inclusion of all	23	0.800	45.8	48.9
Purely quadratic	Vital signs only	6	0.774	13.2	41.4
Purely quadratic	All	25	0.799	55.5	53.9
Purely quadratic	Stepwise inclusion of all	21	0.810	59.3	56.3

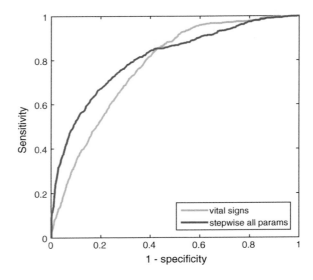

Fig. 22.3 Receiver operating characteristic curves showing the performances of the best algorithms using stepwise inclusion of all parameters, and vital signs alone. These algorithms assumed a quadratic relationship between the predictor variables and the output

alone, demonstrating the benefit of fusing vital signs with additional parameters. In most instances the use of a quadratic relationship resulted in a higher AUROC. Furthermore, stepwise selection of parameters did reduce the number of parameters required, whilst maintaining or improving the AUROC.

Other metrics for comparison of algorithms have been suggested including sensitivity, positive predictive value (PPV) and alert rate [23]. However, these are more difficult to use since each metric varies according to the threshold value. A useful method for comparing algorithms using these metrics is to compare their sensitivities when a threshold is used which provides algorithmic performance in line with clinical requirements. In the case of EWS algorithms, key clinical requirements are that the PPV is at or above a minimum acceptable level, and the alert rate is at or below a maximum acceptable level. In the absence of evidence-based values, for demonstration purposes we used a minimally acceptable PPV of 0.33, indicating that one in three alerts is a true positive, and a maximally acceptable alert rate of 17 %, indicating that one in six observation sets results in an alert. Table 22.2 shows the sensitivities provided by each algorithm when constrained to satisfy these clinical requirements. The PPVs and alert rates at all thresholds are shown in Fig. 22.4 for the best performing algorithms using vital

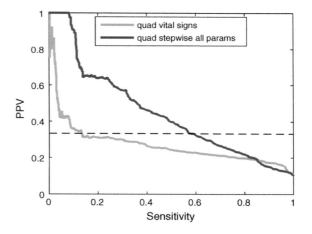

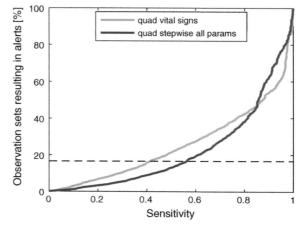

Fig. 22.4 A comparison of the PPVs and alert rates for algorithms using vital signs alone and using all parameters. Exemplary clinical requirements of a PPV ≥ 0.33 and an alert rate ≥17 % are shown by the *dashed lines*. The quadratic algorithm using vital signs alone has a much lower sensitivity of 13.2 % than the equivalent algorithm using stepwise inclusion of all parameters, at 59.3 % when the PPV criterion is met. Similarly, when the alert rate criterion is used, the sensitivity of the vital signs algorithm is 41.4 %, also lower than that of the algorithm using stepwise inclusion of all parameters, at 56.3 %

22.5 Analysis

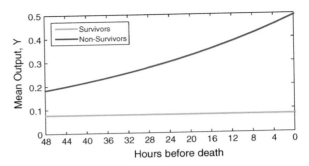

Fig. 22.5 Mean algorithm outputs during the 48 h prior to death on ICU (after exponential smoothing). A lower choice of threshold for alerting results in more advanced warning of deterioration

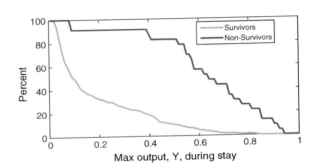

Fig. 22.6 The proportion of survivors and non-survivors who reached each algorithm output value during their ICU stay. A lower choice of threshold for alerting results in more false alerts, and fewer true alerts

signs alone and using stepwise inclusion of all parameters. The highest sensitivities were achieved when using stepwise inclusion of all parameters, with a purely quadratic relationship. The benefit of using additional parameters beyond vital signs is clearly shown by the algorithms' sensitivities at the minimum acceptable PPV, which were 13.2 % when using vital signs alone, and 59.3 % when using stepwise inclusion of all parameters.

In [19] additional visualisations were used to demonstrate the effect of choosing different thresholds. Firstly, the dependent variable of time before death on ICU was used to examine how the output changed with time before death, as shown in Fig. 22.5. This shows that a lower threshold results in more advanced warning of deterioration. Secondly, the proportion of patients who reached each output during their stay was presented, as shown in Fig. 22.6. This suggests that a lower threshold results in more false alerts and fewer true alerts.

22.6 Discussion

The introduction of EHRs has provided opportunity to improve the clinical algorithms used to identify deteriorations. The data fusion algorithms described in this chapter estimate the probability of a patient dying during their ICU stay every 4 h.

The inclusion of additional physiological parameters beyond vital signs alone resulted in improvements in algorithm performance in this study when assessed using the AUROC, as also observed previously [18, 19], and when assessed using the minimum sensitivities corresponding to clinical requirements.

This case study has demonstrated the fundamental steps required to design and evaluate data fusion algorithms for prediction of deteriorations. During pre-processing the required data were extracted from the raw data files, and processed into matrices ready for analysis. It was important to perform this step separately to the analysis to reduce the time required for algorithm design. During this step we identified deficiencies in the dataset. Unfortunately, there is no systematic way to ensure that all deficiencies have been identified. We recommend that firstly the distributions of each variable are inspected to identify obvious discrepancies such as the different units used for temperature in this dataset. Secondly, it is helpful to plot the raw data over time to identify any changes in practice that may have occurred during data acquisition. Thirdly, it is often valuable to seek the guidance of a clinician or database curator at the host institution, or a researcher who has worked with the dataset before.

The results presented here cannot be generalised to a hospital-wide patient population for two reasons. Firstly, the dataset consists of data from critically-ill patients, whereas EWSs are primarily designed to identify deteriorations in acutely-ill patients. Since the disease processes of critically-ill patients are more advanced and they have additional clinical interventions such as mechanical ventilation and organ support, both the baseline physiology and the physiological changes accompanying deteriorations may differ in this population compared to acutely-ill patients. Secondly, death in ICU was used as the dependent variable in this study. Death is the latest possible stage of deterioration, and therefore an algorithm which predicts death may not predict the onset of deteriorations early enough to be of clinical utility in acutely-ill patients.

The choice of statistical methods to assess the performance of EWSs is the subject of debate [23]. The AUROC has often been used to quantify the performance of EWS algorithms, such as in [17]. This statistic is calculated from an algorithm's sensitivities and specificities at a range of threshold values. However, it has been recently suggested that the AUROC is misleading due to the low prevalence of deteriorations [23]. In [23] alternative statistical measures were proposed to account for the clinical requirements of EWS algorithms. Statistical measures should firstly assess the benefits and costs of using EWSs. The benefit is that EWSs can act as a safety net to catch deteriorating patients who have been missed in routine clinical assessments. This requires a high sensitivity (the proportion of EWS assessments of deteriorating patients which do alert). The cost of EWSs is the time taken to respond to false alerts. This cost is relatively small, since the additional clinical assessment triggered by an alert takes only a short amount of time. This means that a high specificity (the proportion of negative tests which are true negatives) is not of great importance. Secondly, it is important to ensure that the positive predictive value (the proportion of alerts which are true) is high enough to prevent caregivers suffering from desensitisation to alerts, which may result in less effective responses to patients who are correctly identified as deteriorating [24]. Thirdly, the alert rate must be manageable to avoid excessive resource utilization. In this case study we presented the AUROC and the maximum sensitivities when algorithms were constrained to a minimally acceptable PPV and a maximally acceptable alert rate [23].

22.7 Conclusions

This case study has demonstrated the potential utility of data fusion techniques to predict clinical deteriorations. Currently identification of deteriorations is achieved using EWSs which take vital signs as inputs. The performance of the data fusion algorithms assessed in this study was improved by increasing the set of inputs to include physiological parameters which are routinely available in EHRs, but are not measured at the bedside.

The fundamental techniques for design and evaluation of data fusion algorithms have been demonstrated. Logistic regression algorithms were used to predict a binary response variable, death in ICU. The use of both linear and quadratic relationships between the predictor and response variables were demonstrated as well as the use of stepwise inclusion of variables. A range of statistical measures were presented for evaluation of algorithms, illustrating the benefits of using alternative statistical measures to the commonly used AUROC.

The results should not be interpreted as representative of the results that could be expected when EWSs are used in acute settings since the study dataset consists of critically-ill patients, and death in ICU was used as the dependent variable. However, the techniques used to design and evaluate algorithms can be easily applied to a wide range of patient settings, providing a basis for further work.

22.8 Further Work

Two particular areas have been identified for further research. Firstly, the work could be repeated using a dataset acquired from acutely-ill, rather than critically-ill patients, and by using a dependent variable other than death. This would facilitate design of algorithms that are generalisable to the target hospital population. Secondly, a range of additional functions could be explored to model the relationship between the predictor variables and the output. More complex functions than the linear or purely quadratic functions such as higher order polynomials or logistic functions may improve performance. In addition it would be prudent to investigate the effect of the inclusion of interaction terms to account for the relationships between predictor variables.

22.9 Personalised Prediction of Deteriorations

The algorithms presented here are limited in scope by the input parameters. Currently they obtain a detailed description of a patient's physiological state from the vital signs and biochemistry values, which make up 23 out of the 25 inputs. However, these parameters provide very little differentiation between individual patients according to their state on admission to hospital. In contrast, additional information present upon hospital admission is used by clinicians during a patient's hospital stay to contextualise physiological assessments.

To illustrate this, consider the response of the algorithms to two fictional 65-year old males, patients A and B. Patient A has a history of hypertension, and a high systolic blood pressure (SBP) prior to hospital admission of 147 mmHg. Patient B has led an active life, has a healthy diet, and has a relatively low SBP prior to admission of 114 mmHg. During their hospital stay, the SBP of both patients is measured to be 114 mmHg. The algorithms cannot distinguish whether this is representative of patient A during a significant deterioration, such as the early stages of hypotension preceding septic shock, or whether it is representative of patient B's usual state in the absence of any deterioration. If the algorithms used a wider range of inputs indicative of patient state prior to admission, such as the presence or absence of co-morbidities (existing medical conditions) including hypertension, they might be able to differentiate between patients A and B in this situation.

This illustrates the potential benefit of incorporating additional inputs indicating co-morbidities. Even greater benefit may be derived by also personalising EWS algorithms according to physiological state prior to admission. Personalised EWS algorithms would not only stratify patients using additional inputs to contextualise physiology, but would also personalise the regression coefficients according to a patient's physiological state measured previously at a time of relative health.

Open Access This chapter is distributed under the terms of the Creative Commons Attribution-NonCommercial 4.0 International License (http://creativecommons.org/licenses/by-nc/4.0/), which permits any noncommercial use, duplication, adaptation, distribution and reproduction in any medium or format, as long as you give appropriate credit to the original author(s) and the source, a link is provided to the Creative Commons license and any changes made are indicated.

The images or other third party material in this chapter are included in the work's Creative Commons license, unless indicated otherwise in the credit line; if such material is not included in the work's Creative Commons license and the respective action is not permitted by statutory regulation, users will need to obtain permission from the license holder to duplicate, adapt or reproduce the material.

Code Appendix

The code used in this case study is available from the GitHub repository accompanying this book: https://github.com/MIT-LCP/critical-data-book. Further information on the code is available from this website. The following key scripts were used to extract data from the MIMIC II database:

- `cohort_selection.sql`: used to identify a cohort of patients for whom data would be extracted.
- `cohort_labs.sql`: used to extract laboratory test results.
- `cohort_vitals.sql`: used to extract vital signs.

Data was extracted in CSV format. Subsequent analysis was performed in Matlab® using `RunFusionAnalysis.m`. It contains the following script:

- `SetupUniversalParams`: used to set universal parameters (in this case, file paths), which are used to load and save files throughout the analysis). These parameters should be adapted when using the code.

It then called the following scripts:

- `LoadData.m`: used to load CSV data into Matlab® for analysis.
- `PreProcessing.m`: performs pre-processing to prepare data for analysis.
- `CreateDataFusionAlgs.m`: creates data fusion algorithms using training data.
- `AnalysePerformances.m`: analyses the performances of data fusion algorithms using validation data.

References

1. Silber JH et al (1995) Evaluation of the complication rate as a measure of quality of care in coronary artery bypass graft surgery. JAMA 274(4):317–323
2. Khan NA et al (2006) Association of postoperative complications with hospital costs and length of stay in a tertiary care center. J Gen Intern Med 21(2):177–180
3. Lagoe RJ et al (2011) Inpatient hospital complications and lengths of stay: a short report. BMC Res Notes 4(1):135
4. Schein RM et al (1990) Clinical antecedents to in-hospital cardiopulmonary arrest. Chest 98(6):1388–1392
5. Franklin C et al (1994) Developing strategies to prevent inhospital cardiac arrest: analyzing responses of physicians and nurses in the hours before the event. Crit Care Med 22(2):244–247
6. Buist MD et al (1999) Recognising clinical instability in hospital patients before cardiac arrest or unplanned admission to intensive care. A pilot study in a tertiary-care hospital. Med J Aust 171(1):22–25
7. Hillman KM et al (2001) Antecedents to hospital deaths. Intern Med J 31(6):343–348
8. Hillman KM et al (2002) Duration of life-threatening antecedents prior to intensive care admission. Intensive Care Med 28(11):1629–1634

9. Whittington J et al (2007) Using an automated risk assessment report to identify patients at risk for clinical deterioration. Jt Comm J Qual Patient Saf 33(9):569–574
10. Smith AF et al (1998) Can some in-hospital cardio-respiratory arrests be prevented? A prospective survey. Resuscitation 37(3):133–137
11. Patient Safety Observatory (2007) Safer care for the acutely ill patient: learning from serious incidents. National Patient Safety Agency, London
12. Whittington J et al (2007) Using an automated risk assessment report to identify patients at risk for clinical deterioration. Jt Comm J Qual Patient Saf 33(9):569–574
13. Royal College of Physicians (2012) National early warning score (NEWS): standardising the assessment of acute-illness severity in the NHS", Report of a working party. RCP, London
14. Goldhill DR et al (2005) A physiologically-based early warning score for ward patients: the association between score and outcome. Anaesthesia 60(6):547–553
15. Paterson R et al (2006) Prediction of in-hospital mortality and length of stay using an early warning scoring system: clinical audit. Clin. Med. 6(3):281–284
16. Churpek MM et al (2012) Predicting cardiac arrest on the wards: a nested case-control study. Chest 141(5):1170–1176
17. Smith GB et al (2013) The ability of the national early warning score (NEWS) to discriminate patients at risk of early cardiac arrest, unanticipated intensive care unit admission, and death. Resuscitation 84(4):465–470
18. Alvarez CA et al. (2013) Predicting out of intensive care unit cardiopulmonary arrest or death using electronic medical record data. BMC Med Inform Decis Mak 13(28)
19. Churpek MM et al (2014) Multicenter development and validation of a risk stratification tool for ward patients. Am J Respir Crit Care Med 190:649–655
20. Maharaj R et al (2015) Rapid response systems: a systematic review and meta-analysis. Crit Care 19(1):254
21. Saeed M et al (2011) Multiparameter intelligent monitoring in intensive care II: a public-access intensive care unit database. Crit Care Med 39(5):952–960
22. Goldberger AL et al (2000) PhysioBank, PhysioToolkit, and PhysioNet: components of a new research resource for complex physiologic signals. Circulation 101(23):E215–E220
23. Romero-Brufau S, Huddleston JM, Escobar GJ, Liebow M (2015) Why the C-statistic is not informative to evaluate early warning scores and what metrics to use. Crit Care 19(1):285
24. Cvach M (2012) Monitor alarm fatigue: an integrative review. Biomed Instrum Technol 46 (4):268–277

Chapter 23
Comparative Effectiveness: Propensity Score Analysis

Kenneth P. Chen and Ari Moskowitz

Learning Objectives
Understand the incentives and disadvantages of using propensity score analysis for statistical modeling and causal inference in EHR-based research.

This case study introduces concepts that should improve understanding of the following:

1. Be aware of different approaches for estimating propensity scores: parametric, non-parametric, and machine learning approaches; and understand the pros and cons of each.
2. Learn different ways of using propensity scores to adjust for pre-treatment conditions, and to assess the balance of pre-treatment conditions among different treatment groups.
3. Appreciate concepts underlying propensity score analysis with EHRs including stratification, matching, and inverse probability weighting (including straight weight, stabilized weight, and doubly robust weighted regression).

23.1 Incentives for Using Propensity Score Analysis

When conducting research with electronic health records (EHRs) or other big data sources, we have access to a large number of covariates [1]. These covariates include patient demographics, physical parameters (e.g., vitals signs and physical examinations), laboratory parameters, home medications, pre-morbid conditions, etc. All these covariates could be confounders when considering the association between an exposure and an outcome. We can use statistical modeling to account for the confounding effect of these covariates and establish an association between the exposure and the outcome of interest [2, 3]. Propensity score analysis is particularly advantageous when dealing with a large number of covariates [1]. The remainder of this chapter assumes a basic understanding of statistics and regression modeling (especially logistic regression).

Adjusting for as many covariates as possible sets the ground for a convincing causal inference by reducing latent biases due to latent variates [4]. However, this results in increased dimension [5]. Although large scale EHRs often have large enough sample size to allow high-dimensional study, dimension reduction is still useful for the following reasons: (i) to simplify the final model and make interpretation easier, (ii) to allow sensitivity analyses to explore higher order terms or interaction terms for those covariates that might have correlation or interaction with the outcome, and (iii) depending on the research question, the study cohort might still be small despite coming from a large database, and dimension reduction therefore becomes crucial for a model to be valid.

23.2 Concerns for Using Propensity Score

Although propensity score analysis has the above mentioned advantages, it is important to understand the theory of propensity score analysis and appreciate its limitations. A propensity score is an 'estimated probability' of one subject being assigned to either the treatment group or the control group given the subject's 'characteristics', or 'pre-treatment conditions'. It is a surrogate for all the covariates that are used to estimate it. It is not hard to imagine that using a single propensity score to represent all characteristics of a subject could introduce bias [6]. Therefore, implementing propensity scores in a statistical analysis model has to take into account the research question, the dataset, and the covariates included in the analysis. Furthermore, results must always be validated with sensitive analyses [7].

23.3 Different Approaches for Estimating Propensity Scores

In a randomized controlled trial, a causal relationship between exposure (treatment) and outcome can be readily determined if the randomization is carried out properly, i.e. if there is no difference in pre-treatment conditions between the two groups. However, in retrospective studies a difference in pre-treatment conditions between the two groups almost always exists. In order to demonstrate comparative effectiveness, causal inference with statistical modeling can be carried out in a number of ways [8, 9]. For propensity score analyses [3, 10], the pre-treatment conditions can be used as predictors in determining the likelihood of a subject being in the treatment group or the control group. In other words, the probability of being in the treatment or control group is a function of pre-treatment conditions. There are a number of ways to generate this function. The most basic one is regression.

When using regression to estimate propensity scores, the outcome of the regression equation is either treatment group or control group, i.e. a binary outcome, and the variables in the regression equation can be a combination of numeric and nominal variables. This is a multivariate logistic regression that can be easily performed using most free or commercial statistical packages. If there is more than one treatment group (e.g., treatment A, treatment B, and control group) [11], then the propensity score can be estimated using a multivariate multinomial logistic regression.

The conventional regression model is a parametric model. Consequently, the estimated propensity score will be subject to any inherent limitations of the parametric model, i.e. model misspecification [12]. It is possible to use a non-parametric model to estimate the propensity score [13], such as regression trees, piecewise approaches, and kernel distributions. However, these methodologies are less established and are likely to require the use of machine learning algorithms [14]. Although non-parametric methods often require machine learning algorithms, machine learning techniques can be applied to both parametric and non-parametric methods. For example, some studies use a genetic algorithm to select variables and model specification for a conventional logistic regression to estimate propensity score [15].

23.4 Using Propensity Score to Adjust for Pre-treatment Conditions

The goal of using propensity score analysis is to create a treatment group and a control group that are indistinguishable from each other in terms of the pre-treatment conditions statistics (e.g., means and standard deviations of numeric variables, distribution of nominal variables). In other words, a treatment group and a control group are created that mimic a post-randomization assignment result of a randomized controlled trial, so that a causal inference can be made. Propensity score analysis is one of the tools to reach this goal [8, 9, 16].

For example, consider one subject that received the study drug or treatment (treatment group) and one subject that received placebo or standard treatment (control group). If they have similar pre-treatment conditions then their chance (probability) of being in the treatment group is the same. Consequently, it is comparable to two identical subjects being randomly assigned to either treatment or control group. When we find two subjects that have similar propensity scores where one actually received treatment and the other actually received placebo, we 'match' them in our final study cohorts before we look at the treatment effect (outcome variable). This process is called "propensity score matching." By doing this, we will have similar propensity score distributions (or pre-treatment conditions distributions) between the treatment and control groups.

If the model used to estimate propensity scores is well-specified [17, 18], we would expect the propensity scores to be representative of subjects' pre-treatment conditions. However, this might not always be the case, so we always look at the group statistics after propensity score matching. Since the ultimate goal is to eliminate the difference in pre-treatment conditions between groups, other methods like propensity score weighting have been proposed to achieve this. More sophisticated machine learning algorithms have also been developed that look at the balance of pre-treatment variables between two groups during the process of estimating a propensity score to ensure a valid model in simulating a randomized controlled trial-like result [19].

In EHR data research, we have access to a large number of pre-treatment covariates that we can extract from the database and use in the propensity score model. Although we cannot use an indefinite number of covariates to simulate a real RCT (which accounts for all unobserved variables), we can gain greater confidence in our conclusion by including more variables [20, 21]. Propensity score analysis is a powerful tool to simplify the final model while allowing a large number of pre-treatment conditions to be included. Figure 23.1 summarizes the above discussion of applying a propensity score model.

We now present a case study that used the MIMIC II database (v.2.26) [22, 23], and focus on the application of propensity scores in the analytic phase. The study was a retrospective cohort study of Intensive Care Unit (ICU) patients who were treated with at least one rate control agent (metroprolol, amiodarone or diltiazem). Propensity score analysis was performed using the following covariates: demographics, vital signs, basic metabolic panels, past medical conditions, disease severity scores, types of admission, and types of ICU. The outcomes measured

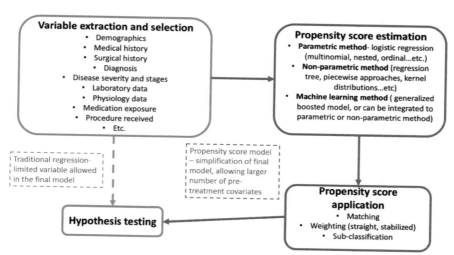

Fig. 23.1 Integration of propensity score analysis into a statistical design

were: (i) whether rate control was achieved by a single agent, or multiple agents (binary outcome); and, for those patients who reached rate control, (ii) the time to reach rate control (continuous outcome).

23.5 Study Pre-processing

In order to identify those patients with atrial fibrillation and rapid ventricular response (Afib with RVR) in the dataset, we used a combination of structured and unstructured data. Specifically, the structured data used included ICD-9 codes (the code for "Atrial Fibrillation" is 427.31) and medication administration data. The unstructured data used included waveform ECG data, serial heart rate (HR) data, discharge summaries and nursing notes. Unfortunately, only a small fraction of patients in the database have waveform data (approximately 2000 out of 32,000 patients). Consequently, we were unable to take full advantage of waveform analysis.

Patients who had Afib with RVR mentioned in their discharge summaries were identified by text searching equivalent keywords in discharge summaries while excluding the past medical history section. Once these patients had been identified we used the serial HR and medication administration data to find the subset of patients who had a HR of over 110 beats per minute (bpm) for more than 15 min and who received at least one of the rate control agents of interest (metoprolol, diltiazem, or amiodarone). Raw data was extracted using the Oracle® variety of SQL and was further processed using Python®, for text-searching discharge summaries, and Matlab®, for processing and plotting serial HR data and establishing temporal relationship between rapid ventricular response and medication administration.

Serial HR data existed for almost every patient in the database. However, contrary to the continuous waveform ECG data, it is only recorded every 5, 10, or 15 min and inconsistently. To make the data more homogenous and easier for plotting and processing, we interpolated the HR every 5 min: during the patient's ICU stay, if a raw HR data was not available for any given 5-min period, a value was interpolated using the two adjacent data points. Because of the infrequent sampling of HR for this data entity, one HR data point above 110 bpm would correspond to an episode of a rapid HR of 5-min duration. We arbitrarily chose a 15-min duration as a significant episode of rapid HR that warrants the algorithm (described below) to bring in more information from other data entity to determine if the tachycardic episode reflected Afib with RVR or another form of rapid rhythm (e.g. sinus tachycardia). This doesn't mean that a patient has to have 15 min of Afib with RVR before the physician decides to treat in clinical practice. Instead, it is a measure to reduce the noise of solitary rapid HRs. One can experiment on implementing different cut-off values and then review the result to determine an appropriate threshold.

After identifying an episode of rapid HR which appeared to last for at least 15 min, we next determined whether the patient received a pharmacologic control agent of interest within 2 h before or after the identified episode. A 2-h window was used because medication data and HR data are two different data entities, and the time stamps they carried might not be aligned exactly. Furthermore, the time stamps associated with medication data might subject to inaccurate data entry by human loggers. This window was arbitrarily determined; a smaller window would have increase specificity but decreased the sensitivity of detecting the cohort of interest, and vice versa for a larger window.

A major criterion for determining the effectiveness of a pharmacologic agent in the control of Afib with RVR is the time until termination of the RVR episode. As this information is not explicitly contained in the database, one has to define when the rate is 'controlled' and then run an algorithm to find the time lapse between the onset and resolution of RVR. The half-life of intravenous metoprolol and dilitazem are each approximately 4 h and, therefore, we defined the resolution of RVR as achieving sustained HR below 110 bpm for 4 h. Although there is no consensus for the definition of RVR resolution, as long as the same definition is used for every subject or sub-cohort, there is a ground for comparison. Our algorithm finds every HR below 110 bpm after the previous identified Afib RVR (episodes of rapid HR that lasted for at least 15 min and were treated by at least one rate control agent) and tested if the ensuing HR data in the following 4 h was below 110 bpm for at least 90 % of the time. The time lapse between the onset and the resolution can then be calculated.

Covariates, including demographics, vital signs, basic metabolic panels, past medical conditions, disease severity scores, types of admission, and types of ICU, were extracted using SQL. We also looked into the patient's home medication and past medical history of Afib. These pieces of information have to be extracted from the "home meds" and "past medical history" sections in the discharge summaries by using natural language processing techniques to text-search in a particular section of a discharge summary. Figure 23.2 is an example that our group used for discussing the analytic model.

Although we identified 1876 patients who were treated for Afib with RVR, only 320 of them received diltiazem as the first rate control agent. Using conventional regression analysis would result in over-fitting because of the small cohort size, and leaving out covariates would likely introduce biases. Propensity score analysis was used to reduce dimensionality. The first step is to estimate the propensity score (probability of being assigned to one treatment group given the pre-treatment covariates). As mentioned earlier, there are several different ways to estimate propensity scores including parametric methods such as multinomial logistic regression, and non-parametric methods such as prediction trees. Machine learning techniques can be implemented to train the propensity score model for optimized prediction. After the propensity score has been estimated, it can be used either as a variable in regression model to match subjects in different treatment groups with similar propensity scores, or to calculate inverse probability weights. When estimating propensity scores, besides optimizing the model to best predict the possible

23.5 Study Pre-processing

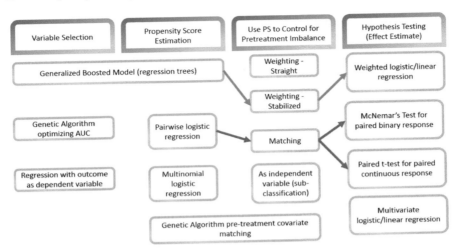

Fig. 23.2 Group discussions of the analytical model. The *green arrows* represent the final model, and the *red arrows* represent the model that was used as sensitivity analysis

treatment assignment given the pre-treatment variables, a newer concept is to estimate propensity scores to balance out pre-treatment covariates after matching or weighting. When using propensity score weighting, one can choose to use either straight weights or stabilized weights. Straight weighting is more susceptible to outliers with very distinct combination of pre-treatment covariates, and will double the cohort size when there are two treatment groups or triple the cohort size when there are three treatment groups. On the other hand, stabilized weighting is less susceptible to outliers, and does not increase the cohort size regardless of the number of treatment groups.

For this study we chose a machine learning algorithm (a generalized boosted model) to build a regression tree for the estimation of propensity scores (a non-parametric method). The reason for not choosing a parametric method is the same as that for not using a conventional regression analysis, as mentioned above. The model iteratively combines many simple regression trees until the pre-determined metrics for assessing between group pre-treatment covariate imbalance (standardized bias or Kolmogorov-Smirnov statistics) reach a minimum.

Extreme weights were eliminated using stabilized weights. Stabilized weights were then implemented in the final weighted regression for hypothesis testing. Depending on the nature of the outcome variable, weighted logistic regression is used for a binary outcome, and weighted liner regression is used for a continuous outcome. Several covariates with higher predictive power (of treatment assignment) were included in the final weighted regression model.

23.6 Study Analysis

In general, propensity score analysis has been used to compare two treatment groups, i.e. treatment versus control group. It is also commonly used for stratification (using propensity score as a covariate in a regression model) and propensity score matching (creating treatment and control groups of similar pre-treatment attribute and thus mimicking randomized trials). However, stratification can only establish association and propensity score matching mainly serves as a way of dimension reduction. Propensity score matching does carry the intention for causal inference, but matching propensity scores of three or more treatment groups requires calculating two or more dimensional distances for each matched group of subjects, which can be mathematically challenging and lacks supporting theory. Therefore, we chose machine-generated regression trees for our propensity score, and used a propensity score weighted regression model for outcome effect. The non-parametric approach avoided the limitations and biases introduced by model specification when using parametric methods. After the propensity score weight was generated, weighted regression was performed. This allows for exploration of interaction terms and adjustment for variables that have heavier effects on the outcomes that could not be fully eliminated by using propensity scores alone.

To validate our model, a series of sensitivity analyses using pair-wise propensity score matching were performed and similar effects of different treatment groups have on the outcomes were observed.

23.7 Study Results

In this single center retrospective cohort study, intravenous metoprolol was the most commonly used rate control agent for the control of Afib with RVR amongst patients in the intensive care unit. Using a novel propensity matching based approach, the effectiveness of metoprolol was compared to two other commonly used pharmacologic agents used for the control of Afib with RVR: diltiazem and amiodarone. With regards to the primary outcome of medication failure (defined as a switch to or addition of a second rate control agent), metoprolol had the lowest overall failure rate. Those patients who received diltiazem (odds ratio OR 1.55, confidence interval CI 1.05–2.3, $p = 0.027$) or amiodarone (OR 1.50, CI 1.1–2.0, $p = 0.006$) as their initial pharmacologic agent were more likely to receive an additional agent prior to the end of the RVR episode. In a secondary analysis of patients who received only one drug during their RVR episode, those who received diltiazem had significantly longer times to resolution of the RVR episode. Similarly, patients who received only diltiazem were also less likely to be controlled at 4 h than those who only received metoprolol (OR 0.59, CI 0.40–0.86, $p = 0.007$).

These results suggest that critically ill patients with Afib with RVR are less likely to require a second pharmacologic agent and more likely to be controlled at

4 h if they receive metoprolol as their initial rate control agent then either diltiazem or amiodarone. This effect seems to be most pronounced when comparing metoprolol to diltiazem.

23.8 Conclusions

While it is widely accepted that Afib with RVR in the ICU is associated with worse outcomes overall, there is no clear consensus with regards to optimal pharmacologic management and practice varies amongst clinicians. Through the use of a three-way propensity matching model, we have compared the most commonly used pharmacologic agents for this phenomenon and found evidence that starting with metoprolol may lead to fewer treatment failures and a more rapid resolution of the RVR episode.

Propensity score theory is more commonly implemented on two-treatment group studies. Estimating propensity score in multiple-treatment group studies and implementing that in causal inference can be statistically and mathematically challenging. In this chapter, we provided an example of multiple-treatment group propensity score analysis using machine-learning algorithm. The concepts explored in this chapter can be easily implemented in any two-treatment group studies. We also provided an example of two treatment group propensity score analysis in the sensitivity analyses of our study by performing pair-wise comparison between different treatment groups. Propensity score analysis can be a powerful way to achieve causal inference and dimension reduction in studies utilizing EHRs.

23.9 Next Steps

The data analysis strategy employed in this project may be particularly helpful in answering a range of research questions in the ICU setting. Critical care clinicians frequently have to select from a range of interventions or pharmacologic agents. As opposed to traditional propensity matching approaches where only two groups are compared, this model allows for the simultaneous comparison of three independent groups. Examples where this analysis approach could be useful include comparing the effectiveness of different vasopressors in the treatment of shock or different sedative agents for intubated patients with ARDS.

Given the degree of clinical equipoise with regards to the treatment of Afib with RVR in the ICU, the above results are powerful in providing some direction to clinicians faced with this complex clinical problem. Still, many questions remain. It is not clear, for instance, whether higher doses of diltiazem may have been more effective and thereby avoided relatively increased rates of treatment failure. We did not look at doses provided in this study. We also did not explore the oral versus intravenous versus combined routes of administration. Atrial fibrillation during critical illness is a common phenomenon whose management requires further investigation.

Open Access This chapter is distributed under the terms of the Creative Commons Attribution-NonCommercial 4.0 International License (http://creativecommons.org/licenses/by-nc/4.0/), which permits any noncommercial use, duplication, adaptation, distribution and reproduction in any medium or format, as long as you give appropriate credit to the original author(s) and the source, a link is provided to the Creative Commons license and any changes made are indicated.

The images or other third party material in this chapter are included in the work's Creative Commons license, unless indicated otherwise in the credit line; if such material is not included in the work's Creative Commons license and the respective action is not permitted by statutory regulation, users will need to obtain permission from the license holder to duplicate, adapt or reproduce the material.

Code Appendix

The code used in this case study is available from the GitHub repository accompanying this book: https://github.com/MIT-LCP/critical-data-book. Further information on the code is available from this website. The following key scripts were used:

- `database_query.sql`: used to extract data from the MIMIC II database.
- `data_extraction.m`: used to extract variables for analysis.
- `propensity_score_analysis.r`: used for propensity score analysis.
- `propensity_score_matching.r`: used for propensity score matching.

References

1. Patorno E et al (2014) Studies with many covariates and few outcomes: selecting covariates and implementing propensity-score-based confounding adjustments. Epidemiology 25(2):268–278
2. Fitzmaurice G (2006) Confounding: propensity score adjustment. Nutrition 22(11–12):1214–1216
3. Austin PC (2011) An introduction to propensity score methods for reducing the effects of confounding in observational studies. Multivariate Behav Res 46(3):399–424
4. Li L et al (2011) Propensity score-based sensitivity analysis method for uncontrolled confounding. Am J Epidemiol 174(3):345–353
5. Toh S, Garcia Rodriguez LA, Hernan MA (2011) Confounding adjustment via a semi-automated high-dimensional propensity score algorithm: an application to electronic medical records. Pharmacoepidemiol Drug Saf 20(8):849–857
6. Guertin JR et al (2015) Propensity score matching does not always remove confounding within an economic evaluation based on a non-randomized study. Value Health 18(7):A338
7. Girman CJ et al (2014) Assessing the impact of propensity score estimation and implementation on covariate balance and confounding control within and across important subgroups in comparative effectiveness research. Med Care 52(3):280–287

References

8. Glass TA et al (2013) Causal inference in public health. Annu Rev Public Health 34:61–75
9. Cousens S et al (2011) Alternatives to randomisation in the evaluation of public-health interventions: statistical analysis and causal inference. J Epidemiol Community Health 65(7):576–581
10. Brookhart MA et al (2013) Propensity score methods for confounding control in nonexperimental research. Circ Cardiovasc Qual Outcomes 6(5):604–611
11. Feng P et al (2012) Generalized propensity score for estimating the average treatment effect of multiple treatments. Stat Med 31(7):681–697
12. Rosthoj S, Keiding N (2004) Explained variation and predictive accuracy in general parametric statistical models: the role of model misspecification. Lifetime Data Anal 10(4):461–472
13. Ertefaie A, Asgharian M, Stephens D (2014) Propensity score estimation in the presence of length-biased sampling: a nonparametric adjustment approach. Stat 3(1):83–94
14. Yoo C, Ramirez L, Liuzzi J (2014) Big data analysis using modern statistical and machine learning methods in medicine. Int Neurourol J 18(2):50–57
15. Hsu DJ et al (2015) The association between indwelling arterial catheters and mortality in hemodynamically stable patients with respiratory failure: a propensity score analysis. Chest 148(6):1470–1476
16. Hernan MA (2012) Beyond exchangeability: the other conditions for causal inference in medical research. Stat Methods Med Res 21(1):3–5
17. Austin PC, Stuart EA (2014) The performance of inverse probability of treatment weighting and full matching on the propensity score in the presence of model misspecification when estimating the effect of treatment on survival outcomes. Stat Methods Med Res
18. Pirracchio R, Petersen ML, van der Laan M (2015) Improving propensity score estimators' robustness to model misspecification using super learner. Am J Epidemiol 181(2):108–119
19. Lee BK, Lessler J, Stuart EA (2010) Improving propensity score weighting using machine learning. Stat Med 29(3):337–346
20. Brookhart MA et al (2006) Variable selection for propensity score models. Am J Epidemiol 163(12):1149–1156
21. Zhu Y et al (2015) Variable selection for propensity score estimation via balancing covariates. Epidemiology 26(2):e14–e15
22. Saeed M et al (2011) Multiparameter intelligent monitoring in intensive care II: a public-access intensive care unit database. Crit Care Med 39(5):952–960
23. Goldberger AL et al (2000) PhysioBank, PhysioToolkit, and PhysioNet: components of a new research resource for complex physiologic signals. Circulation 101(23):E215–E220

Chapter 24
Markov Models and Cost Effectiveness Analysis: Applications in Medical Research

Matthieu Komorowski and Jesse Raffa

Learning Objectives
Understand how Markov models can be used to analyze medical decisions and perform cost-effectiveness analysis.

This case study introduces concepts that should improve understanding of the following:

1. Markov models and their use in medical research.
2. Basics of health economics.
3. Replicating the results of a large prospective randomized controlled trial using a Markov Chain and Monte Carlo simulations, and
4. Relating quality-adjusted life years (QALYs) and cost of interventions to each state of a Markov Chain, in order to conduct a simple cost-effectiveness analysis.

24.1 Introduction

Markov models were initially thoreticized at the beginning of the 20th century by Russian mathematician Andrey Markov [1]. They are stochastic processes that undergo transitions from one state to another. Over the years, they have found countless applications, especially for modeling processes and informing decision making, in the fields of physics, queuing theory, finance, social sciences, statistics and of course medicine. Markov models are useful to model environments and **problems involving sequential, stochastic decisions over time**. Representing such environments with decision trees would be confusing or intractable, if at all possible, and would require major simplifying assumptions [2]. Markov models can be examined by an array of tools including linear algebra (brute force), cohort simulations, Monte Carlo simulations and, for Markov Decision Processes, dynamic programming and reinforcement learning [3, 4].

A fundamental property of all Markov models is their **memorylessness**. They satisfy a first-order **Markov property** if the probability to move a new state to s_{t+1} only depends on the current state s_t, and not on any previous state, where t is the current time. Said otherwise, given the present state, the future and past states are independent. Formally, a stochastic process has the first order Markov property if the conditional probability distribution of future states of the process (conditional on both past and present values) depends only upon the present state:

$$P(s_{t+1}|s_1, s_2, \ldots, s_t) = P(s_{t+1}|s_t)$$

This chapter will provide a brief introduction to the most common Markov models, and outline some potential applications in medical research and health economics. The last section will discuss a practical example inspired from the medical literature, in which a Markov chain will be used to conduct the cost-effectiveness analysis of a particular medical intervention. In general, the crude results of a study are unable to provide the necessary information to fully implement cost-effectiveness analysis, thus demonstrating the value of expressing the problem as a Markov Chain.

24.2 Formalization of Common Markov Models

The four most common Markov models are shown in Table 24.1. They can be classified into two categories depending or not whether the entire sequential state is observable [5]. Additionally, in Markov Decision Processes, the transitions between states are under the command of a control system called the agent, which selects actions that may lead to a particular subsequent state. By contrast, in Markov chains and hidden Markov models, the transition between states is autonomous. All Markov models can be finite (discrete) or continuous, depending on the definition of their state space.

24.2.1 The Markov Chain

The discrete time Markov chain, defined by the tuple $\{S, T\}$ is the simplest Markov model, where S is a finite set of states and T is a state transition probability matrix,

Table 24.1 Classification of Markov models

	Fully observable system	Partially observable systems
Autonomous system	Markov chain (MC)	Hidden Markov model (HMM)
System containing a control process	Markov decision process (MDP)	Partially observable Markov decision process (POMDP)

24.2 Formalization of Common Markov Models

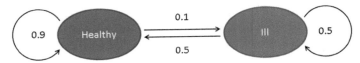

Fig. 24.1 Example of a Markov chain, defined by a set S of finite states {Healthy, Ill} and a transition matrix, containing the probabilities to move from current state s to next state s' at each iteration

Table 24.2 Example of a transition matrix corresponding to Fig. 24.1

		Next state s		Total
		Healthy	Ill	
Initial state s	Healthy	0.9	0.1	1
	Ill	0.5	0.5	1

$T(s', s) = P(s_{t+1} = s' | s_t = s)$. A Markov chain can be **ergodic**, if it is possible to go from any state to every other state in finitely many moves. Figure 24.1 shows a simple example of a Markov Chain.

In the transition matrix, the entries in each column are between 0 and 1 (inclusive) and their sum is 1. Such vectors are called **probability vectors**. The Table 24.2 shows the transition matrix corresponding to Fig. 24.1. A state is said to be **absorbing** if it is impossible to leave it (e.g. death).

24.2.2 Exploring Markov Chains with Monte Carlo Simulations

Monte Carlo (MC) simulations are a useful technique to explore and understand phenomena and systems modeled under a Markov model. MC simulation generates pseudorandom variables on a computer in order to approximate difficult to estimate quantities. It has wide use in numerous fields and applications [6]. Our focus is on the MC simulation of a Markov chain, and it is straightforward once a transition probability matrix, $T(s', s)$, and final time t^* have been defined. We will assume at the index time ($t = 0$), the state is known, and call it s_0. At $t = 1$, we simulate a categorical random variable using the s_0th row of the transition probability matrix $T(s', s)$. We repeat this $t = 1, 2, \ldots, t^* - 1, t^*$ to simulate *one simulated instance* of the Markov chain we are studying. One simulated instance only tells us about one possible sequence of transitions out of very many for this Markov chain, and we need to repeat this many (N) times, recording the sequence of states for each of the simulated instances. Repeating this process many times, allows us to estimate quantities such as: the probability at $t = 5$, that the chain is in state 1; the average proportion of time spent in state 1 over the first 10 time points; or the average length of the longest consecutive streak in state 1 in the first t^* time points.

Using the example shown in Fig. 24.1, we will estimate the probability for someone to be healthy or ill in 5 days, knowing that he is healthy today. MC methods will simulate a large number of samples (say 10,000), starting in s_0 = Healthy and following the transition matrix $T(s', s)$ for 5 steps, sequentially picking transitions to s' according to their probability. The output variable (the value of the final state) is recorded for each sample, and we conclude by analyzing the characteristics of the distribution of this output variable (Table 24.3).

The distribution of the final state at day + 5 for 10,000 simulated instances is represented on Fig. 24.2.

Table 24.4 reports some sample characteristics for "healthy" state on day 5 for 100 and 10,000 simulated instances, which illustrates why it is important to simulate a very large number of samples.

Table 24.3 Example of health forecasting using Monte Carlo simulation

	Instance 1	Instance 2	…	Instance 10,000
Today	Healthy	Healthy	…	Healthy
Day + 1	Healthy	Healthy		Healthy
Day + 2	Healthy	Ill		Healthy
Day + 3	Healthy	Ill		Ill
Day + 4	Healthy	Ill		Healthy
Day + 5	Healthy	Ill	…	Healthy

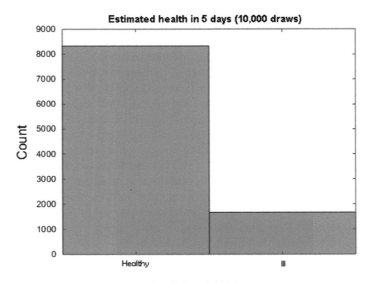

Fig. 24.2 Distribution of the health on day 5, for 10,000 instances

24.2 Formalization of Common Markov Models

Table 24.4 Sample characteristics for 100 and 10,000 simulated instances

	100 simulated instances	10,000 simulated instances
Mean	0.81	0.83
Standard deviation	0.39	0.37
95 % confidence interval for the mean	0.73–0.89	0.83–0.84

By increasing the number of simulated instances, we drastically increase our confidence that the true sample mean falls within a very narrow window (0.83–0.84 in this example). The true mean calculated analytically is 0.838, which is very close to the estimate generated from MC simulation.

24.2.3 Markov Decision Process and Hidden Markov Models

Markov Decision Processes (MDPs) provide a framework for running reinforcement learning methods. MDPs are an extension of Markov chains, which include a control process. MDPs are a powerful and appropriate technique for modeling medical decision [3]. MDPs are most useful in classes of problems involving **complex, stochastic and dynamic decisions like medical treatment decisions**, for which they can find optimal solutions [3]. Physicians will always need to make subjective judgments about treatment strategies, but mathematical decision models can provide insight into the nature of optimal choices and guide treatment decisions.

In Hidden Markov models (HMMs), the state space is only partially observable [7]. It is formed by two dependent stochastic processes (Fig. 24.3). The first is a classical Markov chain, whose states are not directly observable externally, therefore "hidden." The second stochastic process generates observable emissions, conditional on the hidden process. Methodology has been developed to decode the hidden states from the observed data and has applications in a multitude of areas [7].

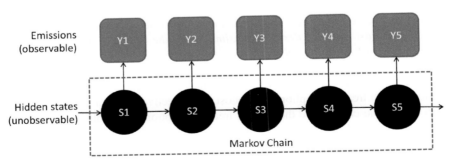

Fig. 24.3 Example of a hidden Markov model (HMM)

24.2.4 Medical Applications of Markov Models

MDPs have been praised by authors as being a powerful and appropriate approach for modeling sequences of medical decisions [3]. Controlled Markov models can be solved by algorithms such as dynamic programming or reinforcement learning, which intends to identify or approximate the optimal policy (set of rules that maximizes the expected sum of discounted rewards).

In the medical literature, Markov models have explored very diverse problems such as timing of liver transplant [8], HIV therapy [9], breast cancer [10], Hepatitis C [11], statin therapy [12] or hospital discharge management [5, 13]. Markov models can be used to describe various health states in a population of interest, and to detect the effects of various policies or therapeutic choices. For example, Scott et al. has used a HMM to classify patients into 7 health states corresponding to side effects of 2 psychotropic drugs [14]. The transitions were analyzed to specify which drug was associated with the least side-effects. Very recently, a Markov chain model was proposed to model the progression of diabetic retinopathy, using 5 pre-defined states, from mild retinopathy to blindness [15]. MDPs have also been exploited in medical imaging applications. Alterovitz has used very large MDPs (800,000 states) for motion planning in image-guided needle steering [16].

Besides those medical applications, Markov models are extensively used in health economics research, which is the focus of the next section of this chapter.

24.3 Basics of Health Economics

24.3.1 The Goal of Health Economics: Maximizing Cost-Effectiveness

This section provides the reader with a minimal background about health economics, followed by a worked example. Health economics intends to maximize "value for money" in healthcare, by optimizing not only clinical effectiveness, but also cost-effectiveness of medical interventions. As explained by Morris: "*Achieving 'value for money' implies either a desire to achieve a predetermined objective at least cost or a desire to maximise [sic] the benefit to the population of patients served from a limited amount of resources*" [17].

Two main approaches can be outlined in health economics: cost-minimization and cost-effectiveness analysis (CEA). In both cases, the purpose is identical: to identify which treatment option is the most cost-effective. Cost minimization deals with the simple case where the several treatment options available have the same effectiveness but different costs. Quite logically, cost-minimization will favor the cheapest option. CEA represents a more likely scenario and is more widely used.

24.3 Basics of Health Economics

In CEA, several options with different costs and different effectiveness are compared. The analysis will compute the relative cost of an improvement in health, and metrics to optimally inform decision makers.

24.3.2 Definitions

Measuring Outcome: Survival, Quality of Life (QoL), Quality-Adjusted Life-Years (QALY)
Outcomes are assessed in terms of enhanced survival (*"adding years to life"*) and enhanced quality of life (QoL) (*"adding life to years"*) [17]. Although sometimes criticized, the concept of Quality-adjusted life-years (QALY) remains of central importance in cost-utility analysis [18]. QALYs apply weights that reflect the QoL being experienced by the patient. One QALY equates to one year in perfect health. Perfect health is equivalent to 1 while death is equivalent to 0. QALYs are estimated by various methods including scales and questionnaires filled by patients or external examiners [19]. As an example, the EuroQoL EQ 5D questionnaire assesses health in 5 dimensions: mobility, self-care, usual activities, pain/discomfort and anxiety/depression.

Cost-Effectiveness Ratio (CER)
The cost-effectiveness ratio (CER) will inform the decision makers about the cost of an intervention, relative to the health benefits this intervention generates. For example, an intervention costing $20,000 per patient and providing 5 QALYs (5 years of perfect health) has a CER of $20,000/5 = $4000 per QALY. This measure allows a direct comparison of cost-effectiveness between interventions.

Incremental Cost-Effectiveness Ratio (ICER)
The incremental cost-effectiveness ratio (ICER) is a measure very commonly reported in the health economics literature and allows comparing two different interventions in terms of "cost of gained effectiveness." It is computed by dividing the difference in cost of 2 interventions by the difference of their effectiveness [20].

As an example, if treatment A costs $5000 per patient and provides 2 QALYs, and treatment B costs $8000 while providing 3 QALYS, the ICER of treatment B will be:

$$\frac{(\$8000 - \$5000)}{3 - 2} = \$3000$$

Said otherwise, it will cost $3000 more to gain one more QALY with treatment B, for this particular medical condition. ICER can inform decision makers about the need to adopt or fund a new medical intervention. Schematically, if the ICER of a new medical intervention lies below a certain threshold, it means that health benefits can be achieved with an acceptable level of spending.

The Cost Effectiveness Plane

The cost-effectiveness plane (CE plane) is an important tool used in CEA (Fig. 24.4). It aims to clearly illustrate differences in costs and effects between different strategies, whether they comprise medical interventions, treatments, or even a combination of the two.

The CE plane consists of a four-quadrant diagram where the X-axis represents the incremental level of effectiveness of an outcome and the Y-axis represents the additional total cost of implementing this outcome. For example, the further right you move on the X-axis, the more effective the outcome. In the upper-right quadrant, a treatment may receive funding if its ICER lies below the maximum acceptable ICER threshold.

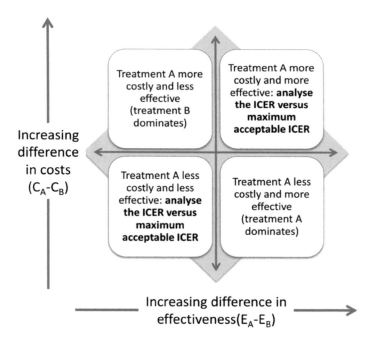

Fig. 24.4 The cost-effectiveness plane, comparing treatment A with treatment B

24.4 Case Study: Monte Carlo Simulations of a Markov Chain for Daily Sedation Holds in Intensive Care, with Cost-Effectiveness Analysis

This example is inspired by the publication by Girard et al. [21], and will allow us to illustrate how to construct and examine a simple Markov Chain to represent a medical intervention, how to relate QALYs and cost of interventions to each state of the Markov Chain, in order to carry out a cost-effectiveness analysis. In this prospective randomized controlled trial, the authors evaluated the impact of daily sedation holds in intensive care on various outcomes such as the number of ventilator-free days, delirium and 28-day mortality. In the ICU, patients frequently undergo mechanical ventilation in the setting of severely impaired consciousness, after heavy surgical procedures, and when suffering from severe respiratory failure. Therapeutically, patients are sedated to maximize their comfort. A growing body of literature, however, has identified the risks of continuous sedation in the ICU, as it is associated with increased mortality, delirium, duration of mechanical ventilation and length of ICU and hospital stay [22]. To strike the right balance between maintaining sedation and mechanical ventilator support as long as the patient needs it, but also moving to extubation as soon as possible, Girard and colleagues proposed actively waking up the patients daily to assess their readiness to come off of the ventilator. The main results are shown in Table 24.5.

In this case study example, we will attempt to approximate those results using a very simple 3-state Markov Chain examined by MC simulation. As an exercise, we will extend the study to CEA. This tutorial will provide the reader with all the tools necessary to implement in other contexts Markov Chain MC simulation methods and simple cost-effectiveness studies.

Most of the study results can be approximated using a very crude 3-state Markov chain (Fig. 24.5), with the following state space: {Intubated, Extubated, Dead}. In this simplistic model, only 7 transitions are possible, and the state 'dead' is absorbing.

Table 24.5 Main results from the original study

	Intervention group	Control group
Ventilator-free days (mean)	14.7	11.6
Ventilator-free days (median)	20.0	8.1
Patients Successfully extubated at 28 days (%)	≈93	≈88
28 day mortality (%)	29	35

Fig. 24.5 The 3-state Markov chain used in this example

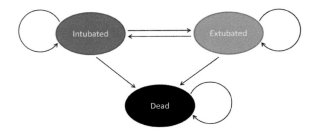

Two different transition matrices can be built by trial-and-error, corresponding to the intervention and control arms of the study (Table 24.6). They correspond to the daily probabilities of transitioning from one state to another. The initial values were selected using a few simple assumptions: the state 'death' is absorbing, the probability to remain intubated or extubated is larger than the probability to change state, the risk of dying while intubated is larger than when extubated, and the total of each row in the transition matrix is one. Another assumption is that the intervention (daily sedation hold) will change the probability of successful extubation and mortality, hence the transition matrix. After each modification, the number of patients in each state was computed for 28 days (results in Table 24.8), so as to try to match the initial study's results as closely as possible.

We can check to see if our code is running correctly by comparing important aspects of the simulation to known theoretical properties of probability theory and Markov Chains. For example, in our example all patients are assumed to be intubated at $t = 0$. Under our Markov model, the waiting time until extubation or death can be determined theoretically, but how to determine this is beyond the scope of this chapter. This waiting time, W^*, is a discrete random variable with a geometric distribution. Geometric distributions have probability mass functions, for a given waiting time, w of $p(w) = (1 - p)p^{(w-1)}$, where p is the probability of remaining intubated. In Fig. 24.6, we compare the number of times we observed different values of w to what we would expect under the true theoretical distribution of W^*, by computing $Np(w)$, where N is the number of simulated instances we computed.

Table 24.6 Transition matrices used in the case study

Intervention group		Next state S'		
		I	E	D
Initial state S	I	0.862	0.12	0.018
	E	0.0088	0.982	0.0092
	D	0	0	1
Control group		Next state S'		
		I	E	D
Initial state S	I	0.878	0.1	0.022
	E	0.01	0.978	0.012
	D	0	0	1

24.4 Case Study: Monte Carlo Simulations of a Markov Chain ...

We can see that our simulation follows very closely to what is theoretically known to be true.

In order to perform CEA, each state must be assigned a value for QALYs and cost. For the purpose of this example, let's also assume the values for QALYs and daily costs shown in Table 24.7.

Table 24.8 shows the results of the first iterations for the control group, when starting with 100 patients intubated (*function* `IED_transition.m`). At each time step, the number of patients still intubated corresponds to the patients who stayed intubated, minus the patients who became extubated (daily probability of 10 %) and those who died (probability of 2.2 %), plus the extubated patients who had to be re-intubated (probability 1 %). After 28 days, the cumulated mortality reaches 35.6 %, and the ratio of patients extubated among the patients still alive is 88.8 %, hence matching quite closely the results of the initial study. At each time step, the sum of the QALYs and costs for all the patients is computed, as well as their cumulative values. The number of QALYs initially increases as more patients become extubated, then decreases as a consequence the number of patients dying.

Table 24.7 Definition of QALY and daily cost for each state

State	I	E	D
QALY	0.5	1	0
Daily cost ($)	2000	1000	0

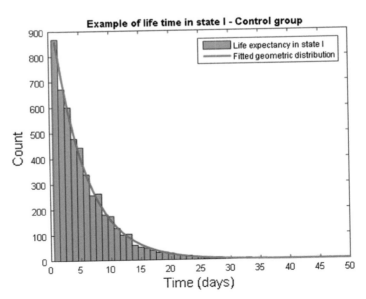

Fig. 24.6 Example of the life expectancy in state "I" in the control group, with fitted geometric distribution. The bar chart represents the distribution of the time spent in the state "intubated" of the Markov chain, before transitioning to another state, for 5000 samples

Table 24.8 Number of patients in each state, QALYs and cost analysis, during 28 iterations (control group)

Day	I	E	D	Extubated/Alive	QALYs	Cumulative QALYs	Daily cost (K$)	Cumulative cost (K$)
0	100.00	0.00	0.00	0.00	50.00	50.00	200.00	200
1	87.80	10.00	2.20	0.10	53.90	103.90	185.60	386
2	77.19	18.56	4.25	0.19	57.15	161.05	172.94	559
3	67.96	25.87	6.17	0.28	59.85	220.90	161.78	720
4	59.92	32.10	7.98	0.35	62.06	282.96	151.95	872
5	52.94	37.38	9.68	0.41	63.85	346.81	143.25	1016
...	...	...	...	...	...	...	...	...
28	7.19	57.21	35.60	0.89	60.80	1863.84	71.59	3184

The following figure represents the ratio of number of patients extubated over number of patients alive, over time and for both strategies (Fig. 24.7). It can be compared to the original figure in the source article.

By simulating the distribution of the average number of ventilator-free days, and its characteristics, can be computed for both strategies (*function* `MCMC_solver.m`). The following Table 24.9 shows examples of patients' states computed using the transition matrix of the control group.

The distribution of ventilator-free days in our 10,000 samples is plotted shown in Fig. 24.8.

The mean and median number of ventilator-free days for both groups is shown in Table 24.10.

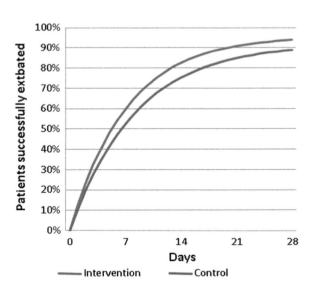

Fig. 24.7 Modelled primary outcome of the study using a Markov chain

24.4 Case Study: Monte Carlo Simulations of a Markov Chain ...

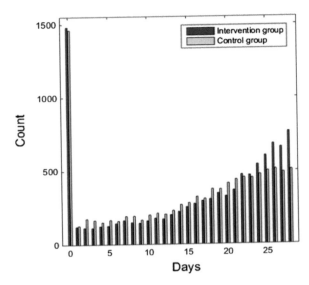

Fig. 24.8 Ventilator-free days for 10,000 samples, for the intervention and control group

Table 24.9 Computing the number of ventilator-free days by Monte Carlo (10,000 simulated instances)

Day	Instance 1	Instance 2	Instance 3	...	Instance 10,000
0	I	I	I		I
1	I	I	I		I
2	I	I	I		I
3	I	I	I		I
4	I	I	I		I
5	I	I	I		I
6	I	I	I		I
7	I	I	I		E
8	E	E	I		E
9	E	E	I		E
10	I	E	I		E
...	...	...	...		...
28	D	D	D		E
Total ventilator-free days	7	3	0	...	22

The cost-effectiveness ratio at 28 day of the both strategies can be computed by dividing the final cumulative cost by the cumulative QALYs (Table 24.11).

The intervention is more expensive but is also associated with health benefits (significantly more QALYs). It belongs to the upper-right quadrant of the CE plane,

Table 24.10 Mean and median number of ventilator-free days for both groups

Number of ventilator-free days	Intervention group	Control group
Mean	17.1	15.9
Median	20	18

Table 24.11 Cost-effectiveness ratio in both groups

	Intervention group	Control group
Cumulative cost (K$)	3213	3184
Cumulative QALYs	2029	1864
Cost-effectiveness ratio ($ per QALY)	1583	1708

where the ICER is used to determine the cost-effectiveness of an intervention. The ICER of this intervention is shown below:

$$ICER = \frac{(3,213,000 - 3,184,000)}{(2029 - 1864)} = 177.3$$

According to this crude analysis, Sedation holds appear to be a very cost-effective strategy, costing only $177 more per additional QALY, relative to the control strategy. Reducing the value (QALY) of the state E from 1 to 0.6 significantly increases the ICER to $1918 per QALY gained, demonstrating the huge impact that the definition of our health states has on the results of the CEA. Likewise, increasing the daily cost of state E from $1000 to $1900 (now only slightly cheaper than state I) leads to a much more expensive ICER of $2041 per QALY gained. Some medical interventions may or may not be funded depending on the assumptions of the model!

24.5 Model Validation and Sensitivity Analysis for Cost-Effectiveness Analysis

An important component to any CEA is to assess whether the model is appropriate for the phenomena being examined, which is the purpose of model validation and sensitivity analyses. In the previous section, we model daily sedation hold as a Markov chain with a known transition probability matrix and costs. Deviations from this model can come in at least two types.

First, the use of a Markov Chain may be inappropriate to describe how subjects transition from the intubation, extubation and death states. It was presumed that this process follows a first-order Markov chain. Given enough real clinical data we can test to see if this assumption is reasonable. For example, given the transition probability matrices above, we can calculate quantities via MC simulation and compare them to values reported in the real data. For instance, the authors report a 28-day mortality rate of 29 and 35 % in the intervention and control groups, respectively. From our simulation study, we estimate these quantities to be 27 and 35 %, which is reasonably close. One can perform formal goodness-of-fit testing as well to better assess if any differences noted provide any evidence that the model may be mis-specified. This process can also be repeated for other quantities, for example, the mean number of ventilator-free days.

In addition to validating the Markov model used to simulate the states and transitions for the system of interest, it is also important to perform a sensitivity analysis on the assumptions and parameters used in the simulation. Performing this step allows one to see how sensitive the results are to slight changes to parameter values. Choosing which parameters values to use in sensitivity analyses can be difficult, but some good practices are to find other parameters (e.g., transition probability matrices) reported in other studies of a similar type. For cost estimates, one may want to try costs reported in other countries, or incorporate important economic parameters like inflation. If using these other scenarios drastically affects the conclusions drawn from the simulation study, this does not necessarily mean that the study was a failure, but rather that there are limits to the generalizability of the simulation study's results. If particular parameters cause great fluctuations this may warrant further investigation into why this is the case. In addition to changing the parameters, one may try to alter the model significantly, by for example, using a higher order Markov model or semi-Markov model in place of a simple first order assumption, but these are advanced topic beyond the scope of this chapter.

The theoretical concepts introduced in the first sections of this chapter were applied to a concrete example coming from the medical literature. We demonstrated how clinical states and transition probabilities could be defined ad hoc, and how the stationary distribution of the chain could be estimated using Monte Carlo methods. The methodology outlined in this chapter will allow the reader to expand the results of other interventional studies to CEA, but countless other applications of Markov models exist, in particular in the domain of decision support systems.

24.6 Conclusion

Markov models have been used extensively in the medical literature, and offer an appealing framework for modeling medical decision making, with potential powerful applications in decision support systems and health economics analysis. They represent relatively simple mathematical models that are easy to grasp by non-data scientists or non-statisticians. Very careful attention must be paid to the verification of a fundamental assumption which is the Markov property, without which no further analysis should be carried out.

24.7 Next Steps

This tutorial hopefully provided basic tools to understand or develop CEA and Markov chains to model the effect of medical interventions. For more information on health economics, the reader is directed towards external references, such as the work by Morris and colleagues [17]. Guidance regarding the use of more advanced Markov models such as MDPs and HMMs is beyond the scope of this book, but numerous sources are available, such as the excellent Sutton and Barto, freely available online [4].

Open Access This chapter is distributed under the terms of the Creative Commons Attribution-NonCommercial 4.0 International License (http://creativecommons.org/licenses/by-nc/4.0/), which permits any noncommercial use, duplication, adaptation, distribution and reproduction in any medium or format, as long as you give appropriate credit to the original author(s) and the source, a link is provided to the Creative Commons license and any changes made are indicated.

The images or other third party material in this chapter are included in the work's Creative Commons license, unless indicated otherwise in the credit line; if such material is not included in the work's Creative Commons license and the respective action is not permitted by statutory regulation, users will need to obtain permission from the license holder to duplicate, adapt or reproduce the material.

Code Appendix

The code used in this case study is available from the GitHub repository accompanying this book: https://github.com/MIT-LCP/critical-data-book. Further information on the code is available from this website. The following functions are provided:

- `health_forecast.m`: This function computes 100 Monte-Carlo simulations of a 5-day health forecast and displays the results.
- `IED_transition.m`: This function computes and displays the proportion of patients in each state (Intubated, Extubated, or Dead), following the transition matrix in the intervention group.
- `MCMC_solver.m`: This function computes 10,000 Monte Carlo simulations for both the control and intervention group, and computes the distribution of ventilator-free days.

References

1. Basharin GP, Langville AN, Naumov VA (2004) The life and work of A.A. Markov. Linear Algebra Appl 386:3–26
2. Sonnenberg FA, Beck JR (1993) Markov models in medical decision making: a practical guide. Med Decis Mak Int J Soc Med Decis Mak 13(4):322–338

References

3. Schaefer AJ, Bailey MD, Shechter SM, Roberts MS (2005) Modeling medical treatment using Markov decision processes. In: Brandeau ML, Sainfort F, Pierskalla WP (eds) Operations research and health care. Springer, US, pp 593–612
4. Sutton RS, Barto AG (1998) Reinforcement learning: an introduction. A Bradford Book, Cambridge, Mass
5. Kreke JE (2007) Modeling disease management decisions for patients with pneumonia-related sepsis [Online]. Available: http://d-scholarship.pitt.edu/8143/
6. Liu JS (2004) Monte Carlo strategies in scientific computing. Springer, New York
7. Zucchini W, MacDonald IL (2009) Hidden Markov models for time series: an introduction using R. Chapman and Hall/CRC, Boca Raton (2Rev Ed edition)
8. Alagoz O, Maillart LM, Schaefer AJ, Roberts MS (2004) The optimal timing of living-donor liver transplantation. Manag Sci 50(10):1420–1430
9. Shechter SM, Bailey MD, Schaefer AJ, Roberts MS (2008) The optimal time to initiate HIV therapy under ordered health states. Oper Res 56(1):20–33
10. Maillart LM, Ivy JS, Ransom S, Diehl K (2008) Assessing dynamic breast cancer screening policies. Oper Res 56(6):1411–1427
11. Daniel PMG, Faissol M (2007) Timing of testing and treatment of hepatitis C and other diseases. Inf J Comput Inf
12. Denton BT, Kurt M, Shah ND, Bryant SC, Smith SA (2009) Optimizing the start time of statin therapy for patients with diabetes. Med Decis Mak Int J Soc Med Decis Mak 29(3):351–367
13. Raffa JD, Dubin JA (2015) Multivariate longitudinal data analysis with mixed effects hidden Markov models. Biometrics 71(3):821–831
14. Scott SL, James GM, Sugar CA (2005) Hidden Markov models for longitudinal comparisons. J Am Stat Assoc 100:359–369
15. Srikanth P (2015) Using Markov chains to predict the natural progression of diabetic retinopathy. Int J Ophthalmol 8(1):132–137
16. Alterovitz R, Branicky M, Goldberg K (2008) Motion planning under uncertainty for image-guided medical needle steering. Int J Robot Res 27(11–12):1361–1374
17. Morris S, Devlin N, Parkin D, Spencer A (2012) Economic analysis in healthcare, 2nd edn. Wiley, Chichester
18. Nord E, Daniels N, Kamlet M (2009) QALYs: some challenges. Value Health 12(Supplement 1):S10–S15
19. Torrance GW (1986) Measurement of health state utilities for economic appraisal. J Health Econ 5(1):1–30
20. Drummond M, Sculpher M (2005) Common methodological flaws in economic evaluations. Med Care 43(7 Suppl):5–14
21. Girard TD, Kress JP, Fuchs BD, Thomason JWW, Schweickert WD, Pun BT, Taichman DB, Dunn JG, Pohlman AS, Kinniry PA, Jackson JC, Canonico AE, Light RW, Shintani AK, Thompson JL, Gordon SM, Hall JB, Dittus RS, Bernard GR, Ely EW (2008) Efficacy and safety of a paired sedation and ventilator weaning protocol for mechanically ventilated patients in intensive care (awakening and breathing controlled trial): a randomised controlled trial. Lancet Lond Engl 371(9607):126–134
22. Roberts DJ, Haroon B, Hall RI (2012) Sedation for critically ill or injured adults in the intensive care unit: a shifting paradigm. Drugs 72(14):1881–1916

Chapter 25
Blood Pressure and the Risk of Acute Kidney Injury in the ICU: Case-Control Versus Case-Crossover Designs

Li-wei H. Lehman, Mengling Feng, Yijun Yang and Roger G. Mark

Learning Objectives
Introduce two different approaches, a case-control and a case-crossover design, to study the effect of transient exposure of hypotension on the risk of acute kidney injury (AKI) development in intensive care unit (ICU) patients.

25.1 Introduction

Acute kidney injury (AKI) refers to a rapid decrease in kidney function, occurring over a period of days. The presence of AKI can be detected using well-established definitions based on serum creatinine rise or urine output reduction [1]. Acute kidney injury has been reported in 36 % of all patients admitted to the intensive care unit ICU [2, 3]. A prior study showed that hospital patients with even very small increases in their serum creatinine (0.3–0.4 mg/dL) have 70 % greater risk of death than patients without creatinine increase [4]. Although the relationship between low blood pressure and kidney function is well documented in an experimental setting based on animal data [5], the association between hypotension and acute kidney injury in a critical care setting is not completely understood.

This chapter describes two different approaches for studying blood pressure and the risk of AKI development in ICU patients using the MIMIC II database [6]. In our first study, we adopted a traditional case-control approach and examined the association between hypotension and AKI by comparing blood pressure measurements of patients who had AKI (case) with patients without AKI (control) [7, 8]. Blood pressure measurements immediately prior to patients' AKI onset were compared with blood pressure measurements of the controls sampled from a similar time window.

In the second study, we adopted a case-crossover design in which each patient serves as his or her own control. Blood pressure measurements immediately prior to each patient's AKI onset were compared with the same patient's blood pressure measurements sampled from an earlier time window while that patient's kidney functions were still stable. In the remainder of the chapter, we highlight the key differences and the design rationale of these two approaches. We applied these analysis techniques to study the relationship between hypotension and AKI development using the MIMIC II database, and present our preliminary findings.

25.2 Methods

25.2.1 Data Pre-processing

Nurse-verified mean arterial blood pressure (MAP) samples, recorded on an hourly basis were used for the analysis. Blood pressure measurements from both invasive arterial line and automated, non-invasive oscillometric methods were included in the study. Our choice of MAP (rather than systolic blood pressure) for blood pressure measurement was motivated by prior work [8] which demonstrated that MAP provided more consistent readings across different measurement modalities in the ICU. Blood pressure measurements were filtered to remove values outside of reasonable physiological bounds (MAP between 20 and 200 mmHg).

25.2.2 A Case-Control Study

In the case-control approach [7], we examined the effect of transient exposure to hypotension (defined as blood pressure falling below specified thresholds) and the risk of AKI development by comparing blood pressure measurements of patients who experienced AKI (case) with patients who never developed AKI in the ICU (control). AKI was defined as an acute increase in serum creatinine ≥ 0.3 mg/dL, or an increase of $\geq 50\,\%$ in serum creatinine within 48 h, based on the Acute Kidney Injury Network (AKIN) definition [1]. Blood pressure measurements (from up to a 48 h window) prior to patients' AKI onset were compared with blood pressure measurements of the controls from a time window prior to the last creatinine measurement time.

Patients were selected from among the adult ICU stays in the MIMIC II [8] database. We examined adult ICU stays (patients ≥ 15 years of age) with at least 2 serum creatinine values. Patients with fewer than 2 serum creatine values in their ICU stay or evidence of end-stage renal disease (ESRD) were excluded.

Among the remaining 16,728 adult ICU stays that had at least 2 creatinine measurements without evidence of end-stage renal disease, AKI occurred in 5207 (31 %). The remaining 11,521 cases were identified as the controls. The average AKI onset time was 2.34 days after ICU admission. For the controls, the last creatinine sample time was, on average, 2.76 days after ICU admission. Figure 25.1

25.2 Methods

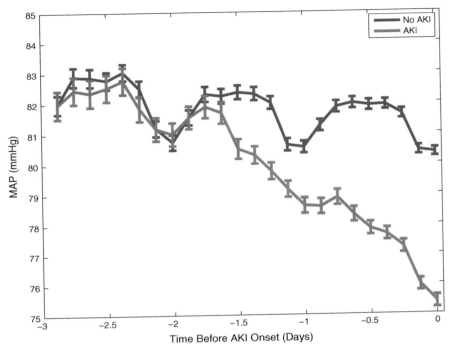

Fig. 25.1 The population mean (and standard error) of median MAP up to 3 days prior to the AKI onset for the AKI cohort, or prior to the last creatinine measurement time for the controls. Mean arterial blood pressure of the AKI cohort diverged from that of the controls during day two prior to the AKI onset, and both cohorts exhibited prominent diurnal variation

plots the population mean and standard error of median MAP up to 3 days prior to the AKI onset for the AKI cohort, or prior to the last creatinine measurement time for the controls. Note that mean arterial blood pressure of the AKI cohort diverged from that of the controls prior to the AKI onset.

We studied the risk of AKI in ICU patients as a function of both the severity and duration of hypotension. Blood pressure features extracted from the target 48-h window were examined as primary predictors for AKI, including the minimum MAP and maximum number of hours that MAP was continuously less than several different thresholds (from 80 to 45 mmHg). Duration of hypotension below a specific threshold was calculated based on linear interpolated blood pressure samples. Hypotensive episodes were considered to begin and end when the interpolated blood pressure values intercepted the target threshold. Hypotensive episodes that were less than one hour apart were merged to form one continuous episode.

Univariate and multivariable logistic regressions were performed to find correlations between hypotension and AKI. Age, SAPS-I, admission creatinine, and the presence (based on ICD-9) of chronic renal failure (585.9), hypertension (401.9), diabetes (250.00), coronary atherosclerosis (414.01), congestive heart failure (428.0), and septic shock (785.52) or sepsis (038) were added as potential confounding factors [9].

Our results indicate that the odds of AKI were related to the severity of hypotension with an odds ratio (OR) of 1.03, 95 % confidence interval (CI) 1.02–1.04 ($p < 0.0001$) per 1 mmHg decrease in minimum MAP ≤ 80 mmHg. Multivariable analysis on hypotension duration involved 3203 patients who had SAPS-I scores and with at least 45 h of blood pressure samples in the target 48-h window. Our results indicate that the duration of time that the patient's MAP was continuously less than or equal to 70, 65, 60, 55, and 50 mmHg were significant risk factors in AKI development. Further, as the extent of hypotension worsened, the incremental risk for AKI from each additional hour of continuous hypotension increased for each 10 mmHg drop in MAP below 80 mmHg. For each additional hour MAP was less than 70, 60, 50 mmHg, the odds of AKI increased by 2 % (OR 1.02, 95 % CI 1.00–1.03, $p = 0.0034$), 5 % (OR 1.05, 95 % CI 1.02–1.08, $p = 0.0028$), and 22 % (OR 1.22, 95 % CI 1.04–1.43, $p = 0.0122$) respectively. As the degree of hypotension worsened, the increased odds for AKI from each additional hour of continuous hypotension more than doubled for each 10 mmHg drop in MAP below 80 mmHg. Our results also suggest that the severity of hypotension significantly shortened the time to the onset of AKI.

25.2.3 A Case-Crossover Design

In the second study, we adopted a case-crossover cohort design to examine the effect of transient exposure to hypotension and the risk of AKI. The case-crossover design was devised to assess the relationship between transient exposures and acute outcomes in situations where the control series of a case-control study is difficult to achieve. In the case-crossover design, subjects serve as their own matched controls defined by prior time periods in the same subject. Given a transient exposure with stable prevalence over time, the case-crossover design uses the difference in exposure rates just before an event (case) with those at other time points in the subject's history (controls) to estimate an odds ratio of the outcome associated with exposure. The case-crossover design was first proposed by Maclure et al. to study the effects of transient changes on the risk of acute events [10]. One advantage of a case-crossover design is that it avoids control selection bias and eliminates between-patient confounding factors [10, 11]. In this study design, the AKI definition is based on hourly urine output (instead of daily creatinine measurements) in order to determine a more precise timing of the acute (oliguria) onset.

Adult patients with normal kidney function (i.e. urine output remaining at 0.5 ml/kg/h or above) during the first 12 h in the ICU, who subsequently developed

25.2 Methods

AKI/oliguria (urine output remains below 0.5 ml/kg/h for at least 6 h) in the ICU were included in the study. The same patients, prior to developing AKI/oliguria, were used as controls. The AKI/oliguria onset was defined as the beginning of the 6-h period when urine output remained below 0.5 ml/kg/h.

The minimum MAP from the 3 h period prior to the AKI onset was used as exposure for the cases. The minimum MAP from a 3-h control period during the first 12 h in the ICU, when the same patient's renal function was still normal, was used as exposure for the controls. Since the blood pressure measurements during the first 6 h patients were in the ICU can be sparse, we chose the control period to be the 7th–9th hour from the beginning of the patients' ICU stays. Blood pressure measurements were filtered to remove outliers as before.

Case-crossover designs are typically analyzed using conditional logistic regression, as it accounts for the matched nature of the data. It is analogous to a matched case-control study, where one compares a 'case' person-moment with a series of 'control' person-moments from different subjects, while in the case-crossover design, the 'control' person-moments are from the same subject. We implemented the latter approach for analyzing case-crossover study data. In addition, time-varying confounding factors (mechanical ventilator, vasopressors, temperature, heart rate, white blood cell count, SpO_2) were included in the multivariable conditional logistic regression model.

The total cohort included 911 adult ICU stays (29.86 % MICU, 21.73 % SICU, 22.94 % CCU, 25.47 % CSRU) from the MIMIC II database. The median time to AKI/oliguria onset was 45 h. The population median of the minimum MAP measurements during the control and case periods were 73 mmHg with an inter-quartile range of [65, 83] mmHg, and 70 [62, 79] mmHg respectively. A paired signed T-test indicates that the minimum MAP during the case period is statistically significantly lower than during the control period (p-value = 0.0001). Our results indicate that the odds of AKI were related to the severity of hypotension with an odds ratio (OR) of 1.035, 95 % confidence interval (CI) 1.024–1.045 ($p < 0.0001$) per 1 mmHg decrease in minimum MAP in multivariable conditional logistic regression after adjusting for temperature, heart rate, SpO_2, white blood cell count, and the use of mechanical ventilation and vasopressors. Furthermore, we performed a similar analysis to understand if the risk of developing AKI increases associated with the worsened hypotension treating the minimum MAP at the binary variable using cutoff of 70, 65, 60, 55, and 50 mmHg. The adjusted odds ratios and 95 % CI for the minimum MAP < 70, MAP < 65, MAP < 60, MAP < 55, and MAP < 50 (vs. when MAP was greater than or equal to the respective thresholds) were 1.854 (1.44–2.38), 1.945 (1.502–2.519), 2.096 (1.532–2.869), 2.002 (1.307–3.065), and 2.107 (1.115–3.982), respectively. These findings are consistent with the results described in the previous section using a case-control study design.

25.3 Discussion

In the study of the association of hypotension with AKI, the case-crossover design is an efficient alternative to the case-control approach. The case-crossover design, based exclusively on the case series, performs within-subject comparisons of blood pressure measurements from the case and the control periods to estimate the rate ratio of the AKI outcome associated with hypotension. This design inherently removes the biasing effects of unmeasured, time-invariant confounding factors from the estimated rate ratio.

Many factors, (including chronic kidney disease, hypertension, diabetes) could potentially contribute to the development of AKI in an ICU setting. In a traditional case-control design, these time-invariant between-patient confounders (as well as the time-varying confounders) would have to be included to adjust for the baseline risk of AKI development. In some cases, these confounding variables can be difficult to determine from a retrospective ICU database. In a case-crossover design, each patient's blood pressure during normal renal function is compared with the same patient's blood pressure immediately prior to AKI onset, so that time-invariant patient characteristics and confounders are eliminated in the analysis. A case-crossover design may be a more efficient approach in investigating the transient effect of exposure (e.g. low blood pressure) on the risk of an acute outcome (e.g. AKI development), when the heterogeneity in the baseline risk may be difficult to account for in the conventional case-control design.

We acknowledge the following limitations in the current study. First, this was a retrospective study, and as such, the incidence of hypotension prior to AKI does not prove a causal mechanism. Second, we did not account for the presence of fluid and several interventions (e.g. contrast agents, NSAIDs, aminoglycosides, ACEI, etc.) that may impair renal function in our multivariable analysis. As part of future work, additional time-varying confounders (such as, usage of Lasix within 6 h, IV fluid, creatinine, time of AKI onset) could be included in the model.

25.4 Conclusions

We have presented two different approaches, a case-control and a case-crossover design, to study the effect of transient exposure to hypotension on the risk of AKI development in ICU patients. Results from multivariable analysis in both studies indicate that hypotension is a statistically significant risk factor in the development of AKI in the ICU. This study serves as an example to illustrate the utility of case-crossover designs to study the association between a risk factor and the subsequent disease development in an EHR-based retrospective clinical analysis.

Open Access This chapter is distributed under the terms of the Creative Commons Attribution-NonCommercial 4.0 International License (http://creativecommons.org/licenses/by-nc/4.0/), which permits any noncommercial use, duplication, adaptation, distribution and reproduction

25.4 Conclusions

in any medium or format, as long as you give appropriate credit to the original author(s) and the source, a link is provided to the Creative Commons license and any changes made are indicated.

The images or other third party material in this chapter are included in the work's Creative Commons license, unless indicated otherwise in the credit line; if such material is not included in the work's Creative Commons license and the respective action is not permitted by statutory regulation, users will need to obtain permission from the license holder to duplicate, adapt or reproduce the material.

Code Appendix

The code used in this case study is available from the GitHub repository accompanying this book: https://github.com/MIT-LCP/critical-data-book. Further information on the code is available from this website.

References

1. Mehta RL, Kellum JA, Shah SV, Molitoris BA, Ronco C, Warnock DG, Levin A (2007) Acute kidney injury network (AKIN): report of an initiative to improve outcomes in acute kidney injury. Crit Care 11:R31
2. Bagshaw S, George C, Dinu I, Bellomo R (2008) A multi-center evaluation of the RIFLE criteria for early acute kidney injury in critically ill patients. Nephrol Dial Transplant 23:1203–1210
3. Ostermann M, Chang R (2007) Acute kidney injury in the intensive care unit according to rifle. Crit Care Med 35:1837–1843
4. Chertow G, Burdick E, Honour M, Bonventre J, Bates D (2005) Acute kidney injury, mortality, length of stay, and costs in hospitalized patients. J Am Soc Nephrol 16:3365–3370
5. Kirchheim HR, Ehmke H, Hackenthal E, Löwe W, Persson P (1987) Autoregulation of renal blood flow, glomerular filtration rate and renin release in conscious dogs. Pflugers Archiv Eur J Physiol 410:441–449
6. Saeed M, Villarroel M, Reisner AT, Clifford G, Lehman LH, Moody G, Heldt T, Kyaw TH, Moody B, Mark RG (2011) Multiparameter intelligent monitoring in intensive care (MIMIC II): a public-access intensive care unit database. Crit Care Med (5):952–960
7. Lehman LH, Saeed M, Moody G, Mark R (2010) Hypotension as a risk factor for acute kidney injury in ICU patients. In: Computing in cardiology 2010. IEEE Computer Society Press, Belfast, pp 1095–1098
8. Lehman LH, Saeed M, Talmor D, Mark RG, Malhotra A (2013) Methods of blood pressure measurement in the ICU. Crit Care Med 41(1):3–40
9. Abuelo G (2007) Normotensive ischemic acute renal failure. N Engl J Med 357:797–805
10. Maclure M (1991) The case-crossover design: a method for studying transient effects on the risk of acute events. Am J Epidemiol 133:144–153
11. Maclure M, Mittleman M (2000) Should we use a case-crossover design. Annu Rev Public Health 21:193–221

Chapter 26
Waveform Analysis to Estimate Respiratory Rate

Peter H. Charlton, Mauricio Villarroel and Francisco Salguiero

Learning Objectives

Use the MIMIC II database to compare the performance of multiple algorithms for estimation of respiratory rate (RR) from physiological waveforms.

1. Extract electrocardiogram (ECG), photoplethysmogram (PPG) and thoracic impedance pneumography (IP) waveforms from the MIMIC II database.
2. Identify periods of low quality waveform data.
3. Identify heart beats in the ECG and PPG signals.
4. Estimate RR from the signals.
5. Improve the accuracy of RR estimation using quality assessment and data fusion.
6. Evaluate the performance of RR algorithms.

26.1 Introduction

Respiratory rate (RR) is an important physiological parameter which provides valuable diagnostic and prognostic information. It has been found to be predictive of lower respiratory tract infections [1], indicative of the severity of pneumonia [2], and associated with mortality in paediatric intensive care unit (ICU) patients [3]. Respiratory rate is measured in breaths per minute (bpm). Current routine practice for obtaining RR measurements outside of Critical Care involves manually counting chest movements [4]. This practice is time-consuming, inaccurate [5], and poorly carried out [6–8]. Therefore, there is an urgent need to develop an accurate, automated method for measuring RR in ambulatory patients. Furthermore, an automated method of measuring RR could facilitate: (i) objective patient-led home-monitoring of asthma; (ii) screening for obstructive sleep apnea; and (iii) screening for periods of

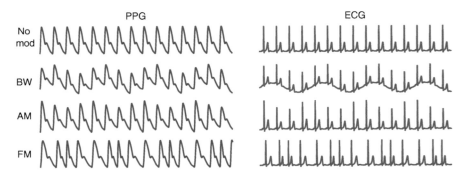

Fig. 26.1 Idealised respiratory modulations of the PPG (*left hand side*) and ECG (*right hand side*). During three respiratory cycles, from *top*: no modulation, baseline wander (BW), amplitude modulation (AM), and frequency modulation (FM). Adapted from [18, 27, 30]

dysregulated breathing during sleep, occasionally seen in advanced congestive heart failure.

A potential solution is to estimate RR from a convenient non-invasive signal which is modulated by respiration and is easily, and preferably routinely, measured. Two such signals are the electrocardiogram (ECG) and the photoplethysmogram (PPG). Both signals exhibit baseline wander (BW), amplitude modulation (AM) and frequency modulation (FM) due to respiration, as shown in Fig. 26.1 (see [9, 10] for further details). Furthermore, both signals can be acquired continuously from ambulatory patients using novel wearable sensors. For example, the SensiumVitals® system (Sensium Healthcare) provides continuous ECG monitoring using a lightweight patch with a battery life of up to five days. The ViSi Mobile® (Sotera Wireless) provides continuous ECG and PPG monitoring using a wrist-worn monitor with additional ECG electrodes. In addition, non-contact video-based technology is being developed for continuous monitoring of the PPG without the need for any equipment to be attached to a patient [11].

Many algorithms have been developed for estimating RR from the ECG and PPG [10, 12], but have not yet been widely adopted into clinical practice. In this case study we demonstrated the application of exemplary techniques to the ECG and PPG. The performance of these techniques was assessed on an example dataset. The case study is accompanied by MATLAB® code, equipping the reader with tools to develop and test their own RR algorithms for estimation of RR from physiological waveforms.

26.2 Study Dataset

PhysioNet's MIMIC II database (Version 3) was chosen for this study since it contains simultaneous ECG, PPG and thoracic impedance pneumography (IP) waveforms [13, 14]. IP signals, usually only measured in critical care, can be

26.2 Study Dataset

Table 26.1 Criteria for determining whether each of the 100 downloaded MIMIC II database records were included in the analysis

Criterion	Percent of records meeting criterion
Contain all the required waveforms (ECG, PPG and thoracic impedance)	76
Contain all the required numerics [heart rate (HR), pulse rate (PR) and respiratory rate (RR)]	64
Required waveforms and numerics last at least 10 min	51

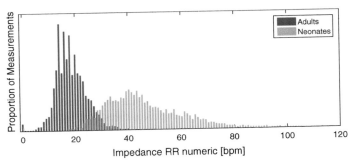

Fig. 26.2 Reference respiratory rate (RR) measurements acquired using thoracic impedance from adults and neonates. The disparity between the distributions of RR measurements acquired from adults (*blue*) and neonates (*red*) prompted a sub-group analysis of these two patient populations

used to estimate reference RRs since individual breaths can be identified as the thoracic impedance increases during inhalation and decreases during exhalation. MIMICII_data_importer.m was used in conjunction with the freely available *WFDB Toolbox*[1] to download the data. One hundred Intensive Care Unit (ICU) stay records, each containing data from a distinct ICU stay, were downloaded.

Records meeting the criteria in Table 26.1 were included in the analysis. The required waveforms and numerics were extracted from the 51 % of records that met these criteria. Each data channel was stored in two vectors of values and corresponding timestamps. This ensured that any gaps in the data due to changes in patient monitoring or data acquisition failures were preserved in the analysis.

Inspection of the dataset revealed a substantial difference in the distributions of IP RR measurements acquired from neonatal and adult patients, as illustrated in Fig. 26.2. This is in keeping with previous findings in [15], in which it was reported that children's RRs decrease from a median of 43 bpm when younger than

---

[1]*WFDB Toolbox* is available from PhysioNet: http://physionet.org/physiotools/matlab/wfdb-app-matlab/.

3 months to a median of 16 bpm when aged 15–18 years. Therefore, we decided to restrict the analysis to adult patients only.

26.3 Pre-processing

The extracted waveforms contained periods of high and low (reliable and unreliable) quality, as shown in Fig. 26.3. This is in keeping with the literature, where it is well reported that physiologic signals can be expected to contain periods of artifact in the Critical Care setting [16]. Each 10 s segment of ECG and PPG data was categorised as either high or low quality using the signal quality indicator (SQI) reported in [17]. This SQI determines the quality of the signal in two steps. Firstly, heart beats are detected to quantify the detected heart rate. Any segments containing physiologically implausible heart rates are deemed to be low quality. Secondly, template matching is used to quantify the correlation between an averaged beat's morphology and that of each individual beat. If the average correlation coefficient across a segment is below an empirical threshold, then the signal quality is deemed to be low (as shown in Fig. 26.4). Low quality segments were eliminated from the analysis.

The RR measurements provided by the clinical monitor were not used as a reference against which to test the accuracy of RR algorithms since they are susceptible to inaccuracies during periods of signal artifact. Instead, reference RRs were extracted from the IP signal, with periods in which reference RRs were unreliable being excluded from the analysis. To do so, the signal was segmented into non-overlapping 32 s windows. Two independent methods were used to estimate RR from each window in line with the methodology presented in [18]. Firstly, Fourier analysis was used to compute the power spectral density of the signal, as described in [19]. A first RR estimate was obtained as the frequency

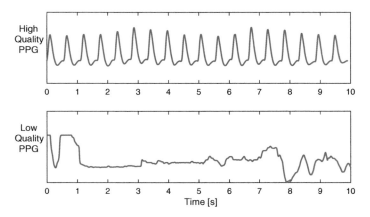

Fig. 26.3 Periods of high and low quality PPG waveform

26.3 Pre-processing

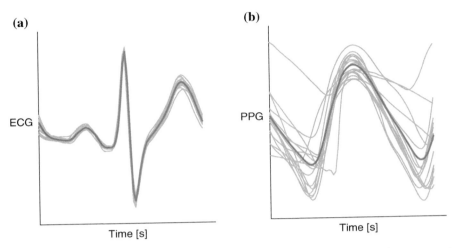

Fig. 26.4 Use of a template-matching signal quality index (SQI) to determine whether a segment of signal is high or low quality. **a** the ECG beats (*grey*) all have a similar morphology to the average beat template (*red*), and the ECG segment is deemed to be high quality. **b** the PPG beats have a highly variable morphology, indicating low signal quality

corresponding to the maximum power within the range of plausible respiratory frequencies (4–60 bpm). Secondly, the "count-orig" method presented in [20] was used to detect individual breaths. A second RR estimate was calculated from the average duration of individual breaths. Count-orig involves normalising the signal, identifying pairs of maxima exceeding a threshold value, and identifying reliable breaths as periods of signal between the pairs of maxima which contain only one minimum below zero. Finally, if the difference between the two RR estimates was < 2 bpm, then the reference RR was calculated as the mean of the two estimates. Otherwise, the window was excluded.

26.4 Methods

A plethora of algorithms have been proposed for estimation of RR from the ECG or PPG. In this case study we implemented exemplary algorithms (using `RRest.m`) which estimate RR by exploiting one of the three fundamental respiratory modulations, modelled on the approach described in [19]. RR algorithms generally consist of two compulsory components and two optional components. The compulsory components are:

- extraction of a respiratory signal (a time series dominated by respiratory modulation) from the raw signal, and
- estimation of RR from the respiratory signal.

Two optional components, quality assessment and fusion, can be used to improve the accuracy of estimated RRs.

Extraction of a respiratory signal is often performed using a feature-based technique, which extracts a time series of beat-by-beat feature measurements. Figure 26.5 shows the steps involved. The first two steps, the elimination of sub-respiratory (<4 bpm) and very high frequencies (>100 Hz and >35 Hz for the

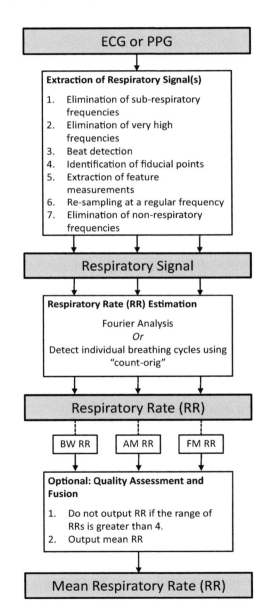

Fig. 26.5 The steps within a respiratory rate (RR) algorithm. Extraction of respiratory signal(s) and RR estimation are compulsory. The third step consisting of quality assessment and fusion is optional

26.4 Methods

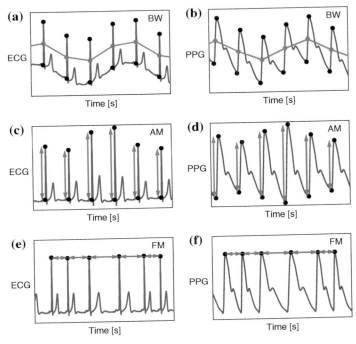

Fig. 26.6 Feature measurement from fiducial points of the ECG and PPG signals. **a** and **b** Measurement of baseline wander (*BW*), the mean of the amplitudes of a beat's peak and trough; **c** and **d** amplitude modulation (*AM*), the difference between the amplitudes of each beat's peak and trough; **e** and **f** frequency modulation (*FM*), the time interval between consecutive peaks

ECG and PPG respectively), are usually not necessary when analysing EHR data since they are often performed by patient monitors prior to signal output. Beat detection was performed in the ECG using a QRS detector based upon the algorithm of Pan, Hamilton and Tompkins [21, 22], and in the PPG using the Incremental-Merge Segmentation (IMS) algorithm [23]. Fiducial points, such as R-waves and pulse-peaks, and Q-waves and pulse troughs, were identified for each beat. Three feature measurements were then extracted from these fiducial points on both the ECG and PPG waveforms as illustrated in Fig. 26.6. The three beat-by-beat time series of feature measurements are sampled irregularly since there is one measurement per heart beat. Since frequency domain analysis requires regularly sampled signals, these signals were resampled at a regular frequency of 5 Hz using linear interpolation. Finally, spurious non-respiratory frequencies introduced in the extraction process were eliminated using band-pass filtering within the range of plausible respiratory frequencies (4–60 bpm). Spurious high frequencies arise due to linear interpolation and spurious low frequencies can be caused by physiological changes.

RR estimation from the ECG and PPG was performed in both the frequency and time domain using the Fourier analysis and breathing cycle detection techniques used to estimate the reference RRs. An additional quality assessment and fusion step, the "Smart Fusion" method [19], was optionally performed in an attempt to increase the accuracy of RR estimates. The first step of "Smart Fusion" is to assess the quality of the RR estimates derived from the three modulations. If the three estimates are within 4 bpm of each other, then a final RR estimate is generated as the mean of the estimates. Otherwise, no output is provided.

26.5 Results

Table 26.2 shows the mean absolute error (MAE) for all methods under analysis. The most accurate algorithm prior to implementing quality assessment and fusion steps had a MAE of 4.28 bpm. This algorithm extracted BW from the PPG and estimated RR using breath detection. Algorithms using BW respiratory signals outperformed those using AM, which in turn outperformed FM algorithms. Furthermore, those using breath detection to estimate RR outperformed those using Fourier analysis.

An improvement in accuracy was observed when the additional quality assessment and fusion step was added to breath detection algorithms. The MAEs for the ECG and PPG decreased from 4.87 to 3.92 bpm, and from 4.28 to 3.36 bpm respectively. This was achieved at the expense of the number of windows from which RRs were estimated. When using this additional step 44 % of ECG windows and 63 % of PPG windows were discarded by the quality assessment. Interestingly, no improvement in accuracy was observed when adding these steps to a Fourier-based algorithm.

It should be noted that a substantial proportion of the data available for analysis was discarded prior to analysis. A reference RR could only be obtained from 10 % of windows. In addition, 44 % of ECG windows, and 30 % of PPG windows were

Table 26.2 The performances of the algorithms applied to the ECG and PPG, measured using the mean absolute error (MAE, measured in breaths per minute, bpm)

Algorithm specification		MAE (bpm)	
Respiratory signal	RR estimation	ECG	PPG
BW	Breath detection	4.87	4.28
AM	Breath detection	4.95	5.58
FM	Breath detection	8.48	7.95
BW	Fourier	7.51	8.18
AM	Fourier	8.69	11.14
FM	Fourier	13.16	12.11
BW, AM, FM	Breath detection + quality assess + fusion	3.92	3.36
BW, AM, FM	Fourier + quality assess + fusion	12.66	10.52

discarded due to low signal quality, likely indicating the presence of movement artifact or sensor disconnection. Consequently, only 6 % of the ECG data, and 7 % of the PPG data were included in the analysis.

26.6 Discussion

RR is widely used in a range of clinical settings to aid diagnosis and prognosis. Despite its clinical importance, it is the only vital sign which is not routinely measured electronically outside of Critical Care. In this case study techniques have been presented for the estimation of RR from two easily and routinely measured physiological signals, the ECG and PPG. There were two important findings. Firstly, the addition of a signal quality and fusion step to the breath-detection algorithms increased accuracy. Secondly, time-domain breath-detection algorithms outperformed the frequency-domain algorithms. This suggests that further research is warranted into time-domain methods, which are far less reliant on the RR being quasi-stationary. If a method is found to perform sufficiently well then it could be used to measure RR during routine physiological assessments to provide early warning of clinical deteriorations.

The dataset used in this case study is a useful resource for further testing of RR algorithms. Its strength is that it contains waveform data from thousands of critically-ill patients, with many datasets lasting hours or days. However, the generalisability of the results is limited by the consisting solely of critically-ill patients. This is particularly significant considering that RR algorithms would most often be used with patients outside of Critical Care. Furthermore, the IP signal gave a reliable reference RR for only 10 % of the time. This resulted in a low number of signal windows being included in the analysis, a significant limitation. Consequently, this case study should be treated as an example of the methodology which could be used to perform a robust study, rather than as a robust study itself. In addition, some uncertainty remained in the reference RRs since they are the mean of two estimates which could differ by up to 2 bpm. When testing algorithms for extraction of clinical parameters from physiological signals, the more accurate the reference value, the better. In this study the measured MAEs are likely to be higher than the true MAEs of the algorithms because of inaccuracies in the reference RR.

A key challenge of waveform analysis is the handling of low quality data. One approach is to detect and exclude low quality data, as performed using the quality assessment and fusion step in this study. A simple template-matching SQI was used here. More complex techniques which fuse the results of multiple SQIs to determine signal quality may improve the performance of RR algorithms in clinical practice [24, 25]. An alternative approach is to refine analysis techniques to ensure they remain accurate even when using low quality data. For instance, in [26] an algorithm is presented for estimation of RR from the ECG during exercise, when the signal is likely to be of low quality.

26.7 Conclusions

This case study demonstrates the potential utility of the ECG and PPG for measurement of RR in the clinical setting. The necessary tools required to design and test RR algorithms are presented, allowing the interested reader to extend this work. The results suggest two particular areas for further algorithmic development. Firstly, the use of signal quality and fusion to improve the accuracy of RR algorithms should be explored further. In the literature much focus has been given to the extraction of respiratory signals and estimation of RR, whereas relatively little research has been conducted into quality assessment and fusion. Secondly, further research should be conducted into the use of time-domain techniques to identify individual breathing cycles. It is notable that in this study the time-domain technique outperformed the frequency-domain technique, whilst in the literature reported time-domain techniques are rarely more sophisticated than peak detection. However, the low data inclusion rate in this study suggests that further investigation is required to ensure that conclusions are robust.

26.8 Further Work

There are two pressing research questions concerning estimation of RR from physiological signals. Firstly, it is not clear which RR algorithm is the most accurate. Until recently validation studies had compared only a few of the many existing algorithms. Comparison between studies is difficult since studies are usually performed on different datasets collected from different populations, using different statistical measures. A recent study evaluated many algorithms on data acquired from young, healthy subjects. Secondly, it is not clear whether the most accurate algorithm performs well enough for clinical use.

Further studies are required to answer such questions. We propose that algorithms should be tested firstly in a healthy population, in ideal operating conditions. This would facilitate assessment of the best possible performance of the algorithms. If any algorithms perform sufficiently well for clinical use, then they could be tested in patient populations in clinical settings. Conversely, if no algorithms perform adequately, then further algorithmic development should be carried out to attempt to improve the performance. The MIMIC II database provides opportunity to test algorithms in a wide range of physiological conditions, such as hyper- and hypotension, and normal and reduced ejection fraction. This may provide insight into the limitations of the algorithms, ensuring that they are only used when in conditions in which they can be expected to perform well.

26.9 Non-contact Vital Sign Estimation

As presented in this chapter, current monitoring systems available to track changes in the vital signs of patients in the clinic or at home require contact with the subject. Most patients requiring regular monitoring find the probes difficult to attach and use properly [28]. The process of recording vital signs, even if it only takes a few minutes, becomes burdensome as it usually has to be performed on a daily basis. The low compliance of patients with wearing sensors is also an obstacle to successful monitoring.

The ideal technology to estimate vital signs would involve sensors with no direct contact with the patient, providing several advantages over traditional methods because no subject participation is required to set the equipment up, it requires no skin preparation, causes no skin irritation, decreases the risk of infection, and has the potential to be seamlessly integrated into the patient's lifestyle.

Several technologies have been proposed for non-contact monitoring of vital signs from Radar-based systems to non-contact ECG using capacitive coupling electrodes. During the last decade, with the cost of digital video cameras continuing to decrease as the technology becomes more ubiquitous, research in non-contact vital sign monitoring has expanded through the use of off-the-shelf video cameras. Video cameras can be found in laptops, mobile phones, set-top boxes and television sets in patients' living room, opening up new possibilities for the monitoring of vital signs.

Video-based vital sign monitoring extends the concepts of traditional photoplethysmography using the multiple photosites present in an imaging sensor to record the blood volume changes associated with the cardiac cycle. These physiological changes result in a waveform known as photoplethysmographic imaging (PPGi), from which vital signals such as heart rate, respiratory rate, oxygen saturation (SpO_2) and other can be estimated [11, 29]. Figure 26.7 shows a 15-s sample of PPGi alongside PPG and IP signals measured using conventional monitoring equipment. The patient was undergoing haemodialysis treatment at the Churchill Hospital in Oxford. During this period the patient had a heart rate of 60 beats/min and a respiratory rate of 15 bpm, both of which can be computed from both the conventional monitoring equipment and the camera using the methods explained in this chapter.

Decades of extensive research from the computer vision community have helped to develop imaging systems that are capable of complex computations (such as face detection, identity access control or other object tracking), are interactive (such as motion/gesture and body tracking in games) and can perform complex 3D reconstruction operations. Therefore, video-based vital sign monitoring has the potential to expand the role vital sign monitoring beyond that which can be met by traditional pulse oximetry.

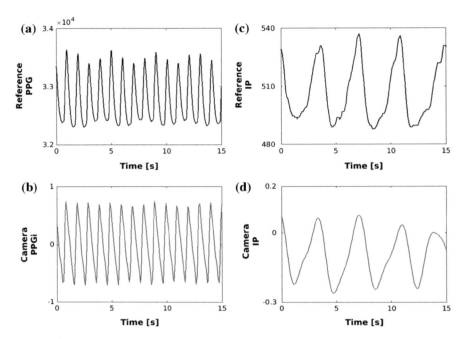

Fig. 26.7 A 15-s sample of data from a patient undergoing haemodialysis treatment at the Churchill Hospital in Oxford. **a** Reference PPG waveform from a Nonin pulse oximeter, **b** extracted photoplethysmographic imaging (PPGi) waveform from a video camera, **c** reference impedance pneumography (IP) respiratory signal, **d** respiratory signal extracted from the PPGi waveform. During the period the patient had a heart rate of 60 beats/min and a respiratory rate of 15 breaths per minute (bpm)

Open Access This chapter is distributed under the terms of the Creative Commons Attribution-NonCommercial 4.0 International License (http://creativecommons.org/licenses/by-nc/4.0/), which permits any noncommercial use, duplication, adaptation, distribution and reproduction in any medium or format, as long as you give appropriate credit to the original author(s) and the source, a link is provided to the Creative Commons license and any changes made are indicated.

The images or other third party material in this chapter are included in the work's Creative Commons license, unless indicated otherwise in the credit line; if such material is not included in the work's Creative Commons license and the respective action is not permitted by statutory regulation, users will need to obtain permission from the license holder to duplicate, adapt or reproduce the material.

Code Appendix

The code used in this case study is available from the GitHub repository accompanying this book: https://github.com/MIT-LCP/critical-data-book. Further information on the code is available from this website. The following key scripts were used:

Code Appendix

- `MIMICII_data_importer.m`: used to extract data from the MIMIC II database.
- `RRest.m`: used to run RR algorithms and assess their performances.

References

1. Shann F, Hart K, Thomas D (1984) Acute lower respiratory tract infections in children: possible criteria for selection of patients for antibiotic therapy and hospital admission. Bull World Health Organ 62(5):749
2. Lim WS, Van der Eerden MM, Laing R, Boersma WG, Karalus N, Town GI, Lewis SA, Macfarlane JT (2003) Defining community acquired pneumonia severity on presentation to hospital: an international derivation and validation study. Thorax 58(5):377–382
3. Pollack MM, Ruttimann UE, Getson PR (1988) Pediatric risk of mortality (prism) score. Crit Care Med 16(11):1110–1116
4. World Health Organization (WHO) (1990) Fourth Programme Report, 1988–1989: ARI Programme for Control of Acute Respiratory Infections. Technical Report, WHO, Geneva
5. Lovett PB, Buchwald JM, Stürmann K, Bijur P (2005) The vexatious vital: neither clinical measurements by nurses nor an electronic monitor provides accurate measurements of respiratory rate in triage. Ann Emerg Med 45(1):68–76
6. Chellel A, Fraser J, Fender V, Higgs D, Buras-Rees S, Hook L, Mummery L, Cook C, Parsons S, Thomas C (2002) Nursing observations on ward patients at risk of critical illness. Nurs Times 98(46):36–39
7. Cretikos MA, Bellomo R, Hillman K, Chen J, Finfer S, Flabouris A (2008) Respiratory rate: the neglected vital sign. Med J Aust 188(16):657–659
8. Hogan J (2006) Why don't nurses monitor the respiratory rates of patients? Br J Nurs 15 (9):489–492
9. Meredith DJ, Clifton D, Charlton P, Brooks J, Pugh CW, Tarassenko L (2012) Photoplethysmographic derivation of respiratory rate: a review of relevant physiology. J Med Eng Technol 36(1):1–7
10. Bailon R, Sornmo L, Laguna P (2006) ECG-derived respiratory frequency estimation. In: Advanced methods and tools for ECG data analysis (Chap. 8). Artech House, London, pp 215–244
11. Tarassenko L, Villarroel M, Guazzi A, Jorge J, Clifton DA, Pugh C (2014) Non-contact video-based vital sign monitoring using ambient light and auto-regressive models. Physiol Meas 35(5):807–831
12. Garde A, Karlen W, Ansermino JM, Dumont GA (2014) Estimating respiratory and heart rates from the correntropy spectral density of the photoplethysmogram. PLoS ONE 9(1): e86427
13. Goldberger AL, Amaral LA, Glass L, Hausdorff JM, Ivanov PC, Mark RG, Mietus JE, Moody GB, Peng CK, Stanley HE (2000) Physiobank, physiotoolkit, and physionet components of a new research resource for complex physiologic signals. Circulation 101(23): E215–E220
14. Saeed M, Villarroel M, Reisner AT, Clifford G, Lehman L, Moody G, Heldt T, Kyaw TH, Moody B, Mark RG (2011) Multiparameter intelligent monitoring in intensive care II: a public-access intensive care unit database. Crit Care Med 39(5):952–960
15. Fleming S, Thompson M, Stevens R, Heneghan C, Plüddemann A, Maconochie I, Tarassenko L, Mant D (2011) Normal ranges of heart rate and respiratory rate in children from birth to 18 years of age: a systematic review of observational studies. Lancet 377 (9770):1011–1018

16. Nizami S, Green JR, McGregor C (2013) Implementation of artifact detection in critical care: a methodological review. IEEE Rev Biomed Eng 6:127–142
17. Orphanidou C, Bonnici T, Charlton P, Clifton D, Vallance D, Tarassenko L (2015) Signal-quality indices for the electrocardiogram and photoplethysmogram: derivation and applications to wireless monitoring. IEEE J Biomed Health Inform 19(3):832–838
18. Pimentel MAF, Charlton PH, Clifton DA (2015) Probabilistic estimation of respiratory rate from wearable sensors. In: Mukhopadhyay SC (ed) Wearable electronics sensors, vol 15. Springer International Publishing, pp 241–262
19. Karlen W, Raman S, Ansermino JM, Dumont GA (2013) Multiparameter respiratory rate estimation from the photoplethysmogram. IEEE Trans Biomed Eng 60(7):1946–1953
20. Schäfer A, Kratky KW (2008) Estimation of breathing rate from respiratory sinus arrhythmia: comparison of various methods. Ann Biomed Eng 36(3):476–485
21. Pan J, Tompkins WJ (1985) A real-time QRS detection algorithm. IEEE Trans Biomed Eng 32(3):230–236
22. Hamilton PS, Tompkins WJ (1986) Quantitative investigation of QRS detection rules using the MIT/BIH arrhythmia database. IEEE Trans Biomed Eng 33(12):1157–1165
23. Karlen W, Ansermino JM, Dumont G (2012) Adaptive pulse segmentation and artifact detection in photoplethysmography for mobile applications. In: Proceedings of the annual international conference of the IEEE engineering in medicine and biology society, vol 2012. EMBS, pp 3131–3134
24. Behar J, Oster J, Li Q, Clifford GD (2013) ECG signal quality during arrhythmia and its application to false alarm reduction. IEEE Trans Biomed Eng 60(6):1660–1666
25. Li Q, Clifford GD (2012) Dynamic time warping and machine learning for signal quality assessment of pulsatile signals. Physiol Meas 33(9):1491–1501
26. Bailón R, Sörnmo L, Laguna P (2006) A robust method for ECG-based estimation of the respiratory frequency during stress testing. IEEE Trans Biomed Eng 53(7):1273–1285
27. Charlton PH, Bonnici T, Tarassenko L, Clifton DA, Beale R, Watkinson PJ (2016) An assessment of algorithms to estimate respiratory rate from the electrocardiogram and photoplethysmogram. Physiol Measur 37(4): 610–626
28. Bonnici T, Orphanidou C, Vallance D, Darrell A, Tarassenko L (2012) Testing of wearable monitors in a real-world hospital environment: what lessons can be learnt? In: 2012 ninth international conference on wearable and implantable body sensor networks, pp 79–84
29. Villarroel M, Guazzi A, Jorge J, Davis S, Watkinson P, Green G, Shenvi A, McCormick K, Tarassenko L (2014) Continuous non-contact vital sign monitoring in neonatal intensive care unit. Healthc Technol Lett 1(3):87–91
30. Addison PS, Watson JN, Mestek ML, Mecca RS (2012) Developing an algorithm for pulse oximetry derived respiratory rate (RR(oxi)): a healthy volunteer study. J Clin Monit Comput 26(1):45–51

Chapter 27
Signal Processing: False Alarm Reduction

Qiao Li and Gari D. Clifford

Learning Objectives
Use a data fusion and machine learning approach to suppress false arrhythmia alarms.

This case study introduces concepts that should improve understanding of the following:

1. Extract relevant features from clinical waveforms.
2. Assess signal quality of clinical data, and
3. Develop a machine learning model, train and validate it using a clinical database.

27.1 Introduction

Modern patient monitoring systems in intensive care produce frequent false alarms which lead to a disruption of care, impacting both the patient and the clinical staff through noise disturbances, desensitization to warnings and slowing of response times [1, 2]. This leads to decreased quality of care [3, 4], sleep deprivation [1, 5, 6], disrupted sleep structure [7, 8], stress for both patients and staff [9–12] and depressed immune systems [13]. Intensive care unit (ICU) false alarm rates as high as 90 % have been reported [14], while only 8 % of alarms were determined to be true alarms with clinical significance [15] and over 94 % of alarms may not be clinically important [16]. There are two main reasons for the high false alarm rate. One is that physiological data can be severely corrupted by artifacts (e.g. from movement), noise (e.g. from electrical interference) and missing data (e.g. from transducer 'pop' leading to impedance or pressure changes and a resultant signal saturation). Figure 27.1 illustrates the bedside monitor 'waveforms' (or high resolution data)

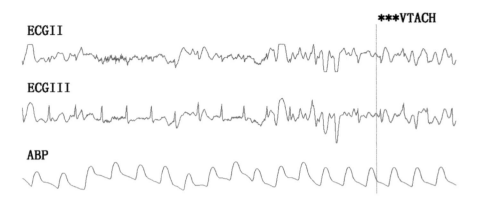

Fig. 27.1 False ventricular tachycardia alarm, 'called' at the point where the vertical line is placed in a 30 s snapshot of two leads of ECG (ECGII an ECGIII) and an arterial blood pressure signal (*ABP*). The alarm is triggered by the strong noise manifesting as high amplitude (±2 mV) oscillations on the ECG at approximately 5 Hz beginning a little over halfway through the snapshot (and a little under 10 s from the vertical VT marker). Note that the ABP continues as normal, with no significant change in rhythm or morphology

recorded around a false ventricular tachycardia alarm (the vertical line indicates the moment at which the monitor triggered the alarm). The alarm is caused by significant noise affecting the electrocardiogram (ECG) leads. However, the regular pulsatile beats present in the arterial blood pressure (ABP) lead clearly indicate this is a false alarm (since the poor pump function during this arrhythmia should cause a significant drop in pulse amplitude and an increase in rate). The other reason for the high rate of false alarms is that univariate alarm algorithms and simple numeric thresholds are predominantly used in current clinical bedside monitors. The reason for this is an historical artifact, in that manufacturers have developed different embedded systems with bespoke hardware and single mode transducers. Univariate alarm-detection algorithms therefore consider a single monitored waveform at a time. The alarm is generally triggered when a variable (e.g. heart rate) derived from the waveform (e.g. ECG) is above or below a preset (or adjustable) threshold for a given length of time, regardless of whether the change is caused by a change in physiological state, by an artifact or by medical interventions, such as moving or positioning the patient, drawing blood and flushing the arterial line, or disconnecting the patient from the ventilator for endotracheal suctioning. Moreover, alarm thresholds are often adjusted in an ad hoc manner, based on how annoying the alarm is perceived to be by the clinical team in attendance. There is little evidence that alarm thresholds are optimized for any population or individual, particularly in a multivariate sense.

Various noise cancellation algorithms such as median filtering [17] or Kalman filtering [18] have been used to suppress false alarms. While transient noise can be removed by median filtering it is brutally non-adaptive. Kalman filtering, on the other hand, is an optimal state estimation method, which has been used to improve heart rate (HR) and blood pressure (BP) estimation during noisy periods and

27.1 Introduction

arrhythmias [18]. However, alarm detection has changed little in decades, with the univariate alarm algorithm paradigm persisting. A promising solution to the false alarm issue comes from multiple variable data fusion, such as HR estimation by fusing the information from synchronous ECG, ABP and photoplethysmogram (PPG) from which oxygen saturation is derived [18]. Otero et al. [19] proposed a multivariable fuzzy temporal profile model which described a set of monitoring criteria of temporal evolution of the patient's physiological variables of HR, oxygen saturation (SpO_2) and BP. Aboukhalil et al. [14] and Deshmane [20] used synchronous ABP and PPG signals to suppress false ECG alarms. Zong et al. [21] reduced false ABP alarms using the relationships between ECG and ABP. Besides calculated physiological parameters, signal quality indices (SQI), which assess the waveform's usefulness or the noise levels of the waveforms, can be extracted from the raw data and used as weighting factors to allow for varying trust levels in the derived parameters. Behar et al. [22] and Li and Clifford [23] suppressed false ECG alarms by assessing the signal quality of ECG, ABP and PPG. Monasterio et al. [24] used a support vector machine to fuse data from respiratory signals, heart rate and oxygen saturation derived from the ECG, PPG, and impedance pneumogram, as well as several SQIs, to reduce false apnoea-related desaturations.

27.2 Study Dataset

A dataset drawn from PhysioNet's MIMIC II database [25, 26] was used in this study, containing simultaneous ECG, ABP, and PPG recordings with 4107 multiple expert-annotated life-threatening arrhythmia alarms [asystole (AS), extreme bradycardia (EB), extreme tachycardia (ET) and ventricular tachycardia (VT)] on 182 ICU admissions. A total of 2301 alarms were found by selecting the alarms when the ECG, ABP and PPG were all available. The false alarm rates were 91.2 % for AS, 26.6 % for EB, 14.4 % for ET, and 44.4 % for VT respectively, and 45.0 % overall. The ICU admissions were divided into two separate sets for training and testing, ensuring that the frequency of alarms in each category was roughly equal through frequency ranking and separating odd and evenly numbered signals. Table 27.1 details the relative frequency of each alarm category and their associated true and false alarm rates. The waveform data from 30 s before to 10 s after the alarm were extracted for each alarm to aid expert verification (since the Association for the Advancement of Medical Instrumentation (AAMI) guidelines require an alarm to respond within 10 s of the initiation of any alarm event [27]). A consensus of three experts was required to label each alarm as true or false. Only data from 10 s before the alarm to the alarm onset were used for automated feature extraction and model classification.

Since the VT alarm was considered the most difficult type of false alarm to suppress, with an associated low false alarm reduction rate and high true alarm suppression rate in literature [14, 20–23, 28], we therefore focus on reducing this

Table 27.1 Distribution of alarms in the dataset and training and test set

Alarm type	Total				Training set				Test set			
	False	True	Total	FA rate (%)	False	True	Total	FA rate (%)	False	True	Total	FA rate (%)
AS	260	25	285	91.2	166	14	180	92.2	94	11	105	89.5
EB	62	171	233	26.6	58	108	166	34.9	4	63	67	6.0
ET	37	220	257	14.4	19	116	135	14.1	18	104	122	14.8
VT	677	849	1526	44.4	306	478	784	39.0	371	371	742	50.0
All	1036	1265	2301	45.0	549	716	1265	43.4	487	549	1036	47.0

false alarm for the rest of the chapter. Interested readers are directed to Li and Clifford [23] for methods to reduce false alarms on the other types of alarms.

27.3 Study Pre-processing

In total 147 features and SQI metrics were extracted from ECG, ABP, PPG, and SpO_2 signals within the 10 s analysis window. These features were generally chosen based upon previous research by the authors and others [14, 20–24, 28–32]. The typical features included HR (extracted from ECG, ABP, and PPG), blood pressure (systolic, diastolic, mean), oxygen saturation (SpO_2), and the amplitude of PPG. Each feature had five sub-features calculated over the 10 s window: including the minimum, maximum, median, variance, and gradient (derived from a robust least squares fit over the entire window). Besides the typical features, the area difference of beats (ADB), the area ratio of beats (ARB) in the ECG, ABP and PPG and thirteen ventricular fibrillation metrics (taken from [29]) were also extracted. The area of each beat was defined to be the area between the waveform and the x-axis, from the start of the ECG beat to 0.6 times of mean beat-by-beat interval (BBi). Note the start of the ECG beat was taken as the position of R peak— 0.2 * BBi. The ADB was calculated by comparing each beat to the median of the beats in the window, as shown in Fig. 27.2. The ADB used four sub-features; the mean ADB of five beats with the shortest beat-to-beat intervals, the maximum of mean ADB of five consecutive beats, the variance and gradient of ADB. The ARB used five sub-features; the ratio between the mean area of five smallest beats and five largest beats of the ECG (ARB_{ECG}), ABP (ARB_{ABP}), and PPG (ARB_{PPG}), the ratio between ARB_{ECG} and ARB_{ABP}, and the ratio between ARB_{ECG} and ARB_{PPG}. The description of the thirteen ventricular fibrillation metrics can be found in Li et al. [29], and included spectral and time domain features shown to allow highly accurate classification of VF. The ECG SQI metrics included thirteen metrics [30], based on standard moments, frequency domain statistics and the agreement between event detectors with different noise sensitivities. The ABP SQI metrics included a signal abnormality index with its nine sub-metrics [31] and a dynamic time warping

27.3 Study Pre-processing

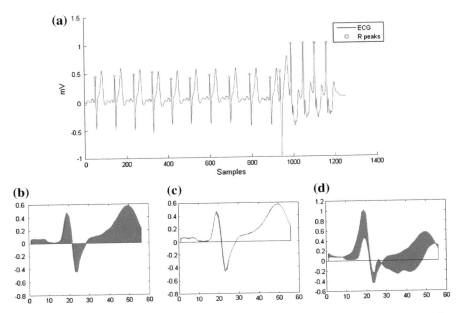

Fig. 27.2 Example of area difference of beats calculation. **a** ECG in a 10 s window. **b** The median beat of the beats in the window (*gray* area shows the area between the waveform and the x-axis). **c** ADB of a normal beat (the first beat, *gray* area shows the ADB). **d** ADB of an abnormal beat (the last beat)

(DTW) based SQI approach with its four sub-metrics [32]. The DTW based SQI resampled each beat to match a running beat template by derived using the DTW. The SQI was then given by the correlation coefficient between the template and each beat. The PPG SQI metrics included the DTW-based SQIs [32] and the first two Hjorth parameters [20] which estimated the dominant frequency and half-bandwidth of the spectral distribution of PPG. While these do not necessarily represent an exhaustive list of features, they do represent the vast majority of features identified as useful in previous studies.

27.4 Study Methods

A modified random forests (RF) classifier, previously described by Johnson et al. [33], was used. The RF [34] is an ensemble learning method for classification that constructs a number of decision trees at training time and outputs the class that is the mode of the classes of the individual trees. The basic principle is that a group of "weak learners" can come together to form a "strong learner." RFs correct for decision trees' defects of overfitting and adding bias to their training set. Each tree selects a subset of observations via two regression splits. These observations are then given a contribution equal to a random constant times the observation's value for a chosen feature plus a random intercept. The contributions across all trees are summed to provide the contribution for a single "forest," where a "forest" refers to a group of trees plus an intercept term. The predicted likelihood function output (L) by the forest is the inverse logit of the sum of each tree's contribution plus the intercept term (27.1). The intercept term is set to the logit of the mean observed outcome.

$$L = \sum_{i=1}^{N} \left((-t_i) * \log\left(\text{logit}^{-1}(s_i)\right) - (1 - t_i) * \log\left(1 - \text{logit}^{-1}(s_i)\right) \right) \quad (27.1)$$

where t_i is the target of the training set, s_i is the sum of tree's contribution, $i = 1\ldots N$ is the number of observations in the training set.

The core of the new RF model we used is the custom Markov chain Monte Carlo (MCMC) sampler that iteratively optimizes the forest. This sampling process constructs the Markov chain by a memoryless iteration process which selects randomly two trees from the current forests and updates their structure. The MCMC randomly samples the observation space by a large user-defined number of bootstrap iterations. After standardizing the training data to a standard normal distribution, the forest is initialized to a null model, with no contributions assigned for any observations.

At each iteration, the algorithm randomly selects two trees in the forest and randomizes their structure. That is, it randomly re-selects first two features which the tree uses for splitting, the value at which the tree splits those features, the third feature used for contribution calculation, and the multiplicative and additive constants applied to the third feature. The total forest contribution is then recalculated and a Metropolis-Hastings acceptance step is used to determine if the update is accepted. The predicted likelihood of the previous forest (L_i) and the likelihood of the forest with the two updated trees (L_{i+1}) were calculated. If $e^{(L_i - L_{i+1})}$ is greater than a uniformly distributed random real number within unit interval, the update is accepted. If the update is accepted, the two trees are kept in the forest, otherwise they are discarded and the forest remains unchanged. After a set fraction of the total number of iterations to allow the forest to learn the target distribution (generally 20 %), the algorithm begins storing forests at a fixed interval, i.e. once every set number of iterations. Once the number of user-defined iterations is reached, the forest is re-initialized as before, and the iterative process restarts. Again, after the set burn-in period, the forests begin to be saved at a fixed interval. The final result of this algorithm is a set of forests, each of which will contribute to the final model classification. The flowchart of the RF algorithm is shown in Fig. 27.3.

27.5 Study Analysis

Fig. 27.3 The flowchart of the random forests algorithm

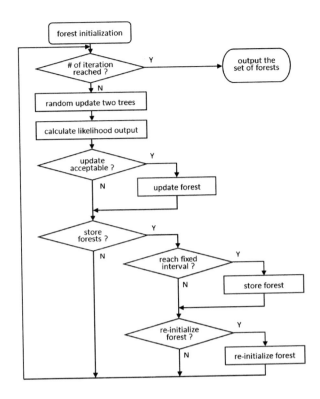

27.5 Study Analysis

The RF model was optimized on the training set and evaluated for out-of-sample accuracy on the test set. During the training phase, a model of 320 forests with 500 trees in each forest was established. The output of the model provides a probability between 0 and 1, which is an estimated value equivalent to a false or true alarm respectively. The receiver operating characteristic (ROC) curve was extracted by raising the threshold on the probability where we switch from false to true from 0 to 1—i.e. the probability greater than the threshold indicates a true alarm and below (or equal) indicates a false alarm. The optimal operating point was selected at the ROC curve when sensitivity equals 1 (no true alarm suppression) with the largest specificity. However, a sub-optimal operating point was also selected with acceptable sensitivity to balance specificity, e.g. sensitivity equals 99 %. (The reason for this is that anecdotally, clinical experts have indicated a 1 % true alarm suppression rate (or increase in true alarm suppression rate) would be acceptable—see discussion in study conclusions.) The model was then evaluated on the test set with the selected operating points.

In the algorithm validation phase, the classification performance of the algorithm was evaluated using 10-fold cross validation. The process sorted the study dataset into ten folds randomly stratified by ICU admissions rather than by the alarms. Then, nine folds were used for training the model and the last fold was used for validation. This process was repeated ten times as one integral procedure, with each of the folds used exactly once as the validation data. The average performance was used for evaluation. We note however, that this may be suboptimal and a voting of all folds may produce a better performance.

27.6 Study Visualizations

The ROC curve on the training set is shown in Fig. 27.4. The optimal operating point (marked by a circle) shows sensitivity 100.0 % and specificity 24.5 %, indicating we suppress 24.5 % of the false alarms without true alarm suppression. The sub-optimal operating point (marked by a star) shows a sensitivity 99.2 % and specificity 53.3 %, indicating a false alarm reduction of 53.3 % with only a 0.8 % true alarm suppression rate. When the model was used on the test set by the optimal

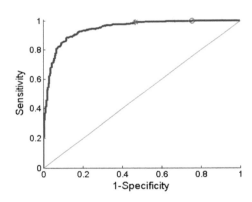

Fig. 27.4 ROC curve for the training set. *Circle* indicates optimal operating point (in terms of clinical acceptability) and *star* a sub-optimal operating point which may in fact be preferable

Table 27.2 Result of 10-fold cross validation of the classification model with different operating points

Operating point (by sensitivity) (%)	Training (on 9 folds)		Validation (on 1 held out fold)	
	Sensitivity (%)	Specificity (%)	Sensitivity (%)	Specificity (%)
99.00	99.06 ± 0.04	56.41 ± 5.60	95.82 ± 5.62	51.68 ± 16.88
99.50	99.56 ± 0.04	49.08 ± 5.37	96.50 ± 5.39	45.19 ± 17.94
99.60	99.66 ± 0.04	43.49 ± 6.45	98.72 ± 2.06	38.14 ± 17.25
99.70	99.75 ± 0.03	39.50 ± 7.39	98.75 ± 2.08	32.07 ± 16.19
99.80	99.87 ± 0.02	34.57 ± 9.02	98.87 ± 2.11	28.16 ± 15.80
100.0	100.0 ± 0.00	27.85 ± 6.17	99.04 ± 2.02	18.10 ± 9.87

operating point, a sensitivity of 99.7 % and a specificity of 17.0 % were achieved, with a sensitivity of 99.5 % and a specificity of 44.2 % for the sub-optimal operating point. The result of 10-fold cross validation with different options of operating points is shown in Table 27.2.

27.7 Study Conclusions

We show here that a promising approach to suppression of false alarms appears to be through the use of multivariate algorithms, which fuse synchronous data sources and estimates of underlying quality to make a decision. False VT alarms are the most difficult to suppress without causing any true alarm suppression since the ABP and PPG waveforms may have morphology changes indicating the hemodynamics changes during VT. We also show that a random forests-based model can be implemented with high confidence that few true alarms would be suppressed (although it's impossible to say 'never'). A practical operating point can be selected by changing the threshold of the model in order to balance the sensitivity and specificity. We note that the best previously reported results on VT alarms were by Aboukhalil et al. [14] and Sayadi and Shamsollahi [28] who achieved false VT alarm suppression rates of 33.0 and 66.7 % respectively. However, the TA suppression rates they achieved (9.4 and 3.8 % respectively) are clearly too high to make their algorithms acceptable for this category of alarm. Compared with our previous studies using some common machine learning algorithms such as support vector machine [22] and relevance vector machine [23], the random forests algorithm, which fused the features extracted from synchronous data sources like ECG, ABP and PPG, provided lower TA suppression rates and higher FA suppression rates. Moreover, a systematic validation procedure, such as k-fold cross validation, is necessary to evaluate the algorithm and we note that earlier works did not follow such a protocol. Without such validation, it is hard to believe that the algorithm will work well on unseen data because of overfitting. This is extremely important to note, that even a 0 % true alarm suppression is unlikely to always hold, and so a small true alarm suppression is likely to be acceptable. In private discussions with our clinical advisors, a figure of 1 % has often been suggested. In the work presented here, we show that with just half a percent of true alarms being suppressed, almost half of the false alarms can be suppressed. This true alarm suppression rate is likely to be negligible compared to the actual number of noise-induced missed alarms from the bedside monitor itself. (No monitor is perfect, and false negative rates of between 0.5 and 5 % have been reported [35].) We also note that the algorithm proposed here used 10 s of data before the alarm only, which meets the 10 s requirement of AAMI standard [27]. In recent work from the PhysioNet/Computing in Cardiology Challenge 2015, it was shown that extending this window slightly can lead to significant improvements in false alarm suppression [36]. Although the regulatory bodies would need to approve such changes, and that is often seen as unlikely, we do note that the 10 s rule is somewhat arbitrary and such work may indeed influence the changes in regulatory acceptance. We note several limitations to our study. First, the number of alarms is still relatively low, and they come from a single database/manufacturer. Second, medical history, demographics, and other medical data were not available and therefore used to adjust thresholds. Finally, information concerning repeated alarms was not used to adjust false alarm suppression dynamically based on earlier alarm frequency during the same ICU stay. This latter point is particularly tricky, since using earlier alarm data as prior information can be entirely misleading when false alarm rates are non-negligible.

27.8 Next Steps/Potential Follow-Up Studies

The issue of false alarms has disturbed the clinical patient monitoring and monitor manufacturers for many years, but the alarm handling has not seen the same progress as the rest of medical monitoring technology. One important reason is that in the current legal and regulatory environment, it may be argued that manufacturers have external pressures to provide the most sensitive alarm algorithms, such that no critical event goes undetected [4]. Equally, one could argue that clinicians also have an imperative to ensure that no critical alarm goes undetected, and are willing to accept large numbers of false alarms to avoid a single missed event. A large number of algorithms and methods have emerged in this area [4, 14, 17–24, 28, 37, 38]. However, most of these approaches are still in an experimental stage and there is still a long way to go before the algorithms are ready for clinical application.

The 2015 PhysioNet/Computing in Cardiology Challenge aimed to encourage the development of algorithms to reduce the incidence of false alarms in ICU [36]. Bedside monitor data leading up to a total of 1250 life-threatening arrhythmia alarms recorded from three of the most prevalent intensive care monitor manufacturers' bedside units were used in this challenge. Such challenges are likely to stimulate renewed interest by the monitoring industry in the false alarm problem. Moreover, the engagement of the scientific community will draw out other subtle issues. Perhaps the three key issues remaining to be addressed are: (1) Just how many alarms should be annotated and by how many experts? (see Zhu et al. [39] for a detailed discussion of this point); (2) How should we deal with repeated alarms, passing information forward from one alarm to the next?; and (3) What additional data should be supplied to the bedside monitor as prior information on the alarm? This could include a history of tachycardia, hypertension, drug dosing, interventions and other related information including acuity scores. Finally, we note that life threatening alarms are far less frequent than other less critical alarms, and by far the largest contributor to the alarm pollution in critical care comes from these more pedestrian alarms. A systematic approach to these less urgent alarms is also needed, borrowing from the framework presented here. More promisingly, the tolerance of true alarm suppression is likely to be much higher for less important alarms, and so we expect to see very large false alarm suppression rates. This is particularly

27.8 Next Steps/Potential Follow-Up Studies

important, since the techniques described here are general and could apply to most non-critical false alarms, which constitute the majority of such events in the ICU. Although the competition does not directly address these four points (and in fact the data needed to do so remains to become available in large numbers), the competition will provide a stimulus for such discussions and the tools (data and code) will help continue the evolution of the field.

Open Access This chapter is distributed under the terms of the Creative Commons Attribution-NonCommercial 4.0 International License (http://creativecommons.org/licenses/by-nc/4.0/), which permits any noncommercial use, duplication, adaptation, distribution and reproduction in any medium or format, as long as you give appropriate credit to the original author(s) and the source, a link is provided to the Creative Commons license and any changes made are indicated.

The images or other third party material in this chapter are included in the work's Creative Commons license, unless indicated otherwise in the credit line; if such material is not included in the work's Creative Commons license and the respective action is not permitted by statutory regulation, users will need to obtain permission from the license holder to duplicate, adapt or reproduce the material.

References

1. Chambrin MC (2001) Review: alarms in the intensive care unit: how can the number of false alarms be reduced? Crit Care 5(4):184–188
2. Cvach M (2012) Monitor alarm fatigue, an integrative review. Biomed Inst Tech 46(4):268–277
3. Donchin Y, Seagull FJ (2002) The hostile environment of the intensive care unit. Curr Opin Crit Care 8(4):316–320
4. Imhoff M, Kuhls S (2006) Alarm algorithms in critical care monitoring. Anesth Analg 102(5):1525–1537
5. Meyer TJ, Eveloff SE, Bauer MS, Schwartz WA, Hill NS, Millman RP (1994) Adverse environmental conditions in the respiratory and medical ICU settings. Chest 105(4):1211–1216
6. Parthasarathy S, Tobin MJ (2004) Sleep in the intensive care unit. Intensive Care Med 30(2):197–206
7. Johnson AN (2001) Neonatal response to control of noise inside the incubator. Pediatr Nurs 27(6):600–605
8. Slevin M, Farrington N, Duffy G, Daly L, Murphy JF (2000) Altering the NICU and measuring infants' responses. Acta Paediatr 89(5):577–581
9. Cropp AJ, Woods LA, Raney D, Bredle DL (1994) Name that tone. The proliferation of alarms in the intensive care unit. Chest 105(4):1217–1220
10. Novaes MA, Aronovich A, Ferraz MB, Knobel E (1997) Stressors in ICU: patients' evaluation. Intensive Care Med 23(12):1282–1285
11. Topf M, Thompson S (2001) Interactive relationships between hospital patients' noise induced stress and other stress with sleep. Heart Lung 30(4):237–243
12. Morrison WE, Haas EC, Shaffner DH, Garrett ES, Fackler JC (2003) Noise, stress, and annoyance in a pediatric intensive care unit. Crit Care Med 31(1):113–119
13. Berg S (2001) Impact of reduced reverberation time on sound-induced arousals during sleep. Sleep 24(3):289–292

14. Aboukhalil A, Nielsen L, Saeed M, Mark RG, Clifford GD (2008) Reducing false alarm rates for critical arrhythmias using the arterial blood pressure waveform. J Biomed Inform 41(3):442–451
15. Tsien CL, Fackler JC (1997) Poor prognosis for existing monitors in the intensive care unit. Crit Care Med 25(4):614–619
16. Lawless ST (1994) Crying wolf: false alarms in a pediatric intensive care unit. Crit Care Med 22(6):981–985
17. Mäkivirta A, Koski E, Kari A, Sukuvaara T (1991) The median filter as a preprocessor for a patient monitor limit alarm system in intensive care. Comput Meth Prog Biomed 34(2–3):139–144
18. Li Q, Mark RG, Clifford GD (2008) Robust heart rate estimation from multiple asynchronous noisy sources using signal quality indices and a Kalman filter. Physiol Meas 29(1):15–32
19. Otero A, Felix P, Barro S, Palacios F (2009) Addressing the flaws of current critical alarms: a fuzzy constraint satisfaction approach. Artif Intell Med 47(3):219–238
20. Deshmane AV (2009) False arrhythmia alarm suppression using ECG, ABP, and photoplethysmogram. M.S. thesis, MIT, USA
21. Zong W, Moody GB, Mark RG (2004) Reduction of false arterial blood pressure alarms using signal quality assessment and relationships between the electrocardiogram and arterial blood pressure. Med Biol Eng Comput 42(5):698–706
22. Behar J, Oster J, Li Q, Clifford GD (2013) ECG signal quality during arrhythmia and its application to false alarm reduction. IEEE Trans Biomed Eng 60(6):1660–1666
23. Li Q, Clifford GD (2012) Signal quality and data fusion for false alarm reduction in the intensive care unit. J Electrocardiol 45(6):596–603
24. Monasterio V, Burgess F, Clifford GD (2012) Robust classification of neonatal apnoea-related desaturations. Physiol Meas 33(9):1503–1516
25. Goldberger AL, Amaral LAN, Glass L, Hausdorff JM, Ivanov PCh, Mark RG, Mietus JE, Moody GB, Peng C-K, Stanley HE (2000) Physiobank, physiotoolkit, and physionet: components of a new research resource for complex physiologic signals. Circulation 101(23):e215–e220
26. Saeed M, Villarroel M, Reisner AT, Clifford G, Lehman L, Moody G, Heldt T, Kyaw TH, Moody B, Mark RG (2011) Multiparameter intelligent monitoring in intensive care II (MIMIC-II): a public-access intensive care unit database. Crit Care Med 39(5):952–960
27. American National Standard (ANSI/AAMI EC13:2002) (2002) Cardiac monitors, heart rate meters, and alarms. Association for the Advancement of Medical Instrumentation, Arlington, VA
28. Sayadi O, Shamsollahi M (2011) Life-threatening arrhythmia verification in ICU patients using the joint cardiovascular dynamical model and a Bayesian filter. IEEE Trans Biomed Eng 58(10):2748–2757
29. Li Q, Rajagopalan C, Clifford GD (2014) Ventricular fibrillation and tachycardia classification using a machine learning approach. IEEE Trans Biomed Eng 61(6):1607–1613
30. Li Q, Rajagopalan C, Clifford GD (2014) A machine learning approach to multi-level ECG signal quality classification. Comput Meth Prog Biomed 117(3):435–447
31. Sun JX, Reisner AT, Mark RG (2006) A signal abnormality index for arterial blood pressure waveforms. Comput Cardiol 33:13–16
32. Li Q, Clifford GD (2012) Dynamic time warping and machine learning for signal quality assessment of pulsatile signals. Physiol Meas 33(9):1491–1501
33. Johnson AEW, Dunkley N, Mayaud L, Tsanas A, Kramer AA, Clifford GD (2012) Patient specific predictions in the intensive care unit using a Bayesian ensemble. Comput Cardiol 39:249–252
34. Breiman L (2001) Random forests. Mach Learn 45(1):5–32
35. Schapira RM, Van Ruiswyk J (2002) Reduction in alarm frequency with a fusion algorithm for processing monitor signals. Meeting of the American Thoracic Society. Session A56, Poster H57

References

36. Clifford GD, Silva I, Moody B, Li Q, Kella D, Shahin A, Kooistra T, Perry D, Mark RG (2006) The PhysioNet/computing in cardiology challenge 2015: reducing false arrhythmia alarms in the ICU. Comput Cardiol 42:1–4
37. Borowski M, Siebig S, Wrede C, Imhoff M (2011) Reducing false alarms of intensive care online-monitoring systems: an evaluation of two signal extraction algorithms. Comput Meth Prog Biomed 2011:143480
38. Li Q, Mark RG, Clifford GD (2009) Artificial arterial blood pressure artifact models and an evaluation of a robust blood pressure and heart rate estimator. Biomed Eng Online 8:13
39. Zhu T, Johnson AEW, Behar J, Clifford GD (2014) Crowd-sourced annotation of ECG signals using contextual information. Ann Biomed Eng 42(4):871–884

Chapter 28
Improving Patient Cohort Identification Using Natural Language Processing

Raymond Francis Sarmiento and Franck Dernoncourt

Learning Objectives

To compare and evaluate the performance of the structured data extraction method and the natural language processing (NLP) method when identifying patient cohorts using the Medical Information Mart for Intensive Care (MIMIC-III) database.

1. To identify a specific patient cohort from the MIMIC-III database by searching the structured data tables using ICD-9 diagnosis and procedure codes.
2. To identify a specific patient cohort from the MIMIC-III database by searching the unstructured, free text data contained in the clinical notes using a clinical NLP tool that leverages negation detection and the Unified Medical Language System (UMLS) to find synonymous medical terms.
3. To evaluate the performance of the structured data extraction method and the NLP method when used for patient cohort identification.

28.1 Introduction

An active area of research in the biomedical informatics community involves developing techniques to identify patient cohorts for clinical trials and research studies that involve the secondary use of data from electronic health records (EHR) systems. The widening scale of EHR databases, that contain both structured and unstructured information, has been beneficial to clinical researchers in this regard. It has helped investigators identify individuals who may be eligible for

---

The two authors contributed equally to this work.

clinical trials as well as conduct retrospective studies to potentially validate the results of prospective clinical studies at a fraction of the cost and time [1]. It has also helped clinicians to identify patients at a higher risk of developing chronic disease, especially those who could benefit from early treatment [2].

Several studies have investigated the accuracy of structured administrative data such as the World Health Organization's (WHO) International Classification of Diseases, Ninth Revision (ICD-9) billing codes when identifying patient cohorts [3–11]. Extracting structured information using ICD-9 codes has been shown to have good recall, precision, and specificity [3, 4] when identifying distinct patient populations. However, for large clinical databases, information extraction can be time-consuming, costly, and impractical when conducted across several data sources [12] and applied to large cohorts [13].

Using structured queries to extract information from an EHR database allows one to retrieve data easily and in a more time-efficient manner. Structured EHR data is generally useful, but may also contain incomplete and/or inaccurate information especially when each data element is viewed in isolation. For example [14], to justify ordering a particular laboratory or radiology test, clinicians often assign a patient with a diagnosis code for a condition that the patient is suspected to have. But even when the test results point to the patient not having the suspected condition, the diagnosis code often remains in the patient's medical record. When the diagnosis code is then viewed without context (i.e., without the benefit of understanding the nuances of the case as provided in the patient's clinical narrative), this becomes problematic because it prohibits the ability of investigators to accurately identify patient cohorts and to utilize the full statistical potential of the available populations. Compared to narratives from clinical notes, relying solely on structured data such as diagnostic codes can be unreliable because they may not be able to provide information on the overall clinical context. However, automated examination of a large volume of clinical notes requires the use of natural language processing (NLP). The domain of study for the automated analysis of unstructured text data is referred to as NLP, and it has already been used with some success in the domain of medicine. In this chapter, we will be focusing on how NLP can be used to extract information from unstructured data for cohort identification.

NLP is a field of computer science and linguistics that aims to understand human (natural) languages and facilitate more effective interactions between humans and machines [13, 15]. In the clinical domain, NLP has been utilized to extract relevant information such as laboratory results, medications, and diagnoses from de-identified medical patient record narratives in order to identify patient cohorts that fit eligibility criteria for clinical research studies [16]. When compared to human chart review of medical records, NLP yields faster results [17–20]. NLP techniques have also been used to identify possible lung cancer patients based on their radiology reports [21] and extract disease characteristics for prostate cancer patients [22].

28.1 Introduction

We considered chronic conditions where both a disease diagnosis and an intervention diagnosis were likely to be found together in an attempt to better highlight the differences between structured and unstructured retrieval techniques, especially given the limited number of studies that have looked at interventions or treatment procedures, rather than illness or disease, as outcomes [14]. The diabetic population was of particular interest for this NLP task because the numerous cardiovascular, ophthalmological, and renal complications associated with diabetes mellitus eventually require treatment interventions or procedures, such as hemodialysis in this case. Moreover, clinical notes frequently contain medical abbreviations and acronyms, and the use of NLP techniques can help in capturing and viewing these information correctly in medical records. Therefore, in this case study, we attempted to determine whether the use of NLP on the unstructured clinical notes of this population would help improve structured data extraction. We identified a cohort of critically ill diabetic patients suffering from end-stage renal failure who underwent hemodialysis using the Medical Information Mart for Intensive Care (MIMIC-III) database [23].

28.2 Methods

28.2.1 Study Dataset and Pre-processing

All data from this study were extracted from the publicly available MIMIC-III database. MIMIC-III contains de-identified [24] data, per Health Insurance Portability and Accountability Act (HIPAA) privacy rules [25], on over 58,000 hospital admissions in the intensive care units (ICU) at Beth Israel Deaconess Medical Center from June 2001 to October 2012 [26]. Aside from being publicly accessible, we chose MIMIC-III because it contains detailed EHR data on critically ill patients who are likely to have multiple chronic conditions, including those with complications from chronic diseases that would require life-saving treatment interventions.

We excluded all patients in the database who were under the age of 18; diagnosed with diabetes insipidus only and not diabetes mellitus; underwent peritoneal dialysis only and not hemodialysis; or those diagnosed with transient conditions such as gestational diabetes or steroid-induced diabetes without any medical history of diabetes mellitus. We also excluded patients who had received hemodialysis prior to their hospital admission but did not receive it during admission. From the remaining subjects, we included those who were diagnosed with diabetes mellitus and those who had undergone hemodialysis during their ICU admission. We extracted data from two primary sources: the structured MIMIC-III tables (discharge diagnoses and procedures) and unstructured clinical notes.

28.2.2 Structured Data Extraction from MIMIC-III Tables

Using the ICD-9 diagnosis codes from the discharge diagnoses table and ICD-9 procedure codes from the procedures table, we searched a publicly available ICD-9 [27] database to find illness diagnosis and procedure codes related to diabetes and hemodialysis as shown in Table 28.1. We used structured query language (SQL) to find patients in each of the structured data tables based on specific ICD-9 codes.

Table 28.1 ICD-9 codes and descriptions indicating a patient was diagnosed with diabetes mellitus and who potentially underwent hemodialysis from structured data tables in MIMIC-III

Structured data table	ICD-9 code and description
Diabetes mellitus	
Discharge diagnosis codes	249 secondary diabetes mellitus (includes the following codes: 249, 249.0, 249.00, 249.01, 249.1, 249.10, 249.11, 249.2, 249.20, 249.21, 249.3, 249.30, 249.31, 249.4, 249.40, 249.41, 249.5, 249.50, 249.51, 249.6, 249.60, 249.61, 249.7, 249.70, 249.71, 249.8, 249.80, 249.81, 249.9, 249.90, 249.91)
	250 diabetes mellitus (includes the following codes: 250, 250.0, 250.00, 250.01, 250.02, 250.03, 250.1, 250.10, 250.11, 250.12, 250.13, 250.2, 250.20, 250.21, 250.22, 250.23, 250.3, 250.30, 250.31, 250.32, 250.33, 250.4, 250.40, 250.41, 250.42, 250.43, 250.5, 250.50, 250.51, 250.52, 250.53, 250.6, 250.60, 250.61, 250.62, 250.63, 250.7, 250.70, 250.71, 250.72, 250.73, 250.8, 250.80, 250.81, 250.82, 250.83, 250.9, 250.90, 250.91, 250.92, 250.93)
Hemodialysis	
Discharge diagnosis codes	585.6 end stage renal disease (requiring chronic dialysis)
	996.1 mechanical complication of other vascular device, implant, and graft
	996.73 other complications due to renal dialysis device, implant, and graft
	E879.1 kidney dialysis as the cause of abnormal reaction of patient, or of later complication, without mention of misadventure at time of procedure
	V45.1 postsurgical renal dialysis status
	V56.0 encounter for extracorporeal dialysis
	V56.1 fitting and adjustment of extracorporeal dialysis catheter
Procedure codes	38.95 venous catheterization for renal dialysis
	39.27 arteriovenostomy for renal dialysis
	39.42 revision of arteriovenous shunt for renal dialysis
	39.43 removal of arteriovenous shunt for renal dialysis
	39.95 hemodialysis

28.2.3 Unstructured Data Extraction from Clinical Notes

The unstructured clinical notes include discharge summaries (n = 52,746), nursing progress notes (n = 812,128), physician notes (n = 430,629), electrocardiogram (ECG) reports (n = 209,058), echocardiogram reports (n = 45,794), and radiology reports (n = 896,478). We excluded clinical notes that were related to any imaging results (ECG_Report, Echo_Report, and Radiology_Report). We extracted notes from MIMIC-III with the following data elements: patient identification number (SUBJECT_ID), hospital admission identification number (HADM_IDs), intensive care unit stay identification number (ICUSTAY_ID), note type, note date/time, and note text.

We used an SQL query to extract pertinent information from all patients' notes that will be helpful in identifying a patient as someone belonging to the cohort, then wrote a Python script to filter the notes by looking for keywords and implementing heuristics in order to refine our search results. As part of our search strategy, we removed the family history sections when searching the clinical notes and ensured that the search for clinical acronyms did not retrieve those that were part of another word. For example, our filters did not retrieve those where "DM" appeared as part of another words such as in 'admission' or 'admit'. Finally, we used cTAKES [28, 29] version 3.2 with access to Unified Medical Language System (UMLS) [30] concepts to use the negation detection annotator when searching the note text. The negation detection feature in cTAKES works by trying to detect which entities in the text are negated. Examples of negation words that may be found in the clinical notes include 'not', 'no', 'never', 'hold', 'refuse', 'declined'. For example, in this case study, if "DM" or "HD" is consistently negated when searching the clinical notes, then the patient should not be considered part of the cohort.

The Metathesaurus [31] in UMLS contains health and biomedical vocabularies, ontologies, and standard terminologies, including ICD. Each term is assigned to one or more concepts in UMLS. Different terms from different vocabularies or ontologies that have similar meanings and assigned with the same concept unique identifier (CUI) are considered UMLS synonyms [32]. In order to identify diabetes mellitus patients who underwent hemodialysis during their ICU stay, we scanned the clinical notes containing the terms "diabetes mellitus" and "hemodialysis". We used the UMLS Metathesaurus to obtain synonyms for these terms because using only these two terms will restrict our search results.

cTAKES is an open-source natural language processing system that extracts information from clinical free-text stored in electronic medical records. It accepts either plain text or clinical document architecture (CDA)-compliant extensible markup language (XML) documents and consists of several annotators such as attributes extractor (assertion annotator), clinical document pipeline, chunker, constituency parser, context dependent tokenizer, dependency parser and semantic role labeler, negation detection, document preprocessor, relation extractor, and dictionary lookup, among others [33]. When performing named entity recognition or concept identification, each named entity is mapped to a specific terminology concept through the cTAKES dictionary lookup component [28], which uses the UMLS as a dictionary.

We refined our query parameters iteratively and searched the clinical notes containing our final query parameters based on UMLS synonyms to diabetes and hemodialysis. These were as follows: (A) include documents that contained any of the following terms: diabetes, diabetes mellitus, DM; (B) include documents that contained any of the following terms: hemodialysis, haemodialysis, kidney dialysis, renal dialysis, extracorporeal dialysis, on HD, HD today, tunneled HD, continue HD, cont HD; (C) finalize the set of documents to be run in cTAKES by only including documents that contained at least one of the terms from group A and at least one of the terms from group B; and (D) exclude documents by using the negation detection annotator in cTAKES to detect negations such as avoid, refuse, never, declined, etc. that appear near any of the terms listed in groups A and B.

28.2.4 Analysis

We manually reviewed all the notes for all patients identified by the structured data extraction method and/or the clinical NLP method as those potentially to have a diagnosis of diabetes mellitus and who had undergone hemodialysis during their ICU stay in order to create a validation database that contains the positively identified patients in the population of MIMIC-III patients. We used this validation database in evaluating the precision and recall of both the structured data extraction method and the clinical NLP method. We compared the results from both methods to the validation database in order to determine the true positives, false positives, recall, and precision. We defined these parameters using the following equation: recall = TP/(TP + FN), where TP = true positives and FN = false negatives; and precision = TP/(TP + FP), where FP = false positives. In this case study, we defined recall as the proportion of diabetic patients who have undergone hemodialysis in the validation database who were identified as such. We defined precision as the proportion of patients identified as diabetic and having undergone hemodialysis whose diagnoses were both confirmed by the validation database.

28.3 Results

In the structured data extraction method using SQL as illustrated in Fig. 28.1, we found 10,494 patients diagnosed with diabetes mellitus using ICD-9 codes; 1216 patients who underwent hemodialysis using ICD-9 diagnosis and procedure codes; and 1691 patients who underwent hemodialysis when searching the structured data tables using the string '%hemodial%'. Figure 28.2 shows the number of patients

28.3 Results

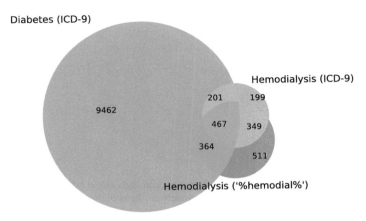

Fig. 28.1 Patients identified by structured data extraction, clockwise from *left* diagnosed with diabetes mellitus using ICD-9 diagnosis codes, underwent hemodialysis using ICD-9 discharge diagnosis and procedure codes, and underwent hemodialysis using the string '%hemodial%'

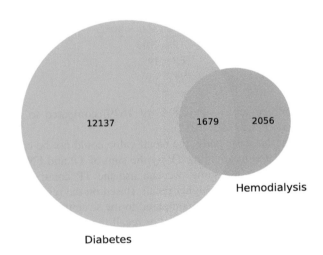

Fig. 28.2 Patients identified by clinical NLP method, from *left* diagnosed with diabetes, diagnosed with diabetes and who underwent hemodialysis, and who underwent hemodialysis

identified using the clinical NLP method: 13,816 patients diagnosed with diabetes mellitus and 3735 patients identified as having undergone hemodialysis during their ICU stay.

There were 1879 patients in the validation database consisting of 1847 (98.3 %) confirmed diabetic patients who had undergone hemodialysis. We identified 1032 (54.9 % of 1879) patients when using SQL only and 1679 (89.4 % of 1879) when using cTAKES. Of these, 832 (44.3 % of 1879) were found by both approaches as illustrated in Fig. 28.3.

Table 28.2 shows the results of the two methods used to identify patient cohorts compared to the validation database. The clinical NLP method had better precision compared to the structured data extraction method. The clinical NLP method also

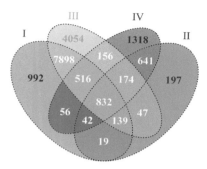

Fig. 28.3 Patients identified by structured data extraction and clinical NLP methods: *I*—diabetes patients found using SQL; *II*—patients who underwent hemodialysis found using SQL; *III*—diabetic patients found using cTAKES and; *IV*—patients who underwent hemodialysis found using cTAKES

Table 28.2 Precision of identifying patient cohorts using structured data extraction and clinical NLP compared to the validation database

Validation database (n = 1879)	Structured data extraction method, positive (n = 1032)	Clinical NLP method, positive (n = 1679)
Positive	TP = 1013	TP = 1666
Negative	FP = 19	FP = 13
Precision	98.2 %	99.2 %

identified fewer FP (0.8 % of 1679) compared to the structured data extraction method (1.8 % of 1032).

In this case study, the recall value could not be computed. But because recall is calculated by dividing TP by the sum of TP and FN, and the denominator for both methods is the same, we can use the TP count as a proxy to determine which method showed a higher recall. Based on the results, we found that more TPs were identified using NLP compared to the structured data approach. Hence, the clinical NLP method yielded a higher recall than the structured data extraction method.

We also analyzed the clinical notes for the 19 patients identified as FP using the structured data extraction method. We found that 14 patients were incorrectly identified as diabetic patients, 3 patients were incorrectly identified as having undergone hemodialysis, and 2 patients were not diabetic nor did they undergo hemodialysis during their ICU stay. In the 13 patients identified as FP when using the clinical NLP method, we also analyzed the clinical notes and found that 5 did not undergo hemodialysis during their ICU stay, 2 had initially undergone hemodialysis but was stopped due to complications, and 6 did not have diabetes (3 did not have any history of diabetes, 1 had initially been presumed to have diabetes according to the patient's family but was not the case, 1 had gestational diabetes without prior history of diabetes mellitus, and 1 was given insulin several times during the patient's ICU stay but was not previously diagnosed with diabetes nor was a diagnosis of new-onset diabetes indicated in any of the notes).

28.4 Discussion

Both the structured data extraction method and the clinical NLP method achieved high precision in identifying diabetic patients who underwent hemodialysis during their ICU stay. However, the clinical NLP method exhibited better precision and higher recall in a more time-saving and efficient way compared to the structured data extraction technique.

We identified several variables that may have resulted in a lower precision when using SQL only in identifying patient cohorts such as the kind of illness and the kind of intervention, the presence of other conditions similar to diabetes (i.e., diabetes insipidus, gestational diabetes), and the presence of other interventions similar to hemodialysis (i.e., peritoneal dialysis, continuous renal replacement therapy). The temporal feature of the intervention also added to the complexity of the cohort identification process.

Extracting and using the UMLS synonyms for "diabetes mellitus" and "hemodialysis" in performing NLP on the clinical notes helped increase the number of patients included in the final cohort. Knowing that clinicians often use acronyms, such as "DM" to refer to diabetes mellitus and "HD" for hemodialysis, and abbreviations, such as "cont" for the word 'continue' when taking down notes helped us refine our final query parameters.

There are several limitations to this case study. Specificity could not be calculated because in order to determine the TN and FN, the entire MIMIC-III database would need to be manually validated. Though it can be argued that the ones in the validation database that were missed by either method could be considered as FN, this may not be the true FN count in MIMIC-III because those that could be found outside of the validation database have not been included. Moreover, since the validation database used was not independent of the two methods, the TP and FP counts as well as the precision and recall may have been overestimated.

Another limitation is the lack of a gold standard database for the specific patient cohort we investigated. Without it, we were not able to fully evaluate the cohort identification methods we implemented. The creation of a gold standard database, one that is validated by clinicians and includes patients in the MIMIC-III database that have been correctly identified as TN and FN, for this particular patient cohort will help to better evaluate the performance of the methods used in this case study. Having a gold standard database will also help calculate the specificity for both methods.

Another limitation is that we focused on discharge diagnosis and procedure events especially in the structured data extraction method. Other data sources in MIMIC-III such as laboratory results and medications may help support the findings or even increase the number of patients identified when using SQL.

Furthermore, although we used a large database, our data originated from a single data source. Comparing our results found using MIMIC-III to other publicly available databases containing EHR data may help to assess the generalizability of our results.

28.5 Conclusions

NLP is an efficient method for identifying patient cohorts in large clinical databases and produces better results when compared to structured data extraction. Combining the use of UMLS synonyms and a negation detection annotator in a clinical NLP tool can help clinical researchers to better perform cohort identification tasks using data from multiple sources within a large clinical database.

Future Work

Investigating how clinical researchers could take advantage of NLP when mining clinical notes would be beneficial for the scientific research community. In this case study, we found that using NLP yields better results for patient cohort identification tasks compared to structured data extraction.

Using NLP may potentially be useful for other time-consuming clinical research tasks involving EHR data collected in the outpatient departments, inpatient wards, emergency departments, laboratories, and various sources of medical data. The automatic detection of abnormal findings mentioned in the results of diagnostic tests such as X-rays or electrocardiograms could be systematically used to enhance the quality of large clinical databases. Time-series analyses could also be improved if NLP is used to extract more information from the free-text clinical notes.

Notes

1. cTAKES is available from the cTAKES Apache website: http://ctakes.apache.org/downloads.cgi. A description of the components of cTAKES 3.2 can be found on the cTAKES wiki page: https://cwiki.apache.org/confluence/display/CTAKES/cTAKES+3.2+Component+Use+Guide [28].

Open Access This chapter is distributed under the terms of the Creative Commons Attribution-NonCommercial 4.0 International License (http://creativecommons.org/licenses/by-nc/4.0/), which permits any noncommercial use, duplication, adaptation, distribution and reproduction in any medium or format, as long as you give appropriate credit to the original author(s) and the source, a link is provided to the Creative Commons license and any changes made are indicated.

The images or other third party material in this chapter are included in the work's Creative Commons license, unless indicated otherwise in the credit line; if such material is not included in the work's Creative Commons license and the respective action is not permitted by statutory regulation, users will need to obtain permission from the license holder to duplicate, adapt or reproduce the material.

Code Appendix

All the SQL queries to count the number of patients per cohorts as well as the cTAKES XML configuration file used to analyze the notes are available from the GitHub repository accompanying this book: https://github.com/MIT-LCP/critical-data-book. Further information on the code is available from this website. The following key scripts were used:

- `cohort_diabetic_hemodialysis_icd9_based_count.sql`: Total number of diabetic patients who underwent hemodialysis based on diagnosis codes.
- `cohort_diabetic_hemodialysis_notes_based_count.sql`: List of diabetic patients who underwent hemodialysis based on unstructured clinical notes.
- `cohort_diabetic_hemodialysis_proc_and_notes_based_count.sql`: Total number of diabetic patients who underwent hemodialysis based on unstructured clinical notes and procedure codes.
- `cohort_diabetic_hemodialysis_proc_based_count.sql`: Total number of diabetic patients who underwent hemodialysis based on procedure codes.
- `cohort_diabetic_icd9_based_count_a.sql`: List of diabetic patients based on the ICD-9 codes.
- `cohort_hemodialysis_icd9_based_count_b.sql`: List of patients who underwent hemodialysis based on the ICD-9 codes.
- `cohort_hemodialysis_proc_based_count_c.sql`: Lists number of patients who underwent hemodialysis based on the procedure label.
- `CPE_physician_notes.xml`: cTAKES XML configuration file to process patients' notes. Some paths need to be adapted to the developer's configuration.

References

1. Kury FSP, Huser V, Cimino JJ (2015) Reproducing a prospective clinical study as a computational retrospective study in MIMIC-II. In: AMIA Annual Symposium Proceedings, pp 804–813
2. Bates DW, Saria S, Ohno-Machado L, Shah A, Escobar G (2014) Big data in health care: using analytics to identify and manage high-risk and high-cost patients. Health Aff (Millwood) 33(7):1123–1131
3. Segal JB, Powe NR (2004) Accuracy of identification of patients with immune thrombocytopenic purpura through administrative records: a data validation study. Am J Hematol 75 (1):12–17
4. Eichler AF, Lamont EB (2009) Utility of administrative claims data for the study of brain metastases: a validation study. J Neuro-Oncol 95(3):427–431
5. Kern EF, Maney M, Miller DR, Tseng CL, Tiwari A, Rajan M, Aron D, Pogach L (2006) Failure of ICD-9-CM codes to identify patients with comorbid chronic kidney disease in diabetes. Health Serv Res 41(2):564–580
6. Zhan C, Eixhauser A, Richards CL Jr, Wang Y, Baine WB, Pineau M, Verzier N, Kilman R, Hunt D (2009) Identification of hospital-acquired catheter-associated urinary tract infections from Medicare claims: sensitivity and positive predictive value. Med Care 47(3):364–369
7. Floyd JS, Heckbert SR, Weiss NS, Carell DS, Psaty BM (2012) Use of administrative data to estimate the incidence of statin-related rhabdomyolysis. J Am Med Assoc 307(15):1580–1582

8. van Walraven C, Austin PC, Manuel D, Knoll G, Jennings A, Forster AJ (2010) The usefulness of administrative databases for identifying disease cohorts is increased with a multivariate model. J Clin Epidemiol 63(12):1332–1341
9. Tieder JS, Hall M, Auger KA, Hain PD, Jerardi KE, Myers AL, Rahman SS, Williams DJ, Shah SS (2011) Accuracy of administrative billing codes to detect urinary tract infection hospitalizations. Pediatrics 128:323–330
10. Rosen LM, Liu T, Merchant RC (2012) Efficiency of International Classification of Diseases, Ninth Revision, billing code searches to identify emergency department visits for blood and body fluid exposures through a statewide multicenter database. Infect Control Hosp Epidemiol 33:581–588
11. Lamont EB, Lan L (2014) Sensitivity of Medicare claims data for measuring use of standard multiagent chemotherapy regimens. Med Care 52(3):e15–e20
12. Bache R, Miles S, Taweel A (2013) An adaptable architecture for patient cohort identification from diverse data sources. J Am Med Inform Assoc 20(e2):e327–e333
13. Sada Y, Hou J, Richardson P, El-Serag H, Davila J (2013) Validation of case finding algorithms for hepatocellular cancer from administrative data and electronic health records using natural language processing. Med Care
14. Abhyankar S, Demner-Fushman D, Callaghan FM, McDonald CJ (2014) Combining structured and unstructured data to identify a cohort of ICU patients who received dialysis. J Am Med Inform Assoc 21(5):801–807
15. Jurafsky D, Martin H (2008) Speech and language processing, 2nd edn. Prentice Hall, Englewood Cliffs, NJ
16. Voorhees EM, Tong RM (2011) Overview of the TREC 2011 medical records track. In: The twentieth text retrieval conference proceedings (TREC 2011). National Institute for Standards and Technology, Gaithersburg, MD
17. Wilbur WJ, Rzhetsky A, Shatkay H (2006) New directions in biomedical text annotation: definitions, guidelines and corpus construction. BMC Bioinform 7:356
18. Buchan NS, Rajpal DK, Webster Y, Alatorre C, Gudivada RC, Zheng C, Sanseau P, Koehler J (2011) The role of translational bioinformatics in drug discovery. Drug Discov Today 16:426–434
19. Nadkarni PM, Ohno-Machado L, Chapman WW (2011) Natural language processing: an introduction. J Am Med Inform Assoc 18:544–551
20. Uzuner Ö, South BR, Shen S, Duvall SL (2011) 2010 i2b2/VA challenge on concepts, assertions, and relations in clinical text. J Am Med Inform Assoc 18(5):552–556
21. Danforth KN, Early MI, Ngan S, Kosco AE, Zheng C, Gould MK (2012) Automated identification of patients with pulmonary nodules in an integrated health system using administrative health plan data, radiology reports, and natural language processing. J Thorac Oncol 7:1257–1262
22. Thomas AA, Zheng C, Jung H, Chang A, Kim B, Gelfond J, Slezak J, Porter K, Jacobsen SJ, Chien GW (2014) Extracting data from electronic medical records: validation of a natural language processing program to assess prostate biopsy results. World J Urol 32(1):99–103
23. Saeed M, Villarroel M, Reisner AT, Clifford G, Lehman LW, Moody G, Heldt T, Kyaw TH, Moody B, Mark RG (2011) Multiparameter intelligent monitoring in intensive care II: a public-access intensive care unit database. Crit Care Med 39(5):952–960
24. Neamatullah I, Douglass MM, Lehman LW, Reisner A, Villarroel M, Long WJ, Szolovits P, Moody GB, Mark RG, Clifford GD (2008) Automated de-identification of free-text medical records. BMC Med Inform Decis Mak 8:32
25. Standards for Privacy of Individually Identifiable Health Information; Final Rule, 45 CFR Parts 160 and 164 (2002) http://www.hhs.gov/ocr/privacy/hipaa/administrative/privacyrule/privruletxt.txt. Last accessed 6 Oct 2015
26. MIMIC. https://mimic.physionet.org/gettingstarted/access. Last accessed 19 Feb 2016
27. The Web's Free 2015 Medical Coding Reference. http://www.icd9data.com. Last accessed 7 Oct 2015

References

28. Savova GK, Masanz JJ, Ogren PV, Zheng J, Sohn S, Kipper-Schuler KC, Chute CG (2010) Mayo clinical Text Analysis and Knowledge Extraction System (cTAKES): architecture, component evaluation and applications. J Am Med Inform Assoc 17(5):507–513
29. Apache cTAKES™. http://cTAKES.apache.org/index.html. Last accessed 3 Oct 2015
30. Lindberg DA, Humphreys BL, McCray AT (1993) The unified medical language system. Meth Inf Med 32(4):281–291
31. Unified Medical Language System® (UMLS®) The Metathesaurus. https://www.nlm.nih.gov/research/umls/new_users/online_learning/Meta_001.html. Last accessed 7 Oct 2015
32. Griffon N, Chebil W, Rollin L, Kerdelhue G, Thirion B, Gehanno JF, Darmoni SJ (2012) Performance evaluation of unified medical language system®'s synonyms expansion to query PubMed. BMC Med Inform Decis Mak 12:12
33. cTAKES 3.2 Component Use Guide. https://cwiki.apache.org/confluence/display/CTAKES/cTAKES+3.2+Component+Use+Guide. Last accessed 7 Oct 2015

Chapter 29
Hyperparameter Selection

Franck Dernoncourt, Shamim Nemati, Elias Baedorf Kassis
and Mohammad Mahdi Ghassemi

Learning Objectives

High Level:
  Learn how to choose optimal hyperparameters in a machine learning pipeline for medical prediction.

Low Level:

1. Learn the intuition behind Bayesian optimization.
2. Understand the genetic algorithm and the multistart scatter search algorithm.
3. Learn the multiscale entropy feature.

29.1 Introduction

Using algorithms and features to analyze medical data to predict a condition or an outcome commonly involves choosing hyperparameters. A hyperparameter can be loosely defined as a parameter that is not tuned during the learning phase that optimizes the main objective function on the training set. While a simple grid search would yield the optimal hyperparameters by trying all possible combinations of hyper parameters, it does not scale as the number of hyperparameters and the data set size increase. As a result, investigators typically choose hyperparameters arbitrarily, after a series of manual trials, which can sometimes cast doubts on the results as investigators might have been tempted to tune the parameters specifically for the test set. In this chapter, we present three mathematically grounded techniques to automatically optimize hyperparameters: Bayesian optimization, genetic algorithms, and multistart scatter search.

To demonstrate the use of these hyperparameter selection methods, we focus on the prediction of hospital mortality for patients in the ICU with severe sepsis. The

---

The original version of this chapter was revised: A chapter author's name Shamim Nemati was added. The erratum to this chapter is available at 10.1007/978-3-319-43742-2_30

© The Author(s) 2016
MIT Critical Data, *Secondary Analysis of Electronic Health Records*,
DOI 10.1007/978-3-319-43742-2_29

outcome we consider is binary: either the patient died in hospital, or survived. Sepsis patients are at high risk for mortality (roughly 30 % [1]), and the ability to predict outcomes is of great clinical interest. The APACHE score [2] is often used for mortality prediction, but has significant limitations in terms of clinical use as it often fails to accurately predict individual patient outcomes, and does not take into account dynamic physiological measurements. To remediate this issue, we investigate the use of multiscale entropy (MSE) [3, 4] applied to heart rate (HR) signals as an outcome predictor: MSE measures the complexity of finite length time series. To compute MSE, one needs to specify a set of parameters, namely the maximum scale factor, the difference between consecutive scale factors, the length of sequences to be compared and a similarity threshold. We show that using hyperparameter selection methods, the MSE can predict the patient outcome more accurately than the APACHE score.

29.2 Study Dataset

We used the Medical Information Mart for Intensive Care II (MIMIC II) database, which is available online for free and was introduced by [5, 6]. MIMIC II is divided into two different data sets:

- the Clinical Database, which is a relational database that contains structured information such as patient demographics, hospital admissions and discharge dates, room tracking, death dates, medications, lab tests, and notes by the medical personnel.
- the Waveform Database, which is a set of flat files containing up to 22 different kinds of signals for each patient, including the ECG signals.

We selected patients who suffered from severe sepsis, defined as patients with an identified infection with evidence of organ dysfunction and hypotension requiring vasopressors and/or fluid resuscitation [7]. We further refined the patient cohort by choosing patients who had complete ECG waveforms for their first 24 h in the ICU. For each patient, we extracted the binary outcome (i.e. whether they died in hospital) from the clinical database. The HR signals were extracted from the ECG signals, and patients with low quality HR were removed.

29.3 Study Methods

We compared the predictive power of the following three sets of features to predict patient outcomes: basic descriptive statistics on the time series (mean and standard deviation), APACHE IV score and MSE. Since these features are computed on time series, for each feature set we obtained a vector of time series features. Once these features were computed, we clustered patients based on these vectors using spectral clustering. The number of clusters was determined using the silhouette values [8]. This allowed us to address the high heterogeneity of the data resulting from the fact

29.3 Study Methods

that MIMIC patients came from different care units. Lastly, for each cluster, we trained a support vector machine (SVM) classifier. To classify a new patient, we computed the distance from each cluster center, and computed the output of each SVM classifier: to make the final decision on the predicted outcome, we computed a weighted average of the output of each SVM classifier, where the weights were the distance from each cluster center. This method of combining clustering with SVM is called transductive SVM. We used the area under the receiver operating characteristic (ROC) curve (AUROC, often named more simply and ambiguously AUC) as the performance metric for the classification. Figure 29.1 illustrates the functioning of transductive SVMs.

MSE may be understood as the set of sample entropy values for a signal which is averaged over various increasing segment lengths. The MSE, y, was computed as follows:

$$y_j^\tau = \frac{1}{\tau} \sum_{i=(j-1)\tau+1}^{j\tau} x_i$$

where:

- x_i is the signal value at sample I,
- j is the index of the window to be computed,
- τ is the scale factor,
- Y is the length of sequences to be compared,
- Z is the similarity threshold.

Additionally, we have the following parameters:

- the maximum scale factor,
- the scale increase, which is the difference between consecutive scale factors,
- the similarity criterion or threshold, denoted r.

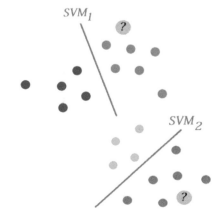

Fig. 29.1 Transductive SVM: clustering is performed first, then a convex combination of the SVM outputs is used to obtain the final prediction probability

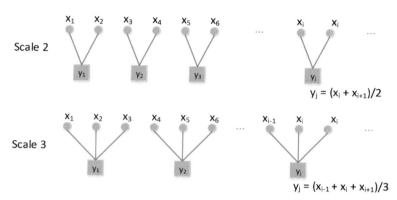

Fig. 29.2 Illustration of various scales from Costa et al. Only scales 2 and 3 are displayed. x_i is the signal value at sample i

Figure 29.2 shows how y is computed for different scales.

To select the best hyperparameters for the MSE, we compared three hyperparameter optimization techniques: Bayesian optimization, genetic algorithms, and multistart scatter search.

Bayesian optimization builds the distribution $P(y_{test}|y_{train}, x_{train}, x_{test})$, where x_{train} is the set of MSE parameters that were used to obtain the y_{train} AUROCs, x_{test} is a new set of MSE parameters, and y_{test} is the AUROC that would be obtained using the new MSE parameters. To put it otherwise, based on the previous observations on MSE parameters and achieved AUROCs, the Bayesian optimization predicts what AUROC a new set of MSE parameters will yield. Each time a new AUROC is computed, the set of MSE parameters as well as the AUROC is added to x_{test} and y_{test}. At each iteration, we can either explore, i.e. compute y_{test} for which the distribution P has a high variance, or exploit, i.e. compute y_{test} for which the distribution P has a low variance and high expectation. An implementation can be found in [9].

A genetic algorithm is an optimization algorithm based on the principle of Darwinian natural selection. A population is comprised of sets of MSE parameters. Each set of MSE parameters is evaluated based on the AUROC it achieved. The sets of MSE parameters with low AUROCs are eliminated. The surviving sets of MSE parameters are mutated, i.e. each parameter is slightly modified, to create new sets of MSE parameters, which form a new population. By iterating through this process, the new sets of MSE parameters yield increasingly high AUROCs. We set the population size of 100, and ran the optimization for 30 min. The first population was drawn randomly.

The multistart scatter search is similar to the genetic algorithm, the only difference residing in the use of a deterministic process to identify the individuals of the next population such as gradient descent.

Figure 29.3 summarizes the machine learning pipeline presented in this section.

29.3 Study Methods

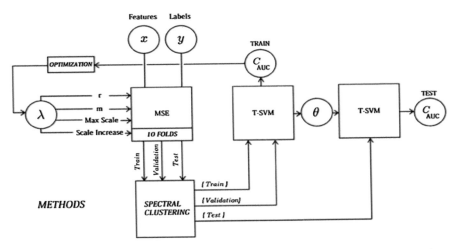

Fig. 29.3 The entire machine learning pipeline. The MSE features are computed from the input x using the parameters r, m, max scale and scale increase. 10 folds are created

The data set was split into testing (20 %), validation (20 %) and training (60 %) sets. In order to ensure robustness of the result, we used 10-fold cross-validation, and the average AUROC over the 10 folds. To make the comparison fair, each hyperparameter optimization technique was run the same amount of time, viz. 30 min.

29.4 Study Analysis

Table 29.1 contains the results for all three sets of features we considered. For the MSE features, Table 29.1 presents the results achieved by keeping the default hyperparameters, or by optimizing them using one of the three hyperparameter optimization techniques we presented in the previous section.

The first set of features, namely the basic descriptive statistics (mean and standard deviation), yields an AUROC of 0.54 on the testing set, which is very low since a random classifier yields an AUROC of 0.50. The second set of features, APACHE IV, achieves a much higher AUROC, 0.68, which is not surprising as the APACHE IV was designed to be a hospital mortality assessment for critically ill patients. The third set of features based on MSE performs surprisingly well with the default values (AUROC of 0.66), and even better when optimized with any of the three hyperparameter optimization techniques. The Bayesian optimization yields the highest AUROC, 0.72.

Table 29.1 Comparison of APACHE feature, time-series mean and standard deviation features, and MSE feature with default parameters or optimized with Bayesian optimization, genetic algorithms, and multistart scatter search, for the prediction of patient outcome

	Max scale	Scale increase	r	m	AUROC (training)	AUROC (testing)
Time series: mean and standard deviation					0.56 (0.52–0.56)	0.54 (0.45–0.60)
APACHE IV					0.77 (0.75–0.79)	0.68 (0.55–0.77)
MSE (defaults)	20	1	0.15	2	0.77 (0.73–0.78)	0.66 (0.60–0.72)
MSE (Bayesian)	17.62 (8.68)	2.59 (0.93)	0.11 (0.07)	2.58 (0.85)	0.77 (0.69–0.79)	0.72 (0.63–0.78)
MSE (genetic)	23.54 (14.34)	2.56 (1.12)	0.18 (0.15)	2.07 (0.70)	0.77 (0.67–0.84)	0.67 (0.44–0.78)
MSE (multi-start)	19.03 (12.57)	2.35 (0.87)	0.18 (0.128)	2.53 (0.87)	0.73 (0.69–0.76)	0.69 (0.53–0.72)

For each MSE parameter we report their cross-fold mean and standard deviation (with standard deviation in parenthesis). For the reported AUROC, we report the 50th percentile in the top half of the cell and the 25th and 75th percentiles in the lower half of the cell

29.5 Study Visualizations

Figure 29.4 provides an insight into the MSE parameters selected by the three hyperparameter selection techniques over the 10-fold cross-validation. Each point represents a parameter value optimized by a given hyperparameter selection technique for a unique data fold. For all 4 MSE parameters, we observe a great variance: this indicates that there is no clear global optimum, but instead there exist many MSE parameter sets that yield a high AUROC.

Interestingly, in this experiment the Bayesian optimization is more robust to the parameter variance, as shown by the confidence intervals around the AUROCs: most AUROCs reached by Bayesian optimization are high, unlike genetic algorithms and multistart scatter search. The two latter techniques are susceptible to premature convergence, while Bayesian optimization has a better exploration-exploitation tradeoff.

We also notice that the max scale and the r values reached by Bayesian optimization have a lower variance than genetic algorithms and multistart scatter search. One might hypothesize that heterogeneity across patients might be reflected more in the scale increase and m MSE parameters than in the max scale and r parameters.

Fig. 29.4 The impact of the MSE parameters on the outcome prediction AUROC

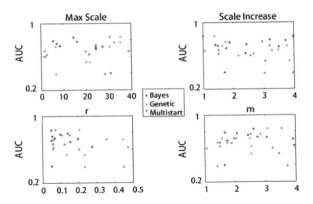

29.6 Study Conclusions

The results of this case study demonstrate two main points. First, from a medical standpoint, they underline the possible benefit of utilizing dynamic physiologic measurements in outcome prediction for ICU patients with severe sepsis: the data from this study indeed suggest that utilizing these physiological dynamics through MSE with optimized hyperparameters yields improved mortality prediction compared with the APACHE IV score. Physiological signals sampled at high-frequency are required for the MSE features to be meaningful, highlighting the need for high-resolution data collection, as opposed to some existing methods of data collection where signal samples are aggregated at the second or minute level, if not more, before being recorded.

Second, from a methodological standpoint, the results make a strong case for the use of hyperparameter selection techniques. Unsurprisingly, the results obtained with the MSE features are highly dependent on the MSE hyperparameters. Had we not used a hyperparameter selection technique and instead kept the default value, we would have concluded that APACHE IV provides a better predictive insight than MSE, and therefore missed the importance of physiological dynamics for prediction of patient outcome. Bayesian optimization seems to yield better results than genetic algorithms and multistart scatter search.

29.7 Discussion

There is still much room for further investigation. We focused on ICU patients with severe sepsis, but many other critically ill patient cohorts would be worth investigating as well. Although we restricted our study to the use of MSE and HR alone, it would be interesting to integrate and combine other disease characteristics and physiological signals. For example, [10] used Bayesian optimization to find the most optimal wavelet parameters to predict acute hypotensive episodes. Perhaps combining dynamic blood pressure wavelets with HR MSE, and even other dynamic data as well such as pulse pressure variation, would further optimize and tune the mortality prediction model. In addition there exist other scores to predict group mortality such as SOFA and SAPS II, which would provide useful baselines in addition to APACHE [11].

The scale of our experiments was satisfying for the case study's goals, but some other investigations might require a data set that is an order of magnitude larger. This might lead one to adopt a distributed design to deploy the hyperparameter selection techniques. For example, [12] used a distributed approach to hyperparameter optimization on 5000 patients and over one billion blood pressure beats. [13, 14] present another large-scale system to use genetic algorithms for blood pressure prediction.

Lastly, a more thorough comparison between hyperparameter selection techniques would help comprehend why a given hyperparameter selection technique performs better than others for a particular prediction problem. Especially, the hyperparameter selection techniques also have parameters, and a better understanding of the impact of these parameters on the results warrant further investigation.

29.8 Conclusions

In this chapter, we have presented three principled hyperparameter selection methods. We applied them to MSE, which we computed on physiological signals to illustrate their use. More generally, these methods can be used for any algorithm and feature where hyperparameters need to be tuned.

ICU data provide a unique opportunity for this type of research with routinely collected continuously measured variables including ECG waveforms, blood pressure waveforms from arterial lines, pulse pressure variation, pulse oximetry as well as extensive ventilator data. These dynamic physiologic measurements could potentially help unlock better outcome metrics and improve management decisions in patients with acute respiratory distress syndrome (ARDS), septic shock, liver failure or cardiac arrest, and other extremely ill ICU patients. Outside of the ICU, dynamic physiological data is routinely collected during surgery by the anesthesia team, in cardiac units with continuous telemetry and on Neurological care units with routine EEG measurements for patients with or at risk for seizures. As such the potential applications of MSE with hyperparameter optimization are extensive.

Open Access This chapter is distributed under the terms of the Creative Commons Attribution-NonCommercial 4.0 International License (http://creativecommons.org/licenses/by-nc/4.0/), which permits any noncommercial use, duplication, adaptation, distribution and reproduction in any medium or format, as long as you give appropriate credit to the original author(s) and the source, a link is provided to the Creative Commons license and any changes made are indicated.

29.8 Conclusions

The images or other third party material in this chapter are included in the work's Creative Commons license, unless indicated otherwise in the credit line; if such material is not included in the work's Creative Commons license and the respective action is not permitted by statutory regulation, users will need to obtain permission from the license holder to duplicate, adapt or reproduce the material.

References

1. Angus DC, Linde-Zwirble WT, Lidicker J, Clermont G, Carcillo J, Pinsky MR (2001) Epidemiology of severe sepsis in the United States: analysis of incidence, outcome, and associated costs of care. Crit Care Med 29(7):1303–1310
2. Saeed M, Villarroel M, Reisner AT, Clifford G, Lehman L, Moody GB, Heldt T, Kyaw TH, Moody BE, Mark RG (2011) Multiparameter intelligent monitoring in intensive care II (MIMIC-II): a public-access ICU database. Crit Care Med 39(5):952–960. doi:10.1097/CCM. 0b013e31820a92c6
3. Goldberger AL, Amaral LAN, Glass L, Hausdorff JM, Ivanov PCh, Mark RG, Mietus JE, Moody GB, Peng C-K, Stanley HE (2000) PhysioBank, PhysioToolkit, and PhysioNet: components of a new research resource for complex physiologic signals. Circulation 101(23): e215–e220 [Circulation Electronic Pages; http://circ.ahajournals.org/cgi/content/full/101/23/e215]
4. Mayaud L, Lai PS, Clifford GD, Tarassenko L, Celi LA, Annane D (2013) Dynamic data during hypotensive episode improves mortality predictions among patients with sepsis and hypotension*. Crit Care Med 41(4):954–962
5. Ng AY, Jordan MI, Weiss Y et al (2002) On spectral clustering: analysis and an algorithm. Adv Neural Inf Process Syst 2:849–856
6. Snoek J, Larochelle H, Adams RP (2012) Practical Bayesian optimization of machine learning algorithms. Adv Neural Inf Process Syst 2951–2959
7. Dernoncourt F, Veeramachaneni K, O'Reilly U-M (2015) Gaussian process-based feature selection for wavelet parameters: predicting acute hypotensive episodes from physiological signals. In: Proceedings of the 2015 IEEE 28th international symposium on computer-based medical systems. IEEE Computer Society
8. Castella X et al (1995) A comparison of severity of illness scoring systems for intensive care unit patients: results of a multicenter, multinational study. Crit Care Med 23(8):1327–1335
9. Dernoncourt F, Veeramachaneni K, O'Reilly U-M (2013c) BeatDB: a large-scale waveform feature repository. In: NIPS 2013, machine learning for clinical data analysis and healthcare workshop
10. Hemberg E, Veeramachaneni K, Dernoncourt F, Wagy M, O'Reilly U-M (2013) Efficient training set use for blood pressure prediction in a large scale learning classifier system. In: Proceeding of the fifteenth annual conference companion on genetic and evolutionary computation conference companion. ACM, New York, pp 1267–1274
11. Hemberg E, Veeramachaneni K, Dernoncourt F, Wagy M, O'Reilly U-M (2013) Imprecise selection and fitness approximation in a large-scale evolutionary rule based system for blood pressure prediction. In: Proceeding of the fifteenth annual conference companion on genetic and evolutionary computation conference companion. ACM, New York, pp 153–154
12. Knaus WA et al (1981) APACHE-acute physiology and chronic health evaluation: a physiologically based classification system. Crit Care Med 9(8):591–597
13. Costa M, Goldberger AL, Peng C-K (2005) Multiscale entropy analysis of biological signals. Phys Rev E 71:021906
14. Costa M, Goldberger AL, Peng C-K (2002) Multiscale entropy analysis of physiologic time series. Phys Rev Lett 89:062102

1

Erratum to: Secondary Analysis of Electronic Health Records

MIT Critical Data

Erratum to:
MIT Critical Data, *Secondary Analysis of Electronic Health Records*, DOI 10.1007/978-3-319-43742-2

The book was inadvertently published without the addition of Edward Moseley in the list of chapter authors in chapter 6 and Shamim Nemati in the list of chapter authors in chapter 29. The erratum book and the chapter has been updated.

Open Access This chapter is distributed under the terms of the Creative Commons Attribution-NonCommercial 4.0 International License (http://creativecommons.org/licenses/by-nc/4.0/), which permits any noncommercial use, duplication, adaptation, distribution and reproduction in any medium or format, as long as you give appropriate credit to the original author(s) and the source, a link is provided to the Creative Commons license and any changes made are indicated.

The images or other third party material in this chapter are included in the work's Creative Commons license, unless indicated otherwise in the credit line; if such material is not included in the work's Creative Commons license and the respective action is not permitted by statutory regulation, users will need to obtain permission from the license holder to duplicate, adapt or reproduce the material.

The updated original online version for this chapter can be found at
10.1007/978-3-319-43742-2_6
10.1007/978-3-319-43742-2_29

MIT Critical Data (✉)
Massachusetts Institute of Technology, Cambridge, MA, USA
e-mail: leoanthonyceli@yahoo.com

© The Author(s) 2016
MIT Critical Data, *Secondary Analysis of Electronic Health Records*,
DOI 10.1007/978-3-319-43742-2_30

9783319437408

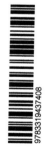

Katja Brandis
Seawalkers
Ein Riese des Meeres

Bücher von Katja Brandis im Arena Verlag:
Woodwalkers. Carags Verwandlung
Woodwalkers. Gefährliche Freundschaft
Woodwalkers. Hollys Geheimnis
Woodwalkers. Fremde Wildnis
Woodwalkers. Feindliche Spuren
Woodwalkers. Tag der Rache
Woodwalkers & Friends. Katzige Gefährten

Seawalkers. Gefährliche Gestalten
Seawalkers. Rettung für Shari
Seawalkers. Wilde Wellen

Khyona. Im Bann des Silberfalken
Khyona. Die Macht der Eisdrachen

Gepardensommer
Koalaträume

Katja Brandis, Jahrgang 1970, hat Amerikanistik, Anglistik und Germanistik studiert und als Journalistin gearbeitet. Schon in der Schule liehen sich viele Mitschüler ihre Manuskripte aus, wenn sie neuen Lesestoff brauchten. Inzwischen hat sie zahlreiche Romane für Jugendliche veröffentlicht, zum Beispiel *Khyona, Gepardensommer, Floaters – Im Sog des Meeres* oder *Ruf der Tiefe*. Die begeisterte Taucherin hat in den Meeren dieser Welt schon unvergessliche Begegnungen mit Haien, Delfinen und Rochen erlebt. Sie lebt mit Mann, Sohn und drei Katzen, von denen eine ein bisschen wie ein Puma aussieht, in der Nähe von München.

Katja Brandis

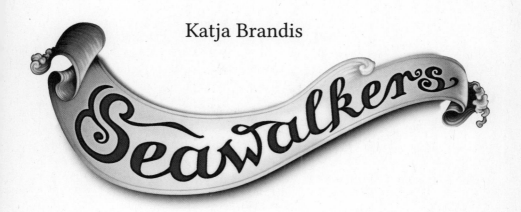

Ein Riese des Meeres

Zeichnungen von Claudia Carls

Arena

Für Sonja

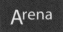

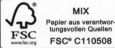

1. Auflage 2021
© 2021 Arena Verlag GmbH,
Rottendorfer Str. 16, 97074 Würzburg
Alle Rechte vorbehalten
Dieses Werk wurde vermittelt durch die
Autoren- und Projektagentur Gerd F. Rumler (München).
Cover und Innenillustrationen: Claudia Carls

Gesamtherstellung: Westermann Druck Zwickau GmbH
Printed in Germany

ISBN 978-3-401-60528-9
Besuche den Arena Verlag im Netz:
www.arena-verlag.de

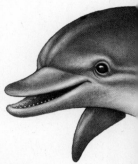

Es ist ein tolles Gefühl, dass wir unsere Schule zurückerobern konnten und dank Lucys Freund genug Geld haben, um die Hurrikan-Schäden an der Schule zu reparieren. Aber Mrs Lennox hat es leider geschafft, meine Lieblingslehrerin Miss White loszuwerden. Und noch wissen wir nicht, was Ellas Mutter mit diesen Haikämpfen zu tun hat oder was sie noch für fiese Dinge plant. Wird sie noch einmal versuchen, Mr Clearwater als Schulleiter zu entmachten? Ich hoffe nicht, denn im Moment fühlen wir uns alle sehr wohl an der Blue Reef Highschool ...

Schreck in der Morgenstunde

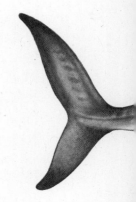

Als der schrille Ton mich um vier Uhr früh aus dem Schlaf riss, wusste ich im ersten Moment nicht, was los war. Während mein Gehirn so gemächlich hochfuhr wie ein sehr, sehr alter Laptop, kapierte ich nach und nach, dass das ein Alarm sein musste. Nur was für einer? Das Geräusch veränderte sich, erst war es hoch und durchdringend gewesen, nun wurde es zirpend und anschließend zu einem dumpfen Wummern, bevor sich das hohe Pfeifen wiederholte. Es kam ganz aus der Nähe!

Unter meinem oberen Stockbett regte sich was. Das braune Schnäuzchen und die gespitzten, blattförmigen Ohren meines Mitbewohners kamen zum Vorschein. *Oje,* sagte Jasper-das-Gürteltier, er klang nervös. *Das habe ich schon lange nicht mehr gehört!*

»Was ist das?«, fragte ich und spürte eine Gänsehaut auf meinen bloßen Armen.

Das heißt, dass sich 'n Seawalker im Schlaf versehentlich verwandelt hat, erklärte Jasper aufgeregt, er deutete mit der Nase auf den roten Knopf an der Seite seines Bettes.

Deswegen pennen wir in Zweibettzimmern, damit der Nichtverwandelte den Alarmknopf drücken kann, das weißte doch.

Stimmt, das wusste ich eigentlich. »Schnell, wir müssen helfen!« Hektisch warf ich die Decke von mir herunter und krabbelte zum Rand meines Bettes. Ich angelte mit dem Fuß nach der Leitersprosse, verfehlte sie, stürzte ab und klatschte auf den Boden wie irgendwas Überreifes von einem Obstbaum.

Noch immer gellte der Alarm durch die Nacht. Was war, wenn es Shari passiert war, dem tollsten Delfinmädchen der Welt? Wie lange würde sie außerhalb des Wassers durchhalten? Deutlich länger als zum Beispiel Juna in ihrer zweiten Gestalt als Falterfisch oder Zitteraal Leonora. Mehr als eine Minute hatten die nicht.

Ich stieß die Tür auf, stolperte nach draußen und blickte mich um. Natürlich waren Jasper und ich nicht die Einzigen, die den Alarm gehört hatten. Von allen Seiten strömten aufgeregte Schüler auf die Hütte zu, an deren Seite ein rotes Licht rotierte. Es war die Hütte Nr. 2, genau neben uns! Weil ich noch nicht wirklich wach war, erreichten Mr Clearwater und Mr García die Hütte trotzdem vor mir, sie mussten sofort vom Hauptgebäude losgerannt sein. Instinktiv schaute ich mich nach Miss White um, unserer jungen Lehrerin für Kampf und Überleben und genau die Richtige für so eine Situation. Mist, die war ja nicht mehr da.

»Schnell! Es ist Carmen passiert!« Eine Zweitjahresschülerin mit dunklen Locken – Enya, in zweiter Gestalt ein roter Neon – stand in der geöffneten Tür und winkte uns hektisch heran. »Zum Glück bin ich von den seltsamen Geräuschen aufgewacht, aber ich weiß nicht, wie lange sie schon ...«

Unser Schulleiter stürzte an ihr vorbei, dicht gefolgt von zwei Jungs (Chris und Barry), mir und unserem Verwandlungslehrer.

Ich ... krieg ... keine ... Luft, hörte ich Carmen stöhnen, eine andere Zweitjahresschülerin. Sie war gerade ein großes Hammerhaiweibchen und es war ein krasser Anblick, wie dieses fast drei Meter lange graue Meerestier in der unteren Koje eines Doppelstockbettes zappelte. Carmens Brustflossen ragten bis auf den Boden, ihr T-förmiger Kopf rammte ständig die Querbalken des Bettes und ihre peitschende Schwanzflosse fetzte gerade eins von Enyas abstrakten Aquarellen von der Wand. Stücke eines zerbissenen Kissens flogen herum wie Konfetti.

Obwohl wir wussten, dass Carmen in Lebensgefahr war, zögerten wir. Die Zähne in ihrem panisch schnappenden Maul sahen ganz schön groß aus. Sicher würde es Carmen nachher furchtbar leidtun, wenn sie jemandem eine Hand abbiss. Aber es gibt Situationen, in denen eine Entschuldigung einem nicht so rasend viel bringt.

»Alles gut, Carmen, wir helfen dir«, sagte Jack Clearwater und wagte sich nah genug an sie heran, um die Hand auf ihren Rücken legen zu können. »Halt still und mach das Maul zu, ja?«

Farryn García hastete zu Carmens Kopf, ein Tablet in den Händen, auf dem er ein Bild ihrer stämmigen rotblonden Mädchengestalt aufgerufen hatte. Er hielt es vor eins ihrer Haiaugen, die weit auseinander, sozusagen an den Querbalken des T-Kopfes saßen. »Versuch, dich zu konzentrieren, Carmen. Ich weiß, das ist nicht leicht ...«

Genau, weil ich nämlich gerade ersticke!, brüllte Carmen in unsere Köpfe. *Bringt mich ins Meer, macht schon!*

»Okay. Ganz ruhig, wir haben das gleich«, sagte Jack Clearwater und warf uns Helfern einen Blick zu. »Erst müssen wir sie aus dem Bett auf den Boden kriegen.« Er und Mr García packten Carmen um den Bauch und zogen sie zu sich hin, ich kletterte über ihren Rücken ins Bett und schob von der anderen Seite.

»Es gibt Erfahrungen, die macht man nur einmal im Leben – hoffentlich«, ächzte Chris und packte unsere Mitschülerin an der Rückenflosse, Barry zerrte an der Schwanzwurzel und wurde dadurch hin- und hergeschleudert. Aber er hielt eisern fest und beschwerte sich nicht mal, als er gegen das Bettgestell knallte.

Kurz darauf hatten wir Carmen aus ihrer Koje herausgewälzt und konnten sie tragen. Ein Dutzend Hände packten mit an, darunter die von Finny (gut erkennbar an ihrem Geisternetz-Armband) und von Noah. Eine erschrocken dreinblickende Shari mit verwuschelten blonden Haaren, die wie ein Vogelnest aussahen, hielt die Tür auf. Dann stapften wir durch den Sand, so schnell wir konnten.

Carmen war unglaublich schwer und ihre schleifpapierraue Haut, die ich so auch von mir kannte, schrappte uns die Hände auf. Aber keiner von uns ließ los. Aufgeregt wuselte Jasper vor uns in Richtung Meer und rief *Hier entlang, hier entlang!*, als hätten wir nicht selbst Augen, die im Dunkeln sehen konnten. Sogar Ella half mit und schob neugierige Schüler weg, die im Weg standen.

Oh bitte, bitte, beeilt euch!, japste Carmen und erleichtert spürte ich die ersten kleinen Wellen über meine Zehen lecken. Wir wateten so weit hinein, bis das Wasser uns bis zum Bauch reichte, dann schoben Barry, unser Rochenmädchen Finny, die anderen Schüler und ich Carmen ins Meer hinein.

Sie ging unter wie ein Stein.

»Hab ich gesagt, ihr sollt loslassen?«, schimpfte Mr García. »Ihre Muskeln sind steif, es dauert noch einen Moment, bis sie wieder schwimmen kann.«

Selbst für mich war es ein nicht allzu tolles Gefühl, mit einem vor Angst durchdrehenden Hai im Meer zu sein. Carmens

Hammerkopf war jetzt genau in Höhe meiner Schienbeine. Aber das war mir inzwischen egal und den anderen anscheinend auch, denn niemand flüchtete. Grimmig packten wir sie wieder um den Bauch und schoben sie voran, damit Wasser durch ihre Kiemen strömen konnte. Das Salzwasser brannte auf meinen übel aufgeschürften Händen, aber ich achtete nicht darauf.

»Das wird schon, wir kriegen das hin«, murmelte Barry und tätschelte Carmens Rücken. Verdutzt blickte ich ihn an. Moment mal, das war doch Barry, oder? Der große, dünne Typ mit den kalten Augen und den kackbraunen Haaren, der ständig mit Ella herumhing? Zusammen mit Toco der übelste Typ der Blue Reef Highschool?

Nach und nach erholte sich Carmen und nach ein paar Minuten bewegte sie sich wieder ruhig durchs Wasser. *Uff, das fühlt sich gut an – danke,* keuchte sie. *Meine Pulsrate geht schon wieder runter. Echt peinlich, dass mir das passiert ist, obwohl ich schon im zweiten Jahr bin! Ich ... manchmal will ich nicht wahrhaben, dass ich eine Seawalkerin bin, und wäre lieber ganz normal ... vielleicht liegt es daran?*

»Vielleicht macht sich dein Hai-Ich dann absichtlich bemerkbar und fordert sein Recht, das kann sein«, meinte Mr García. »Wir besprechen es bei Gelegenheit unter vier Augen, okay?«

»Jetzt bin ich erst mal froh, dass wir dich gerettet haben, Carmen.« Jack Clearwater klatschte sich lächelnd mit uns ab und Farryn García schlug uns auf die Schulter. »Toll gemacht, Leute.«

Wir stapften an den Strand zurück. Ich war unfassbar erleichtert, dass Carmen nichts passiert war. Obwohl sie nicht viel mit anderen Leuten zu tun haben wollte und lieber ihre Fitnesszeitschriften las, mochte ich sie irgendwie, seit sie sich bei der Reparatur der Schule nach dem Hurrikan so reingehängt hatte. Dass sie manchmal lieber »normal« wäre, konnte ich gut verstehen. Auch ich war nicht immer glücklich mit meiner Haigestalt.

Chris blickte auf seine blutenden Hände. »Oh Mann, Haie. Hätten sich nicht Olivia oder Enya verwandeln können? Die hätte ich mit einer Hand tragen können.«

»Ich kann mir das mit Enya gut vorstellen«, meinte Shari fröhlich. »Morgens ist das andere Bett leer und in Carmens Wasserglas schwimmt ein kleiner, rotblau gestreifter Fisch, der nervös ›Nicht austrinken, nicht austrinken!‹ ruft.«

»Unrealistisch«, sagte Blue und sah mich von der Seite an. »Bei einem Hai wie Carmen läuft das eher so: Morgens fragt sie jemand: ›Wo ist eigentlich deine Mitbewohnerin?‹, und sie sagt: ›Weiß nicht, aber ich hatte einen ganz komischen Traum!‹«

Ich winkte ab. »Rote Neons sind doch kein ernsthaftes Fressen, die sind nur halb so lang wie mein Daumen.«

»Genau, die sind eher Food-Deko«, meinte Finny.

Immerhin hatten Neons keine Zähne, Dornen, Klingen, Nesselzellen ... die meisten Meerestiere fasste man besser nicht an, wie uns Miss White in Kampf und Überleben eingeschärft hatte. Wo war eigentlich unsere neue Lehrerin für dieses Fach, diese Miss Bennett? Schließlich entdeckte ich sie im Pulk der neugierigen Schüler, sie schaute besorgt zu, was wir taten, und wirkte ein bisschen ratlos.

»Na toll«, raunte ich Noah und Shari zu und wies mit dem Kinn in Richtung der neuen Lehrerin.

Shari murmelte: »Miss White hätte ganz vorne an Carmens Kopf mit angepackt.«

»Oder sie sogar allein getragen«, behauptete ich und fühlte, wie Traurigkeit mich überschwemmte. Wo konnte meine Lieblingslehrerin sein? Es war ein Schock gewesen, was Ellas Mutter über sie offenbart hatte, klar. Aber wieso war Miss White nicht geblieben, um mit uns zu reden, uns zu erklären, ob sie früher wirklich als Kopfgeldjägerin für Kriminelle gearbeitet hatte und warum?

Kurz darauf standen Noah, Finny, Chris und ich in der Schlange vor dem Krankenzimmer, wo die schlecht gelaunte Mrs Misaki einem Helfer nach dem anderen eine Heilsalbe und große wasserfeste Pflaster verpasste. »So, jetzt am besten zwei Tage nicht verwandeln«, empfahl sie uns.

Pflaster mit Muränenspucke – ein ganz neues Patent, lästerte unser Papageifisch Nox aus dem Aquarium und Mrs Misaki blickte noch ein bisschen finsterer drein.

»Nachher haben wir die erste Stunde Kampf und Überleben bei Miss Bennett«, meinte Finny. »Was meint ihr, zeigt sie uns, wie man sich bei Gefahr aufbläst? Das will ich sehen, wie *du* das machst, Tiago.«

Ich musste grinsen. Miss Bennet war in zweiter Gestalt ein Igelfisch, deren einzige Verteidigung war das Aufpumpen ihres Stachelkörpers. »Ein aufgeblasener Tigerhai? Willst du mich als Schwimmtier benutzen oder was?«, fragte ich.

Skeptisch hatte Noah zugehört. »Denkt dran, Leute – man kann auch stark, mutig und eine gute Kämpferin sein, ohne eine Raubkatze, ein Wolf oder ein Hai zu sein.«

»Stimmt«, meinte ich. »Oder ein Alligator oder eine riesige Python.« Ich war froh, dass die krawallige Reptilien-Sonderklasse inzwischen aufgelöst worden war, weil die meisten meiner neuen Mitschüler in die Everglades-Sümpfe zurückgekehrt waren (nicht alle von ihnen freiwillig). Auch Jerome und Tomkin hatten sich auf den Rückweg dorthin gemacht. Nur Polly, ein nettes Alligatormädchen, und Tino, ein Pythonjunge, waren geblieben und inzwischen Teil unserer Klasse.

»Du bist dran, Tiago«, verkündete Mrs Misaki und ich hörte auf, über Reptilien nachzudenken – sich von dieser Muräne verarzten zu lassen, tat ordentlich weh.

Zum Glück war es nur ein Kratzer. Kein Vergleich zu der Harpunenwunde, die der Bullenhai gehabt hatte. Ich dachte noch oft daran, wie wir vergeblich versucht hatten, ihn gesund zu pflegen. Ob die illegalen Taucher-gegen-Hai-Kämpfe weitergingen, obwohl wir einen davon unterbrochen hatten? Garantiert. Die Kerle, die diese Arenakämpfe veranstalteten, hatten höchstens eine Pause gemacht, nachdem wir die Polizei eingeschaltet hatten.

Ich hätte wetten können, dass sie schon einen neuen Ort dafür gesucht hatten und wieder Kämpfe planten, auf die reiche Leute wetten konnten. Es fiel mir schwer, den Gedanken zu ertragen, dass vielleicht schon jetzt wieder wilde Meerestiere gequält wurden. Hatte die Polizei schon etwas herausgefunden?

Die anderen schlurften zum Frühstück, aber ich ging noch einmal in Jaspers und meine Hütte. Finny hatte ihren Vater Nick Greyson gebeten, sich in die Ermittlungen einzuklinken, und er war es, dessen Nummer ich nun wählte. Ganz spontan, weil mir diese Sache keine Ruhe ließ. »Hallo, Mr Greyson, hier ist Tiago von der Blue Reef Highschool. Gibt's was Neues wegen der Haikämpfe?«

»Ah. Guten Morgen, Tiago.« Ich hörte jemanden gähnen. Ups. Erst jetzt kam ich auf die Idee, auf die Uhr zu schauen.

Erst halb sieben! Und dabei hatte mir Finny erzählt, dass ihr Vater die Abendschicht auf dem Revier hatte.

»Oh, habe ich Sie geweckt? Das tut mir ...«

»Schon okay. Ich darf dir leider nicht viel über die Ermittlungen sagen, aber es sieht so aus, als würde der Kerl, der das Glasbodenschiff gemietet hat, mit einer Geldstrafe davonkommen. Er hat behauptet, er hätte nur eine kleine Rundfahrt veranstaltet, die etwas aus dem Ruder gelaufen sei.«

»Sonst nichts? Und die Leute, die dort waren, was ist mit denen?«

»Carl Bittergreen ist ja ein alter Bekannter von uns. Er hat überall seine Finger drin, Drogen, Schutzgeld, das volle Programm. Wir sammeln weiter Beweise gegen ihn, aber diese Tierkampf-Sache ist nicht ganz oben auf unserer Prio-Liste, fürchte ich. Wieso interessiert es euch eigentlich so sehr, dass diese Leute Haie killen?«

»Äh ...« Ich konnte ihm nicht sagen, dass ich selbst ein Hai war – er hatte keine Ahnung, dass Seawalker existierten. »Ich, ähm, finde es einfach nicht okay, wenn Tiere gequält werden, und das auch noch zum Spaß.«

»Versteh ich. Üble Sache. Sag bitte meiner Tochter schöne Grüße von mir und sie soll bitte ab und zu lernen, kannst du ihr das ausrichten?«

Ziemlich ernüchtert legte ich auf. Nein, das würde ich Finny ganz bestimmt nicht ausrichten, sonst machte ich mich ja total zum Deppen.

Gerade wollte ich mich ebenfalls auf den Weg zur Cafeteria machen, da spürte ich etwas. Jemand berührte meine Gedanken, jemand, den ich kannte. Moment mal ... war das etwa Steve, mein älterer Bruder, der als Tigerhai lebte?

Ja genau, ich bin's, meldete sich Steve in meinem Kopf. *Hüb-*

sche Lagune habt ihr und diesmal ist zum Glück weniger los. Was ist, kommst du ins Wasser?*

Klar! Bin gleich bei dir. Ich freute mich total, dass er hier war. Hastig riss ich mir die Klamotten vom Leib und rannte in die Lagune. Einen Moment lang schwammen wir friedlich nebeneinander, ein Menschenjunge und ein fünf Meter langer Tigerhai. Hätte irgendein Tourist das gesehen, wären Steve und ich wahrscheinlich in den Abendnachrichten aufgetaucht und jede Menge Badegäste hätten vorerst keinen Zeh mehr ins Wasser gesteckt.

Schön, dich zu sehen, sagte ich zu Steve. *Warst du zufällig in der Gegend?*

Nicht ganz zufällig, meinte Steve. *Was meinst du, gibt's noch irgendwas, was wir gegen die illegalen Haikämpfe tun können? Das Ganze lässt mir keine Ruhe.*

»Mir auch nicht«, antwortete ich laut, dachte nach ... und hatte tatsächlich eine Idee. *Die Kerle brauchen für die Kämpfe Glasbodenschiffe oder -boote. Davon kann es nicht unendlich viele geben. Wie wäre es, wenn du in nächster Zeit an der Küste patrouillierst und abcheckst, was mit den Glasbodenbooten passiert, die es in der Gegend gibt?*

He, du bist ja gar nicht so blöd, Bruderherz. Steve wandte sich mir zu und knuffte mich sanft mit der Schnauze. *Mach ich. Ab und zu komme ich vorbei und halte dich auf dem Laufenden, okay?*

Sehr cool, sagte ich. Am liebsten hätte ich meinen Bruder umarmt, doch das ließ ich lieber sein – eine Haihaut-Abschürfung am Tag reichte mir.

Kämpfen wie ein Igelfisch

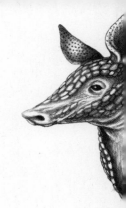

Das Thema dieser illegalen Haikämpfe ließ mir keine Ruhe ... und ich dachte oft daran, was Mr García versprochen hatte: Lydia Lennox' Gedanken zu sondieren, um herauszufinden, was sie darüber wusste ... und vor allem, ob sie mich als Hai erkannt hatte und wirklich hätte sterben lassen. Besser, wir hielten diesen Plan vorerst geheim.

»He, warum schlingst du denn das Frühstück in dich rein, als hättest du drei Tage gehungert?«, fragte Shari verblüfft.

»Das ist nich' gesund, so schnell zu essen«, ermahnte mich Jasper.

»Ich werd's überleben«, meinte ich nur, brachte meinen Teller weg und marschierte in die Verwandlungsarena, wo wir gleich unsere erste Stunde haben würden. Ich wusste, dass Mr García immer vor uns dort war, und das war meine Chance, allein mit ihm zu reden.

Er lächelte, als er mich reinkommen sah. »Na, Tiago? Hast du dich schon von der Carmen-Aktion erholt?« Unser Lehrer war ein Delfin-Wandler, der mir erstaunlich ähnlich sah – wir waren beide schlank und groß, auch die braune Haut und die schwarzen Haare hatten wir gemeinsam.

»Hab ich ... aber darum geht's mir gerade nicht, sondern um

diese fiesen Haikämpfe«, sagte ich schnell und erzählte ihm von meinem Gespräch mit Steve.

»Guter Plan.« Mr García nickte, blickte sich um und senkte die Stimme. »Du willst wahrscheinlich wissen, wann ich versuche, die Lennox zu sondieren, oder?«

Schweigend nickte ich.

»Ich habe am Montagnachmittag einen Termin mit ihr in Miami, angeblich um über Ellas Leistungen zu reden.«

»So bald schon?« Mein Herz legte einen Trommelwirbel ein. »Aber das wird gefährlich. Können Sie ... irgendjemanden mitnehmen, der Sie schützt, wenn etwas schiefgeht?«

Miss White hätte ihn verteidigen können, aber wir wussten nicht einmal, wo sie war.

»Jack kommt mit, also keine Sorge«, sagte Farryn García.

»Okay«, brachte ich heraus. Doch, ich machte mir weiterhin Sorgen. Jack Clearwater war kein Kämpfer – konnte er im Notfall wirklich helfen?

Nach und nach trudelten die anderen ein und ich setzte mich auf einen der wasserfesten Stühle in der Mitte, als sei alles wie sonst. Jasper und Shari setzten sich neben mich und ich merkte, wie ich allmählich ruhiger wurde.

Natürlich war das heiße Thema in dieser Verwandlungsstunde der Hammerhai-Zwischenfall. »Enya hat es genau richtig gemacht – sie hat erst kurz nach Carmen geschaut, dann den Alarm ausgelöst und sich anschließend um ihre Mitbewohnerin gekümmert. In der Menschenwelt sollte man es ebenso machen, wenn man einen Verletzten findet«, sagte Mr García. »Warum ist das so wichtig? Ella, du weißt das doch sicher, oder?«

Ella, in erster Gestalt blond mit grünen Augen, in zweiter Gestalt Tigerpython, lackierte sich gerade mit voller Konzentration die Fingernägel. Aber anscheinend hatte sie trotzdem zugehört. »Weil die Helfer ein paar Minuten brauchen, bis sie da sein können«, antwortete sie, ohne aufzuschauen, und pustete einen grellpinken Nagel trocken.

»Genau«, sagte unser Verwandlungslehrer.

»Wieso klingt der Alarm eigentlich so seltsam, manchmal tief und manchmal hoch?«, wagte ich zu fragen.

Sofort schossen die Arme von Blue, Shari und Mara – in zweiter Gestalt Seekuh – in die Höhe. Mara kam dran. »Damit wir ihn alle hören können, auch diejenigen, die gerade als Tier unterwegs sind«, erklärte sie mir. »Wale und Seekühe können tiefe Töne besser wahrnehmen ...«

»... und Delfine hohe«, unterbrach sie Shari. »Dieser Alarm war schön pfeifig, den hätte ich sogar als Großer Tümmler unter Wasser bemerkt.«

Es war herrlich, mehr über ihre Welt zu erfahren, ich hätte ihr stundenlang zuhören können. Doch Mr García hatte andere Pläne. »So, Leute, wir machen jetzt die Zweierübung *Erste Hilfe bei ungeplanten Verwandlungen,* macht euch bitte bereit.«

Ich schielte zu Shari hinüber – ob sie auch gerade daran dachte, wie oft ich ihr schon bei so etwas geholfen hatte? Ja offensichtlich, denn sie lächelte verschmitzt zurück. Mir wurde warm ums angeblich so kalte Knorpelfischherz.

»Tiago, du übst mit ...«, begann Mr García und ich hielt die Luft an. »... Juna«, fuhr er fort. Ich versuchte, nicht enttäuscht zu sein, und unsere zierliche Klassensprecherin mit den glatten dunkelblonden Haaren bekam ganz große, erschrockene Augen.

»Hast du tatsächlich noch Angst vor mir?«, fragte ich sie und sie schüttelte energisch den Kopf. »Du würdest bestimmt nichts fressen, was mal in einer Toilette geschwommen ist, oder?«, flüsterte sie mir zu und ich musste lachen.

Wir bekamen es prima hin. Als sie sich in einen weiß-gelben Falterfisch verwandelte, sprintete ich in Rekordtempo los, um einen Eimer Meerwasser zu besorgen und sie hineinzustecken. Als ich dran war und als Tigerhai japsend auf dem Boden lag, pustete sie mir Luft in die Kiemen, was zwar überhaupt nichts half, aber lieb von ihr war.

Während ich darauf wartete, dass sie »Rettung organisierte«, schaute ich mich in der Verwandlungsarena um und hätte beinahe mit all meinen Reißzähnen gegrinst. Chris jagte hinter einem fliegenden Fisch her, weil Izzy nicht in der Stimmung war, sich von ihm retten zu lassen. Lachmöwe Daphne blickte genervt drein, während Olivia sie aus ihrem T-Shirt zu befreien versuchte, ohne ihr einen Flügel zu brechen. Ella und Lucy hatten sich versehentlich gleichzeitig verwandelt und bildeten ein Knäuel aus Krake und Riesenschlange. Tino tat so, als müsste er Polly beruhigen, obwohl sie als Alligatorweibchen wohlig in der Sonne döste.

Als wir uns alle von unseren Rettungen erholt hatten, war die Stunde bei Miss Bennett dran. Gespannt drängten Jasper und ich uns als Erste aus der Verwandlungsarena raus an den Strand, denn der Kampfunterricht fand üblicherweise in der Lagune statt. Erstaunt sahen wir, dass Miss Bennett – heute in einem einteiligen hellgrünen Badeanzug – halb hinter einer Palme versteckt, hektisch in einem Buch blätterte. Als sie uns sah, zuckte sie zusammen, stopfte das Buch hinter einen Busch, straffte die Schultern und versuchte ein Lächeln. »Ah, hallo ... wer seid ihr beiden noch mal?«

Inzwischen hatte ich mich daran gewöhnt, mich hier in der Schule als »Tiago Anderson, Tigerhai« vorzustellen. Der Hai war ein Teil von mir, ob ich wollte oder nicht. Jasper, gerade ein nicht sehr großer Junge mit Brille und braunen Strubbelhaaren, schob sofort nach: »Jasper Tillmann, Neunbinden-Gürteltier«, und reckte den Hals, um einen Blick auf das geheimnisvolle Buch werfen zu können.

Unauffällig stellte unsere neue Lehrerin sich ihm in den Weg. »Na, ihr seid ja ein ungewöhnliches Paar«, bemerkte sie.

Paar? Was genau meinte sie damit? Toco, Barry und Ella, die inzwischen ebenfalls am Strand aufgetaucht waren, prusteten los, sie liebten Witze auf meine Kosten. Aber weil Jasper auch lachte, verzog ich ebenfalls die Mundwinkel.

Als auch die anderen Schüler eingetroffen waren, stellte sich Ivy Bennet vor uns auf. Sie war ungefähr so alt wie meine Mutter und hatte mittellange mittelbraune Haare, die mit Spangen hochgesteckt waren. Auf ihrem Gesicht klebte ein verkrampftes Lächeln. »Herzlich willkommen«, sagte sie. »Das war ja ein Schreck heute Morgen, was? Ich hoffe, ihr seid trotzdem richtig wach. Wir machen erst mal eine Übung in Menschengestalt. An wem kann ich sie euch zeigen?« Nervös warf sie einen Seitenblick auf Noemi, deren schwarzes Fell in der Sonne schimmerte.

An mir, schlug unser Panthermädchen fröhlich vor, erhob sich und wetzte ihre Krallen an der nächstbesten Palme.

Miss Bennett wich einen Schritt zurück. »Ähm, danke. Wer meldet sich noch?«

»Ach, machen Sie es ruhig mit mir – ich bin Alligator und heiße Toco«, sagte unser blasser, rothaariger Schläger vom Dienst, spannte seine Armmuskeln an und blickte sich um, um abzuchecken, ob auch alle ihn bewunderten. Das klappte nur bei Polly.

Miss Bennett schluckte. »Gut. Komm bitte langsam auf mich zu, ja?«

Grinsend stapfte Toco auf sie zu. Wir warteten alle gespannt, was passieren würde. Er kam nicht weit. Miss Bennett trat ihm mit dem bloßen Fuß das vorgereckte Bein seitlich weg und Toco ging zu Boden. »Haha, guter Trick«, meinte er, klopfte sich den Sand ab und stand auf. »Ich trete auch gerne Leute.«

Miss Bennett lächelte; sie wirkte erleichtert, dass es geklappt hatte. »Diese Übung kommt aus dem Judo und heißt Fußfeger.« Sie wandte sich an alle. »Stellt euch jetzt bitte zu zweit auf und macht sie nach.«

»Na, dann los.« Jasper grinste mich treuherzig an. »Ich besieg dich, wirste schon sehen!«

»Mach nur.« Ich grinste zurück.

Er schaffte es tatsächlich, mich in den Sand zu schicken, aber gleich darauf revanchierte ich mich.

Ungefähr eine Viertelstunde lang traten wir uns gegenseitig eifrig gegen die Schienbeine und verpassten uns blaue Flecken.

»Okay, das reicht, vielen Dank.« Ivy Bennett klatschte in die Hände, und als wir sie anblickten, ging sie in Richtung Meer und marschierte ins türkisfarbene Wasser hinein. »Folgt mir bitte. Wir machen eine Übung in zweiter Gestalt und ...«

Sie kreischte auf, riss die Arme hoch und machte einen Satz. Wir reckten neugierig die Hälse. Oha, da bewegte sich etwas im Wasser, ein hellbrauner Schatten unter der Oberfläche, der hastig davonglitt. Um sich spritzend, hastete Miss Bennett zurück an Land.

»Alles okay?«, rief Juna, lief zu unserer zitternden Lehrerin und berührte sie am Arm.

»Ich glaube, sie ist auf einen Stachelrochen getreten«, sagte Shari mitleidig. »Na, der hat sich bestimmt erschreckt.«

Nestor rief: »Sie haben den Rochen-Schlurf vergessen, Miss Bennett.« Unser Klassenstreber war gnadenlos – wenn Lehrer einen Fehler machten, wies er sie jedes Mal darauf hin. Kam total gut an. Bei den Schülern jedenfalls.

Finny drückte Shari ihre Sonnenbrille und ihren Geisternetz-Armreif in die Hand, rannte ins Wasser und verwandelte sich dort in eine Art zwei Meter breiten schwarzen Pfannkuchen – ihr Teufelsrochen-Ich. *Mal schauen, ob unter Wasser jemand verletzt ist.*

»Was in aller Welt ist der Rochen-Schlurf?«, erkundigte sich Izzy, unser Neuzugang aus Kalifornien.

»In Florida gibt's viele Rochen, sie liegen gut getarnt auf dem Sand oder knapp darunter«, erklärte ihr Chris, der neben ihr gegen eine Palme lehnte und auf einem Grashalm herumkaute. »Deshalb sollte man schlurfen, wenn man durchs Flachwasser geht, also die Füße kaum heben. Das wirbelt Sand auf – der Rochen merkt, dass du kommst, und haut ab.«

He, das zu sagen wäre mein Job gewesen, beschwerte sich Finny. *Dem Rochen, den sie getreten hat, ist übrigens nichts passiert.*

»Also, Kinder, achtet bitte in Zukunft darauf, so durchs Wasser zu gehen«, verkündete eine sehr blasse Miss Bennett. Sie räusperte sich ein paarmal, zupfte ihren Badeanzug zurecht und ging zögerlich zurück in die Lagune. Diesmal mustergültig schlurfend. »So, jetzt bitte alle verwandeln, wir arbeiten in zweiter Gestalt weiter.«

Es war ein ziemliches Durcheinander, als alle gleichzeitig ins Wasser wateten und sich verwandelten. Neben mir wälzte sich eine Seekuh durch die Brandung, während Linus – ein Seepferdchen – ihr hastig auszuweichen versuchte. Ralph kreuzte als Riffhai durch die Lagune, Polly stand als Mensch mit Alligatorkopf am Strand. Shari ruderte verzweifelt als Delfin mit zwei Menschenarmen statt Brustflossen herum, wobei Noah ihr gut zuredete. Blue hatte ihre eigenen Probleme, weil sie vergessen hatte, vor dem Verwandeln ihre Drei-Flossen-Kette auszuziehen (was ihr eigentlich nicht ähnlich sah).

Bildet jetzt bitte eine Reihe!, rief unsere Kampflehrerin, als wieder etwas mehr Ordnung eingekehrt war. Sie war nun ein nicht sehr großer, gelb-braun gefleckter Fisch mit eckigem Kopf und Glupschaugen. Die Stacheln, die ihren Körper bedeckten, waren stromlinienförmig angelegt.

Ich manövrierte meinen Tigerhaikörper neben Finny und Shari, erwartungsvoll beobachteten wir unsere neue Lehrerin. Niemand bewegte eine Flosse oder schwatzte von Kopf zu Kopf, weil wir alle sehr gespannt waren.

Aber nicht darauf, was Miss Bennett nun sagen würde. Sondern ob sie merken würde, dass Nox sich gerade von hinten an sie heranpirschte.

So, würdet ihr jetzt bitte ..., begann sie.

Nox stupste den Igelfisch von hinten kräftig mit dem Schnabel an.

Unsere neue Kampflehrerin quiekte auf, begann, panisch Wasser zu schlucken, und blähte sich zu einem weiß-hellbraunen Stachelball auf, an dem hier und da winzig wirkende Flossen hingen.

Ich weiß, es war nicht sehr nett. Schließlich konnte sie nichts dafür. Aber sie sah einfach zu putzig aus.

Wir applaudierten, so gut man das mit Flossen kann.

Danach war die Stunde etwas früher zu Ende und Miss

Bennett hastete völlig aufgelöst zu ihrer Hütte. Dabei vergaß sie, das hinter der Palme versteckte Buch mitzunehmen. Neugierig schauten Jasper, Shari und ich es uns an. Es war ein Exemplar von *Judo für Dummies*.

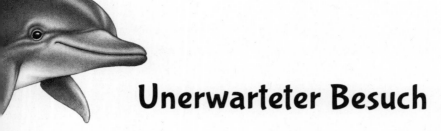

Unerwarteter Besuch

Als Jack Clearwater von der verpatzten Kampfstunde erfuhr, war er sauer. Auf uns!

»Leute, könnt ihr euch bitte benehmen?«, schimpfte er uns in der Mittagspause, als wir bis zu den Knien im Wasser der Cafeteria standen. »Wisst ihr eigentlich, wie schwer es ist, eine Seawalker-Lehrerin zu finden?«

Betretenes Schweigen in der Klasse. Dann sah ich, wie Juna aufstand, unsere Klassensprecherin. »Es tut uns leid«, sagte sie und gab ihr Bestes, um zerknirscht auszusehen. »Wäre es denn irgendwie möglich ...«, sie zögerte, »... Miss White zurückzuholen?«

Jack Clearwaters Gesichtsausdruck veränderte sich, nun sah er einfach nur traurig aus.

Mir fiel wieder ein, dass er mehr als nur eine Lehrerin verloren hatte.

»Die Chancen stehen leider schlecht, fürchte ich«, sagte er. »Findet euch bitte mit der Situation ab und verzichtet darauf, Miss Bennett das Leben schwer zu machen, ja?«

Ich wollte mich nicht mit der Situation abfinden. Was für eine Chance hatte ich denn ohne Miss Whites Privatstunden? Irgendwann würde mich wieder die Wut packen, ich hatte meine Gefühle noch längst nicht perfekt im Griff! Außerdem fehlte sie mir.

Lustlos schlangen die Delfine, Jasper, Finny und ich das Essen in uns hinein, ein Risotto mit Frischkäse und Lachs.

»Als Kampflehrerin ist diese Frau ein schlechter Witz, wieso hat Mr Clearwater sich die Stunde nicht mal angeschaut?«, schimpfte Finny, die mit uns in unserem rot-weißen Lieblings-Tischboot saß.

»Genau, und jetzt sin' wir schuld, dabei hat Nox das gar nich' böse gemeint«, fügte Jasper betrübt hinzu.

Stimmt – wenn ich es böse gemeint hätte, hätte ich sie in den Hintern gebissen, erklang es aus dem Wasser neben unserem Boot.

»Ihr wollt Miss White auch zurück, oder?« Finny blickte in die Runde. »Sie war hart drauf, klar, aber das war irgendwie okay, wisst ihr, was ich meine?«

Ich musste grinsen. »Du meinst, dass sie dich an deinem Rochenschwanz gepackt und im Kreis geschleudert hätte, wenn du ihr frech gekommen wärst?«

»Genau!«

»Wenn wir wenigstens wüssten, wo sie hingeschwommen ist«, sagte Shari bedrückt. »Vielleicht könntest du sie überreden, dass sie zurückkommt, Tiago. Dann reden wir in Ruhe darüber, was sie früher getan hat.«

»Genau, das kannste bestimmt!« Jasper war begeistert. Er wusste das mit den geheimen Privatstunden.

In meiner Kehle war ein dicker Kloß. Es fühlte sich an, als würde das Risotto nicht mehr hindurchpassen. »Vielleicht«, brachte ich heraus.

»Bestimmt! Sie mag dich«, meinte auch Finny. »Aber nicht so sehr wie Jack natürlich. Am besten richtest du ihr aus, dass er sie vermisst. Muss er ja nicht selbst gesagt haben. Man sieht ihm das an, oder?«

Ich nickte. »Aber hallo. Vorhin sah er aus wie ein gestrandetes Schiff.«

Oh, hey, ein Hai, der zu poetischen Vergleichen neigt, zog Nox mich auf.

»Vergleiche kann ich auch«, meinte Noah und schob sich eine Gabel Risotto in den Mund. »Ein Orca, der hier in Florida durch die Gegend schwimmt, müsste doch auffällig sein wie ein ... ein knallpinkes Kreuzfahrtschiff!«

»Könnten wir nicht einfach herumfragen, wer sie gesehen hat?«, schlug Blue vor.

Aus guten Ideen sollte man gleich was machen, sonst werden sie ranzig. Ich ließ mein Risotto im Stich und watete quer durch die Cafeteria rüber zu dem Boot, in dem ein paar Zweitjahresschüler saßen, darunter Carmens Retterin Enya und Jamie, als Tier ein Einsiedlerkrebs. Garantiert hatte er das Schneckenhaus, in dem er in zweiter Gestalt wohnte, so wie immer in der Hosentasche. Aber diejenige, die ich ansteuerte, war die zierliche Shelby, eine Brandseeschwalbe und begeistertes Mitglied unserer Fliegerstaffel.

Doch ich kam nicht bei ihr an, denn in diesem Moment tauchte jemand am Eingang der Cafeteria auf, genau am Rand der trockenen Zone beim Schuhregal. Es war eine schlanke blonde Frau im weißen Kostüm und mit High Heels – als Tier war sie eine hellgelbe Python, doch mit ganz normal dunklen Augen, ein richtiger Albino war sie nicht (die hatten eine rote Iris). Die meisten Leute hätten nur eine attraktive Geschäftsfrau gesehen. Ich sah einen wandelnden Albtraum. Zum Glück waren wenigstens ihre Bodyguards, die Tigerzwillinge, nirgendwo in Sicht.

»Ella, Schatz, ich bin gekommen, um dich abzuholen!«, verkündete Lydia Lennox und winkte fröhlich in Richtung ihrer Tochter.

Ella wirkte verblüfft – und nicht sehr erfreut. »Aber ich hab doch noch Unterricht?«

»Ach, lass den sausen, ich habe Tickets für ein Musical heute Abend, da müssen wir uns rechtzeitig stylen und auf den Weg machen.« Es schien Mrs Lennox überhaupt nicht zu stören, dass Mr Clearwater und die anderen Erwachsenen am Lehrertisch alles hören konnten.

»Mum, das geht echt nicht, dass du einfach so hier in der Schule auftauchst«, sagte Ella. Wahrscheinlich war ihr dieser Auftritt vor ihren Freunden megapeinlich. Ich fand es mutig von ihr, dass sie ihrer Mutter widersprach.

»Stell dich bitte nicht so an!« Mrs Lennox' Ton war schärfer geworden. »Los, pack deine Sachen, du hast dich doch bestimmt schon auf das Musical gefreut, oder? Die Karten waren nicht billig!«

»Moment mal«, sagte unser junger Schulleiter und stand auf. »Ella hat recht, sie hat noch Unterricht und ...« Lydia Lennox beachtete ihn nicht. »Wo ist eigentlich dein Verwandlungslehrer! Ah, da ist ja der liebe Farryn.«

Mein Verwandlungslehrer erhob sich ebenfalls, er wirkte auf der Hut. »Was gibt's, Lydia?«, fragte er vorsichtig.

»Diesen Termin am Montag, den brauchen wir nicht. Ella kann sich ganz hervorragend verwandeln und sie ist so klug, dass sie leicht Klassenbeste werden könnte.«

Verdammt! Wie sollte Mr García sie sondieren, wenn sie jetzt den Termin absagte?

»Du willst also nichts über ihren genauen Lernstand wissen?« Noch gab Farryn García nicht auf. »Die anderen Eltern wären froh über eine solche Gelegenheit, ausführlich über ihr Kind zu reden.«

Mit hängenden Armen und hilflosem Blick stand Ella dabei

und hörte zu. Über das Lob ihrer Mutter schien sie sich nicht zu freuen, wahrscheinlich war ihr klar, dass sie weit davon entfernt war, Klassenbeste zu werden.

»Ihr Lernstand?« Lydia Lennox winkte ab. »Ich bitte dich, natürlich will ich das, aber wir bereiten gerade einen großen Prozess vor und arbeiten in der Kanzlei bis spät in die Nacht.«

Aha. Aber dafür, in ein Musical zu gehen, war noch genug Zeit?

»Ella wird mir alles erzählen, was wichtig ist. Das wirst du doch, oder, mein Juwel?« Zärtlich lächelte sie Ella an. »So, und jetzt komm schon, wir müssen los!«

Ella gab auf. »Okay, ich pack meine Sachen. Komme gleich.«

Meine Gefühle waren gerade dabei, mich in Stücke zu reißen. Ein Teil von mir wollte fliehen, unbedingt und so schnell wie möglich. Schließlich war Lydia Lennox nicht nur eine raffinierte Anwältin, die jedem das Wort im Mund verdrehte, sondern auch eine riesige Python, die mich schon einmal fast erwürgt hatte. Der andere Teil von mir regte sich gerade tierisch auf, weil bei ihrem Anblick diese ganze Sache mit den Arenakämpfen in mir hochkam. Mrs Lennox hatte einfach zugeschaut und nicht eingegriffen, als ich in zweiter Gestalt beinahe getötet worden wäre!

Dieser Teil gewann. Bevor ich genau wusste, was ich tat, war ich schon auf den Füßen und watete auf meine Feindin zu. Sekunden später standen wir uns an der Rampe gegenüber, der den Trocken- vom Nassbereich trennte.

Ich starrte ihr direkt ins etwas kantige Gesicht, das von welligen dunkelblonden Haaren umrahmt wurde. Ihre Augen waren eisblau.

»Sie waren dort, auf dem Schiff.« Meine Worte kamen wie von selbst. »Sie haben irgendeinen Cocktail getrunken und mit den anderen Leuten zugeschaut, wie ein bezahlter Taucher mit einer Harpune auf einen Hai schießt. Einen Hai, der einfach nur in Ruhe gelassen werden wollte!«

Die vollen, violett geschminkten Lippen verzogen sich spöttisch. »Du bist so ein zartes Seelchen. Machst dir solche Sorgen wegen ein paar Haien! Fast alle Menschen hassen Haie und freuen sich, wenn sie dezimiert werden.«

»Sie haben gewusst, dass ich es bin, der da in die Arena gezerrt wurde! Ich war nur ein paar Meter entfernt – Sie haben mich erkannt, aber mir trotzdem nicht geholfen!«

Lydia Lennox schüttelte mitleidig den Kopf und wandte sich an Mr Clearwater, der hastig herangewatet war. »Ihr Schüler scheint an Verfolgungswahn zu leiden, er braucht offensichtlich Hilfe. Soll ich Ihnen einen guten Psychiater empfehlen?«

Am liebsten hätte ich heftig gegen die Wand getreten oder etwas durch die Gegend geschleudert. Aber dann hörte ich in mir die vertraute Stimme von Miss White. *Lass dich von ihr nicht reizen – wenn du deine Wut zeigst, hat sie ihr Ziel erreicht. Überrasch sie lieber, tu etwas, womit sie nicht rechnet!*

Obwohl Miss White wahrscheinlich Hunderte von Meilen entfernt war, half sie mir noch. Irgendwie schaffte ich es, ruhig stehen zu bleiben. Was konnte ich tun, um sie zu überraschen? Mit dem nächsten Wimpernschlag fiel mir etwas ein. Obwohl es mich unglaubliche Anstrengung kostete, lächelte ich Mrs

Lennox ins Gesicht. »Es gibt da ein paar Dinge, die Sie nicht wissen. Lassen Sie sich ruhig davon überraschen, wie das mit den Arenakämpfen für Sie und Ihre Mafiafreunde ausgeht.«

Treffer. Eine Millisekunde lang schaute sie verblüfft drein, bis sie sich wieder gefangen hatte und zurücklächelte. »Na, da bin ich aber gespannt. Kleiner Tipp: Falls du öffentlich irgendwelche Verdächtigungen äußerst, braucht ihr einen guten Anwalt, du und dein Onkel. Weil ihr dann nämlich eine Millionen-Dollar-Klage wegen Rufschädigung am Hals habt.«

Darauf fiel mir keine Antwort ein. Mein Gehirn war auf einmal genauso ausgedörrt wie mein Mund.

»Mrs Lennox, Sie können Ella noch nicht mitnehmen«, mischte sich unser junger Schulleiter ein. »Aber Sie können gerne hier warten, bis der Unterricht endet. Dauert auch nicht mehr lange, sie hat nur noch Menschenkunde und ...«

»Ach Blödsinn! Komm, Ella, wir gehen«, unterbrach ihn Lydia Lennox.

»Warte mal«, unterbrach sie Ella, die inklusive Handtasche am Eingang der Cafeteria erschienen war. »Hast du Tiago bei diesen Haikämpfen nun erkannt oder nicht? Das würde mich auch interessieren.«

»Nein, ich habe ihn selbstverständlich nicht erkannt, für mich sieht ein Hai aus wie der andere«, sagte ihre Mutter gereizt.

Dann zerrte Mrs Lennox Ella förmlich mit sich. Sie kam nicht mal mehr dazu, sich von ihren Fans Barry, Toco und Daphne zu verabschieden.

Plötzlich tat Ella mir leid. Meine Eltern waren schlimm, aber immerhin mischten sie sich nicht so in mein Leben ein und überließen meine Erziehung Johnny.

»Alles in Ordnung, Tiago?«, fragte mich Jack Clearwater besorgt.

»Jaja, geht schon«, brachte ich irgendwie heraus. Konnte sie mich und Johnny wirklich verklagen? Bestimmt. Meine Beine waren so weich, dass ich nur mit Mühe zu den Tischbooten zurückwaten konnte.

Mit gedämpfter Stimme sagte Mr García zu mir: »Ich versuche, einen neuen Termin bei ihr zu bekommen oder sie sonst wie abzufangen. Das war nur ein kleiner Rückschlag ... wir kriegen das hin, okay?«

Ich nickte und lächelte ihm dankbar zu.

Auf halbem Weg zu Shari und meinen anderen Freunden, die die Szene erschrocken beobachtet hatten, fiel mir etwas ein und ich änderte die Richtung.

Neugierig blickten mir die Zweitjahresschüler entgegen. Shelby hatte mittellanges schwarzes Haar, eine braune Haut und feine Gesichtszüge. Neben ihr saß Maris, ein Albatros, als Mensch ein schlaksiger, schüchterner Junge mit abstehenden Ohren. Die beiden hingen oft zusammen herum. Sie probierten gerade die selbst gebackenen Mandelmuffins, die Alligator-Wandlerin Polly stolz herumreichte – Backen war ihr großes Hobby, und falls man sie suchte, dann am besten erst mal in der Küche. Allerdings hatte sie großes Heimweh nach den Everglades, ich war nicht sicher, ob sie an unserer Schule bleiben würde.

»Könnte ich euch, ähm, um einen Gefallen bitten?«, fragte ich unsere Vogel-Wandler und erklärte ihnen, dass wir vorhatten, Miss White zu suchen, und dass wir verhindern wollten, dass noch einmal diese illegalen Haikämpfe stattfanden. »Könntet ihr bei Gelegenheit losfliegen und ein paar Leute fragen, ob sie Miss White gesehen haben und vielleicht sogar wissen, in welche Richtung sie geschwommen ist?«

»Kein Problem«, sagte Shelby sofort, sie war zum Glück sehr

hilfsbereit. »Ich könnte am Wochenende ein paar Erkundungsflüge machen – bist du dabei, Maris?«

»Meine Flügel sagen ganz laut Ja«, rief ihr Freund.

In mir spulte sich noch einmal die Begegnung mit Lydia Lennox ab und mir wurde klar, dass wir Miss White noch aus einem anderen Grund dringend brauchten. Sie war unsere stärkste Verbündete gegen die Machenschaften der Lennox und ihrer fiesen Freunde. Eine Kämpferin der Extraklasse. Sie war vielleicht die Einzige, die uns helfen konnte, diese scheußlichen Arenakämpfe zu beenden. Auch wenn Haie von vielen Leuten gefürchtet wurden, sie hatten ein Recht darauf, in Ruhe gelassen zu werden!

»Zu diesen Haikämpfen: Könntet ihr bitte außerdem nach großen Jachten Ausschau halten, die an abgelegenen Orten ankern und dort Netze auswerfen?«

»Gute Idee!« Shelbys Augen glänzten.

»Wir schnappen diese Kerle«, sagte ich grimmig.

Muschelpläne und Buffets

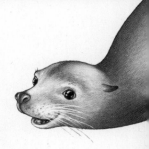

Ich verabschiedete mich von den Zweitjahresschülern und kehrte zu meinen Freunden zurück. Shari umarmte mich. »Das war echt mutig – ich dachte, jeden Moment macht sie eine Fischfrikadelle aus dir! Aber du bist keine Schnauzenlänge zurückgewichen!« Gespannt blickte sie mich aus ihren warmen braunen Augen an und fingerte an ihrer Drei-Flossen-Kette herum. »Was sind denn diese Dinge, die die Lennox nicht weiß?«

»Ähm ... das hab ich mir leider nur ausgedacht.« Ich gab ein verlegenes Pseudolachen von mir, das die Sache noch peinlicher machte.

Meine Freunde blickten betreten drein.

»Oh«, sagte Finny und kämmte sich mit den Fingern die blauen Haare durch. »Und ich dachte, du hättest am Wochenende irgendetwas total Gefährliches vor, was den Schurken demnächst das Wasser unter den Flossen wegzieht ...«

Von Mr Garcías Plan, die Lennox zu sondieren, durfte ich ihnen nichts erzählen. Falls etwas darüber durchsickerte, konnten wir die Aktion vergessen. Einmal war der Termin ja schon geplatzt.

»Etwas Gefährliches habe ich schon vor – aber nicht gefährlich für mich«, erklärte ich und Jasper ging prompt darauf ein: »Was meinste denn damit?«

»Johnny und ich werden zum ersten Mal in zweiter Gestalt zusammen ins Meer gehen. Er hatte bisher Angst davor, weil Tigerhaien Zackenbarsch ziemlich gut schmeckt.«

Finny, Shari, Jasper und Chris starrten mich an. »Oh wow«, sagte Chris. »Aber wehe, ihm fehlt nachher eine Flosse! Wir erwarten, dass du Bericht erstattest.«

Das versprach ich natürlich. Und musste mitbekommen, dass sich meine Pläne schon während der nächsten Stunden in der ganzen Klasse herumsprachen.

»Wetten, er frisst seinen Onkel versehentlich?«, hörte ich Barry mit einem hämischen Seitenblick auf mich behaupten. »Haie sind unberechenbar ...«

Ich warf ihm einen finsteren Blick zu. Was für ein Blödsinn! Johnny war mein Ersatzvater und das mit dem »gefährlichen Vorhaben« hatte ich nur so dahingesagt. Auch als Tigerhai, wenn meine Instinkte stärker waren als an Land, würde ich lieber sterben, als ihm eine Schuppe zu krümmen.

Es gab da noch etwas, das ich den anderen nicht gesagt hatte. Ich würde nicht irgendwo mit Johnny schwimmen, sondern an einem ganz besonderen Ort. Doch den behielt ich lieber für mich, sonst hätte ich auch gleich verraten können, welche Überraschung wir für meine beste Freundin geplant hatten.

Bei nächster Gelegenheit nahm ich Juna beiseite. »Hast du schon mit den anderen gesprochen wegen der neuen Muscheln für Shari?« Beim Hurrikan war ihre Sammlung am Grund der Bucht zerstört worden und ich wollte auf keinen Fall, dass unser Delfinmädchen deswegen traurig war.

»Ja, viele aus der Klasse wollen mitmachen und ihr eine Muschel schenken«, flüsterte Juna, nachdem sie sich zweimal umgeschaut hatte.

»Cool. Machen wir Montag die feierliche Übergabe? Gleich beim Frühstück?«

Das Lächeln passte fast nicht mehr auf Junas Gesicht. »Du hast es aber eilig. Wetten, du hast die schönste Muschel von allen für sie?«

Ich spürte, wie mir das Blut ins Gesicht stieg. Ahnte sie, was Shari mir bedeutete? »Noch nicht. Aber bestimmt bald.«

Wir planten am Wochenende einen Ausflug an die Westküste von Florida, zu Sanibel Island. Dessen Strände waren berühmt für die vielen Muschelschalen, die dort angespült wurden. Auf Sanibel würde ich garantiert genau das richtige Geschenk für Shari finden. Eigentlich hätte ich es auch am Meeresboden suchen können, schließlich war ich ein Seawalker. Doch mein Haimaul hätte auch den tollsten Fund in einen Haufen Trümmer verwandelt. Meine Flossen in der Tiefe zu Händen teilzuverwandeln, traute ich mich noch nicht. Wenn ich dabei einen Fehler machte, fand ich mich womöglich in Menschengestalt am Meeresboden wieder. Nicht lustig!

Doch noch vor dem Wochenende gab es eine andere »Übergabe« – die Delfine waren nämlich der Meinung, dass sie unserer meistens mies gelaunten Schulsekretärin schon viel zu lange keinen Streich mehr gespielt hatten. Deshalb hatten sie sich zwischendurch in die Werkstatt unserer Schule verzogen. Nun erzählte Noah: »Wir haben etwas für Mrs Misaki gebastelt – wer kommt mit und schaut zu, wie wir es ihr geben?«

Natürlich wollte der größte Teil der Klasse mit. Neugierig folgten wir Shari, Blue und Noah, die feierlich etwas trugen. Es sah aus wie ein auf einem Holzblock angebrachter goldener Fisch, wofür sollte der denn gut sein?

Mrs Misaki schaute misstrauisch drein, als sich eine große Horde Schüler in ihr Reich, das Sekretariat, drängte. Feierlich trat Shari vor und reichte ihr den goldenen Fisch. »Wir haben abgestimmt und Sie zur besten Schulsekretärin in Südflorida gewählt!«, sagte sie und strahlte Mrs Misaki an. »Hier ist Ihr Preis.«

Die anderen und ich versuchten, nicht zu verwundert dreinzuschauen. Das mit der Abstimmung musste irgendwie an uns vorbeigegangen sein. Sonst hätten wir sie eher zum Schüleralbtraum des Jahres gewählt.

Nachdem sich Mrs Misaki von der Verblüffung erholt hatte, sah sie tatsächlich geschmeichelt aus. »Also wirklich ... seid ihr sicher ... das ist nett von euch.« Sie betrachtete den goldenen Fisch von allen Seiten und stellte ihn dann auf ihren Schreibtisch, wo wir ihn alle einen Moment lang bewunderten. Dann wurden wir rausgescheucht. »Husch, husch, hier wird hart gearbeitet, schließlich habe ich jetzt einen Ruf zu verlieren!«

Brav zogen wir ab.

Als wir alle wieder im Erdgeschoss waren, prusteten Blue, Noah und Shari los.

»Der Fisch ist eine tote Meeräsche, die wir mit Goldspray angesprüht haben«, berichtete Noah. »Aber sah doch gut aus, oder?«

Finny kicherte. »In ein paar Tagen zeigt sie dann ihr wahres Gesicht. Geld und Gold stinken nicht, heißt es. Aber manchmal eben doch.«

»Mal schauen, wie lange Mrs Misaki durchhält, bis sie den Preis wegschmeißt«, sagte Shari mit einem breiten Grinsen.

Wir waren uns einig, dass das ein cooler Streich war. Juna und ich tauschten einen Blick. Eins war klar, unsere Muschelgeschenke für Shari würden deutlich haltbarer und wohlriechender sein!

Als Johnny mich am Wochenende mit unserem klapprigen Chevrolet abholte, spürte ich, dass er nervös war. »Na, alles klar?«, brummte er.

Ich entschied, ihm lieber nichts von der angedrohten Klage zu erzählen – dafür berichtete ich ihm von der chaotischen Kampfstunde und dass wir dringend Miss White zurückbrauchten.

»Ja, ich glaub auch«, meinte Johnny, er wirkte ein bisschen unentspannt.

»Und bei dir – alles okay? Keine Sorge, ich werde mich richtig vollfressen, bevor wir zusammen ins Meer gehen. Vielleicht finden wir ein *All-you-can-eat*-Buffet.« Ich versuchte, ihn beruhigend anzulächeln, doch er starrte auf den Highway und umklammerte das Lenkrad.

Wir übernachteten in unserer neuen Bleibe bei Sally im Stadtteil Coconut Grove und nahmen dort am nächsten Morgen ihren Enkel an Bord, meinen Wandler-Freund Rocket. Er würde als unser Assistent mitkommen auf die Expedition. »Hab ich schon gesagt, dass ich Muschelsammeln hasse?«, begrüßte er mich. »Hat bestimmt was mit meiner zweiten Gestalt zu tun. Meine Rattenart sammelt nichts.«

»Delfine und Haie normalerweise auch nicht«, sagte ich fröhlich. »Super, dass du keine Muscheln suchen willst, dann kannst du meinen Sammelbeutel tragen.«

»Vergiss das mal ganz schnell, Alter!«, kam es sofort zurück.

»Und nächstes Mal fahren wir zum Kennedy Space Center, klar?«

»Klar«, sagte ich gehorsam.

Während der Fahrt erzählte ich Rocket von den Arenakämpfen mit wilden Haien und dass wir versuchen wollten zu verhindern, dass so was noch mal stattfand.

»Arenakämpfe?«, fragte er verblüfft. »Mit Gladiatoren oder so?«

»So ähnlich ... die Gladiatoren sind Profitaucher ohne Gewissen. Jedenfalls haben sie kein Problem damit, einem Hai, der ihnen nichts getan hat, eine Harpune zu verpassen.«

»Fies! Und woher kriegen sie die Haie?«

»Die kann man fangen. Je größer, desto besser, ist mein Eindruck.«

Noch kannte ich Rocket nicht wirklich gut. Hätte ja sein können, dass er jetzt »Cool, gibt's einen Film von diesen Kämpfen auf YouTube?« rief. Aber das tat er zum Glück nicht.

»Eklig«, sagte er. »Könnt ihr diese Fights stoppen?«

»Weiß ich noch nicht. Erst mal müssen wir rausfinden, wo und wann weitere stattfinden«, meinte ich. »Zwei Vogel-Wandler aus der Schule – eine Seeschwalbe und ein Albatros – halten für mich Ausschau.«

»Hm.« Rocket kratzte sich an der Stirn. »Wäre es nicht noch besser, wenn sie mehr tun würden, als Ausschau zu halten? Ich könnte 'ne Minikamera organisieren, die man auf einem Tier festschnallen kann. So ein Ding, mit dem Vögel filmen, wo sie langfliegen.«

Ich war sofort begeistert. »Du meinst, falls sie was finden, könnten sie es sofort filmen, sodass wir endlich mehr Beweismaterial haben? Cool! Geht das denn so einfach? Und bis wann kannst du die Ausrüstung besorgen?«

Er nickte. »Eine Seeschwalbe ist ein bisschen klein für eine Kamera, aber dafür kann ein Albatros ordentlich was tragen, der hat ja größere Flügel, als unsere Arme lang sind. Ich bring was mit, wenn ich das nächste Mal vorbeikomme.«

»Also bald?« Ich war wild darauf, etwas gegen diese Tierquäler zu unternehmen.

»Sehr bald«, versprach er.

Den Rest der Fahrt erzählten Rocket und ich uns schlechte Witze und fachsimpelten über die *Star-Wars*-Raumschiffe, die sich Rocket als Modelle bauen wollte.

Nach ein paar Stunden Fahrt konnten wir in einem kleinen Hotel unsere Zimmer beziehen – Ventilator an der Decke, pastellfarbene Überdecken über den Betten und geflochtene Korbstühle. Das kleine, mit dunklem Holz dekorierte Restaurant war gemütlich. »Wenigstens haben die hier nicht wie in dem Lokal neulich einen ausgestopften Fisch an der Wand hängen«, sagte ich.

Die Bedienung trug einen dampfenden Teller vorbei und servierte ihn unseren Tischnachbarn. »So, Ihr Zackenbarsch mit Limettensoße!«

Johnnys Miene verfinsterte sich. »Miesen Appetit«, wünschte er unseren verblüfften Nachbarn.

Sanibel Island hatte breite helle Sandstrände, die von Millionen weißer, brauner und bunter Muscheln gepunktet waren. Natürlich nahm Rocket genau wie alle anderen Touristen sofort die typische Haltung ein – gebückt, den Blick auf den Boden geheftet. »Schau mal, die hier! Ist die nicht cool?« Begeistert zeigte er mir einen seiner Funde.

»Ja, die ist gut. Aber hattest du nicht eigentlich vor, an deinen Zeichnungen für eine Marsstation weiterzuarbeiten?«, stichelte ich, bewunderte kurz das Gehäuse seiner Meeresschnecke und scannte dann wieder den Bereich vor meinen Füßen nach Beute.

Mein Sammelbeutel füllte sich und schließlich fand ich das ultimative Stück – eine große sahneweiße und gelb getupfte Meeresschnecke, deren viele Stacheln sie wie eine Orchideenblüte wirken ließen.

»Oh wow«, flüsterte ich, nahm sie in beide Hände und stellte mir vor, wie Shari dreinschauen würde, wenn ich sie ihr überreichte. Ehrfürchtig brachte ich meinen Fund in meinem Rucksack unter, sicher in ein T-Shirt gewickelt, damit nicht etwa eine Ecke abbrach.

»Du magst dieses Mädchen wirklich, was?« Rocket schaute mich von der Seite an.

Boah! Wenn das so weiterging, wusste es wirklich bald jeder. Außer Shari hoffentlich.

Während wir am Flutsaum stöberten, kundschaftete Johnny entlang des Bowman Beach Stellen aus, an denen wir später unbeobachtet zusammen ins Meer gehen konnten.

»Hab was gefunden, etwas nördlich – da sind um diese Uhrzeit keine Leute mehr und wir haben Deckung durch ein paar Bäume und Büsche«, berichtete er, als die Sonne schon sank. Leider doch kein *All-you-can-eat*-Buffet, aber wir hatten belegte Brote mitgenommen. »He, lass auch was für uns übrig, Fressmaschine!«, beschwerte sich Rocket, als ich drei davon verschlungen hatte.

»Jaja, chill mal«, gab ich zurück und bewarf ihn mit einer Handvoll Chips. Ob satt oder nicht, natürlich würde ich meinem »Onkel« nichts tun!

Trotzdem klopfte mein Herz schnell, als Johnny und ich uns auszogen und ins Flachwasser wateten. Es war so weit.

Sharis Überraschung

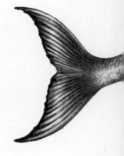

Viel Glück! Und mach nichts, was dir später leidtut, okay?«, raunte mir Rocket zu, als er unsere Klamotten einsammelte. »Und Ihnen viel Spaß, Mr Marisol. Wow ... hübsch!«

Danke, sagte Johnny, der sich gerade in einen halben Meter langen, korallenroten und mit hellblauen Punkten getupften Fisch verwandelt hatte. *Juwelenzackenbarsch, falls es euch interessiert. Ah, da ist mein Nachtisch!* Er riss das breite Maul auf und ein verblüfftes Fischchen, das nichts ahnend über den Sandboden geschwommen war, wurde hineingesaugt. Harmlos war auch Johnny nicht!

Als *ich* mich verwandelte und meine Rückenflosse durch die Wellen stieß, sagte niemand etwas von »hübsch«. Rocket, der bis zu den Knien im Meer gestanden hatte, watete hastig an Land und mein »Onkel« paddelte mit seinen fächerförmigen Flossen rückwärts. Ich versuchte, nicht gekränkt zu sein.

Bis später, du wartest auf uns, ja?, meinte ich zu Rocket.

Dann schwammen Johnny und ich nebeneinander los, hinein in die blaue Wildnis.

Wir waren ein ungleiches Paar, das im Meer einigen Aufruhr verursachte. Ein Schwarm silberner Fische, der gerade Algen von einem Felsen abweidete, stob davon, als er uns sah. Ein anderer Meeresbewohner wühlte sich blitzartig in den Sand und hoffte wohl, sich so unsichtbar zu machen.

Haha, ich weiß noch genau, wo er ist, berichtete ich. *Die Energieströme in seinen Muskeln kann er nicht verstecken.*

Solche Haisinne sind echt praktisch, sagte Johnny. *Du kannst froh sein über deine zweite Gestalt. Und es ist toll, dass wir endlich mal zusammen im Meer sind, Tiago.*

Leider konnte ich mit meinem Haimaul nicht lächeln. *Ja, finde ich auch.*

Während wir in etwa fünf Meter Tiefe über den geriffelten Sandboden und Seegrasfelder schwammen, spürte ich, dass Johnny sich immer mehr entspannte. Schön. Ist ja auch irgendwie unnatürlich, wenn dein Erziehungsberechtigter Angst vor dir hat!

Als wir in eine felsigere Gegend kamen, fragte er vergnügt: *Wie wäre es mit ein bisschen Wellness?*

Äh, was?, fragte ich zurück.

Da vorne ist eine Putzstation, meinte er und schwamm voraus. *Ich zuerst, dann du!*

Ein Dutzend fingerlanger, hellblau-schwarz gestreifter Fischchen schwamm auf Johnny zu, als er sich dem Felsen näherte.

Johnny-der-Zackenbarsch blieb im Wasser stehen, spreizte Kiemen und Flossen und öffnete das Maul. Eifrig machte sich die Putzerfischkolonne daran, ihm Parasiten und lose Schuppen vom Leib zu picken, was ihnen offenbar schmeckte. Sogar in sein Maul trauten sie sich.

Aaah, das tut gut ... und kostet keinen Cent, sagte Johnny nach einer Weile, wackelte mit den Flossen und gab so anscheinend das Signal, dass die Putzer sich zurückziehen sollten. *Willst du auch?*

Es kitzelte, als die Fischchen an meinen Kiemenschlitzen arbeiteten. Aber ich beherrschte mich und schaffte es, nicht versehentlich das Maul zuzuklappen und die kleinen Dienstleister runterzuschlucken.

Als meine Tigerhai-Gestalt wieder blitzsauber war, zeigte mir Johnny, wie er als Zackenbarsch unter felsigen Überhängen lauerte, bis Beute vorbeikam. Kurz, wir hatten jede Menge Spaß und kehrten müde, aber zufrieden und mit reicher Muschelbeute nach Miami zurück.

Als ich am Montag beim Frühstück davon erzählte, wie gut unser erstes gemeinsames Schwimmen geklappt hatte, freuten sich Shari, Blue und Noah für mich und Jasper klopfte mir stolz auf den Rücken. »Hab ich eh nicht gedacht, dass du Johnny was tun würdest«, versicherte er mir. »Genauso wenig, wie Miss White *dich* fressen würde.«

Miss White. Noch immer wussten wir nichts darüber, wo sie war und was mit ihr passiert war. Ich schaute mich in der Cafeteria nach Shelby und Maris um, doch die beiden waren nirgendwo in Sicht.

»So, Leute!« Als die anderen zu ihren Tellern zurückkehren wollten, klatschte Juna in die Hände. »Ich würde sagen, es ist Zeit für eine meerige Überraschung.«

Wir beobachteten alle Shari, aber sie blickte nur ratlos drein – gut!

Hastig aß ich auf und rannte so wie ein Dutzend andere aus unserer Klasse los. Die Fundmuschel für Shari lag noch in meiner Hütte, ich hatte sie in eine blaue Serviette gewickelt, etwas Schöneres hatte ich nicht. Als ich zurückkam, warteten meine Klassenkameraden schon in der Cafeteria, alle hielten verstohlen etwas in den Händen ... und schon zum zweiten Mal an diesem Morgen schauten alle mich an. Im Mittelpunkt zu stehen, war nicht so mein Fall, aber diesmal war es immerhin ein besserer Anlass. Feierlich ging ich auf Shari zu.

»Was ist?«, fragte sie. »Warum guckst du, als wäre dir gerade eine Garnele in die Kiemen gekrochen?«

»Shari, wir haben alle mitbekommen, dass deine Muschelsammlung in der Lagune durch den Hurrikan verloren gegangen ist«, begann ich. »Also haben wir uns gedacht, ähm, genauer gesagt ich, aber die anderen waren gleich dafür – na ja, egal, jedenfalls haben wir uns gedacht, dass du vielleicht gerne ein paar neue hättest.« Ich gab ihr die eingewickelte Muschel, die ich auf Sanibel Island entdeckt hatte.

Es war einfach nur genial wunderbar, wie ihre Augen aufleuchteten, als sie die Muschel auswickelte. »Oh, die ist aber meerig«, sagte sie und strahlte mich an. »So eine habe ich noch nie gesehen!«

Ach, ich schon, verkündete Lucy, glitt aus ihrem Tonkrug-Versteck und überreichte Shari mit einem ihrer acht Arme eine gestreifte, längliche Blitzschnecke. Finny hatte irgendwo eine große, wie ein Leopardenfell gefleckte Kauri aufgetrieben, Noah eine rosafarbene Kammmuschel. Linus überreichte ihr mithilfe seiner winzigen Kinder ein kleines weißes Schneckenhaus – »Sorry, mehr konnte ich als Seepferdchen nicht tragen, auch das hier war schon sauschwer« – und Nox schwamm mit einer kleinen gelben Muschel im Schnabel auf sie zu und schob sie Shari in die Hand. *Ich selbst steh ja nicht auf dieses Pissgelb, aber ich hab irgendwo gehört, das ist deine Lieblingsfarbe.*

Shari musste lachen. »Danke, danke, danke, ihr seid alle so süß!«

Bald hatte sie in einem Körbchen, das eigentlich für Frühstücksbrötchen gedacht war, eine bunte Sammlung. Aus dem Augenwinkel beobachtete ich Nestor und Chris, von denen ich wusste, dass sie für Shari schwärmten. Was würden die zu bieten haben? Zum Glück präsentierte ihr Nestor nur das Gehäuse einer Blitzschnecke. Aber dann kam Chris mit seinem Geschenk, das er bisher hinter seinem Rücken versteckt hatte. Eine Riesenflügelschnecke, außen beige-weiß-braun, innen zartrosa gefärbt.

Shari riss die Augen auf. »Wow«, sagte sie und drehte das gewaltige Ding ehrfürchtig in den Händen. »Die kommt ganz in die Mitte meiner Sammlung. Bei der großen Welle, damit wird der Boden der Lagune aussehen, als würde dort eine Königin wohnen!«

»Dann passt es ja«, meinte Chris und lächelte sie an. Dieser Schleimbeutel!

Ich war nicht wirklich am Boden zerstört. Okay, ein bisschen schon. Neben diesem Hammerding sahen alle anderen Geschenke – meins eingeschlossen – mickrig aus. Als das Muschelhorn ertönte und uns zur ersten Stunde rief, war ich erleichtert, dass ich abhauen und die ganze Überraschungsaktion hinter mir lassen konnte.

Doch Shari watete auf mich zu, erwischte mich am Arm und zog mich zu sich. »Hiergeblieben«, murmelte sie und umarmte mich. »Danke, Tiago. Deine Muschel finde ich am allerbesten – weil sie von dir ist!«

Oh mein Gott, bedeutete das, dass ich für sie mehr geworden war als ein guter Freund? Leider war ich zu feige, um nachzufragen. Stattdessen freute ich mich einfach und genoss jede Sekunde dieser Umarmung. Leider war sie viel zu schnell wieder vorbei und alle hasteten zum Unterricht. Auch die Zweitjahresschüler, unter denen weder Shelby noch Maris waren. Waren die etwa immer noch auf Expeditionsflug?

Aus dem Augenwinkel sah ich etwas aufblinken und wartete noch einen Moment, bevor ich den anderen folgte. Deshalb

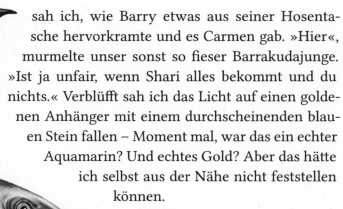

sah ich, wie Barry etwas aus seiner Hosentasche hervorkramte und es Carmen gab. »Hier«, murmelte unser sonst so fieser Barrakudajunge. »Ist ja unfair, wenn Shari alles bekommt und du nichts.« Verblüfft sah ich das Licht auf einen goldenen Anhänger mit einem durchscheinenden blauen Stein fallen – Moment mal, war das ein echter Aquamarin? Und echtes Gold? Aber das hätte ich selbst aus der Nähe nicht feststellen können.

Normalerweise war Carmen ziemlich schroff, und zwar zu allen. Ich wartete gespannt darauf, wohin sie den Klunker schleudern und welche Sprüche sie Barry entgegenknallen würde. Aber es kam nur ein »Oh! Ist das wirklich für mich?« und – nein, ich irrte mich nicht! – ein rosa Schimmer überzog ihre Wangen.

Mit der Welt stimmte irgendwas nicht.

»Was glotzt du denn so?«, fuhr Barry mich an, der gemerkt hatte, dass ich die Übergabe beobachtet hatte. »Bist du neidisch oder was, Dreckshai?«

Na ja, okay, manches änderte sich auch nicht.

Am Nachmittag wollte ich noch ein bisschen in der Lagune entspannen, am besten mit Shari – doch daraus wurde nichts. Als Erstes kam Shelby in ihrer Gestalt als Seeschwalbe aufgeregt auf mich zugeflattert, dann sah ich auch Maris, den Albatros, über mir kreisen. Atemlos landete Shelby auf meiner Schulter, ein winziges Geschöpf aus weißen Federn mit schwarzem Schopf.

»Ihr habt geschwänzt, oder? Habt ihr was herausgefunden?«, fragte ich aufgeregt.

Ja, wir haben einiges herausgefunden, sagte Shelby, die kaum still halten konnte, sie pickte mir sogar gegen das Ohr. *Wir haben fedrig viel herausgefunden!*

»Finden irgendwo wieder Haikämpfe statt?« Mein Puls legte einen Trommelwirbel hin. »Oder wisst ihr, wo Miss White ist?«

Nein, aber wir wissen, wohin sie geschwommen ist – ein paar Leute haben sie gesehen, informierte mich Shelby. *Und vor gar nicht langer Zeit!*

»Ihr seid der Hit, Leute! Wo?« Mit vor Eile ungeschickten Fingern rief ich auf meinem Handy eine Landkarte auf.

Mit dem Schnabel zeichnete Shelby von unten nach oben eine Linie auf das Display. *Hier entlang die Küste hoch nach Norden. Und in dieser Gegend hier könnte sie immer noch sein.*

Ich musste nicht lange darüber nachdenken, was ich jetzt tun wollte – nein, tun *musste*. »Danke – und behaltet das für euch, ja?«, rief ich den Mitgliedern unserer Fliegerstaffel zu, denn Ella sollte möglichst nichts davon erfahren. Dann ließ ich Shelby von meiner Schulter abheben ... und rannte los.

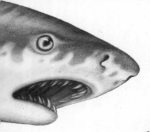

Jede Menge Zähne

Ich rannte in den ersten Stock hoch zu Mr Clearwater, denn ich war absolut sicher, dass den die Neuigkeiten interessieren würden. Tatsächlich, als ich hervorsprudelte. »Die Fliegerstaffel hat herausgefunden, wo Miss White hingeschwommen ist!«, leuchteten seine Augen auf. Aber seine Stimme klang nüchtern, als er sagte: »Hätte ich sowieso gedacht, dass sie nach Norden unterwegs ist. Orcas mögen kaltes Wasser.«

»Bitte, können Sie mir erlauben, dass ich dorthin schwimme und sie suche?« Es regte mich auf, dass er so ruhig hinter seinem Schreibtisch sitzen blieb. Sie bedeutete ihm doch auch was, wieso machte er sich nicht sofort auf den Weg? Vermutlich war er noch sauer auf sie.

»Na gut. Das Problem ist nur, dass ihr morgen den Test in Sei dein Tier habt«, meinte Jack Clearwater. »Den musst du mitschreiben, sonst schadet das deiner Note ... und damit deinem Stipendium, daran muss ich dich ja sicher nicht erinnern.«

Ich schluckte. »Natürlich bin ich rechtzeitig zurück. Versprochen.«

Dann raste ich wieder nach unten und ging auf die Suche nach Shari. Doch die war nirgendwo zu finden, weder auf dem Schulgelände noch in der Lagune. »Ach, die ist mit den anderen Delfinen rausgeschwommen, sie wollen mal wieder ihrem Hobby frönen und Leute retten, glaube ich«, sagte Finny, die gerade mit aufgeschlagenem Sei-dein-Tier-Lehrbuch am Strand lag und dabei *Stressed Out* von den *Twenty One Pilots* hörte. Ihre Haare glänzten in der Sonne azurblau. »Was gibt's denn? Irgendwo ein Fisch in Not?«

»Sie ist kein Fisch und wahrscheinlich auch nicht in Not, aber es gibt trotzdem Neuigkeiten«, sagte ich und erzählte ihr, was die Fliegerstaffel über Miss White herausgefunden hatte.

Finny sprang auf. »Bin dabei. Nichts wie los! Je länger wir warten, desto weiter weg ist sie wahrscheinlich.«

Ich zögerte noch. Eigentlich wollte ich nicht ohne Shari losschwimmen, ich wusste, dass auch sie Miss White mochte und für jedes Abenteuer zu haben war. Außerdem gehörten wir zusammen. Aber was war, wenn Shari erst spät in der Nacht zurückkam? Dann war es zu spät, Miss White suchen zu gehen.

»Okay«, sagte ich, noch immer hin- und hergerissen. »Let's go. Wir müssen schließlich morgen früh zurück sein und den Test mitschreiben.«

Ich verabschiedete mich von Jasper, der natürlich bettelte: »Kannste mich nicht mitnehmen?«

»Wir werden sehr schnell schwimmen, dabei kann ich kein Boot ziehen«, sagte ich entschuldigend. »Nächstes Mal, okay?«

Dann liefen Finny und ich in die Lagune und verwandelten uns, ihren schwarzen Bikini und meine Badeshorts würde schon irgendjemand herausfischen. Als Teufelsrochen und Tigerhai schossen wir durchs Wasser, finster entschlossen und voller Energie. Sobald wir ein bisschen weiter draußen waren, die Küste aber noch sehen konnten, wandten wir uns nach Norden. Mein breiter Tigerhaikopf pflügte in fünf Meter Tiefe durchs Wasser, während ich in stetem Rhythmus die Schwanzflosse von einer Seite zur anderen schlug.

Finny strahlte jede Menge gute Laune aus. *Ziemlich cool,*

mit dir im Meer zu sein ... so zu zweit, meine ich, schickte sie mir in den Kopf.

Ja, äh, bisher ist es ein schöner Ausflug, meinte ich und schaute sie von der Seite an. Mir fiel ein, was der Pumajunge Carag mir gesagt hatte. Dass noch jemand außer Shari an der Schule mich besonders mochte. Um Himmels willen, hatte er etwa Finny gemeint? Und war es ein Zufall, dass ihre Flossenspitze eben beim Schwimmen meine berührt hatte? Ja bestimmt.

Keine Ahnung, warum Finny und ich zusammenzuckten, als ein Pfeifen durchs Wasser hallte. Für mich war es ein freudiger Schreck. So klangen Delfine!

Sofort wendete ich, um mich umschauen zu können.

Es waren Shari und Chris, die in einem Höllentempo auf uns zuschwammen. *Oh, hey, toll, dass ihr hier seid,* begrüßte ich sie freudig.

Doch Shari wirkte nicht ganz so vergnügt wie sonst. *Wieso hast du mich nicht gefragt, ob ich mitwill? Jasper hat mir erzählt, dass ihr zu zweit losgeschwommen seid!*

Ich konnte dich nicht finden, rechtfertigte ich mich.

Aha, und es war dir zu lang, ein paar Minuten zu warten, bis ich zurückkomme? Ich war nur an der nächsten Landzunge. Shari klang enttäuscht. Sie schaute von Finny zu mir. *Ist es euch überhaupt recht, dass wir mitkommen? Oder wollt ihr lieber alleine sein?*

Nein, nein, wie kommst du darauf? Ich war entsetzt. Da hatte ich mir ja was eingebrockt. *Bitte kommt mit, es ist toll, dass ihr uns eingeholt habt.*

Na gut. Shari klang ein bisschen besänftigt. Trotzdem war die Atmosphäre angespannt, während wir zu viert weiterschwammen.

Habt ihr eigentlich schon für Sei dein Tier gelernt? Elegant tauchte Chris-der-Seelöwe neben uns entlang und schoss dann kurz nach oben, um Luft zu holen.

Nicht genug, gestand ich und von Finny kam nur ein Ächzen. Sharis einzige Antwort war ein Lachen – schließlich war sie als Delfin aufgewachsen.

Lach du ruhig, sagte Chris. *Aber was ist, wenn sie dich zum Beispiel fragen, was Tümmler in Florida von denen in den kalten Gewässern rund um Großbritannien unterscheidet?*

Äh ..., gab Shari von sich. *Vielleicht sind sie runder, weil sie eine dickere Fettschicht brauchen?*

Ganz gut geraten, meinte ich. *Sie sind größer und massiger, ich habe gelesen, dass sie länger als drei Meter werden. Meist haben sie auch eine dunklere Farbe.*

Meine drei Freunde starrten mich an. Chris stupste mich in die Flanke. *Stimmt. Aber woher weißt denn du so was?*

Ich hab mir, äh, ein paar Bücher über Delfine durchgelesen, gestand ich. Zum Glück fragte niemand, wieso. Es war sehr praktisch, dass man als Hai nicht rot werden konnte.

Wir könnten uns gegenseitig abfragen! Shari jagte hoch zur Meeresoberfläche, sprang und tauchte in einem Blasenschwall wieder ein. *Dann können wir Miss White suchen und gleichzeitig lernen. Wie klingt das?*

Einwandfreie Idee, sagte Finny, die ihre gute Laune wiedergefunden hatte. *He, Tiago, wie viele Zähne benutzt ein Tigerhai?*

Da musste ich raten. *Im aktiven Gebiss ... äh, so um die fünfzig? Wenn mir einer von denen ausfällt, rückt ein neuer nach, das jedenfalls weiß ich.*

Ich zähl schnell mal nach, sagte Chris, schwamm vor mich und tat so, als wolle er in mein Maul spähen.

Nicht nötig, er hat ziemlich genau achtzig, meinte unser Rochenmädchen.

Soso, und wieso weißt DU das, Plattfisch? Chris drehte eine Pirouette um Finnys Rochengestalt.

Ähm ... ICH hab Bücher über Haie gelesen. Finny klang verlegen.

Soso. Wie es aussah, war an meinem Verdacht was dran. Ich musste unbedingt mit ihr reden und ihr erklären, dass meine Gefühle für sie rein freundschaftlich waren. O Gott.

Ach echt, Bücher über Haie? Aber was ..., begann Chris und Finny klatschte ihm die Flossenspitze über den Rücken. Sah nicht ganz versehentlich aus.

Ups, das tut mir sooo leid!

Ach, meinte Chris und brachte sich in Sicherheit. *Jetzt bist du dran, du blauhaariges Scheusal. Wieso ist deine Rochenoberseite schwarz und dein Bauch weiß?*

Soll das 'ne schwere Frage sein?, schoss Finny zurück. *Tarnung halt. Durch meinen dunklen Rücken bin ich fast unsichtbar, wenn man von oben auf mich draufguckt und unter mir tiefes Wasser ist. Wenn man aus der Tiefe hochschaut, bin ich gegen den hellen Himmel auch schwer zu sehen.*

Ich war froh über Sharis Idee mit dem Lernen-beim-Schwimmen, das lenkte uns ab. Außerdem hatte ich das Lernen wirklich nötig!

Allmählich wurde das Wasser kühler, wir kamen immer weiter nach Norden. Die Sonne sank unter den Horizont, aber das machte nichts, auch im Licht der Sterne sahen wir noch genug. Gerade hatte Shari Chris eine besonders knifflige Frage gestellt, nämlich warum Kalifornische Seelöwen manchmal Sand vom Meeresboden fressen, da bemerkten wir einen fremden bräunlich gelben Hai in der Nähe. Obwohl er kleiner war als ich, schwammen meine Freunde und ich unwillkürlich dichter nebeneinander. Es war mir peinlich, es zuzugeben, aber manchmal war ich ein bisschen misstrauisch meinen Artgenossen gegenüber.

So einen nennen die Menschen Zitronenhai, die sind nicht besonders bissig, meldete Shari.

Außer wenn sie sauer sind, fügte Finny hinzu und ich konnte sie fast grinsen sehen.

Haha. Shari verdrehte die Augen, anscheinend hatte sie Finny noch nicht ganz verziehen. *Tiago, magst du mit ihm reden? Vielleicht hat er Miss White gesehen, während sie durch sein Revier geschwommen ist.*

Ich? Mit ihm reden?, meinte ich verblüfft. *Wie denn? Das ist ein Tier.*

Ja und? Chris kundschaftete voraus, vermied aber, dem Zitronenhai wirklich nahe zu kommen. *Man kann die Sprache seiner eigenen Tierart von Geburt an, stimmt doch, oder, Shari? Alle anderen Tiersprachen muss man sich in den Kopf prügeln.*

Stimmt, bestätigte meine Freundin. *Wahrscheinlich spricht der da einen Haidialekt, den du gut verstehen kannst, Tiago.*

Oh. Wenn ich das bei meinem Abenteuer mit dem weißen Hai gewusst hätte! Also schwamm ich auf meinen Artgenossen zu und achtete darauf, ganz entspannt zu schwimmen und die Flossen nicht zu senken ... Dass ich das machte, bevor ich angriff, war mir schon aufgefallen. *Hallo, Fremder, wie geht's?*

Der Hai glotzte mich an.

An deiner Stelle würde ich es nicht in Gedanken probieren, sagte Shari.

Ähm, stimmt. Ich versuchte es noch mal und diesmal klappte es. Aber weil wir uns hauptsächlich in Bewegungen verständigten, dauerte es eine Weile, bis ich aus ihm raushatte, was ich wissen wollte. *Er sagt, hier ist tatsächlich ein Meerestier entlanggekommen, das noch 'ne Ecke größer war als ich*, meldete ich meinen Freunden triumphierend. *Anscheinend ist das nur einen Sonnenaufgang her, wenn ich ihn richtig verstanden habe.*

Shari wurde ganz aufgeregt. *Das muss Miss White gewesen sein!*

Ein echt wichtiger Hinweis ... ich würde diesen Hai am liebsten abknutschen!, jubelte Finny.

Welchen von beiden?, fragte Chris und hätte dafür beinahe noch einen Flossenschlag abbekommen.

Im Eiltempo schwammen wir weiter nach Norden, denn es war schon spät. Mitternacht, schätzte ich. Wie lange, bis wir umkehren mussten? So langsam wurde ich nervös. *Wenn wir nicht bald umdrehen, wird's arg knapp mit der Zeit*, sagte ich schließlich zu den anderen.

Shari sah mich beunruhigt aus ihren dunklen Delfinaugen an. *Aber wir können doch nicht aufgeben, wenn Miss White vielleicht ganz in der Nähe ist!*

Mach dich mal locker, Tiago, was ist schon dabei, wenn du mal zu spät kommst?, meinte Chris.

Hä, Moment mal? Plötzlich stand ich als verkrampfter Streber da! Zum Glück sagte Finny: *Sorry, Pelztierchen, aber ich jedenfalls muss diesen Test mitschreiben. Und wenn sich Tiago zu locker macht, verliert er sein Stipendium, klar?*

Jaja, schon gut, wir kehren bald um, murmelte Chris und ich schickte Finny ein lautloses Danke.

Kurz darauf merkten wir, dass wir uns alle getäuscht hatten. Das große Meerestier, das der Hai meinte, war sehr wahrscheinlich nicht Miss White gewesen. Sondern etwas von einem ganz anderen Kaliber.

Das merkten wir, als wir beinahe mit ihm zusammenstießen.

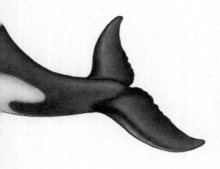

Wave

Wie aus dem Nichts tauchte eine gigantische Gestalt aus dem blauen Dunst des Meeres auf und wurde schnell größer. Eine Gestalt mit dunkelgrauer Haut, einer hubbeligen Schnauze und endlos langen Brustflossen. Wir stoben auseinander – Finny und Chris nach links, Shari und ich nach rechts –, damit der Buckelwal uns nicht über den Haufen schwamm.

He, du Meerespanzer, du denkst wohl, du hast die Vorfahrt eingebaut!, schimpfte Finny.

Mir blieb das Maul mit den ziemlich genau achtzig Zähnen offen stehen, als eine Jungenstimme durch unseren Kopf schallte. *Panzer? Vorfahrt? Keine Ahnung, was das sein soll. Ich hab euch halt nicht gesehen. Nichts passiert, oder?*

Du ... du bist ein Seawalker, stammelte ich.

Bin ich? Ja, ich glaub schon, das Wort hab ich irgendwo schon mal gehört, kam es fröhlich zurück. *Ich bin übrigens Wave. Trägt das Wasser euch gut heute?*

Oh ja, danke. Shari hatte sich als Erste wieder von der Überraschung erholt. *Bist du allein hier? Ich dachte, Wale mögen Gesellschaft genauso gerne wie wir Delfine.*

Ach, das geht schon. Wenn alles klappt, habe ich bald jede Menge Gesellschaft. Der Wal klang unternehmungslustig. *Ich bin auf dem Weg zu 'ner Schule, von der mir jemand erzählt hat. Hab leider den Namen vergessen. Blue irgendwas.*

Die kennen wir, auf die gehen wir! Shari drehte fast durch vor Begeisterung, sprang ein paarmal, schwamm an Waves Seite und passte ihre Bewegungen seinen an. Ihr Delfinkörper wirkte winzig neben diesem Koloss. *Es ist sehr meerig dort, du wirst sehen.*

Ein Buckelwal-Wandler wollte auf unsere Schule gehen? Krass! Seine gewaltigen Flossen, oben grauschwarz und unten weiß, wedelten durchs Wasser neben mir, die Druckwelle hätte mich beinahe auf die Seite geworfen. Ich versuchte, ihn mir in der Lagune vorstellen, in der Verwandlungsarena oder in der Cafeteria. Was dabei herauskam, war eine Art Katastrophenfilm.

Wisst ihr, wie man dahin kommt?, erkundigte sich Wave. *Ich kenn mich hier nicht aus, ist nicht ganz auf meiner üblichen Wanderroute.*

Wir müssen sowieso zurück und können dir den Weg zeigen, antwortete ich eifrig, weil es inzwischen wirklich spät war. In meinem Kopf blinkten schon rote Warnhinweise.

Aber nur, wenn du nicht versuchst, uns plattzumachen, Großer, sagte Finny.

Der Buckelwal schwenkte den massigen Kopf in ihre Richtung. *Du hast das gesagt, oder? Ach, ich mag Rochen. Meine Freunde und ich packen die oft mit der Schnauze und schleudern sie übers Meer, weil sie so gut fliegen.*

Wale spielten mit anderen Tieren Frisbee? Das verschlug nicht nur mir die Sprache.

Wave prustete los. *Nur Spaß! Natürlich machen wir so was nicht. Aber ist eigentlich 'ne gute Idee.*

Finny guckte ein bisschen verdutzt drein. Vielleicht war es das erste Mal, dass sie selbst verulkt worden war und nicht jemanden verulkte.

Wehe – sonst spiele ICH Gewichtheben mit Bartenwalen!, gab sie zurück, als sie sich von der Überraschung erholt hatte.

Nein, nein, oh, bitte nicht, bettelte Wave und musste noch mehr lachen.

In der Zwischenzeit hatte ich gewendet und schwamm wieder in Richtung Schule; ich war furchtbar enttäuscht, dass wir Miss White nicht gefunden hatten, aber mit etwas Glück würden wir sie beim nächsten Versuch entdecken. Jetzt mussten wir dringend zurück.

Kommt, Leute, lasst uns Gas geben, sagte ich zu den anderen.

Gas geben?, fragte Wave, der sich offensichtlich mit der Menschenwelt überhaupt nicht auskannte. *Egal, was das ist, ich kann es noch nicht machen, erst brauche ich einen Happen zu essen.*

Etwas hilflos folgten wir ihm, als er ohne jede Eile ein bisschen durch die Gegend schwamm und schließlich einen Schwarm kleiner Fische entdeckte. Wave tauchte ab, rauschte senkrecht nach oben und riss dabei sein Maul auf, wobei sich seine Kehle mit all dem einströmenden Meerwasser ausdehnte wie ein Ballon. Dieses Maul war wirklich gigantisch und für die Hälfte der Fischchen der letzte Anblick ihres Lebens.

Wave presste das Wasser wieder aus seinem Maul und schluckte seine Beute. An der Oberfläche prustete er einen Strahl feuchte Luft aus seinem Blasloch und tauchte dann gemächlich ab für einen weiteren Anlauf.

Ich glaube, der weiß gar nicht, was beeilen heißt, flüsterte Shari uns zu. *Mir ging das früher auch so, ich hatte ja keine Uhr und wusste nicht mal, was Zeit ist.*

Spielerisch drehte sich Wave in der Tiefe um sich selbst, wir sahen seinen weißen Bauch und seine meterlangen Brustflossen aufblitzen. Ein fünfundzwanzig Tonnen schwerer Tänzer des Meeres.

Meinst du, wir können ihn irgendwie dazu bringen, bald mit uns zu kommen?, fragte Chris, anscheinend wurde selbst Mr Lässig langsam unruhig.

Falls du zufällig Zehn-Kilo-Bonbons mit Fischgeschmack zu bieten hast ..., meinte ich.

Ich glaube, ihr unterschätzt ihn alle, sagte Finny, sie klang ein bisschen trotzig. Bevor uns eine Antwort einfiel, stürzte sie sich todesmutig in den Strudel aus ganz viel Wal und immer weniger panischen Fischen.

Hey, Wave!, rief sie und schwamm auf eins seiner großen dunklen Augen zu. *Wenn wir nicht gleich losschwimmen, bekomme ich Ärger in der Schule.*

Wieso hast du das nicht gleich gesagt?, meinte Wave, klappte das Maul zu und presste eine Flutwelle daraus hervor. Dann gesellte er sich zu uns und schwamm uns nach, als wir uns Richtung Süden wandten. Endlich kamen wir voran.

Es ist so toll, dass ihr Humor habt, meinte Wave. *Meine Eltern würden einen Witz nicht mal erkennen, wenn sie ihn gerade verschlucken.*

Ich hatte tausend Fragen an ihn, schließlich hatte ich noch nie mit einem Buckelwal geredet. Aber Shari kam mir zuvor. *Hast du dich schon mal verwandelt?*

Ja, ein paarmal heimlich nachts an einem Strand, berichtete unser neuer Freund. *Diese Menschengestalt ist so komisch – ich hatte keine Schwanzflosse mehr, sondern zwei BEINE, könnt ihr euch das vorstellen?*

Wir versicherten ihm, dass wir uns das sehr gut vorstellen konnten.

Die Welt der Menschen ist total interessant, schwärmte Shari. *Es gibt darin so viele Dinge zu entdecken wie Sardinen in einem Schwarm. Du musst unbedingt mal tagsüber an Land, unser Schulleiter gibt dir Sachen zum Anziehen.*

Bin schon gespannt, meinte Wave. *Wieso wart ihr überhaupt so weit weg von der Schule?*

Ich schwamm etwas näher an ihn heran. *Wir suchen jemanden. Eine Frau, die in zweiter Gestalt ein Orca ist. Hast du sie vielleicht sogar gesehen?*

Nein, ich selbst nicht, antwortete Wave. *Aber ich hab gehört, dass meine Eltern einer Orca-Seawalkerin begegnet sind und sich gewundert haben, dass sie so weit südlich lebt. Sie hat gesagt, dass sie noch nicht lange dort ist. Ihr Revier war in der Nähe eines Hafens mit einer Insel.*

Wie elektrisiert blickten wir uns an. Wie viele weibliche Seawalker-Schwertwale konnte es in dieser Gegend geben? *Er könnte die Stadt Charleston meinen,* sagte Finny aufgeregt. *Wenn wir daheim sind, schauen wir auf einer Karte nach!*

Obwohl Wave ähnlich schnell schwamm wie wir, mussten wir hin und wieder auf ihn warten und entsetzt sah ich, dass schon die Sonne aufging. Und wir waren noch ein ganzes Stück von der Schule entfernt! Der Test war leider ausgerechnet in der ersten Stunde.

Zeig mal, wie schnell du schwimmen kannst, forderte Finny unseren neuen Freund heraus und zum Glück sprang Wave darauf an. Da Shari und Chris nun endlich richtig aufdrehen konnten, brachte uns das Rennen ein gutes Stück voran. Endlich kamen wir in Gedankenreichweite der Schule. Chris hatte von uns das größte Talent für Fernrufe, deshalb überließen wir es ihm, unseren Schulleiter zu benachrichtigen. *Mr Clearwater, hier sind Shari, Finny, Tiago und Chris,* trompetete er so laut hinaus, dass uns fast der Kopf platzte und selbst Wave zusammenzuckte. *Wir haben Miss White leider nicht gefunden, dafür aber einen neuen Schüler ...*

Bringt ihn bitte in mein Büro, kam als Antwort zurück.

Äh, das wird nicht gehen. Warum, werden Sie selbst merken, wenn Sie ihn sehen.

Na gut, ich fliege euch entgegen, antwortete unser Schulleiter etwas irritiert. *Bringt ihn bitte zur Boje über unserem Hausriff. Und beeilt euch, der Unterricht fängt gleich an!*

Shari stieß einen erschrockenen Pfiff aus.

Wir ließen Wave an der Boje zurück, verabschiedeten uns hastig von ihm und versprachen, ihm bald wieder Gesellschaft zu leisten. Dann legten wir ein unglaubliches Tempo vor, als wir zurückdüsten zur Schule. Obwohl ich ziemlich erledigt war, kam ich knapp hinter Shari und den anderen in der Lagune an.

Am Schulstrand erwartete uns zu unserer Überraschung ein zierliches, hübsches Mädchen in knallbuntem Kleid – Izzy. »Hier sind eure Klamotten!«, sagte sie, lächelte Chris an und reichte ihm seine Sachen.

»Äh, danke«, antwortete er verblüfft.

Auch unsere Klamotten hatte Izzy schon bereitgelegt. Wir zerrten sie uns über, sprinteten zum Hauptgebäude und platzten tropfend ins Klassenzimmer. Dort lagen schon die Aufgaben des Tests auf den Tischen. Schweigend und konzentriert, beugten sich die anderen darüber, manche fingen schon an zu schreiben. Schnell glitt Izzy wieder an ihren Platz und tat, als sei sie nie weg gewesen.

»Na, das war wirklich auf den letzten Drücker!«, sagte Miss Bennett, die neben den anderen Fächern von Miss White auch Sei dein Tier übernommen hatte. »Ich hatte nicht mehr mit euch gerechnet!«

»Wir mit uns auch nicht«, murmelte Finny, während sie sich keuchend auf einen freien Stuhl fallen ließ. Ihre nassen blauen Haare tropften das vor ihr liegende Blatt voll, doch das war zum Glück wasserfest wie die meisten Sachen hier an der Schule.

Aufgeregt vertiefte ich mich in die Aufgaben. Nur da zu sein, brachte nichts, wenn man im Test selbst versagte. Und das durfte ich auf keinen Fall!

Zu groß für die Schule?

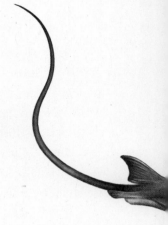

Schon bei der ersten Frage bekam ich große Augen. Aber nicht vor Angst, sondern weil mir solche wunderbaren Zufälle in meiner normalen Schule nie passiert waren. Zur Sicherheit las ich mir die Frage noch mal durch, aber sie lautete immer noch: *Erkläre, was es bringt, dass dein Tigerhaikörper oben grau ist und unten weiß. Wie lautet der Begriff für diese Farbgebung? Und wozu dienen deine Streifen?*

Yeah! Einmal tief durchatmen und dann das hinschreiben, was Finny über sich gesagt hatte. Weil Tigerhaie im flacheren Wasser unterwegs waren, war mein Rücken wahrscheinlich grau und nicht so wie ihrer schwarz. Bei den Streifen musste ich raten, aber dann dachte ich daran, wie ich manchmal über geriffelten Sandboden schwamm, über den ein Sonnenlicht-Muster tanzte. Ah, ebenfalls Tarnung! Das war bestimmt auch der Fachbegriff, um den es ging. Schnell hinschreiben.

Ran an die nächste Frage, sie war leider kniffliger. *Wie viele Kiemenschlitze hast du und gibt es auch Haie, die mehr haben?*

Es wäre auch zu schön gewesen, wenn sie nach der Zahl meiner Zähne gefragt hätte. Auf diese verdammten Kiemenschlitze hatte ich nie geachtet. Kurz überlegte ich, ob ich mich unauffällig teilverwandeln und mir dann über den Hals tasten sollte, aber das war mir zu riskant und galt vielleicht auch als Schummeln. Ich versuchte, mir mein Hai-Ich vorzustellen, hörte aber sofort damit auf, als ein verdächtiges Kribbeln durch meinen Körper lief. Es hätte mir gerade noch gefehlt, gleich als Raubfisch auf dem Fußboden zu zappeln!

Zum Glück hatte ich tatsächlich ein bisschen was gelernt und so fiel mir der seltene Sechskiemer-Hai ein, der in der Tiefsee lebte. Ich tippte bei normalen Haien auf fünf Kiemenschlitze auf jeder Seite und spürte, dass das richtig war. Uff. Noch zwei Fragen übrig.

Ich brütete gerade über der letzten Frage *(welche Gefahr ist die größte, mit der Haie derzeit zu kämpfen haben, und wie kann man sie abwenden?)*, als Miss Bennett verkündete: »So, liebe Kinder, die Zeit ist um, bitte gebt eure Bögen ab!«

»Oh nein!«, stöhnte Shari und raufte sich die blonden Locken. Das hatte sie sich erst vor Kurzem angewöhnt, weil sie gesehen hatte, wie es jemand in einer Fernsehshow gemacht hatte. Als Delfin hatte sie ja keine Haare gehabt.

»Bitte, bitte geben Sie uns noch ein paar Minuten.« Chris setzte seinen schönsten Bettelblick auf, mit dem er als Seelöwe wahrscheinlich von allen Seiten Fischhäppchen zugeworfen bekam.

»Na gut. Fünf Minuten extra für alle, die mitgesucht haben«, sagte Ivy Bennett und bekam von mir dafür einen dicken Pluspunkt. Vielleicht war sie doch keine so üble Lehrerin, obwohl sie von Kampf und Überleben keine Ahnung hatte!

»Das ist unfair, wieso kriegen die Verlängerung und wir nicht?«, motzte Ella und Daphne fügte ein »Genau!« hinzu. Auch Nestor blickte unwirsch drein. Mara sagte natürlich nichts. Weil sie durch ihre zweite Gestalt als Seekuh so langsam war, bekam sie sowieso jedes Mal zwanzig Minuten Extraverlängerung.

Mit der »Gefahr« für Haie war vermutlich eher nicht diese Sache mit den Arenakämpfen gemeint, obwohl die mir so oft durch den Kopf ging. Ich schrieb hastig einen Absatz über die hundert Millionen Haie, denen Fischer jedes Jahr die Flossen abhackten, weil die Leute in Asien unbedingt Suppe daraus kochen wollten. Als Lösung fiel mir nur »Schutzgebiete einrichten« ein. Dann waren die fünf Minuten auch schon um und mit letzter Kraft drückte ich Miss Bennett mein Blatt in die Hand. Geschafft.

Von der anschließenden Stunde Spanisch bekam ich nicht allzu viel mit, weil ich ständig an Wave denken musste. Hatte das Treffen mit Mr Clearwater geklappt? Durfte der junge Wal in Zukunft auf die Blue Reef High gehen? In der Pause hatten wir vier, die unseren Gast schon kannten, es eilig, wieder ins Wasser zu kommen und zu Wave hinauszuschwimmen.

»Wo wollt ihr denn schon wieder hin?«, fragte Jasper verblüfft.

»Einen Buckelwal-Wandler besuchen«, erklärte Shari, und als sich das herumsprach, stürzten sich nicht vier Leute ins Meer, sondern alle, die als Tier weit genug rausschwimmen oder -fliegen konnten. Also ziemlich viele, es war ein ziemliches Gedränge im Wasser. Die anderen inklusive Jasper quetschten sich in unser Schnellboot *Powerfish,* mit dem Mr García sie netterweise rausfahren wollte, damit sie nichts verpassten.

»Wir machen die Verwandlungsstunde einfach dort«, meinte er. Wieso hatte ich ihn früher eigentlich nicht gemocht? Er hatte nur versucht, mich vor mir selbst zu warnen, und damit absolut recht gehabt.

Wir fanden Wave am Riff, wo er sich im Wasser treiben ließ und ab und zu einen Atemstrahl in die Luft blies. Sein schiefergrauer, fast schwarzer Rücken glänzte im Sonnenlicht. Mr Clearwater saß als Weißkopf-Seeadler in der Nähe auf der Boje.

Beide sahen nicht übermäßig fröhlich aus. Oje, was hatte das zu bedeuten?

Hi, wir sind die Schüler der Blue Reef High und kommen zum Hallosagen, begrüßte ihn Tan Li, ein Wasserschildkrötenjunge, Klassensprecher der Zweitjahresleute.

Schön, dass du zu uns gefunden hast, ergänzte Farryn García und schickte unserem Gast eine Welle warmer Willkommensgefühle.

Ja genau! Es ist uns eine Ehre! Izzy war offensichtlich hin und weg. Sie war gerade ein handlanger silbriger Fisch und sah neben Wave aus wie eine Mücke neben einem Elefanten.

Darf ich dich anfassen?, fragte Jasper, er hatte ganz große Augen.

Klar, mach nur, sagte Wave. Jasper beugte sich so weit über die Bordwand, dass ich ihn wahrscheinlich in fünf Sekunden aus dem Wasser ziehen musste, und legte Wave die Hand auf die riesige hubbelige Schnauze. »Wow! Fühlt sich an wie schwarzes Gummi!«

Nox schwamm währenddessen eifrig um Wave herum und betrachtete ein paar helle Seepocken, die sich auf seiner Haut angesiedelt hatten. *Äh, da wächst was auf dir, hast du das schon gewusst?*

Wenn du so langsam schwimmen würdest wie ich, dann hättest du so was auch, kam es trocken zurück. *Stört nicht sehr.*

Wave wirkte freundlich, aber ungewohnt kurz angebunden. *Alles in Ordnung?,* fragte ich ihn besorgt und Shari und die anderen Delfine blieben dicht neben ihm.

Ich musste ihm leider sagen, dass wir ihn nicht in der Blue Reef High aufnehmen können, informierte uns Jack Clearwater.

Sofort brach unter und über Wasser ein Protestchor los. »Was?« *Warum nicht?* »Aber er ist doch so cool!« *Bitte lassen Sie ihn doch, Mr Clearwater!*

Es tut mir auch furchtbar leid, aber Wave ist sehr unerfahren in Verwandlung, meinte unser junger Schulleiter. *Wenn er sich in unseren Gebäuden versehentlich verwandelt, sind die hinüber ... und das will ich nicht riskieren. Wir haben sie nach dem Hurrikan gerade erst wieder instand gesetzt.*

Das brachte die anderen zum Schweigen, weil es leider ziemlich logisch war.

Ich bin also zu groß für euch, sagte Wave und ich spürte seine Enttäuschung. *Tja, das ist nicht zu ändern. Kann ich verstehen. Also mach ich mich mal wieder auf den Weg.*

An seiner Stelle wäre ich auch eingeschnappt gewesen. Was konnte er denn für seine zweite Gestalt?

Furchtbar schade, seufzte Finny, sie wirkte geknickt.

Shari fügte hinzu: *Besuch uns bitte mal, wenn du wieder in der Gegend bist, ja?*

Mach ich, sagte Wave und berührte Finny, die als Rochen um ihn herumflatterte, ganz sanft mit der Schnauze. *Ich wünsche euch noch viele Sonnenaufgänge.*

Als er die gewaltige Schwanzflosse auf und ab bewegte und seine flügelartigen Brustflossen durchs Wasser schnitten, entfernten sich panikartig alle kleineren Wandler aus seiner Nähe. Aber Wave bewegte sich so geschickt und vorsichtig, dass er weder das Boot noch einen der Schüler berührte.

Finny, Shari, Chris und ich eskortierten Wave noch ein Stück, dann verabschiedeten auch wir uns. Und sahen, dass Finny noch einmal dicht zu ihm schwamm. Ich hörte, wie sie ihm etwas zuflüsterte, aber es war zu leise, um es zu verstehen.

Was lief da?

Der Rest des Ausflugs ans Riff bestand aus Verwandlungsübungen im offenen Wasser. Keiner von uns konnte sich besonders gut konzentrieren, wir wollten eigentlich nur über Wave reden.

»Total schade, dass er nicht in unsere Klasse gehen darf«, sagte ich, als wir gegen Mittag wieder zurück am Strand waren und zur Cafeteria pilgerten.

»Aber vielleicht darf er sie sich mal anschauen?«, meinte Finny und grinste breit. Dann setzte sie ihre Sonnenbrille auf, versenkte die Hände in den Taschen ihrer Shorts und schlenderte zum Buffet.

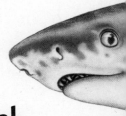

Liebesbriefe und Seeigel

»Was könnte Finny vorhaben?«, fragte ich Shari. »Die hat doch was vor!«

Shari zuckte die Schultern. »Frag mich doch so was nicht. Ich kann nicht *alle* Gedanken lesen, weißt du? Und wieso lächelst du gerade so verkrampft?«

»Verkrampft? Wieso verkrampft? So sehe ich immer aus, wenn ich Hunger habe«, behauptete ich und lud mir gleich drei Fischburger auf den Teller. Immerhin hatte ich gestern das Abendessen und heute das Frühstück verpasst und mich außerdem ein paarmal verwandelt.

Es war sehr, sehr gut, dass Shari nicht meine Gedanken lesen konnte, sonst wäre ich für sie nur noch einer ihrer vielen Verehrer. Irgendeine nervige innere Stimme erinnerte mich daran, dass ich noch mit Finny reden und ihr vorsichtig klarmachen musste, dass mein Herz schon vergeben war. Aber dafür gab es bestimmt einen besseren Moment, ja, ganz sicher. Morgen oder in einer Woche oder in zwanzig Jahren.

Das ließ mich komischerweise wieder an Miss White denken. Hatte sie wirklich mal als Kopfgeldjägerin gearbeitet? Vielleicht würde ich sie nie danach fragen können. Vielleicht stimmte es ja gar nicht, was Ellas Mutter uns erzählt hatte, oder Miss White hatte zwingende Gründe dafür gehabt? Aber bei einem war ich mir sicher – sie hätte nie bei so etwas Scheußlichem wie diesen unfairen Taucher-gegen-Hai-Kämpfen mitgemacht! Wenn wir es schafften, sie zurückholen, würde sie mir helfen, diese Verbrechen zu verhindern.

Bevor die nächste Stunde – Geografie bei Mrs Pelagius – begann, konnte ich noch schnell nachschauen, wo diese Stadt Charleston lag, von der Finny dachte, dass dort vielleicht Miss White war. »Könnte passen«, flüsterte Jasper, nachdem er das Satellitenbild genau gemustert hatte. »Jedenfalls gibt's einen Hafen und eine Insel mitten darin, so wie Wave es gesagt hat.«

»Ey, in Charleston bin ich aufgewachsen!«, rief Ralph, der schräg neben uns saß. »Was willst du da? Ist hübsch dort, aber abends nix los.«

»Kennst du noch irgendwelche Wandler dort?«, fragte ich ihn hoffnungsvoll.

»Ja klar, mein einer Dad ist ein Dachs und der andere Dad eine Sardine.«

Ich zuckte nur ganz kurz mit der Augenbraue, dann fiel mir ein, dass andere Jugendliche auch erst mal erstaunt waren, wenn sie mitbekamen, dass meine »Tante« Jenny sich zu einem »Onkel« namens Johnny gewandelt hatte. »Könnte dein Sardinen-Dad mal nachforschen, ob dort im Meer seit kurzer Zeit eine Schwertwal-Wandlerin lebt? Und wenn ja, kann er ihr sagen, sie soll mich bitte anrufen?«

Das kam mir zwar irgendwie lächerlich vor – in Filmen lief es nie so, wenn jemand gefunden werden sollte. Aber ich riss trotzdem ein Stück aus einer Heftseite und kritzelte meine Handynummer darauf.

Stolz reichte Polly zum Nachtisch einen duftenden Zitronenkuchen herum. Doch ausgerechnet ihr Sumpfkumpel, der kleine Python-Wandler Tino – der in unsere Klasse ging, aber dort meistens wenig sagte –, lehnte ab. »Ich hatte doch schon vorgestern was zu essen«, meinte der kleine Schlangen-Wandler. »Frag mich morgen noch mal.« Typisch Python! Schlangen konnten Riesenportionen verdauen, dafür brauchten viele von ihnen nur einmal im Monat Futter. Als die Sumpfschüler zu uns gekommen waren, hatten sie sich den Bauch vollgeschlagen, jetzt fasteten sie wieder.

»Morgen ist nichts mehr da, Kleiner«, murmelte Chris und schnappte mir das letzte Stück Kuchen knapp vor der Nase weg.

Geografie hatten wir diesmal in großer Runde, weil bei den Zweitjahresschülern sonst eine Stunde ausfallen würde. Wir drängten uns im größten Klassenzimmer, dem K7, und wurden von Mrs Pelagius zu den verschiedenen Meeren und Ozeanen abgefragt. Während Finny gerade versuchte, alle Meere zu nennen, die Farben im Namen hatten, fiel mir auf, dass Barry einen Zettel schrieb und versuchte, ihn in Richtung unseres Haimädchens zu schnippen.

»Schwarzes Meer, äh, Rotes Meer ... es gibt kein Grünes Meer, oder?«

Nein, sagte Mrs Pelagius und schwamm hinüber zu Barrys Zettel, der keine guten Flugeigenschaften gezeigt und kurz vor seinem Ziel ins Wasser gefallen war. Carmen angelte danach, kam aber nicht ganz dran. Gespannt beobachteten wir das Drama.

Nur Millisekunden bevor Carmen ein wenig aufstand und ihre Finger zugreifen wollten, erwischte Mrs Pelagius den Zettel in ihrem Schildkrötenschnabel. *Lies das bitte vor,* befahl sie Lucy, die den Zettel mit drei ihrer acht Arme auffaltete.

Da steht »Carmen, du bist der Hammer!«, berichtete Lucy.

Zwei Schulklassen grölten vor Lachen. Unser Hammerhaimädchen und Barry sahen aus, als würden sie sich am liebsten unsichtbar machen und das den Rest des Tages bleiben. Ich lachte auch, aber eigentlich fand ich es süß. Dass sich unser Klassenfiesling verliebt hatte, machte ihn mir fast schon sympathisch.

Nach Geografie hatten wir an dem Tag noch Menschenkunde. Fast alle von uns (sogar Ella) zeigten Jack Clearwater die kalte Schulter wegen der Sache mit Wave. Niemand meldete sich, wenn Mr Clearwater etwas fragte.

»Na gut, ihr wollt nicht mitmachen ... okay, dann gibt's jetzt was, was ihr eigentlich erst später bekommen solltet. Ivy Bennett und ich haben uns etwas für euch überlegt.« Er holte einen Stapel Umschläge aus seiner Tasche.

Die Zweitjahresschüler beugten sich gespannt nach vorne, anscheinend kannten sie das schon. Ich, Jasper und Shari tauschten einen ratlosen Blick. Doch wir fanden schnell raus, was die Umschläge bedeuteten, eine Minute später hatte nämlich jeder von uns einen in der Hand und durfte ihn öffnen.

Lernexpedition
Teilnehmer: Toco, Shari, Tiago
Auftrag: Informationen zum Thema »Meeresschutz« in der Key Largo Highschool abgeben
Zeitraum: Irgendwann in dieser Woche an einem Nachmittag

Zusammen mit Shari! Genial! Der Auftrag selbst klang harmlos. Ein Klacks. Aber es war Pech, dass Toco dabei sein sollte. Der hasste mich und würde garantiert versuchen, mir und Shari die Note zu ruinieren.

Aufgeregt tuschelnd, zeigten sich die anderen ihre Aufträge. »Wer auch immer sich das ausgedacht hat, hat sie nicht mehr alle!«, verkündete Ella wütend. Wie sich herausstellte, sollten sie, Juna und Linus einen Seeigel fangen und hier in der Schule dazu bringen, dass er über einen Bleistift und wieder zurück kroch.

»Das passt – du bist schließlich selbst der reinste Seeigel, Ella«, meinte Noah mit einer Verbeugung und einem Lächeln; ein Gentleman selbst dann, wenn er jemanden beleidigte.

Normalerweise wären ihr jetzt ihre Verehrer zu Hilfe gekommen und hätten versucht, Noah mit drohenden Blicken einzuschüchtern. Aber Toco starrte noch immer mit mürrischer Miene auf seinen Auftrag – wahrscheinlich konnte er noch nicht fassen, dass er mit mir zusammenarbeiten sollte – und Barry himmelte ja seit Neustem jemand anders an. Also erledigte Ella das mit den finsteren Blicken selbst, unterstützt von unserem kleineren Python-Wandler Tino, der Ella toll fand.

»Was sollst *du* machen?«, fragte ich Lucy.

Ralph, Nestor und ich sollen einem Zweiarm helfen, dem der Hurrikan an der Küste großviel kaputt gemacht hat, erzählte Lucy gut gelaunt. *Unter Wasser aufräumen kann ich gut, Spaß macht das!*

»Kann man dich mieten?«, fragte Finny.

»Aufräumen? Spaß?« Daphne schaute Lucy an, als kapiere sie die Welt nicht mehr. »Na, da gehe ich doch lieber shoppen. Schaut mal, Leute, mein Kleid ist von Balenciaga – ganz neu!«

»Wow, was hat das denn gekostet?«, fragte Leonora.

»Ach, ist doch nicht so wichtig.« Daphne winkte ab.

Ich wunderte mich kurz, weil ich wusste, dass ihre Mutter als Angestellte in einem Supermarkt arbeitete und ihr Vater hauptsächlich als Möwe lebte. Doch dann kam Shari in meine Richtung und ich blendete alles andere aus. Meist interessierte ich mich für das, was Daphne erzählte, ungefähr so sehr wie eine Seegurke für das aktuelle Kinoprogramm.

Shari hatte mich erreicht und strahlte mich an. »Cooler Auftrag, oder? Ich war noch nie in einer Menschenschule, meinst du, ich schaffe es, mich nicht zu verraten?«

»Klar schaffst du das«, versicherte ich ihr.

»Der Auftrag ist unglaublich öde und wahrscheinlich bekommst du zwischendurch Flossen, Delfin-Girl.« Feindselig starrte Toco uns ins Gesicht und rempelte nebenbei Ralph an, als der an ihm vorbeiging. »Am besten gehen wir heute Nachmittag, dann haben wir es hinter uns. Oder seid ihr anderer Meinung?«

»Nein«, sagte ich knapp. Während Ralph Toco einen bösen Blick zuwarf, tastete ich nach dem Handy in der Tasche meiner Badeshorts. Ralph und ich nickten uns zu. Er würde die Botschaft an seine Eltern überbringen und die würden hoffentlich Miss White fragen, falls sie es tatsächlich war. Mehr konnte er nicht tun.

Auch die Zweitjahresschüler bekamen Umschläge – wie wir herausfanden, war es ihr Job, uns auf unseren Missionen heimlich zu überwachen. Schon begannen manche, flüsternd zu diskutieren, wie sie das am besten anstellen konnten.

»Wenn ich jemanden sehe, der uns überwacht, mache ich ihn platt«, kündigte Toco den Zweitjahresleuten mit drohendem Blick an, während wir alle die Klasse verließen.

Oh prima. Das konnte wirklich nett werden.

Hi, Tiago! Das war mein Bruder Steve, wahrscheinlich war er wieder in der Lagune.

»Wartet ihr kurz?«, bat ich die anderen und rannte runter zum Strand. Ja, dort kreuzte seine Rückenflosse durchs Wasser, ein graues Dreieck, das ich längst nicht mehr fürchtete. *Was hast du rausgefunden, Steve?*

Dass es hier in der Gegend sehr leckere Zackenbarsche gibt. Haha, nein, nur Spaß. Ich wollte dir durchgeben, dass ich sieben Glasbodenboote und -schiffe gefunden habe, die behalte ich im Auge.

Anscheinend hatte mein Bruder einen Hang zu schlechten Witzen. Aber egal. *Oje, das sind wirklich viele,* gab ich erschrocken zurück. Die konnte er doch niemals ständig kontrollieren. Wir brauchten dringend die Minikamera, die Rocket mir versprochen hatte. Und eine neue Gelegenheit, Mrs Lennox zu sondieren.

»Tiago? Wo bleibst du?«, rief Shari und rasch verabschiedete ich mich von Steve. Jetzt war es erst mal Zeit für unsere Lernexpedition.

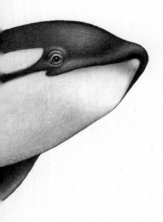

Eine rollende Überraschung

Ich fragte mich, wann eigentlich Miss Whites schwarzer BMW vom Parkplatz verschwunden war. Hatte den jemand für sie abgeholt? Sie war ja als Schwertwal weggeschwommen, da hatte sie auch ihre Sachen nicht mitnehmen können. Was war aus denen geworden? Keine Ahnung, und Mr Clearwater zu fragen, traute ich mich nicht.

Es war nicht weit bis zu der normalen Highschool von Key Largo, wir überlegten erst, ob wir zu Fuß gehen sollten, liehen uns dann aber doch ein paar der Schulfahrräder.

Shari hatte gerade erst das Radfahren gelernt und fand das Anfahren immer noch ziemlich schwierig. »Aaah, Hilfe, ich falle gleich um!«, quietschte sie, während sie auf abenteuerliche Art vom Parkplatz auf den ungeteerten Weg schlingerte.

»Weitertreten!«, rief ich. »Je schneller du bist, desto leichter wird es!«

Das hätte ich vielleicht nicht sagen sollen. Shari trat in die Pedale wie wild und schoss davon.

Toco und ich pedalten hastig hinterher und schafften es ganz knapp, sie abzufangen, bevor sie direkt vor einem SUV auf die Straße düste. Der hupte wütend und durch die Scheibe sahen wir, dass der Fahrer ziemlich eindeutige Mundbewegungen machte.

Toco zeigte ihm den hochgereckten Mittelfinger. Dann raunzte er unser Delfinmädchen an: »Sag mal, hast du einen Todeswunsch oder was?«

»Nö wieso?«, fragte Shari, sie war wieder bestens gelaunt. »Ich hab's mir überlegt, eigentlich macht Rad fahren doch ziemlich viel Spaß.«

»Ja schon, aber wenn du einem Auto in die Quere kommst, siehst du anschließend aus wie Finny als Rochen«, meinte ich. »Fahr mir einfach hinterher, okay?«

»Okay«, sagte Shari und lächelte mich an.

Beim nächsten Anfahren fiel sie um und klemmte sich dabei den Fuß ein. Aber sie jammerte nicht, sondern biss sich nur kurz auf die Lippe, richtete ihr Rad wieder auf und folgte mir, während wir auf dem Seitenstreifen an der Tankstelle und dem Burgerladen vorbei nach Key Largo reinfuhren. Toco blieb ein Stück hinter uns, vielleicht waren wir ihm peinlich.

Die normale Highschool war ein flaches Gebäude mit gepflegtem Rasen und einem Fahnenmast, an dem die amerikanische Flagge wehte. Neugierig betrachtete Shari die Schule. »Haben die auch einen Privatstrand, so wie wir?«

»Vermutlich nicht«, sagte ich und dachte an meine alte, von Maschendraht umzäunte Schule in Miamis übelstem Viertel Liberty City. Ich war dermaßen froh, dass ich da nicht mehr hingehen musste. »Was jetzt? Wahrscheinlich sollten wir erst mal das Sekretariat suchen, oder?«

»Logisch«, brummte Toco, hängte sich den Rucksack mit unserem mitgebrachten Material über eine Schulter und warf mir einen verächtlichen Blick zu. »Gut, dass man dir nicht ansieht, dass du 'n blutrünstiger Meeres-Mülleimer bist.«

»Ich bin was?« Schon spürte ich, wie sich in mir die Wut regte. Noch immer hatte ich das Problem, dass ich unglaublich schnell rotsah und durchdrehte, wenn andere nur ein bisschen ärgerlich geworden wären. Aber Miss White hatte mir ein paar Tricks beigebracht, mit denen ich mich in solchen Fällen ablenken konnte. Ich atmete ein paarmal tief und begann, meine Atemzüge zu zählen. Es half.

Aber Toco war noch nicht fertig mit mir.

»Tigerhaie fressen alles, was sie vor die Schnauze kriegen«, legte Toco nach, seine Augen funkelten. »Sogar Autoreifen und so einen Scheiß. Die sind einfach zu dämlich, Dreck von richtiger Beute zu unterscheiden.«

Wenn die Leute so über uns dachten, wunderte es mich nicht, dass sie sich zum Spaß anschauten, wie Taucher uns angriffen und verletzten! Ich starrte ihm in die blassblauen Augen. »Entweder du hörst jetzt auf, so einen Mist zu reden, oder ...«

»Leute, habt ihr eigentlich schon gewusst, dass wir auch eine Note für Zusammenarbeit bekommen?« Shari trat zwischen uns.

»Meinst du wirklich, jemand beobachtet uns gerade, Shari?« Ich schaute mich um, sah aber niemanden.

Auch Toco checkte die Umgebung ab. »Blödsinn, das behauptet Clearwater doch nur. Das ist so, wie wenn überall Schilder mit *Videoüberwachung* hängen, obwohl keine Kamera da ist.«

»Egal«, sagte Shari. »Du hast jedenfalls kein Recht, Tiago zu beleidigen, ist das klar?«

Toco warf ihr einen gehässigen Blick zu, hielt den Mund und zockelte düster brütend hinter uns her, als wir zum Eingang der Schule gingen. Unser ganz eigener Troll, toll!

Im Sekretariat wurden wir von einer Frau mit sportlichem Kurzhaarschnitt, die ein T-Shirt mit dem Schullogo trug, freundlich begrüßt. Ich erklärte, weshalb wir hier waren, und bekam zur Antwort: »Ah ja, ich weiß, wem ihr das Material am besten gebt.«

»Einem Biologielehrer?«, fragte ich, doch die Frau schüttelte den Kopf. »Nein, Daisy Cousteau. Sie leitet bei uns die Meeresschutz-AG. Ich rufe sie gleich mal aus, sie übt gerade Baseball.«

Es gab hier eine Meeresschutz-AG? Ich war beeindruckt. Ohne es zu wissen, schützten diese Leute *uns*.

Da im Sekretariat einiges los war, gingen wir raus in den Gang, um zu warten.

Wenige Minuten später kam dort ein schlankes, sonnengebräuntes Mädchen mit dunkelbraunen Locken und Sommersprossen auf uns zu … aber nicht auf ihren eigenen Füßen. Shari stieß einen Laut der Überraschung aus.

»Was ist?«, fragte ich. »Hast du noch nie einen Rollstuhl gesehen? Das ist ein Ding, mit dem man …«

»Ich weiß – hatten wir mal in Menschenkunde«, zischte Shari mir zu. »Aber merkst du denn nicht, dass sie …«

Daisy hatte uns erreicht und Shari bekam den Satz nicht zu Ende. Geschickt wendete das Mädchen, das einen blauen Hoody und bequeme Hosen trug, ihren Rollstuhl, den Baseballschläger hatte sie quer über ihre Beine gelegt. Sie begrüßte Shari und mich mit einem Lächeln. »Hallo! Ihr seid die Leute von dieser anderen Schule, oder? Schön, dass ihr da seid.«

Nachdem Shari und ich uns vorgestellt hatten, spähte Daisy an uns vorbei und musterte Toco, der noch immer mürrisch Abstand von uns hielt. »Gehört er auch zu euch?«

Wir wandten uns alle zu ihm um, aber es war Shari, die antwortete. »Er hat zwar vorhin ein paar blöde Sprüche über Tiago abgelassen, aber ja, er gehört zu uns«, sagte sie fest.

Etwas geschah in Tocos Gesicht, ich kann nicht genau beschreiben, was. Aber als er zu uns kam, schaffte er es sogar, die Mundwinkel nach oben zu ziehen. »Toco McBride. Hi.«

Währenddessen rätselte ich, was Shari mir hatte sagen wollen. Was sollte ich merken? Moment mal, war diese Daisy etwa ein Woodwalker oder Seawalker? Leider war mein Gespür dafür ziemlich schwach. Ich versuchte, dicht neben Daisy zu gehen, während sie uns, fröhlich plaudernd und dabei ihren Rollstuhl an den Schwungrädern vorantreibend, in die Cafeteria begleitete. Leider war ich zu abgelenkt von den neuen Eindrücken, um viel zu spüren.

»In meiner AG versuchen wir, die Leute dazu zu bringen, weniger Einwegplastik zu benutzen«, erzählte Daisy. »Dann gerät es nicht ins Meer und schadet Fischen, Schildkröten, Delfinen und allen anderen.«

»Haien zum Beispiel«, ergänzte ich.

»Gab es nicht mal einen berühmten Meeresforscher, der Cousteau hieß?«, fragte Toco und erstaunt blickten Shari und ich ihn an. In der Schule war er nicht gerade einer, der mit Wissen glänzte.

Daisy strahlte. »Ja, und ich bin seine Urenkelin«, sagte sie stolz. »Aber natürlich setze ich mich nicht nur deswegen für das Meer ein, ich mag es einfach! Trotz allem.«

»Sehr cool«, sagte ich, während wir uns an der Theke Limos holten – natürlich in Glasflaschen und ohne Plastikstrohhalm, sonst hätte Daisy uns bestimmt ihren Baseballschläger übergezogen.

Als ich Daisy ihre Flasche reichte, berührten sich fast unsere Finger und Aufregung durchströmte mich. Ja, sie war ein Wandler!

Shari, Toco und ich tauschten einen Blick und ich merkte,

dass auch die anderen das aufregend fanden. Und so kurz nach Wave!

»Was meinst du mit ›Trotz allem‹?«, fragte Shari.

Daisy deutete auf ihren Rollstuhl. »Na ja, wegen dem Meer sitze ich in dem hier.«

Ich verschluckte mich an meiner Limo. »Was?!«

»Wir haben Urlaub in Südamerika gemacht und da hat mich beim Baden eine Qualle erwischt ... das Gift hat irgendwie die Nerven in meinen Beinen geschädigt, die Ärzte wissen nicht genau, wie und warum«, erzählte Daisy. »Ich kann auf Krücken kurze Strecken gehen, aber es ist ziemlich mühsam. Zweimal die Woche muss ich zur Therapie.«

»Fies«, sagte ich und versuchte, mir vorzustellen, wie es wäre, nicht gehen zu können. »Wird das irgendwann wieder besser?«

»Eher nicht«, meinte Daisy und tastete nach dem goldenen Engel mit ausgebreiteten Flügeln, den sie um den Hals trug. »Aber jetzt erzählt mal von euch, seid ihr auch Klima- und Naturschützer?«

»Klar«, sagte Toco und wir sahen ihn schon wieder verdutzt von der Seite an. »Was?«, knurrte er. »Dachtet ihr, mir ist egal, ob die Erde sich in einen dampfenden Klumpen verwandelt?« Dafür bekam er ein strahlendes Lächeln von Daisy.

Toco wandte schnell den Blick ab, fummelte an seinem Rucksack herum, versuchte, die Unterlagen rauszuzerren, blieb damit stecken und zerstörte beinahe den Reißverschluss, während er es mit Gewalt versuchte. Dabei zerknickte er mindestens ein Drittel der Meeresschutz-Broschüren, die wir hier abgeben sollten. Shari und ich stöhnten.

»Ach, nicht schlimm, ich bügele die einfach, dann sieht man das nicht mehr«, versprach Daisy und bewunderte die Broschüren, die eine Arbeitsgruppe an unserer Schule entworfen und Mr Clearwater ausgedruckt hatte.

Während sie mehr über ihre AG erzählte, fiel es ihr zum Glück nicht auf, dass wir sie alle drei anstarrten. Was für ein Tier konnte sie in zweiter Gestalt sein? Ich sah keinen offensichtlichen Hinweis darauf. Sie war klein und dünn ... vielleicht ein ... äh ... verdammt, ich hatte einfach zu wenig Ahnung von Fischarten. Ein Hering?

Toco hatte ausgetrunken und pfefferte seine Glasflasche in Richtung Mülleimer, obwohl garantiert Pfand darauf war. Leider war er nicht sehr treffsicher und die Flasche zerschellte auf dem Boden in ungefähr zehntausend Stücke. Uninteressiert blickte Toco in eine andere Richtung.

Unsere Gastgeberin wirkte erschrocken. »Ups«, sagte sie. »Aber nicht schlimm. Die Kassiererin gibt dir bestimmt Kehrschaufel und Handbesen, damit du das wegräumen kannst.«

Natürlich tat Toco, als hätte er nichts gehört. Oh Mann! Shari und ich starben tausend Tode vor Verlegenheit.

»Mach schon – bitte!«, flüsterte Shari.

Gnädigerweise stand unser Alligator-Wandler auf, aber statt zu den Scherben schlenderte er zum Ausgang. Auf halbem Weg holte ich ihn ein und packte ihn am Arm. »Hier geht's lang«, zischte ich ihm zu und zwang ihn zu einer anderen Richtung.

Toco wollte sich losreißen, aber inzwischen wusste ich, wie stark ich war, und ließ nicht locker. Es half natürlich, dass er diesmal alleine war, ohne Kumpels, die ihm halfen. Während Shari Daisy ablenkte, drehte ich dem vor Wut fast platzenden Toco den Arm auf den Rücken. Dann tat ich so, als wolle ich ihm helfen, die Reste der Flasche aufzusammeln, und hoffte, dass Daisy nicht bemerkte, dass ich ihn in Wirklichkeit nach unten drückte. Zum Glück brachte uns gerade jemand eine Kehrschaufel.

»Los – auch Reptilien können ihren eigenen Dreck wegräumen«, kommandierte ich.

Toco drehte den Kopf, um mir einen hasserfüllten Blick zuwerfen zu können. »Vergiss es!«

»Wenn du es nicht machst, sage ich Ella, du warst den ganzen Tag total *nett* zu uns.«

»Okay, okay!« Sofort griff Toco nach der Kehrschaufel. Kurz darauf war die Schweinerei beseitigt. Ich atmete auf und sah, dass Shari ebenso erleichtert war.

»So, ich muss wieder zum Baseballtraining«, meinte Daisy, nahm ihren Schläger mit beiden Händen und tat so, als würde sie einen Ball übers Feld dreschen. »Ich bring euch noch raus, ja?«

Als Daisy neben uns zum Ausgang rollte, fragte Shari betont beiläufig: »Was ist eigentlich dein Lieblingstier?« Toco und ich spitzten die Ohren.

»Ich habe zwar zwei Katzen, aber am meisten liebe ich Delfine!«, erklärte unsere neue Bekannte und betrachtete ein bisschen neidisch Sharis Flossenkette. »Mein Zimmer daheim ist tapeziert mit Delfinpostern.«

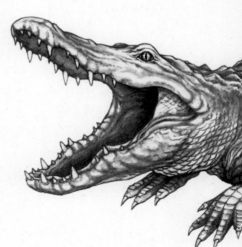

»Gute Wahl«, sagte Shari und blickte so selbstzufrieden, dass ich ihr einen Rippenstoß verpasste.

»Ja, sind schon tolle Tiere, nur manchmal ein bisschen wirrköpfig«, zog ich sie auf. »Wir haben drei davon an der Schule, sie schwimmen meistens in unserer Lagune herum und denken darüber nach, wie sie Spaß haben können.«

»Echt jetzt? Ihr habt zahme *Delfine?*« Völlig begeistert blickte Daisy uns an. »Kann ich mal vorbeikommen und mit ihnen schwimmen? Manchmal stelle ich mir vor, dass ich auch ein Delfin bin und mühelos durch die Wellen gleite ...«

»Komm uns doch mal besuchen«, sagten Shari und Toco fast gleichzeitig.

»Wenn meine Eltern es erlauben.« Daisy runzelte die Stirn. »Meine Mutter ist ein bisschen, äh, überbehütend und will nicht, dass ich ins Wasser gehe. Absolut verständlich nach dem, was mir mit dieser Qualle passiert ist, oder?«

»Absolut«, sagte ich.

Als wir aus dieser Schule raus waren, fingen wir alle gleichzeitig an zu reden.

»Sie ist ein Wandler! Ist das nicht der Hummer?«, schwärmte Shari.

»Hammer«, korrigierte ich, aber keiner hörte zu.

»Ich wette, sie ist eine Korallennatter, das sind wirklich hübsche kleine Schlangen«, brummte Toco, unser Reptil vom Dienst.

»Dagegen spricht aber, dass sie Delfine besonders mag«, widersprach ich. »Meint ihr, Mr Clearwater hat irgendwie erfahren, dass sie eine von uns ist? Vielleicht hat er uns gerade deswegen hingeschickt.«

»Keine Ahnung, am besten, wir fragen ihn«, sagte Shari und tanzte vor lauter Aufregung um unsere Fahrräder herum, was ihr seltsame Blicke der im Eingangsbereich herumstehenden menschlichen Schüler einbrachte. »Ich hoffe nur wirklich, dass sie kein Delfin ist.«

»Warum?«, fragte ich verblüfft.

»Ist doch klar.« Sharis Miene verdüsterte sich schlagartig. »Mr García hat uns doch erklärt, wie so was funktioniert. Wenn sie als Mensch gelähmt ist, ist sie das als Delfin auch. Und wenn sie bei ihrer ersten Verwandlung mit gelähmter Schwanzflosse zu schwimmen versucht ...«

Auf meinem Arm hatte sich eine Gänsehaut gebildet, die Härchen standen nach oben wie winzige Ausrufezeichen.

»... dann ertrinkt sie wahrscheinlich«, vollendete ich den Satz.

»Algenschleim!«, sagte Toco. »Hoffentlich besucht sie uns bald. Bevor ihr irgendwas passiert.«

Da waren wir uns ausnahmsweise einig.

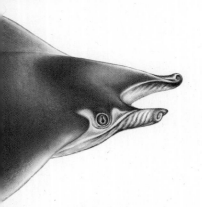

Schrott!

»Nein, ich wusste nichts davon. Wie heißt sie? Daisy Cousteau?« Jack Clearwater – gerade in einer Besprechung mit Mr García – wirkte höchst interessiert an unserer Entdeckung. »Ich versuche rauszukriegen, wo ihre Eltern wohnen und ob die auch Wandler sind. Vielleicht lässt es sich irgendwie einrichten, dass Daisy auf die Blue Reef gehen darf.«

»Das wäre meerig.« Shari klang noch immer besorgt.

Seit wir wieder in unserer Schule waren, wirkte Toco deutlich wortkarger als noch während unserer Expedition. »Haben Sie uns eigentlich bespitzeln lassen?«, fragte er nun so aggressiv wie eh und je.

»Bespitzeln? Das ist ein hässliches Wort«, meinte Mr Clearwater. »Natürlich seid ihr überwacht worden. Sonst wäre ich für die Note ja rein auf euren Bericht angewiesen. Übrigens Glückwunsch, Shari, dass du diesmal keine Verwandlungspanne hattest.«

»Aber ... wir haben niemanden gesehen«, sagte ich ein bisschen verwirrt.

Unsere Lehrer begannen beide zu grinsen. »Vincent ist gerade in der Eingangshalle und unterhält sich mit unserer Seeanemone Miss Monk, glaube ich«, erklärte unser Verwandlungslehrer. »Ihr könnt ihm gerne mal Hallo sagen.«

Die anderen marschierten gleich los und verschwanden die

Treppe hinunter, aber ich zögerte und blieb stehen. Es gab noch etwas, das mir auf der Seele lag. »Mr García ... haben Sie schon eine Idee, wie Sie das mit Lydia Lennox doch noch hinkriegen könnten? Der Termin ist ja geplatzt ...«

»Wird nicht leicht, einen neuen Termin bei ihr zu bekommen.« Farryn García runzelte die Stirn. »Außer, sie will mal selbst etwas von uns oder hat irgendwelche Pläne mit unserer Schule. Dann hätte ich bestimmt eine Chance, nah genug an sie herankommen.«

»Du willst es wirklich durchziehen?« Unser junger Schulleiter wirkte nicht begeistert. »Sei um Himmels willen vorsichtig. Wenn wir dich auch noch verlieren, kann ich den Laden hier dichtmachen.«

»Wird schon klappen«, meinte Mr García. »Glaub mir, Tiago, ich bin zwar ein Delfin, aber genauso daran interessiert, dass diese Haikämpfe aufhören. Ich finde es widerlich, Tiere für so etwas zu missbrauchen.«

»Das ist es«, sagte ich und gestand: »Außerdem habe ich Angst, dass sie noch mal meinen Bruder schnappen ... oder meinen Vater, der ist schließlich auch ein Tigerhai.«

»Oder dich.« Mr García musterte mich. »Darauf sollten wir es nicht ankommen lassen. Wir müssen diese Kämpfe stoppen.«

Da waren wir absolut einer Meinung!

»Schau mal, Neuigkeiten über Lydia Lennox' Kumpel Carl Bittergreen.« Er zeigte mir einen Zeitungsartikel. Schnell überflog ich ihn. Die Polizei wusste, dass Bittergreen unter anderem den Drogenschmuggel in Miami organisierte, doch nachdem ein Zeuge gegen ihn tot aufgefunden worden war, steckten sie mit ihren Ermittlungen in der Sackgasse.

Was für ein Widerling. Auf dem Zeitungsfoto war er mit

Lydia Lennox zu sehen, ein dritter Mann – jung, mit kantigem Gesicht und selbstsicherem Blick – stand neben den beiden. »Wer ist das denn?«, fragte ich Mr García.

»Patrick Blennon, der wichtigste Assistent von Mrs Lennox. Ein Woodwalker, soweit ich weiß«, sagte Mr García. »Kann gut organisieren und hat keinerlei Gewissen. Er passt wirklich gut zu ihr.«

Ich bedankte mich für die Infos und zischte ab in die Eingangshalle, wo Shari und Toco gerade mit einem dünnen Jungen mit ungesunder Gesichtsfarbe sprachen. »Das hier ist Vincent, er meint, wir hätten das ganz gut gemacht mit der Lernexpedition«, stellte Shari ihn vor und trat ein Stück zurück. »Willst du raten, was er ist? Rätst du nie!«

»Kleiner Tipp – *Ssssssssh!*«, meinte Finny, die sich zu uns gesellt hatte.

Das ersparte mir das Raten. »Du bist ein Moskito-Wandler?«, fragte ich fasziniert.

Vincent nickte, kam auf mich zu und schüttelte mir die Hand. Auch ich ging unauffällig rückwärts, weil er mir dabei ein wenig zu nah gekommen war. Außerdem hatte er Mundgeruch.

»Ihr habt Glück, dass ich eine männliche Stechmücke bin und kein Blut saugen muss«, meinte er. »Sonst hätte ich eure Daisy ein bisschen angezapft, haha, und keiner von euch hätte es gemerkt.«

Toco holte aus, um ihm die Faust ans Kinn zu knallen. Doch Vincent konnte den Schlag blocken und gleichzeitig ausweichen. Man merkte, dass er schon einige Zeit Kampfunterricht bei Miss White hatte!

»Na, na«, sagte Finny zu unserem Alligatorjungen. »Das finde ich jetzt ein bisschen übertrieben. Wer ist Daisy?«

Wir erklärten es ihr und natürlich war sie begeistert. »Cool, ich bin gespannt, was sie ist!«, sagte sie. »Aber erst mal müssen wir uns natürlich um Wave kümmern. Soll ich euch Bescheid geben, wenn er uns hier in der Schule besucht?«

»Wave kommt zu Besuch?«, fragte ich erfreut. »Aber Mr Clearwater hat doch ...«

Finny legte einen Finger auf ihre Lippen, denn gerade kamen unsere Lehrer die Treppe herunter.

Mehr erfuhren wir erst lange nach dem Abendessen. Genauer gesagt, erst dann, als uns eine leise Stimme aus dem Tiefschlaf riss.

»Hey, ihr! Wave ist da. Kommt ihr?«

Ich blinzelte mit schlafverklebten Augen in die Dunkelheit und sah Finnys Silhouette in der halb geöffneten Tür. Noch bevor ich antworten konnte, flüsterte Jasper, der heute als Junge schlief: »Kannste drauf wetten! Gib uns noch 'n Sekündchen.«

Hastig sprangen wir aus unseren Betten, zerrten uns T-Shirts über und schlichen auf bloßen Füßen über den Strand zum Hauptgebäude. Ein halbes Dutzend Leute standen schon dort, darunter Shari und ihre Delfinfreunde, Chris, Izzy ... und ein Junge, den ich nicht kannte. Auf den ersten Blick sah er mit seinen blauen Badeshorts aus wie einer von uns, aber mir fiel auf, dass ich das T-Shirt aus unserer schuleigenen Kleiderkiste kannte und er es verkehrt herum anhatte.

»Darf ich vorstellen?« Finny hatte ein ultrabreites Grinsen im Gesicht. »Das ist Wave in erster Gestalt.«

»Sehr meerig bei euch«, sagte der Junge, der nur wenig größer war als Finny und ich, aber dafür breitere Schultern hatte.

Er sah ein bisschen indianisch aus mit seinen langen braunen Haaren, die einen Kupferschimmer hatten, und seinen ein bisschen schräg stehenden, dunklen Augen. Staunend wie ein Kind, blickte er sich um, musterte die Gebäude, unsere Hütten, seine eigenen Füße. »Und ihr seid wirklich alles Wandler hier in der Schule?«

»Sogar die Lehrer und der Koch«, bestätigte Finny fröhlich. »Soll ich dir jetzt zeigen, wie es drinnen aussieht? Das packst du, oder?«

»Ach bestimmt«, sagte Wave. Sein Optimismus war mir ein bisschen unheimlich, schließlich hatte er sich noch nicht oft verwandelt. Aber ich fand es auch toll, dass er ein so großes Selbstvertrauen hatte. Davon hätte ich mir zu gerne ein Scheibchen abgeschnitten.

»Ich habe vom Meer aus schon oft Häuser gesehen, aber ich konnte mir nie vorstellen, wie es drinnen aussieht«, meinte Wave, als Blue ihm die Tür aufhielt und Izzy, Chris und ich uns hinter ihm durchdrängten in die kniehoch geflutete Cafeteria. »Jetzt weiß ich, dass sie innen nass sind – das hätte ich nicht gedacht.«

»Nur hier bei uns, normale Menschen mögen das nicht so«, meinte Chris. »Die haben daheim lieber trockene Füße.«

»Warum?«, fragte Wave verständnislos und betrachtete das Schuhregal am Eingang der Cafeteria. Noah reichte ihm seine Flip-Flops. »Hier, probier mal an. Wenn sie dir passen, schenke ich sie dir.«

Sie passten und Wave flappte mit schuhgeschmückten Füßen weiter. In der Eingangshalle bewunderte er das Aquarium – Miss Monk hauchte ihm tentakelwedelnd ein *Hallo* zu – und besonders die Tische und Stühle. »Was macht man damit?«, fragte er und sofort demonstrierten es ihm Finny, Izzy und ich, indem wir uns setzten. Wave begann zu lachen. »Ist das witzig! Wenn ich das meinen Eltern erzähle, werden sie sich totlachen. Vielleicht denken sie auch nur, dass ihr verrückt seid.«

Er ließ sich so schwer auf einen der Stühle fallen, dass ein Stuhlbein einknickte und er auf dem Boden landete. »Muss das so sein?«, fragte er verwirrt.

»Äh, nein, alles okay?«, fragte Finny und reichte ihm eine Hand, um ihn hochzuziehen.

»Hm, Riffe sind eindeutig stabiler als eure komischen Sachen hier«, meinte Wave, während er sich wieder aufrichtete. »Aber ich habe auch noch nie versucht, mich auf eins draufzusetzen.«

Währenddessen nahmen Chris und ich den kaputten Stuhl in Augenschein.

»Kein Problem, das reparieren wir morgen«, sagte ich und lauschte nervös in die Dunkelheit, ob einer der Lehrer den Krach gehört hatte – die meisten hatten eine kleine Wohnung im ersten Stock. »Ein paar Tropfen Holzkleber und die Lehrer merken nicht, dass er jemals kaputt war.«

»Wo kommt man denn dahin?«, fragte Wave und schaute sich die Treppe an. Er setzte einen Fuß auf die erste Stufe, anscheinend fasziniert davon, dass man so irgendwo hinaufgelangen konnte.

»Zu anderen Zimmern, in denen Leute arbeiten können«, erklärte Finny. »Komm, ich zeige sie dir ...«

Ich öffnete den Mund, wollte Finny warnen, dass das vielleicht keine gute Idee war. Aber schon schlichen die beiden die Treppe hoch und alle anderen folgten ihnen. Mit einem mulmigen Gefühl im Bauch schlich ich hinterher, weil ich natürlich nicht verpassen wollte, wie jemand, der bisher als Buckelwal gelebt hatte, unsere Welt entdeckte.

Stolz zeigte Finny ihrem neuen Bekannten die Bibliothek. Es

dauerte eine Weile, bis wir ihm erklärt hatten, was ein Buch war.

»Die Seiten sehen aus wie Fächerkorallen, nur kleiner«, meinte Wave, während er ein Lexikon durchblätterte. Dann riss er ein Stück von der Seite ab, steckte es sich in den Mund und kaute.

»Was machst du?«, schrie Finny auf und riss ihm das Lexikon weg. »Du hast gerade die Stichworte von *Riesenmuschel* bis *Riemenfisch* verschlungen!«

»Oh, tut mir leid. Ich wollte dich nicht traurig machen. Nur probieren, ob man davon im Notfall satt werden könnte.« Besorgt blickte Wave auf Finny hinab.

»Ich hab mal gelesen, dass Buckelwale eine Tonne Fisch am Tag verputzen«, mischte ich mich ein und die anderen sahen ein bisschen geschockt aus. Tausend Kilo! Das war ungefähr so viel wie zweitausend richtig dick belegte Pizzas.

»Aber nur im Sommer, wenn wir ganz weit im Norden sind«, versicherte uns Wave. »Im Winter, wenn wir ins warme Wasser schwimmen, fressen wir ein halbes Jahr lang *gar nichts*. Na ja, ab und zu einen kleinen Fischschwarm, wenn wir zufällig einem begegnen.«

Falls uns das beruhigen sollte, wirkte es nicht so richtig.

»Der würde unser Riff ruck, zuck leer fressen«, flüsterte Izzy besorgt.

»Nenn ihn nicht ›der‹, er heißt Wave. Und so was würde er nie tun«, gab Finny ein bisschen trotzig zurück.

Wave widersprach nicht weiter, was wahrscheinlich daran lag, dass er nicht mehr zuhörte. Er war schon mit seinen nächsten Erkundungen beschäftigt. Im Computerraum rätselte er, was da für graue Dinger herumstanden, und konnte auch mit unserer Erklärung, dass es sich um Laptops handelte, nichts anfangen. »Ist das auch etwas, worauf man sich setzen kann?«

»*Nein!*«, riefen fünf Leute gleichzeitig.

Blue bekam allmählich Schnappatmung. »Man kann sie auch nicht essen!«

»Wir müssen es ihm zeigen, sonst kann er sich das nicht vorstellen«, sagte Jasper eifrig, wieselte zu einem der Laptops und schaltete ihn ein.

Ganz schlechte Idee. Irgendjemand hatte nämlich, nachdem wir Wave kennengelernt hatten, einen neuen Bildschirmhintergrund eingestellt. Genau – einen Buckelwal!

»Oh ... bin ich das?«, fragte Wave und schaute genauer hin. Ich sah, wie ein Schauer durch seinen Körper lief, und ahnte entsetzt, dass er gerade ein Verwandlungskribbeln spürte.

»Raus! Wir müssen ihn rausbringen, schnell!«, rief ich, packte Wave am Arm ... und spürte, wie dieser Arm seine Form veränderte, flach und knotig wurde. Auf einmal fühlte er sich an wie Hartgummi. Ich hatte nicht mal mehr Zeit, »Achtung!« zu rufen. Schon pflügten Waves Arme, die sich plötzlich in meterlange Flossen verwandelt hatten, durch den Raum.

Auf der Suche nach dem Ausgang drehte Wave sich um sich selbst ... und fegte dabei alle drei Laptops von den Tischen, es krachte und splitterte. Seine eine Flossenspitze fetzte eine Pinnwand herunter, die andere warf einen Stuhl um. Izzy, Chris und ich warfen uns in Deckung unter die Computertische, Finny drückte sich gegen die Wand und Jasper rollte sich als Gürteltier in einer Ecke zusammen, seine Klamotten lagen überall verstreut.

Natürlich waren ungefähr zehn Sekunden später sämtliche Lehrer vor Ort, außerdem eine empörte Mrs Misaki im Nachthemd und ein verschreckt wirkender Hausmeister, halb Krake, halb Mensch. Sie fragten nicht lange, was hier los war, das sahen sie selbst. Auch dass ein paar Tropfen Holzkleber diesmal nicht reichen würden.

Jack Clearwaters Lippen waren zusammengepresst, ich merkte, dass er wütend war, aber erstaunlicherweise blieb er freundlich. »Ganz ruhig, Wave«, sagte er zu dem jungen Buckelwal-Wandler, der schwer atmete, wilde Augen hatte und noch immer nach einem Ausgang suchte. »Atmen. Gleichmäßig atmen. Halt still, nicht bewegen.«

Er legte Wave beide Hände auf die (noch halbwegs menschlichen) Schultern und blickte ihm in die Augen. »Alles gut. Wir bringen dich hier raus.« Unser Schulleiter wandte sich an uns. »Hat jemand ein Foto von ihm in kompletter Menschengestalt?«

»Ja ich.« Finny reichte ihm ihr Handy mit dem Schnappschuss eines lächelnden, leicht indianisch wirkenden Jungen darauf.

»Schau es dir an, Wave. Das bist du, so siehst du aus. Spürst du das Kribbeln? Ganz ruhig.«

Nach fünf Minuten intensiver Betreuung waren die Arme unseres Besuchers wieder geschrumpft und Mr García und Miss Bennett eskortierten Wave ins Meer zurück.

Mr Clearwater blieb bei uns im Computerraum und stemmte die Arme gegen die Hüften. »Finny, das hast du organisiert, richtig? War dir nicht klar, dass ihn das vollkommen überfordern würde?«

»Es tut mir leid«, sagte Finny zerknirscht. »Aber es hat ihm so viel Spaß gemacht, sich hier alles anzuschauen.«

»Das kann ich mir vorstellen! Aber jetzt habe ich hier drei wasserdichte Speziallaptops, von denen jeder mal tausend Dollar gekostet hat und die jetzt nur noch Schrott sind! Dafür hast du dir einen Verweis mehr als verdient, Finny.«

»Ja stimmt«, flüsterte unsere Rochen-Wandlerin und ich sah Tränen in ihren Augen glänzen.

Wir ließen alle die Köpfe hängen. Dreitausend Dollar! So viel Geld hatte keiner von uns, das war klar. »Sind die nicht versichert?«, wagte ich zu fragen und kassierte dafür einen strengen Blick.

»Nicht gegen unfreiwillige Verwandlungen!«

Jasper schmiegte sich als Gürteltier an Shari, die völlig geschockt wirkte von dem, was passiert war. *Ist noch was übrig von dem Gold, das Lucys Freund Leon für uns hochgeholt hat?*

»Das Geld habe ich für die Reparatur der Hurrikanschäden ausgegeben. Und das Wrack liegt so tief, dass wir es selbst nur schwer erreichen können, um Nachschub zu holen. Auf weiteres Gold sollten wir also nicht zählen.« Langsam schien Mr Clearwaters Zorn zu verrauchen, er seufzte. »Ab ins Bett mit euch, morgen überlegen wir uns eine Lösung. Notfalls muss ich eben betteln gehen. Beim Rat oder bei … irgendwelchen reichen Wandlern.«

Nicht bei Mrs Lennox! Bitte nicht! Der Gedanke war mir unerträglich.

Niedergeschlagen schlichen wir zurück zu unseren Hütten.

Wave?, hörte ich Shari in Gedanken rufen, aber es kam keine Antwort. Der junge Buckelwal war wieder unterwegs.

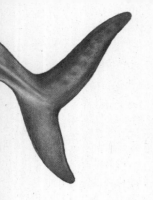

In dunkle Tiefen

Auf dem Weg zu unseren Hütten machten wir einen Abstecher zur Lagune und ließen uns davon trösten, dass kleine Wellen unsere Beine umspülten. Hoffentlich ging es Wave gut – war er schon auf seiner weiten Wanderschaft? Würde er nach diesem Schock überhaupt noch mal versuchen, sich zu verwandeln?

Plötzlich ergriff Shari das Wort. »Ich will nicht, dass Mr Clearwater bei irgendjemandem betteln muss, nur weil wir etwas angerichtet haben. Wie wäre es, wenn wir noch mehr Gold aus dem Wrack hochholen und es ihm geben?«

»Gute Idee eigentlich, aber Lucys bester Freund Leon – dieser Tieftaucher – ist wieder zurück in Kalifornien«, wandte Chris ein.

»Dem guten alten Kalifornien!« Izzy seufzte. »Leider ein paar Tausend Meilen weit weg.«

»Vielleicht schaffen wir es auch ohne Leon«, wandte ich ein.

Genau, haltet eben ein bisschen länger die Luft an, Leute, sagte Nox. *Wie schwer kann das sein?*

»Was weißt *du* denn darüber, du buntes Kleintier?«, fragte Shari.

»Jetzt gib bloß nicht mit deinen Kiemen an«, legte Chris nach.

»Eins ist klar, ich bin dabei.« Ich hob die Hand. »Es ist an der Zeit herauszufinden, wie tief so ein Tigerhai kommt. Wer macht noch mit?«

»Ich natürlich, schließlich ist das Ganze meine Schuld.« Finny reckte den Arm.

Shari sah enttäuscht aus. »Bei mir macht es keinen Sinn, Große Tümmler tauchen nicht besonders tief.« Auch Noah schüttelte den Kopf. »Sorry, aber dreihundert Meter sind ein bisschen *too much*. Oder eher, nicht nur ›ein bisschen‹.«

Zu unserer Überraschung war es die sonst so ruhige Blue, die sich meldete. Sie blickte entschlossen drein. »Ich bin ein Hochseedelfin. Wahrscheinlich komme ich ziemlich weit runter, auch wenn ich außer Übung bin.«

Und ich! Wir waren tausend Meter tief, Leon und ich. Lucy war längst von ihrer Lernexpedition zurück, ich fühlte, wie ihre Krakenarme sich um meine Beine ringelten und ganz zart meine Zehen betasteten.

»Super«, sagte ich und lächelte meine Freunde aufmunternd an. »Wir schaffen das und haben ruck, zuck das Geld für neue Laptops zusammen, ihr werdet sehen.«

Dankbar lächelte Finny zurück. Sie hatte hoffentlich nicht ernsthaft gedacht, wir würden sie mit diesen dreitausend Dollar Schulden alleine lassen?

Ich war zwar müde – schließlich hatte ich mir schon die letzte Nacht um die Flossen geschlagen –, aber als die anderen sofort rausschwimmen wollten, sagte ich nichts, sondern zog mich einfach aus und stellte mir mein Hai-Ich vor, um mich zu verwandeln.

Shari brauchte drei Anläufe, viel gutes Zureden und fast zwanzig Minuten für ihre Verwandlung. Das war auch gut so, denn während dieser Zeit fiel Jasper noch ein, dass wir fast die Ausrüstung vergessen hätten. Er rannte zurück und holte aus dem Fundus der Schule einen Leinenbeutel, eine kleine Pressluftflasche und einen Hebeballon.

»Was ist das denn?« Neugierig betastete Shari den schlaffen Ballon, der ungefähr viermal so groß war wie das beliebte Modell für Kinder. Er bestand aus gummiertem Stoff.

Damit kann man Ding hochholen, informierte sie Lucy. *Man muss ihn nur festhaken und Luft in den Ballon reinblasen, dann schwebt er nach oben. Mit Ding!*

»Ach so«, sagte Noah. »Sieht aus, als würde sogar ein Hörnchen reinpassen. Wenn Holly hier wäre, müssten wir sie wahrscheinlich mit Gewalt davon abhalten, mit auf Tiefseeexpedition zu gehen.« Er bekam einen ganz sehnsüchtigen Blick.

Wir einigten uns schnell auf ein Team. Finny, die zwar mies in Geografie war, aber dafür lustigerweise einen guten Ortssinn hatte, würde uns an die richtige Stelle führen. Blue konnte wie die anderen Delfine Objekte mit Schallwellen »durchleuchten« und feststellen, welche Klumpen Gold waren. Lucy würde die Brocken in den Sammelbeutel heben, den Hebeballon dranhaken und die Pressluft aufdrehen. Und ich? Ich war der große Beschützer, der die anderen beim Ab- und Auftauchen sichern sollte.

»Es wird mir eine Ehre sein«, schwafelte ich geschmeichelt.

»Jaja, schon gut – packen wir's an«, sagte Finny.

Unsere Delfin-Wandler umarmten sich und drückten in ihrem Maori-Gruß Stirn und Nase aneinander, Shari zog mich einfach zu ihnen und schon berührte Blues Nasenspitze meine.

Nachdem Shari es endlich geschafft hatte, sich zu verwandeln, ging es los. In ihrer Rochengestalt führte uns Finny zu der Stelle, die uns Leon gezeigt hatte. Dort lag eine der vielen Galeonen, mit denen die Spanier damals Gold aus der Neuen Welt nach Spanien gebracht hatten. Das Schiff selbst war längst verrottet – Holz zersetzt sich unter Wasser irgendwann – und seine Metallteile überkrustet, aber angeblich noch zu erkennen.

Unwillkürlich wollte ich ein paarmal tief einatmen, aber als Hai hatte ich das natürlich nicht nötig.

Möge Tangaroa mit euch sein!, rief Noah, als Lucy nach unten schoss, einen ihrer acht Arme um die Pressluftflasche geklammert.

Genau, und lasst euch nicht von irgendwas fressen, empfahl uns Shari, die uns ein Stück begleitete, aber schon bald umkehrte.

Wir versuchen es, gab ich ein bisschen beklommen zurück und hielt mich in der Nähe der anderen. Ich war noch nie richtig tief runtergegangen und fragte mich, wie ich damit zurechtkommen würde. Und wem wir dort unten begegnen würden. Klar, ich hatte in meiner alten Schule Sachbücher über die Tiefsee durchgeschmökert, aber in ein paar Minuten wirklich dort zu sein, war eine ganz andere Nummer. Obwohl, galten dreihundert Meter überhaupt schon als Tiefsee? Bestimmt nicht – und ich machte mir hier ganz umsonst ins Hemd.

Juchhu ... ab nach unten! Blue, ein schlanker, gestreifter Delfin, tauchte Lucy pfeilschnell hinterher, den Hebeballon in der Schnauze. Auch ich richtete den Kopf steil nach unten. Es war tröstlich, dass meine feinen Haisinne die Bewegungen der anderen neben mir wahrnahmen.

Dunkel war es sowieso schon, aber in den oberen Wasserschichten hatten meine Augen noch das schwache Mond- und Sternenlicht aufgefangen. Nun wurde es immer finsterer und kälter. Nicht sehr angenehm. Außerdem drückte das Wasser immer heftiger gegen meinen Körper. Erst fiel mir das kaum auf, aber dann immer stärker.

Ich versuchte, nicht an die vielen Tausend Tonnen Wasser zu denken, die von oben auf mich herabpressten.

Wir sind auf etwa hundertfünfzig Meter, schätze ich, sagte Blue, ein Schatten in der Dunkelheit.

Ist dir noch wohl, Tiago?, wollte Lucy wissen.

Geht so, gestand ich ... aber dann sah ich etwas, was mich von meiner Beklommenheit ablenkte. Vor uns jede Menge blaue Lichter, es wirkte wie eine außerirdische Großstadt von oben. Ein Meer aus Licht, das aus vielen kleinen Leuchtpünktchen bestand.

Wow, was ist das?, fragte ich.

Mhmm, Laternenfische, sagte Blue. *Und ausgerechnet jetzt habe ich das Maul voll!*

Lass bloß nicht den Hebeballon los, sagte ich zu ihr.

Wir tauchten ein in den leuchtenden Schwarm. Die Lichter waren um uns herum, wichen vor uns zurück, flossen um uns herum, als die Laternenfische versuchten, Abstand zu uns zu halten. Der Anblick verzauberte mich so sehr, dass ich vergaß, wie unangenehm der Druck war. Ich drehte und wendete mich, badete im blauen Schein.

Wohin will Tiago?, fragte Lucy erstaunt, während sie und Blue weiter abtauchten.

Keine Ahnung, er schwimmt, als wäre er besoffen, meinte Blue.

Ich bin nicht besoffen, protestierte ich. *Aber es wäre nett, wenn mir jemand sagen könnte, wo oben und unten ist ...*

Oh Mann, Haie!, kam es zurück, dann zeigten meine Freunde

mir den Weg. Sie hatten es eilig, klar, auch Blue konnte nicht ewig die Luft anhalten. Aber als ich etwas Überraschendes spürte, bremste ich trotzdem ab. War hier etwas oder jemand? Meine Sinne meldeten mir, dass wir nicht mehr allein waren. Als Hai kann man keine Gänsehaut bekommen, aber dafür hatte ich plötzlich Schluckauf. Als Hai. Total peinlich.

Was ist?, fragte Blue beunruhigt.

Wir werden beobachtet, sagte ich, jetzt ganz in meiner Rolle als Bodyguard. Vorsichtig schwamm ich einen Kreis, um herauszufinden, woher dieses Gefühl kam. Blue stieß währenddessen Klicklaute aus, um zu orten, ob außer uns noch jemand in der Gegend herumhing.

Meine empfindlichen Haiaugen erfassten ein blaues Leuchten in der Nähe – was war das denn? Neugierig schwamm ich auf den Leuchtpunkt zu, der hin und her zuckte.

Nicht!, rief Lucy.

Plötzlich erhellte rötliches Licht die unmittelbare Umgebung – und was ich sah, verschlug mir die Sprache.

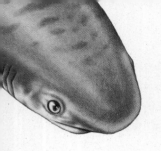

Unheimliche Begegnung

Ich sah ein grauenhaft aussehendes Wesen. Es hatte nadelspitze, glasartige Fangzähne, die so groß waren, dass sie nicht mehr in seinen Kopf passten, und große weiße Zombie-Glotzaugen. Das blaue Licht kam von einer Art länglichem Schwanz, der aber an seinem Kinn befestigt war, das rote Licht von irgendwelchen Organen an seinem Kopf. Und leider hing dieses Albtraumtier nur eine Handlänge von meiner Schnauze entfernt im Wasser und starrte mir grimmig ins Gesicht.

Ich erschrak so sehr, dass ich versuchte rückwärtszuschwimmen. Was nicht gut klappte.

Blue schrie auf. *Tiago! Was machst du?*

Aaaaah! Mein Gezappel hatte mich in die Gegenrichtung treiben lassen. Gleich würde ich mit diesem Fisch mit den Riesenzähnen zusammenstoßen. Netterweise versuchte er auszuweichen, aber mit seinen mickrigen Flösschen war er nicht gerade ein schneller Schwimmer.

Wir prallten zusammen und ich sah Sterne. Aber nicht, weil der Zusammenstoß so wehgetan hatte, sondern weil dieser ganze seltsame Fisch aufleuchtete. Eine Orgie aus pulsierenden Lichtern.

Du kannst jetzt wieder ruhig werden, Tiago, sagte Lucy. *Denk dran, fünfmal größer bist du als dieser Viperfisch!*

Das stimmte. Als er direkt vor meiner Schnauze gewesen war, hatte er riesig ausgesehen, aber als er nun hastig davonflösselte, sah ich, dass er kaum armlang war. Ups. Hoffentlich erzählten die anderen nicht weiter, wie sich ihr Beschützer eben angestellt hatte.

Wenn du hier irgendwo ein Licht siehst ... nicht hinschwimmen, meistens ist es ein Köder, schärfte uns Lucy ein und ein bisschen belämmert folgten Blue und ich ihr weiter nach unten.

Aber nicht besonders weit. Der Wasserdruck fühlte sich inzwischen an, als würde mich eine Schraubzwinge einquetschen. Kurz darauf gab ich auf. *Fürchte, ich muss umkehren*, sagte ich zu Lucy und Blue.

Oh ... bist du sicher?, fragte Blue. *Von hier aus ist es bestimmt nicht mehr weit zum Meeresboden.*

Sorry, presste ich hervor, drehte um und schwamm hastig nach oben. Mist! Jetzt konnte ich nur hoffen, dass meine Freunde es schafften, sonst konnten wir die neuen Laptops vergessen. Daumen drücken ging als Hai leider nicht.

Oben angekommen, musste ich Shari und Finny beichten, dass ich es nicht bis zum Schatzwrack geschafft hatte. *Nicht schlimm*, versuchte Shari mich zu trösten, schwamm dicht neben mich und stupste mich mit der Schnauze an. *Was war das vorhin für ein Gedankengeschrei bei euch da unten?*

Ich habe mich vor einem kleinen, leuchtenden Fisch erschreckt, gestand ich, weil Blue es ihr sowieso erzählen würde.

Shari pfiff vor Begeisterung. *Oooh, ein leuchtender Fisch? Wieso hast du mir keinen mitgebracht? Meine Nachttischlampe ist kaputt!*

Er hatte leider was dagegen, mitgenommen zu werden, erklärte ich. *Und seine Zähne waren größer als meine.*

Wir hörten auf herumzufrotzeln, als uns ein schwacher Fernruf von Blue erreichte. *Wir sind unten und haben das Wrack gefunden, aber ich muss blöderweise auch wieder hoch! Tut mir echt leid, Lucy ... schaffst du alles Weitere alleine? Hier ist der Hebeballon.*

Schaff ich schon, Flossenfreundin, hörte ich Lucy antworten.

Kurz darauf schoss Blue zurück zu uns an die Oberfläche und atmete erst mal ausgiebig. Wir mussten noch unendlich lange warten, bis Lucy endlich aus der Tiefe rief: *So! Ich schicke euch was hoch.*

Wir jubelten, als der Hebeballon an die Oberfläche ploppte. Shari schnappte sich den schweren Leinenbeutel und triumphierend schwammen wir zurück zur Schule. Der tropfende, verkrustete Inhalt erwies sich leider zum größten Teil als normale Steine, die Lucy versehentlich eingepackt hatte. Aber es waren auch ein paar verkrustete Klümpchen Gold dabei. Als wir sie bei Mr Clearwater abgaben, war er beeindruckt. »Könnte für neue Laptops reichen. Respekt, Leute.«

»Yay! Geschafft!« Finny drückte uns alle erleichtert und Lucy umkrakte uns mit allen acht Armen. Aber sie wirkte sehr matt und zog sich gleich in ihren Tonkrug unter Wasser zurück, um auszuruhen.

»Oft können wir ihr so was nicht zumuten, das ist klar«, sagte Shari besorgt.

Da wussten wir noch nicht, was uns am nächsten Tag bevorstand.

»Einen Viperfisch habt ihr gesehen? Ich glaube, über den steht hier was drin.« Nestor hatte ein paar brandneu wirkende

Naturbücher zu unserem Tisch-Boot mitgebracht und gerade blätterten wir den Band *Tiefsee* durch, bis wir das richtige Monster fanden.

Beeindruckt betrachteten meine Freunde das Foto. »Der pikt sich ja selbst in die Nase mit seinen Zähnen«, meinte Jasper erstaunt.

»Ich vermute, er hat keine Nase«, sagte ich und las mir den Text durch. »Wow, hört mal zu ... ›Der Viperfisch kann Tiere fressen, die größer sind als er selbst‹!«

Erschrocken schauten alle mich an.

»Hey, Leute, Tiago ist *dreieinhalb Meter* lang, schon vergessen? Das wäre ungefähr so, als würde *ich* versuchen, ihn runterzuschlucken«, sagte Finny.

»Viel Erfolg«, war das Einzige, was mir dazu einfiel.

Shari strich bewundernd über die Fotoseiten. »Tolle Bücher übrigens, Nestor. Sind die aus der Bibliothek?«

»Nein, das sind meine.« Stolzgeschwellt zeigte Nestor ihr gleich noch drei andere, ebenfalls nagelneue Bildbände, die er zum Frühstück mitgebracht hatte. Die sahen echt teuer aus.

Ich freute mich nach all den Aufregungen, dass wir nun ein bisschen ganz normalen Unterricht hatten. In Englisch und Mathe meldete ich mich so oft wie möglich, um ein paar mündliche Pluspunkte zu sammeln, und freute mich, als Miss Bennett in Gewässerkunde kurz vorbeischaute, um uns den Sei-dein-Tier-Test zurückzugeben. Auf meinem Blatt prangte eine Zwei plus. Ich freute mich enorm. Die Eins hatte ich nur verfehlt, weil ich den Fachbegriff für die oben dunkle, unten helle Körperzeichnung nicht gewusst hatte (ich hätte *Gegenschattierung* hinschreiben müssen).

In Gewässerkunde nahmen wir das Seegras durch und erfuhren, dass es fünfunddreißigmal so viel Kohlendioxid aufnehmen und speichern konnte wie dieselbe Fläche Regenwald. Ein echter Geheimtipp gegen die Klimakatastrophe!

»Und es schmeckt sogar noch gut«, verkündete Mara, Seekuh in zweiter Gestalt. »Ich hab schon ganz viel davon abgeweidet ...«

Zwei Dutzend entsetzte Blicke trafen sie.

»... aber wenn man es frisst, wächst es wieder nach, ganz ehrlich!«, versicherte Mara erschrocken und zum Glück nickte Mrs Pelagius. »Das stimmt.«

Als wir uns zum Mittagessen aufmachten, stöhnte Chris: »Und jetzt Kampf und Überleben bei Miss Bennett – das wird wieder so dermaßen langweilig ...«

»Superöde!«, sagte Noah.

»Und es bringt noch nicht mal was«, beschwerte sich Blue.

»Gibt's irgendwas Neues von Miss White?«, fragte mich Juna hoffnungsvoll, als sie an unserem Tisch-Boot vorbeikam. Ich konnte nur den Kopf schütteln und beschloss, dass ich heute, wenn wir den Unterricht hinter uns hatten, noch einmal losschwimmen würde, um meine Lieblingslehrerin zu suchen.

Doch dazu kam es nicht, nach dem Mittagessen war es mit dem ruhigen Schultag vorbei. Kaum hatten wir uns nach dem Essen wieder bei der Lagune vor einer unsicher wirkenden Miss Bennett versammelt, kam mit langen Schritten Mr Clearwater aus dem Hauptgebäude zu uns. Er sah sehr ernst aus und war ungewöhnlich schick gekleidet – bisher hatte ich ihn nur an den Besuchstagen mit einem weißen Hemd, Jeans und richtigen Schuhen gesehen. »Chris und Finny, kommt ihr bitte mit mir?«

»Oh! Haben diese beiden etwas angestellt?«, fragte Miss Bennett verblüfft.

»Ausnahmsweise mal nicht, ich brauche sie für eine Sondermission«, sagte Jack Clearwater knapp. »Es gibt ein Problem.«

»Was denn für eins?«, fragte Ella und klang dabei endgelangweilt.

»Gerade habe ich einen Anruf bekommen. Wave ist von der Polizei verhaftet worden.«

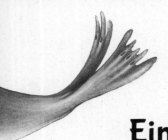

Ein Wal im Gefängnis

»Zieht euch schnell was Ordentliches an, wir fahren zum Polizeirevier«, bat unser Schulleiter die erschrocken dreinblickenden Auserwählten.

»Ist er ... ist Wave denn in Ordnung?«, fragte Shari und Finny war ganz blass geworden. Der Rest der Klasse lauschte atemlos.

»Keine Ahnung«, antwortete Jack Clearwater. »Es hieß nur, sie hätten einen jugendlichen Straftäter geschnappt, der sich weigere, mehr zu sagen als seinen Vornamen. Aber er hat die Officers zum Glück gebeten, unserer Schule Bescheid zu geben.«

»Straftäter?« Chris schüttelte den Kopf. »Aber Wave ist doch ein total netter Kerl, was soll der denn getan haben?«

»Bitte, Mr Clearwater, lassen Sie noch Tiago mitkommen«, bettelte Finny. »Und Shari! Schließlich haben die beiden Wave mit entdeckt, er vertraut ihnen.«

»Es sollte möglichst nicht die ganze Klasse dort auf dem Polizeirevier antanzen«, meinte Mr Clearwater und warf mir einen Blick zu. »Und was ist, wenn du dort eine Verwandlungspanne hast, Shari?«

»Werde ich nicht – ich habe geübt, ganz ehrlich!«

»Na gut, Shari und Tiago sind dabei.«

Chris sah nicht begeistert aus, als mein Name fiel. Wahrscheinlich hatte er gehofft, diese Sondermission zusammen mit Shari durchziehen zu können, ohne dass ich dabei störte.

»So, jetzt aber Beeilung«, drängte Jack Clearwater. »Ihr wisst, in welcher Gefahr Wave ist, oder?«

Wir nickten. Mein Mund war ganz trocken, als ich daran dachte, wie unerfahren Wave noch bei Verwandlungen war. Stichwort Computerraum! Wenn er sich in der Zelle, in die sie ihn vermutlich gesperrt hatten, plötzlich in einen Buckelwal verwandelte, würde das nicht nur Schlagzeilen machen, sondern ihn auch umbringen.

»Sollen wir ein paar Eimer Wasser mitnehmen? Damit wir ihn anfeuchten können, so wie ihr es mit mir gemacht habt bei diesem Miami-Ausflug?«, fragte Shari.

»Ja gut, aber viel nützen wird es nicht«, sagte Mr Clearwater und strich sich abwesend durch das hellblonde Haar. »Was einen Großwal an Land tötet, ist sein eigenes Gewicht ... und ein um ihn herum einstürzendes Haus wird nicht gerade helfen.«

»Sein eigenes Gewicht?«, fragte ich verblüfft.

»Das kenne ich auch«, meldete sich Shari zu Wort. »Im Wasser bin ich schwerelos. Aber wenn ich an Land komme, fühle ich mich, als wäre mein Körper mit Steinen gefüllt. Ein ganz blödes Gefühl ...«

»... und bei einem so gewaltigen Tier wie einem Wal leiden dabei die Organe.« Jack wandte sich an unsere Rochen-Wandlerin. »Finny, du hast ein Foto von Wave als Mensch. Kannst du es mir weiterleiten, jetzt gleich? Ich drucke es aus, sodass wir es mitnehmen können.«

»Klar.« Schon tippte Finny wie wild auf ihr Handy ein.

Die anderen und ich rasten zu unseren Hütten, um uns hastig in unsere schicksten Sachen zu werfen. Dann sprangen wir in unseren dunkelblauen Kleinbus. »Falls einer von euch ein Bild von einem Buckelwal dabeihat, ist das *jetzt* der Moment, es aus dem Wagen zu werfen«, sagte Mr Clearwater. »Und nehmt das Wort ›Wal‹ bitte gar nicht erst in den Mund!«

Wir nickten.

Er fuhr schweigend und konzentriert, so schnell, wie die Geschwindigkeitsbegrenzung es gerade noch erlaubte. Trotzdem schien es endlos zu dauern, bis wir endlich vor dem Polizeirevier in Miami ankamen, einem schlichten, hellbraun gestrichenen Klotz.

»Ist das Revier das, auf dem dein Vater arbeitet?«, fragte ich Finny neugierig. »Vielleicht kann er uns helfen ...«

»Ja, es ist genau das Revier, aber er hat heute erst ab achtzehn Uhr Dienst«, sagte sie und setzte sich eine Basecap auf, die den größten Teil ihrer blauen Haare verbarg. »Oh Mann, ich kann es noch gar nicht glauben! Wave, hier drinnen!«

Shari wirkte völlig fertig. »Der arme Kerl, er weiß bestimmt nicht mal, was Polizei ist. Ich konnte mir darunter auch erst nichts vorstellen, als ich an Land gekommen bin.«

Wir durften zu einer Empfangstheke gehen, an der uns ein Officer mit hellbraunem Uniformshirt und dunkelbrauner Krawatte begrüßte. »Das ist der Sergeant, der gerade Dienst hat«, flüsterte Finny uns zu.

»Guten Tag, Sir, ich bin Jack Clearwater, Leiter der Blue Reef Highschool«, sagte unser Schulleiter. »Wir sind wegen Wave hier.«

»In welcher Beziehung stehen Sie zu dem Angeklagten?«, fragte der Cop. »Geht er auf Ihre Schule?«

»Nein, noch nicht, aber er wollte sich dafür bewerben, dafür war er in der Gegend«, gab Jack zurück, während wir uns ein bisschen eingeschüchtert, aber aufmerksam lauschend im Hintergrund herumdrückten. »Was hat er denn getan?«

»Er wurde von einer Überwachungskamera gefilmt, wie er

in einem Snackshop mehrere Muffins mitgenommen und gegessen hat, ohne sie zu bezahlen.«

Ich war erleichtert. Das war keine schlimme Sache, vielleicht konnten wir ihn gleich mitnehmen und er würde mit einer Verwarnung davonkommen.

Doch der Sergeant war noch nicht fertig. »Der Inhaber hat versucht, ihn festzuhalten, und dabei hat der Junge ihn verletzt.«

»Oh *shit*«, flüsterte Finny und das war ungefähr auch das, was mir durch den Kopf ging. Jetzt war mir auch klar, wieso sie Wave in eine Zelle gesteckt hatten.

»Wie schlimm verletzt?«, fragte Jack Clearwater und ich spürte, dass auch er geschockt war.

»Platzwunde am Kopf, Hämatome am Schienbein und andere Prellungen«, sagte der Sergeant und klang sehr streng dabei. »Danach konnte der Täter fliehen, aber eine unserer Streifen hatte seine Beschreibung und konnte ihn etwas später in der Nähe schnappen.« Er blätterte in seinen Papieren. »Wie lautet der Nachname des Jungen? Wir brauchen seine Personalien!«

Ich verkrampfte mich. Natürlich hatte Wave keinen Nachnamen, aber wie sollten wir das diesen Polizisten klarmachen, ohne das Geheimnis der Woodwalker zu verraten?

»O'Connor«, erwiderte Jack Clearwater, ohne mit einer Wimper zu zucken. »Er ist vor fünfzehn Jahren in Florida geboren worden. Mehr weiß ich leider nicht. Aber wenn wir ihn sehen dürfen, können wir den Rest bestimmt aus ihm rauskriegen.«

Wir versuchten alle, uns nicht anmerken zu lassen, wie verblüfft wir waren. Eiskalt log unser Schulleiter die Polizei an, das war echt krass!

»Moment«, sagte der Cop und ging eine junge, dunkelhaarige Kollegin holen. Die begleitete uns in einen anderen Teil des Gebäudes, in dem sich viele grau gestrichene Türen aneinanderreihten. In jede waren ein Guckloch und eine Klappe eingebaut.

Die Polizistin schloss uns auf und wir drängten uns alle in die Zelle. Wave saß auf einer Pritsche, den Kopf in die Hände gestützt.

Als wir hereinkamen, blickte er überrascht auf ... ich sah, dass er sich freute. »Oh, ihr seid hier! Der großen Welle sei Dank! Es ist schrecklich hier, wieso muss ich hier drinbleiben?«

Shari, Finny und wir Jungs versuchten erst mal ungeschickt, ihn zu umarmen, was er nicht gewohnt zu sein schien.

»Wir bekommen dich raus, du wirst schon sehen«, versicherte ihm Finny.

Wave lächelte schwach. »Warum bin ich hier?«, fragte er noch einmal.

»Du hast etwas getan, was die Menschen nicht gut finden«, versuchte unser Schulleiter, Wave zu erklären. »In Läden darf man sich nur etwas nehmen, wenn man dem Besitzer Geld dafür gibt.«

»Puh, das wusste ich nicht«, schnaubte Wave. »Ich war neugierig und bin an Land gegangen, um mir die Menschenwelt anzusehen. Nachdem ich ein paar Anziehsachen gefunden hatte, dachte ich in einem anderen Haus, das ist ja toll, hier stehen lauter Sachen herum, die essbar riechen. Also habe ich sie gegessen. Als der Mann mich festgehalten hat, bin ich wohl, äh, irgendwie in Panik geraten.«

»Wäre ich bestimmt auch«, versuchte ich, ihn zu beruhigen, zog ein paar Scheine und Münzen hervor und zeigte sie ihm.

»Schau mal, das benutzen wir für so einen Austausch. Dollars, Cents.«

Fasziniert drehte Wave die Münzen in den Fingern. »Die glänzen wie Fischschuppen – hübsch. Wie komme ich von hier aus ins Meer zurück? Meine Haut ist schon ganz trocken, das ist bestimmt nicht gesund.«

»Moment, das haben wir gleich«, sagte Shari, die noch immer einen Eimer trug. Sie eilte zum kleinen, in die Wand eingebauten Waschbecken und zapfte ein paar Liter. Bevor Jack Clearwater sie stoppen konnte, hatte sie Wave das Ganze schon über den Kopf geschüttet.

»Danke – fühlt sich gut an!« Selig schloss der triefende Wave die Augen, während seine Haare und Kleider den Boden volltropften. Unwillkürlich verkrampfte ich mich – bei mir hatte das Meerwasser damals eine Verwandlung ausgelöst. Das hier war Süßwasser, aber trotzdem ...

»Hier! Schau das an, schnell!« Hastig drückte Jack Clearwater unserem Freund das ausgedruckte Foto in die Hand, das er in seinem Büro in Plastik eingeschweißt hatte. »Denk dran, du bist ein Mensch, und ...«

»He, was soll das?« Ein Schlüsselbund rasselte, dann knallte die Tür auf. »Sie können doch hier nicht alles unter Wasser setzen!«

»Sorry, wir wollten unserem Freund nur etwas zu trinken geben.« Shari lächelte die Polizistin an. »Dabei ist mir der Eimer aus der Hand gerutscht.«

»Er wollte aus dem Eimer trinken?«, fragte die Polizistin.

»Unter drei Liter fängt er gar nicht erst an«, behauptete Chris und empört schnaubend zog die Polizistin ab, um einen Wischmopp zu holen.

Sehr, sehr angespannt beobachteten wir alle Wave und hofften, dass das Wasser ihn nicht »triggern« würde. Wenn seine Haut gleich dunkelgrau wurde und zu glänzen begann, hatte nicht nur Wave ein Problem – ein plötzlich hier auftauchender Buckelwal würde alle, die in seiner Nähe waren, zerquetschen!

»Du bist ein Mensch, Wave«, wiederholte Mr Clearwater eindringlich, auch er beobachtete den jungen Wandler. »In zweiter Gestalt passt du hier nicht rein, klar, oder?«

»Klar – ich versuche, mich zu beherrschen«, sagte Wave, strich sich das lange Haar zurück und versuchte noch mal ein Lächeln. Es fiel ziemlich kläglich aus.

»Du heißt Wave O'Connor und bist fünfzehn Jahre alt. Wiederhol das!«

»Wave Okonner, fünfzehn Jahre«, wiederholte Wave mit einem Funken Neugier. »Haben Sie sich das ausgedacht?«

»Ja – es ist ein irischer Name, weil viele Polizisten in Amerika irischer Abstammung sind. Hilft vielleicht ein bisschen. Ich versuche, dir einen Pass zu organisieren. Einen Beweis, dass du ein Mensch bist.«

»Haha, wenn die wüssten«, sagte Wave und zum ersten Mal sah sein Lächeln echt aus. »Danke, dass ihr versucht, mich rauszuholen.« Er stand auf und diesmal war er es, der ungeschickt versuchte, uns zu umarmen. »Wenn ich wieder frei bin, schwimmen wir zusammen, ja?«

»Wir schwimmen zusammen«, bestätigten Chris und ich, Finny brachte nur ein ein ersticktes »Machen wir« heraus. Dann war es Zeit zu gehen.

»Gibt es eine Kaution?«, fragte Jack Clearwater die junge, sportlich wirkende Polizistin. »Wie viel Geld müssten wir hinterlegen, damit der Junge bis zu seiner Verhandlung freikommt?

»Moment, ich schaue nach«, sagte sie mit einem verständnisvollen Lächeln und tippte etwas auf ihrem Computer. »Ich fürchte, dafür sind 20.000 Dollar festgelegt worden. Wird das nicht gezahlt, muss der Junge wohl erst mal unser Gast bleiben.«

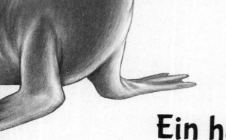

Ein haariger Plan

Mir fiel vor Schreck gar nichts mehr ein. 20.000 Dollar wollten die von uns?

»Ist das viel?«, fragte Shari verunsichert.

»Ja, es ist viel«, stöhnte Finny, während wir im Schockzustand das Polizeigebäude verließen. »Es dient als Sicherheit. Erscheint Wave brav zur Gerichtsverhandlung, bekommen wir das Geld nach der Verhandlung zurück. Flieht er, behalten sie die Kohle.«

Chris verzog das Gesicht. »Schön und gut, dass man die Kohle zurückbekommt, aber erst mal muss man so viel Geld haben und dalassen!«

»Ich muss dringend telefonieren«, murmelte Jack Clearwater. Anscheinend war es das Schicksal unserer Schule, immer wieder zu wenig Kohle zu haben! Aber vielleicht gab es eine Lösung. Ich musste nicht lange herumrätseln, wen unser Schulleiter anrufen wollte, ich erfuhr es eine Minute später: seine Mutter Lissa Clearwater, die unsere Partnerschule in den Rocky Mountains leitete.

»Mum, sorry, dass ich dich aus dem Unterricht reißen muss, aber wir haben hier ein Problem ... du erinnerst dich an den Buckelwal-Wandler, von dem ich dir erzählt hatte?« Schnell berichtete unser Schulleiter ihr von der Verhaftung und fuhr fort: »Wir brauchen so schnell wie möglich einen Ausweis und eine Geburtsurkunde für einen Wave O'Connor, fünfzehn Jahre. Das Foto schicke ich dir gleich. Ja, eine Ausweiskopie per Mail wäre super.« Er schwieg einen Moment, hörte zu und fuhr dann fort: »Kann der Rat etwas zur Kaution beisteuern? Einen Anwalt brauchen wir auch. Alles klar, ich warte, bis du zurückrufst.«

Mit einem tiefen Seufzer lehnte sich Jack Clearwater im Fahrersitz zurück.

Wahrscheinlich sah er meinen fragenden Blick, denn er erklärte: »Meine Mutter kennt ein paar sehr gute Fälscher, die uns mit Papieren für Wandler versorgen, die als Tier aufgewachsen sind. Sie schickt den Ausweis per Eilkurier zu uns.«

Daran hatte ich noch gar nicht gedacht. Aber Shari nickte stolz. »Ich hab auch so einen Pass bekommen. Wie heiß ich noch mal mit Nachnamen?«

Jack Clearwater musste lächeln. »Seaborn, ›die im Meer Geborene‹. Und als Geburtstag hast du dir den 16. März ausgesucht, damit du Sternzeichen Fisch bist.«

»Stimmt, ja!« Shari schlug sich mit der flachen Hand gegen die Stirn. »Es gab ja leider kein Sternzeichen Delfin und Fische fresse ich nun mal richtig gerne.«

»Du willst dein Sternzeichen *essen*?«, fragte Finny.

Bevor wir weiter darüber diskutieren konnten, mischte sich Chris ein: »Was ist mit dieser blöden Kaution? Die können wir uns nie und nimmer leisten!«

»Wegen der ruft sie den Rat an«, erklärte unser junger Schulleiter und nahm einen Schluck aus seiner Wasserflasche. »Dessen Job ist es ja, Wandlern in Schwierigkeiten zu helfen. Und David Johnson, der Ratsvorsitzende, ist selbst Anwalt. Keine Sorge, wir kriegen Wave da raus, okay?«

Ich versuchte, daran zu glauben. Aber Sorgen machte ich mir

trotzdem. Schließlich war unser neuer Freund gerade in tödlicher Gefahr. Selbst wenn er sich tagsüber beherrschen konnte, was war, wenn er sich nachts versehentlich verwandelte, so wie Carmen neulich?

Unser Schulleiter startete den Motor und wir machten uns auf den Rückweg nach Key Largo. Auf dem Weg dorthin klingelte sein Handy und er reichte mir das Gerät rüber, weil er beim Fahren nicht telefonieren konnte.

»Hallo?«, fragte ich ein bisschen schüchtern. »Hier ist Tiago Anderson.«

»Ah, hallo, Tiago. Hier ist Lissa Clearwater. Mein Sohn kann gerade nicht rangehen, oder? Stell mal laut, damit er mithören kann. David sagt, der Rat übernimmt die Hälfte der Kaution. Aber er selbst kann Wave nicht vertreten, weil er für Florida keine Anwaltszulassung hat. Ob ihr euch an Lydia Lennox wenden könntet, sie sei schließlich die Mutter einer Schülerin bei euch.«

Sämtliche Insassen des Busses stöhnten gleichzeitig auf.

»Ich hab eine bessere Idee«, sagte Finny plötzlich mit fester Stimme. »Ich habe eine ähnliche Statur wie er. Wenn ich mich verkleide, um auszusehen wie er – Langhaarperücke, breitere Schultern und so weiter –, dann kann ich behaupten, dass das Ganze eine Verwechslung war. Dass ich das bin auf der Videoaufzeichnung. Dass ich die Muffins geklaut und den Ladenbesitzer getreten habe.«

»Das würdest du tun? Aber ...« Jack Clearwater umklammerte das Lenkrad.

Finny war rot im Gesicht vor Aufregung. »Klar, ich würde Ärger kriegen, aber ich würde nicht sterben, so wie Wave, wenn etwas schiefgeht. Außerdem bin ich jünger als er und die Tochter eines Polizisten, das zählt vielleicht ein bisschen mehr als ein irischer Nachname.«

»Bitte, Mr Clearwater, Sie müssen ihr das erlauben.« Sharis braune Augen wirkten ganz dunkel vor Sorge. »Wegen dieser Kaution machen Sie sich mal bitte keine Sorgen. Blue und Lucy holen einfach noch mehr Gold hoch.«

Ich sagte nichts, hatte aber Zweifel, ob wir das noch einmal schafften.

Schon wieder klingelte das Handy. »Hm, die Schule ...«, meinte Jack Clearwater mit gerunzelter Stirn und gab mir zum zweiten Mal das Gerät.

»Hier ist Farryn«, hörte ich. »Ich wollte nur Bescheid sagen, dass ich gerade die Tierärztin anrufen musste. Lucy ist ohnmächtig geworden.«

Unser junger Schulleiter trat das Gaspedal durch.

Wir hasteten in die Cafeteria und fanden dort schon eine Menge Schüler vor, die neugierig um eins der Tisch-Boote herumstanden – alle in Menschengestalt, denn bestimmt wusste die Tierärztin nicht, was das hier wirklich für eine Schule war. Mitten auf dem Tisch, dort wo normalerweise Teller mit Pfannkuchen und Lachsröllchen standen, lag heute stattdessen eine rote Pazifische Riesenkrake. Eine, die im Moment eine eher graue Haut hatte. Oh nein, war Lucy etwa ... nein, ich sah, wie ihre Arme sich schwach ringelten!

Eine Frau mit auberginefarben gefärbten Haaren beugte sich über sie und tastete sie ab. »Ist sie in letzter Zeit tief getaucht?«, fragte sie. »Oder wissen Sie das nicht? Ihre Tiere dürfen ja frei ins Meer, soweit ich gehört habe.«

Blue umklammerte ihre Kette mit den drei Delfinflossen. »Ja, sie ... äh, sie war ungefähr in dreihundert Meter Tiefe.«

»Ah.« Die Tierärztin runzelte die Stirn. »Anscheinend ist sie dabei zu schnell hochgekommen, das schädigt das Gewebe, wenn auch nicht so heftig wie bei Tauchern, die Pressluft geatmet haben.«

Zweiarm hat recht, ich war nicht vorsichtig genug, meldete sich Lucy schwach zu Wort. *Dumm war ich, dumm!*

»Am besten lassen Sie sie in den nächsten drei Wochen nicht ins Freiwasser, damit sie auf keinen Fall taucht«, fuhr die Tierärztin fort, die nichts gehört hatte. »Hier ist ein Stärkungsmittel. Zweimal täglich nach der Fütterung.«

»Danke«, sagte unser junger Schulleiter und streckte die Hand danach aus. Doch schon hatte Mrs Misaki – die auch unsere Sanitäterin war – es der Tierärztin aus der Hand geschnappt und eingesteckt. »*Ich* mache das, Mr Clearwater. Davon verstehen Sie nichts.«

»Das ist wahr«, antwortete unser Schulleiter und verzichtete heldenhaft darauf, die Augen zu verdrehen.

Als die Besucherin gegangen war, strich ich Lucy betroffen über die samtweiche Haut. »Gute Besserung, es tut mir echt leid«, sagte ich und viele andere murmelten ähnliche gute Wünsche.

»Wird schon wieder.« Joshua, unser Koch, nahm den Körper unserer Mitschülerin auf die Arme und trug ihn behutsam zurück zu ihrem Versteck.

»Das war's mitm Gold, ohne Lucy kriegen wir es niemals hin, noch mehr hochzuholen«, sagte Jasper betrübt und putzte seine Brille an seinem T-Shirt.

Sämtliche Lehrer zogen sich zu einem Krisengespräch in den ersten Stock zurück, in dem es garantiert um Wave ging. Die Delfine, Finny, Jasper und ich hockten uns an den Strand, schauten zu, wie Barry Carmen im Sand eingrub, und diskutierten über Wave.

»Also, ich bin für Finnys Plan, sich zu verkleiden und als Wave auszugeben«, sagte Shari. »Wer noch?«

All unsere Arme sausten nach oben.

Dass wir dabei nicht die Einzigen waren, merkten wir, als Jack Clearwater und Mr García mit langen Schritten auf uns zukamen, den Blick auf Finny gerichtet.

»Hast du das mit deinem Vorschlag wirklich ernst gemeint?«, fragte Mr García. »Wenn das klappt, bekommst du einen Orden.«

»Was soll ich mit einem Orden?« Finny zog die Augenbrauen hoch. »Ich hab eh schon zu viel Zeug gehortet. Manche würden sagen, ich bin ein Messie, obwohl das natürlich nicht stimmt.«

»Dann verkauf den Orden doch«, sagte ich.

»Aber nur, wenn mir gar nichts anderes einfällt. Logisch hab ich das ernst gemeint, Mr García. Wir müssen Wave da rausholen!«

»Dann sollten wir keine Zeit verlieren«, sagte unser Schulleiter. »Kannst du in einer halben Stunde so weit sein?«

»Muss reichen!«, rief Finny, sprang auf und rannte los.

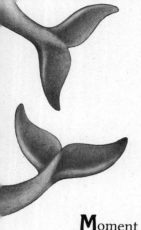

Wave mal zwei

Moment mal, stimmte mit meinen Augen was nicht? Das war eindeutig Wave, der da vor mir stand. Ein breitschultriger Junge mit langem braunem Haar, das in der Sonne einen Kupferschimmer bekam, dunkelbraunen Augen und langer Nase. Er trug Hosen und ein langärmeliges Shirt.

»Äh, bist du das, Finny?«, fragte Jasper verunsichert.

»So was in einer halben Stunde machen zu müssen, ist eine Zumutung«, sagte der Junge mit Finnys Stimme. »So lange brauche ich normalerweise allein für das Make-up!«

»Wie hast du das mit den Augen gemacht?«, staunte Leonora. »Die sind doch normalerweise blaugrau?«

»Das ging am schnellsten – gefärbte Kontaktlinsen«, meinte Finny, hob die Hand, um sich an der Nase zu kratzen, und überlegte es sich im letzten Moment anders. Vielleicht weil sonst Teile dieser Nase abfallen würden.

»Nichts wie los.« Jack Clearwater klapperte mit den Autoschlüsseln. »Du darfst dir eine Begleitung aussuchen.«

»Tiago«, sagte Finny sofort. Das war mir ein bisschen peinlich. Ich musste eindeutig bald mit ihr reden – und nicht erst in zwanzig Jahren.

»Schon wieder Tiago? Das ist unfair«, beschwerte sich Juna. Sie neigte nicht zum Schmollen, aber diesmal war sie kurz davor. »Ich bin immerhin Klassensprecherin!«

»Wave ist noch nicht in unserer Klasse, Falterfischchen«, sagte Finny, drückte Juna an sich und winkte mir mitzukommen. Weil ich mal wieder Hunger hatte, verschlang ich gerade einen Müsliriegel. Das ersparte mir eine Antwort, ich folgte ihr einfach.

Diesmal begleitete uns Mr García zum Auto, anscheinend war er mit von der Partie. »Ich hätte Tiago sowieso gebraucht – ich habe nämlich gerade einen Termin mit Lydia Lennox in Miami vereinbart.«

»Oh«, rief ich überrascht. »Wie haben Sie sie denn dazu bekommen?«

»Es war kein Trick dabei, sie hat gleich Ja gesagt. Wir treffen uns am Abend an der Strandpromenade, dabei versuche ich, sie zu überreden, dass sie Wave – oder Finny, je nachdem – verteidigt und die Hälfte der Kaution übernimmt. Vielleicht könnte ich sie danach ganz vorsichtig sondieren, das wird sie sicher nicht mitkriegen.«

Das Essen fiel mir aus dem Gesicht. »Sie tun es wirklich?«

»Wir müssen das klären«, sagte Mr García. »Und nicht nur, weil ich es dir versprochen habe, Tiago. Eine andere Gelegenheit bekommen wir wahrscheinlich nicht.« Er verzog das Gesicht. »Aber es ist ein Risiko. Falls sie sich einverstanden erklärt, uns zu helfen, sollten wir sie nicht gerade wütend machen, sonst platzt womöglich der Deal.«

Ich spürte, wie Angst in mir hochkroch, kalt wie frisch aus dem Tiefkühler. »Das wird gefährlich, vor allem, wenn sie die Tigerzwillinge dabeihat!«

»Ach echt«, sagte Finny. »Du kannst auch hierbleiben und Lego spielen.«

Das traf meinen Stolz. »He, was denkst du von mir? Ich bin ein Tiger- und kein Katzenhai!«

»Fast schade, Katzenhaie sind echt niedlich.«

»Mir kommt es komisch vor, dass sie diesem Treffen gleich zugestimmt hat«, sagte ich alarmiert zu Mr García. »Diese Frau hat doch irgendwelche Hintergedanken!«

»Garantiert«, stimmte Mr García zu. »Bin gespannt, welche.«

»Können wir jetzt endlich losfahren?«, fragte Finny.

Genau das machten wir.

Während Finny und unser Schulleiter auf den vorderen Sitzen alle Details ihrer Aktion absprachen, taten ich und mein Verwandlungslehrer eine Sitzreihe weiter hinten das Gleiche. Ich sollte mich in der Nähe halten, aber in Deckung bleiben, damit Mrs Lennox mich nicht sah und Verdacht schöpfte, dass es bei diesem Treffen um mehr ging als die Kaution. Falls sie etwas behauptete, was nicht stimmte, konnte ich meinen Lehrer per Gedankenflüstern (was niemand abhören konnte) sofort auf die Widersprüche hinweisen.

»Für diesen Job brauchen wir eindeutig Verstärkung«, sagte ich, zückte mein Handy und rief Rocket an. »Denkst du an die Minikamera? Die brauchen wir dringend, um diese Sache mit den illegalen Haikämpfen aufzuklären.«

»Klar, weiß ich. Ich habe das Ding schon besorgt und bringe es so bald wie möglich bei euch vorbei.«

»Super. Sag mal, hast du heute Abend schon was vor?«

»Ja, zusammen mit Logan fünf oder sechs Leute verprügeln und anschließend noch Pizza essen. Und du?«

»Haha, sehr witzig«, sagte ich. »Ich hab einen besseren Job für dich und Pizza gibt es vielleicht trotzdem. Wenn wir das Ganze überleben.«

»Klingt gut, worum geht's?«, fragte Rocket.

Ich erklärte es ihm und beschrieb ihm, wo wir uns treffen würden.

»Da bringe ich doch gleich mal Logan mit«, sagte Rocket

und legte auf, bevor ich »Moment mal!« rufen konnte. Logan war der Schläger, der dafür gesorgt hatte, dass ich bei meinem ersten Besuch in der Blue Reef Highschool ausgesehen hatte wie frisch aus der Notaufnahme.

Den Rest der Fahrt über probten wir das Gedankenflüstern, damit ich nachher nicht durch einen dummen Fehler eine Katastrophe auslöste. Als wir vor dem Polizeirevier ankamen, war ich erschöpft von all dem Wispern, bei dem ich mich maximal konzentrieren musste. Aber das Adrenalin sorgte dafür, dass ich hellwach war. Würden die Cops Finny die Show glauben? Wenn ja, dann konnten wir Wave vielleicht heute noch mitnehmen und ins Meer zurückbringen!

Der Sergeant an der Theke erkannte Mr Clearwater wieder. »Was vergessen?«, fragte er ... und bekam große Augen, als er Finny-alias-Wave sah. »Na, so was, wer ist denn ...«

»Es kann sein, dass bei dieser Sache mit Wave eine Verwechslung vorliegt«, unterbrach ihn Jack Clearwater. Er wirkte völlig ruhig, aber ich sah, dass er schwitzte.

»Sieh an.« Der Cop musterte Finny noch immer verblüfft.

»Ich will mich freiwillig stellen«, sagte Finny laut und deutlich. »Es sollte eine Mutprobe sein, dass ich in diesem Laden die Muffins gegessen habe. Ja, ich weiß, echt dämliche Idee. Und dann habe ich Panik bekommen, als der Ladenbesitzer mich festgehalten hat. Es tut mir wirklich total leid!«

»Das heißt, wir haben den Falschen aufgegriffen?« Nun sah der Cop doch ein wenig misstrauisch drein.

»Wie hat Wave O'Connor reagiert, als die Polizisten ihn verhaftet haben?«, fragte Jack Clearwater. »Wirkte er schuldbewusst?«

»Nein, er war völlig überrascht«, mischte sich ein anderer Officer ein, der sich zu uns gesellt hatte.

»Na also, sehen Sie.« Jack Clearwater versuchte, triumphierend zu klingen, aber ich hörte die Erleichterung in seiner Stimme. Er hatte richtig geraten.

»Ich dachte wirklich, der Junge wäre das gewesen auf der Videoaufzeichnung«, meinte der Sergeant vom Dienst. »He, Dave, hol mal den Kerl aus Zelle 5, ja?« Er wandte sich an Finny. »Du hast ganz recht, das war eine miese Idee mit diesem Ladendiebstahl, so was ist kein Scherz. Wie heißt du? Ausweis, bitte!«

Es funktionierte! Finny feierte es, indem sie eine meisterhafte Schlechtes-Gewissen-Show ablieferte. Ihre ganze Gestalt atmete Reue. »Finny Greyson«, sagte sie. »Wie heißt der Ladenbesitzer? Ich muss mich noch bei ihm entschuldigen, dass ich ihn gegen das Schienbein getreten habe.«

Ich wunderte mich, dass sie verstohlen auf die Uhr blickte, die im Revier an der Wand hing. Hatte sie es eilig?

»Finny Greyson? Moment mal, bist du etwa die Tochter von Patrolman Nick Greyson?«

Finny biss sich auf die Lippe. Es war ein kritischer Moment und wir wussten es alle. »Ja. Pa wird dermaßen wütend auf mich sein ...«

»Das fürchte ich auch!«, sagte der Sergeant. »Ach, da kommt schon mein Kollege mit dem Jungen. Wissen Sie, wie wir seine Erziehungsberechtigten erreichen, damit sie ihn hier abholen?«

»Nicht nötig, ich habe hier eine Vollmacht, dass ich ihn abholen darf, und eine Kopie seines Ausweises.« Jack Clearwater präsentierte ein frisch gefälschtes Schreiben und öffnete auf seinem Handy die Ausweiskopie. Mit einem Nicken gab ihm der Polizist beides zurück, nachdem er es geprüft hatte.

Fast geschafft! Gleich hatten wir unseren Buckelwal raus

aus dem Knast und damit außer Lebensgefahr! Innerlich jubelte ich. Da war Wave schon. Er ging neben der Polizistin her, freute sich offensichtlich, uns zu sehen, und musterte verblüfft Finny in ihrer Verkleidung. »Oh, seit wann gibt es mich zweimal? Ist der da etwa auch ein ...«

Zum Glück brachte ihn ein scharfer Blick unseres Schulleiters zum Schweigen. »Das da ist Finny. Sie war es, die die Muffins in Wirklichkeit gestohlen hast, während du ganz friedlich die Straße entlanggegangen bist.«

Blöd war Wave zum Glück nicht. »Ach so«, sagte er nur.

Wieder blickte Finny auf die Uhr und ich merkte, wie sie immer nervöser wurde. Hä?

Dann fiel mir ein, was sie vorhin erzählt hatte.

Um achtzehn Uhr würde die Schicht ihres Vaters hier im Revier beginnen. Und inzwischen war es fünf Minuten vor sechs.

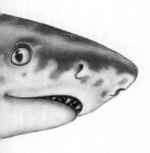

Abgeschminkt

Ich sah, wie Finny zusammenzuckte, als ein hochgewachsener Mann mit langem Hals, vorstehendem Adamsapfel und Segelohren quer durch das Großraumbüro hinter der Theke ging. Leider waren wir beide nicht die Einzigen, die bemerkt hatten, dass Nick Greyson seine Schicht begonnen hatte.

»Hey, Nick, kommst du mal kurz rüber?«, rief der Sergeant, der uns betreute. »Hier ist jemand, dem du vielleicht Hallo sagen möchtest.«

Finnys Vater wandte sich um und blickte erstaunt drein. »Wieso? Wer denn?«

Der Sergeant grinste, aber nur kurz. »Schau dich um und sag es mir. Es wird dir nicht gefallen, fürchte ich.«

Etwas ratlos kam Nick Greyson heran und blickte sich um. »Ihr habt Zwillinge da? Tja, das ist interessant, aber was ...« Nicht nur ich sah, dass es bei ihm klick machte. »Finny! Spielt ihr beide in einem Theaterstück mit?« Noch immer verwirrt, schaute er zwischen Wave und seiner Tochter hin und her. Dann bemerkte er unseren Schulleiter und schüttelte ihm die Hand. »Tag, Mr Clearwater.«

Bisher hatte ich nur mit Mr Greyson telefoniert, gesehen hatte ich ihn nie. Deshalb war ich erstaunt, wie völlig anders Finnys Vater war als seine Tochter. Eher steif und förmlich, nicht der Typ, der schnell Freunde gewann.

»Hi, Dad«, sagte Finny mit einem gezwungenen Lächeln. »Schön, dich zu sehen.«

Nick Greyson nickte ihr zu, dann wandte er sich mit gerunzelter Stirn an seinen Kollegen. »Also, was läuft hier? Finny hat doch nicht etwa Ärger, oder, Stan?«

»Ich habe gestern ein paar Muffins in einem Laden geklaut.« Finny ließ den Kopf hängen, ihr langes Perückenhaar verbarg fast ihr Gesicht. »Ja, ich weiß, dumm von mir.«

Sein Kollege wurde wieder nüchtern-förmlich. »Außerdem hat sie leider den Ladenbesitzer verletzt. Er hat Anzeige erstattet.«

»*Jesus!* Du hast was?« Nicks Greysons Gesicht rötete sich. Seine Augen schienen unsichtbare Harpunen auf seine Tochter abzuschießen, Jack Clearwaters Adlerblick war nichts dagegen.

»Hast du doch gehört«, murmelte Finny.

Sie tat mir total leid. Was sie aushalten musste, hätte ich nicht mal unserer immer schlecht gelaunten Muräne Mrs Misaki gewünscht, und das alles nur, weil Finny Wave retten wollte. Wieso war *ich* eigentlich nie so edel und gut?

Schuldbewusst hatte Wave das alles angehört, er trat einen Schritt vor und öffnete den Mund, um etwas zu sagen. O Gott, wollte er etwa alles gestehen, damit Finny nicht länger leiden musste? Ich trat ihm auf den Fuß und flüsterte: »Mund halten. Finny weiß, was sie tut, okay?«

Wave warf mir einen finsteren Blick zu und plötzlich sah er älter aus als die fünfzehn, die er angeblich war. Überhaupt nicht mehr kindlich. »Das ist nicht recht«, sagte er.

Die Strafpredigt war noch im vollen Gange, sogar der andere Cop wirkte beeindruckt. Schließlich wandte sich Nick Greyson an seinen Kollegen. »Sag mal, Stan, könnten wir die

Sache nicht auf sich beruhen lassen? Du hast ja gehört, es war nur ein dummer Streich. Sie wird sich bei dem Ladenbesitzer entschuldigen und ich zahle ihm ein Schmerzensgeld. Und wir treffen uns bald mal auf ein Bier oder zum Grillen, okay?«

Es fühlte sich an, als würden wir darauf warten, ob irgendwo in unserer Nähe der Blitz einschlug. Bitte, bitte, sag Ja, trinkt fünf Kästen Bier und grillt zwei Dutzend Steaks, betete ich, aber der Sergeant wirkte noch unentschlossen. »Eigentlich kein Problem, ich kenne ja deine Finny, die ist nicht verkehrt. Wir müssten nur das Protokoll irgendwie ...«

Nick Greyson nahm ihm das Protokoll aus der Hand ... und stutzte. »Moment mal! Das hat alles heute um Viertel nach zehn am Vormittag stattgefunden?«

»Wird wohl stimmen, wenn es da steht«, antwortete Finny. »Hab halt Schule geschwänzt, mach ich vielleicht einmal im Jahr oder so.«

»Das kann nicht sein.« Greysons Stimme klang, als wäre sie aus Gusseisen. »Ich habe dich in der ersten Pause auf dem Festnetztelefon in deiner Schule angerufen, um dir zu sagen, dass du an deine Impfung denken sollst. Und eure Sekretärin hat dich ans Telefon geholt. Du kannst also kaum eine Dreiviertelstunde später in Miami etwas geklaut haben.«

Manchmal kann man Leuten ja die Gedanken vom Gesicht ablesen. In diesem Fall stand sowohl Finny als auch Mr Clearwater in großen neonfarbenen Buchstaben SHIT! auf die Stirn geschrieben. Und mir selbst wahrscheinlich auch.

Unser Bluff war aufgeflogen. Auch Wave schien kapiert zu haben, dass etwas gewaltig schieflief.

»Darüber reden wir noch, junge Dame«, sagte Nick Greyson, ergriff Finny am Arm und rupfte ihr mit der anderen Hand die

Perücke ab. Darunter blitzte es azurblau auf, als ihre normalen Haare zum Vorschein kamen. »Du kommst jetzt erst mal mit in die Umkleide und wischst dir diese Schminke aus dem Gesicht. Ich bringe meine Tochter selbst zur Schule zurück, Mr Clearwater, machen Sie sich keine Mühe.«

Finny warf mir einen wilden Blick zu, dann wurde sie weggezogen und hatte kaum Zeit, sich von uns zu verabschieden.

Auf einmal begann Wave zu singen. Es war ein Lied ohne Worte und erinnerte mich an einen indianischen Gesang, den ich mal in einem Video gehört hatte. Seine Augen verließen Finny keine Sekunde lang und jeder von uns wusste, dass es ein Lied für sie war.

Finny wandte sich um, blickte Wave an ... und ich sah, wie ihre Augen sich mit Tränen füllten. Doch leider hatte auch Mr Greyson sich umgewandt. »Stan, lässt du den Jungen in seine Zelle zurückbringen? Wir klären das später.«

Ruhig, voller Würde, ließ sich Wave von zwei Polizisten abführen.

»Gib nicht auf«, sagte Jack Clearwater schnell zu ihm. »Und denk an das, was ich dir gesagt habe!«

Wave nickte stumm, seine Augen blickten in die Ferne. Ich glaube, er sah uns nicht in diesem Moment – er sah die Tiefen der Meere.

»Viel Glück!«, rief ich ihm hinterher, dann war er außer Sicht in einem der Flure.

Niedergeschlagen verließen mein Schulleiter und ich das Polizeirevier.

»Oh Mann«, sagte ich frustriert, während wir zurückgingen zum Auto. »Wir hatten ihn schon fast ... und jetzt haben wir weder Wave noch Finny!«

Jack Clearwater seufzte tief. »Das war sehr tapfer von ihr.

Hoffentlich hält Wave durch. Nicht auszudenken, wenn er in dieser Zelle stirbt.«

»Mr Greyson weiß nicht, dass seine Tochter und seine Frau Wandler sind, oder?« Ich zögerte. »Das heißt, wir müssen ihm verschweigen, was Wave für ein Problem hat.«

»Genau.« Unser Schulleiter klang ein bisschen verbittert.

Ich strengte mich richtig an und brachte es fertig, nur ein paar meiner Zähne teilzuverwandeln. Während Jack dabei war, Mr García – der im Auto gewartet hatte – Bericht zu erstatten, rief ich in Gedanken: *Finny? Kannst du mich hören? Geht's dir gut?*

Nicht wirklich, kam sofort zurück. *Ich habe zwei Wochen Hausarrest in der Blue Reef. Außerdem Handyverbot, Fernsehverbot, Internetverbot, Schokobrunnenverbot ...*

Oh Mann, stöhnte ich.

... ach ja, und Perückenverbot, fügte Finny hinzu.

Falls Mr Clearwater das wirklich durchsetzt, werden wir dich alle verwöhnen – es wird dir kaum auffallen, was du nicht darfst, versprach ich ihr.

Ach, du bist so süß, sagte Finny und Mr Clearwater erkundigte sich: »Darf ich fragen, warum du gerade rot wirst, Tiago?«

»Nein«, murmelte ich und verwandelte meine Zähne zurück. Dann dachte ich darüber nach, was wir noch für unseren gefangenen Buckelwal tun konnten. Leider fiel mir ungefähr so viel ein wie einem Hering, der Vorschläge für den Weltfrieden machen soll.

»Wir haben keine Wahl mehr«, sagte Mr García. »Jetzt müssen wir mit Lydia Lennox verhandeln. Sie ist eine erfahrene

Strafverteidigerin, sie paukt den Jungen schneller raus, als der Staatsanwalt ›Piep!‹ sagen kann.«

»Und sie hat mehr als genug Geld, um die andere Hälfte der Kaution zu übernehmen«, ergänzte Jack Clearwater. »Vielleicht solltest du mit dem Sondieren besser abwarten. Nicht dass es dir deine Verhandlungen mit ihr verpatzt.«

Mein Verwandlungslehrer zögerte. »Stimmt. Ich schaue mal, ob sich eine Gelegenheit ergibt, sonst lasse ich es sein. Aber die Sondierung ist auch wichtig, Jack.«

»Ja, ist sie«, bekräftigte ich. Was war, wenn schon die nächsten Haikämpfe organisiert wurden, während wir uns hier unterhielten? Nein, sie hatten sicher nicht noch mal meinen Bruder Steve gefangen. Das passierte nur in meinen Albträumen, dort aber fast jede Nacht. Ich musste ihn suchen gehen, um sicher zu sein!

»Fast niemand, der sondiert wird, merkt etwas davon«, beruhigte uns Mr García. »Es ist bald so weit. Ich würde vorschlagen, du wartest mit der Karre in der Nähe, Jack – falls du einen Parkplatz findest. Besser, sie sieht dich nicht.« Seine weißen Zähne leuchteten auf, als er grinste. »Bei euren letzten Treffen lief es ja nicht allzu gut zwischen euch.«

»Was ist mit mir?«, fragte ich mit klopfendem Herzen.

»Du versteckst dich in der Nähe, sodass du auf jeden Fall in Reichweite meiner Gedanken bist.«

Wir waren zu früh dran. Als wir den Ocean Drive entlangfuhren, hoffte ich, dass Rocket schon in der Nähe war. Ich strengte mich richtig an und schaffte es, nur ein paar meiner Zähne teilzuverwandeln. Dann rief ich: *Rocket, bist du da? Hast du noch ein paar Leute mitgebracht?*

Ah, Tiago, du alter Knorpelfisch! Ja, wir sind zu dritt. Wo sollen wir warten?

Ich nannte ihnen die Stelle, die ich mit Mr García vereinbart hatte, und stieg dort aus. »Du hältst dich von der Lennox fern, verstanden?«, schärfte unser Verwandlungslehrer mir ein.

»Ja, ich weiß, mich kann sie auch nicht leiden.« Ich lächelte schief. »Beruht auf Gegenseitigkeit. Passen Sie auf sich auf, ja?«

»Mach ich. Du auch.« Wir lächelten uns zu und wieder fiel mir auf, wie ähnlich wir uns sahen. Die gleiche nussbraune Haut, die gleiche Statur. Das gab mir einen Stich. Warum konnten meine echten Eltern nicht ein bisschen mehr so sein wie Farryn García?

Natürlich sah ich Rockets Freund Logan sofort, als ich ausstieg – einen breitschultrigen blonden Typ mit beeindruckenden Armmuskeln. Er war nicht hübscher geworden, seit ich ihn das letzte Mal gesehen hatte. Jemand hatte ihm die Nase geplättet, sie war noch geschient und verbunden, was ihn aussehen ließ, als hätte er einen Wattebausch statt eines Riechorgans.

Lando, mein alter Kumpel, war auch da und lächelte mir zu, während er in respektvoller Entfernung von Logan an einer Palme lehnte. Er hatte einen schwarz glänzenden Darth-Vader-Helm unter dem Arm. »Na ja, ich dachte, der ist praktisch, wenn ich irgendwas unerkannt machen soll«, meinte er verlegen und ich lächelte zurück.

»Echt unauffällig. Aber vielleicht stoßfest. Falls es 'ne Keilerei gibt.«

»Klar gibt's eine«, sagte Logan und stieß mich gegen die Schulter. »Auch gerne mit dem Loser hier.«

»Nein, nicht mit dem«, schimpfte ihn Rocket aus. »Und sag ihm nicht, dass er gewachsen ist, seit du ihn das letzte Mal gesehen hast. Sonst klingst du wie deine eigene Oma.«

Ich schaute mich nach Rocket um, sah seine schmale Gestalt aber nirgendwo. Anscheinend war er in zweiter Gestalt und hatte nur seinen Mund teilverwandelt. Keine Ahnung, wie er das seinen Freunden erklärt hatte, dass sie es mit einer körperlosen Stimme zu tun hatten.

Du siehst mich nicht, ich bin gerade 'ne Ratte, Alter, kicherte mein Freund. *Graubraun wie der Straßenbelag, schnell wie 'ne DSL-Verbindung. Keine Sorge, niemand hat was mitgekriegt, als ich mich verwandelt habe, und du rätst nie, wo ich gerade hocke. Und, wann kommt die Lennox?*

Sie ist schon da, sagte Mr Garcías klare, durchdringende Gedankenstimme. *Ruhig jetzt. Es geht los.*

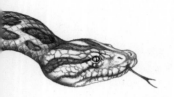

Tief in Gedanken

Ich hatte gerade noch Zeit, mich in ein Touri-Geschäft in der Nähe zu ducken und zwischen quietschbunten Handtüchern, Luftmatratzen und Tassen mit *Miami*-Schriftzug und Delfinbildern zurückzuziehen.

Sehen konnte ich aus dieser Entfernung – mehr als fünfzig Meter – durchs Schaufenster höchstens den Rücken von Mrs Lennox, wenn ich viel Glück hatte. Aber Mr García schickte mir und wahrscheinlich auch Rocket und Mr Clearwater einen Gedankenstrom von dem, was er sagte und hörte. Anscheinend hatte er sich an irgendeiner unauffälligen Körperstelle teilverwandelt.

Er konnte das verdammt gut, die Bilder waren so gestochen scharf und farbig, dass ich völlig darin eintauchte und fast vergaß, was um mich herum geschah. Dagegen war jede VR-Brille Dreck. Ich konnte sogar das schwere, süßliche Parfum riechen, als sich Lydia Lennox – einen Kaffeebecher in der Hand – neben meinen Verwandlungslehrer auf die Bank am Rand der Strandpromenade setzte.

Ich fragte mich, wo Rocket gerade war. Als Mr García sich umblickte, sah ich nirgendwo eine Ratte.

»Eben habe ich mich mal wieder mit Carl getroffen, Carl Bittergreen, er ist so ein wunderbarer Mensch und wir sind ein so großartiges Team«, schwärmte Mrs Lennox und nickte einem jungen Mann mit kantigem Gesicht zu, der mir bekannt vorkam. War das nicht ihr Assistent?

»Brauchen Sie mich noch, Mrs Lennox?«, fragte er.

»Nein, Patrick, du kannst zurückfahren in die Kanzlei, organisiere bitte alles für morgen«, kommandierte Mrs Lennox und winkte ihn weg.

»Zum Thema Bittergreen ... wenn es stimmt, was in der Zeitung steht, hat dieser ›wunderbare Mensch‹ seine Finger in so ziemlich allen verbotenen Geschäften hier in Miami«, hörte ich Mr García sagen. »Außerdem lässt er Leute umbringen, die ihm nicht in den Kram passen.«

Lydia Lennox lachte. »So was würde ich an deiner Stelle nicht zu laut sagen, er hört so was nicht gerne. Reden wir lieber darüber, warum du hier bist, lieber Farryn. Ihr braucht mal wieder meine Hilfe, richtig?« Sie nippte gut gelaunt an ihrem Becher und beobachtete Touristen und Einheimische, die im kleinen Park zwischen Stadt und Strand entlangschlenderten.

»Weil ihr nicht alleine klarkommt?«

Ich konnte förmlich fühlen, wie Mr García die Zähne zusammenbiss. »Normalerweise kommen wir blendend klar«, sagte er. »Aber du weißt selbst, dass es manchmal nicht ganz leicht ist, wenn neue Wandler die Menschenwelt entdecken.«

»Meinst du etwa diese wunderbaren jungen Leute, die aus dem Sumpf zu euch gekommen sind und ...«

»... und die Blue Reef High besetzt haben, bis wir sie zurückerobern konnten? Nein, die meine ich nicht. Wir haben gerade einen Buckelwal-Wandler zu Gast.«

Lydia Lennox lachte. »Ach! Seid froh, dass es kein Blauwal ist, die werden locker doppelt so groß. Hat er eure Schule schon eingerissen?«

»Er hat erst mal geschafft, sich verhaften zu lassen, weil er nicht wusste, was Geld ist.« Mr García seufzte. »Liebe Lydia, wärst du eventuell bereit, ihn zu vertreten? Es würde dich bestimmt nicht viel Zeit kosten.«

»Ach, gar kein Problem, lieber Farryn«, sagte Mrs Lennox und lächelte meinen Verwandlungslehrer an. »Der Rat hat mich auch schon deswegen angerufen.«

»Genau – der Rat, bei dem du mich netterweise angeschwärzt hast«, meinte Farryn García und lächelte zurück. »Was übrigens nichts genutzt hat, weil ich dort besser vernetzt bin als du. Aber zurück zum Thema ...«

»Ja genau! Ihr braucht auch ein bisschen Kaution, schätze ich? Das lässt sich machen.«

»Du willst nicht mal wissen, wie viel es ist?«

Wieder lachte Lydia Lennox. Allmählich wurde mir das unheimlich. Wenn sie so gut gelaunt war, gab es dafür einen Grund ... und ich war ziemlich sicher, dass der uns nicht gefallen würde! »So viel wird es bei einem Kleinkriminellen schon nicht sein.«

»Wave ist kein Kleinkrimineller, deshalb wollen wir ihn ja rausholen. Aber schön zu hören, dass du nicht an Geldknappheit leidest, liebe Lydia.« Mr García ließ den Blick schweifen. Er und ich entdeckten gleichzeitig die Tigerzwillinge, zwei junge Frauen mit Modelfigur, langen rötlich braunen Haaren und geschmeidigen Bewegungen. Eine von ihnen – war es Latisha oder Natasha? – tat so, als wollte sie sich gerade die sandigen Füße an einer Duschsäule am Rand der Promenade abspülen. Die andere schlenderte auf dem Rasen zwischen den Palmen herum und tat, als würde sie sich mit ihrem Handy beschäftigen. Aber ich wusste, dass die beiden ihre Chefin mit einem Sprung erreichen konnten.

»Jedenfalls ist es großartig, dass du uns helfen willst«, fuhr

Mr García fort. »Na, dann gebe ich dir jetzt die Kontaktdaten von …«

»Moment«, meinte Lydia Lennox. Sie lächelte noch immer. »Es gibt eine Bedingung.«

Mr García und ich verkrampften uns gleichzeitig.

»Kann ich dir helfen?« Ich zuckte zusammen. Die Stimme war aus der wirklichen Welt gekommen, der Welt des Souvenirgeschäfts, in dem ich mich versteckt hielt. Angestrengt blinzelte ich, versuchte, den Gedankenstrom zu ignorieren. Eine Verkäuferin blickte mich fragend an. Anscheinend war ich nicht so unauffällig gewesen, wie ich mir gewünscht hätte.

»Äh … haben Sie dieses T-Shirt noch in anderen Größen?«, stammelte ich und wollte nur eins: wieder zurück in den Gedankenstrom und hören, was die Bedingung war, die Lydia Lennox uns stellte.

»Was brauchst du? M oder L?« Die Verkäuferin wühlte im Stapel der dunkelblauen Shirts mit dem lachenden Delfin und der Aufschrift *Miami*. »Hm, wo ist es nur … ich bin sicher, wir haben noch eins in L … ach hier!«

Sehr erleichtert stellte ich fest, dass es eine Umkleidekabine gab. Es war mir egal, ob die Verkäuferin es seltsam fand – ich stürzte mich hinein und riss den Vorhang zwischen uns. Endlich allein. Ich lehnte mich an die Sperrholzwand der Kabine und schloss die Augen. Sofort war ich wieder drin.

»… ziemlich heftig«, sagte Mr García gerade, er klang aufgewühlt. »Du wirst verstehen, dass ich das erst mit Jack besprechen muss.«

»Ja natürlich, das verstehe ich.« Lydia Lennox suppte der Charme aus allen Poren. »Ihr werdet bestimmt einsehen, dass es zum Besten der Schule ist.«

Was? Was war die Bedingung gewesen? Ich ging fast die

Wände dieser Umkleidekabine hoch. Vielleicht spürte es mein Verwandlungslehrer durch unsere Verbindung, denn er sagte: »Aber wir müssten natürlich einen anderen Schulleiter suchen, wenn Jack zurücktreten soll.«

Großer Gott, wieder einmal versuchte sie, Jack Clearwater loszuwerden! Aber das würden die anderen Lehrer nie akzeptieren ... oder?

»Ich wüsste da schon jemanden«, sagte die Lennox selbstgefällig. Oje – ich war sicher, dass ihre Wahl uns nicht gefallen würde.

»Ach wirklich.« Farryn García dachte einen Moment lang nach und ich spürte, dass er nicht an diesen Deal glaubte. Der Preis war zu hoch. Aber das sagte er nicht, stattdessen fuhr er fort: »Ich spreche mit Jack über deine Bedingungen. Dann melden wir uns wieder bei dir.«

Würde Jack Clearwater wirklich zustimmen zurückzutreten? Sicher nicht. Wir würden das Geld für Waves Kaution irgendwie anders auftreiben müssen.

»Einen schönen Tag noch, Lydia.« Mr García stand auf und reichte Lydia Lennox die Hand. Als sich ihre Finger berührten, strömte plötzlich ein Tornado von neuen Bildern auf mich ein. Keuchend sackte ich auf den Boden der Umkleidekabine. Er hatte es riskiert, er hatte mit der Sondierung begonnen! *Eine weiße Luxusjacht auf türkisem Meer. Gesichter, noch mehr Gesichter, Cocktailgläser, un-*

ter Wasser wendet ein Hai abrupt, Blut wie eine graue Wolke im Wasser, Lachen ... Ich fühlte mich, als würde mein Kopf platzen, während fremde Gedanken sich in meine krallten. Wahrscheinlich stieß ich ein Ächzen aus, vielleicht auch ein Wimmern.

»Alles in Ordnung?« Das war die Verkäuferin, ich hörte sie aus weiter Ferne. »Soll ich dir eine andere Größe bringen?«

Gerade versuchte ich, meiner trockenen Kehle irgendeine Antwort abzuringen, als der Bilderstrom ganz plötzlich abriss.

»Aufhören, *sofort!*«, hörte ich Lydia Lennox zischen, ihre Stimme klang wie eine Kreissäge. »Du Dreckskerl hast wohl gedacht, du kommst damit durch? Tja, ich bin besonders geschult, so was zu bemerken! Das wirst du büßen! Auf die Hilfe und das Geld könnt ihr jetzt lange warten, ihr glaubt nicht wirklich, dass mein Angebot noch steht nach dieser bodenlosen Frechheit?«

Rocket! Wo bist du? Ich konnte nur hoffen, dass ich wirklich gedankenflüsterte, jedenfalls strengte ich mich an wie nie zuvor. *Mr García ist in Schwierigkeiten!*

Ich bin auf der Palme genau über den beiden, erwiderte mein Freund. *Ja, das sehe ich, dass er in Schwierigkeiten ist, oh shit, gleich haben ihn diese beiden Tiger-Girls erreicht ...*

Ich riss den Vorhang der Umkleidekabine zur Seite, warf der verblüfften Verkäuferin das T-Shirt entgegen und raste aus dem Laden. *Kannst du dich nicht Mrs Lennox in den Nacken fallen lassen?*

Spinnst du?, kam es von Rocket zurück. *Ich würde sofort als Snack enden! Zeit für die andere Ablenkung.*

»Passt das nicht? Ich könnte dir noch eins in XL bringen!«, rief die Verkäuferin mir hinterher.

Ich hastete über die Strandpromenade am Ocean Drive. Da

der Gedankenstrom abgebrochen war, versuchte ich irgendwie, mit eigenen Augen zu erkennen, was gerade geschah. *Mr García, was ist los?*

Ich glaube, sie hat vor, mich als Geisel zu nehmen, sagte mein Verwandlungslehrer grimmig. *Jack, kannst du mich abholen? Beeil dich!*

Oh Mann ... ich brauche mindestens vier Minuten, bis ich mit dem Auto bei dir bin, erwiderte Jack Clearwater. *Versuch, ins Meer zu entkommen!*

Mach ich, aber die Chancen stehen nicht gut, gab Mr García zurück und ich lief noch ein bisschen schneller.

Logans Hose

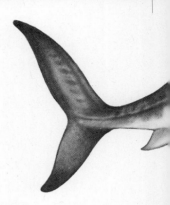

Doch je näher ich kam, desto verblüffter war ich. Obwohl Rocket nicht da war, hatte er Logan anscheinend klare Anweisungen gegeben. Aber welche? Verblüfft sah ich, dass der Schlägertyp keine Anstalten machte, Mr García zu helfen, der sich unauffällig in Richtung Meer zu bewegen versuchte. Logan versuchte auch nicht, die Tigerzwillinge dumm anzumachen. Stattdessen griff er keine zwei Meter von Mrs Lennox und meinem Lehrer entfernt *Lando* an. Was zum Teufel sollte das?

Lando war kleiner als Logan und die totale Couch-Potato. Seine Idee von Sport war, sich im Fernsehen die Basketball-Playoffs anzuschauen. Als Logan begann, ihn zu schubsen, ihm eklige Bezeichnungen an den Kopf zu werfen und ihm die Faust in den Magen zu rammen, wirkte er wie ein Hamster, der es mit einem Kampfhund zu tun hat. Schwächlich, mit weit aufgerissenen Augen, wehrte er sich, während Logan ihn am Hemd packte, und versuchte gleichzeitig, seinen Darth-Vader-Helm nicht fallen zu lassen.

Zum Glück schrie ich nicht, dass Logan aufhören sollte. Weil es nämlich funktionierte, was die beiden da aufführten. Latisha und Natasha versperrten Mr García den Weg zum Meer, aber statt ihn sofort zu packen, machten sie sich daran, erst mal diese beiden nervenden Teenager zu verscheuchen, die sich direkt neben ihrer Chefin prügelten und ihr dabei fast auf die Füße fielen. »Zieht ab, aber ein bisschen flott!«, herrschte eine der Woodwalkerinnen Logan an.

»Mach den Kerl meinetwegen fertig, aber woanders – los, los!«, knurrte die andere und trat Logan drohend entgegen. Der schien immun gegen ihren Killerblick. »Lady, das hier geht Sie nix an, gehen Sie doch selber weg!«

Wow, der hatte Mut! Andererseits wusste er nicht, was die beiden für eine zweite Gestalt hatten. Einen Moment dachte ich, die Zwillinge würden ihn mit einem Karateschlag zu Boden schicken, aber es erregt ja Aufsehen, wenn jemand halb tot herumliegt. Also griff die eine Wandlerin nur Logans Ellenbogen und drückte zu, anscheinend an einer Stelle, wo es richtig wehtat. Dann raunte sie ihm etwas zu und schob ihn weg. Bitterböse Beleidigungen murmelnd, räumte Logan das Feld. Mein Kumpel Lando stand währenddessen herum und beobachtete mit großen Augen, was geschah.

Leider konnten sich Lydia Lennox' Bodyguards jetzt Farryn García zuwenden. Er war losgesprintet, um sich als Delfin ins Meer zu retten, doch die Tigerzwillinge glitten heran und fingen ihn ab.

»Ich warne dich, Lydia«, sagte Mr García kalt. »Du erinnerst dich, dass ich Ratsmitglied bin? Ein Schritt weiter und du hast sämtliche Woodwalker und Seawalker Nordamerikas gegen dich.«

»Ach, meinst du wirklich?«, fragte Lydia Lennox sehr freundlich und gab den Tigerzwillingen ein Signal. Ich ahnte, dass die beiden ihre Finger zu messerscharfen Krallen teilverwandelten.

Verzweifelt blickte ich mich nach einem der schwarz-weißen Polizeiautos um, die doch sonst überall in Miami unterwegs waren. Nur leider gerade nicht hier und nicht jetzt.

In den nächsten Sekunden passierten sehr viele Dinge.

Ich rannte los.

Die Tigerzwillinge packten Farryn García, und weil wir noch in Verbindung waren, spürte ich seine Schmerzen selbst, als sie ihm die Krallen in die Arme gruben.

Lando setzte seinen Darth-Vader-Helm auf, senkte den Kopf und lief los.

Rocket huschte in seiner Rattengestalt die Palme herunter und auf Lydia Lennox zu.

Logan zog seinen Hosenschlitz auf.

Wahrscheinlich war Latisha – ich war mir ziemlich sicher, dass sie es war – nicht darauf vorbereitet, von einem Weltraumschurken gerammt zu werden. Ebenso wenig wie Lydia Lennox darauf, dass eine Ratte sie in den Hintern biss. Oder Natasha, von einem jugendlichen Schläger angepinkelt zu werden. Kurz darauf war in dem sonst so friedlichen Strandpark so einiges los.

Latisha taumelte und ließ Farryn García los, zog ihm dabei allerdings die Krallen über den Arm. Brüllend vor Wut, stürzte sich Natasha auf Logan, ohne noch weiter auf den Gefangenen oder ihre Chefin zu achten. Lydia Lennox sprang mit einem Aufschrei hoch, ihre Hände flogen zu ihrem gebissenen Körperteil.

Inzwischen waren ziemlich viele Menschen stehen geblieben und beobachteten neugierig, was geschah. Manche fragten Farryn García, ob sie ihm helfen konnten, andere hatten schon die Handys am Ohr und waren dabei, die Polizei zu rufen. Ich schob sie freundlich weg und half meinem Lehrer, dessen blutüberströmte Arme fies aussahen, durch die Menge zu kommen. Zur Straße! Verzweifelt blickte ich mich um, sah aber keinen Wagen, den ich kannte.

Jack, wo bist du?, hörte ich Mr García in Gedanken rufen. *Wir brauchen dich JETZT!*
Bin gleich bei euch, kam es grimmig zurück.
Nimm das, Tussi!, hörte ich währenddessen Rocket rufen. Ich wandte mich um und sah, wie er noch schnell eine der Tigerzwillinge biss und dann die nächstbeste Palme hochsprintete. *Haha, Tiger können ja vieles, aber nicht klettern – viel Spaß mit den Cops, ich seh sie schon anrücken!*
Auch ich hörte schon die Sirene. Im selben Moment, in dem Rocket wieder seine Palme hochzischte und Logan und Lando in verschiedene Richtungen davonjagten, fuhr mit Höllentempo Mr Clearwaters Privatauto vor. Wir rissen die Türen auf und warfen uns hinein. Kaum waren die Türen zu, fuhr unser junger Schulleiter los.
»Also, Alisha hätte es geschafft, die Reifen ordentlich quietschen zu lassen«, presste Mr García hervor und inspizierte seine blutenden Arme. Zum Glück war unsere Verbindung wieder unterbrochen. Aber ich wusste auch so, wie er sich fühlte, weil ich die Krallen der Tigerzwillinge auch schon mal abbekommen hatte.
»Weiß ich«, sagte Jack Clearwater und warf ihm einen besorgten Seitenblick zu. »Krankenhaus oder Schule?«
»Schule, bitte«, antwortete Mr García. »Du hast gehört, was sie vorgeschlagen hat, oder? Sie wusste offensichtlich schon Bescheid über unser Problem mit Wave. Durch Ella, schätze ich.«
Währenddessen kramte ich den Auto-Verbandskasten heraus und ließ ihn leider gleich darauf fallen, weil mir noch immer die Hände zitterten und Mr Clearwaters Kurventechnik verbesserungswürdig war. Verbandspäckchen, eine Schere, Klebeband, Desinfektionsmittel und ungefähr tausend andere

Dinge verteilten sich auf der Rückbank. »Tiago! Das hier ist kein Pflasterweitwerfen«, schimpfte Mr García.

Irgendwie schaffte ich es, meinen Verwandlungslehrer während der Fahrt nach Key Largo notdürftig zu verarzten.

»Es tut mir wirklich leid«, sagte Mr García und ließ den Kopf gegen die Nackenstütze zurücksinken. »Ich hab's vergeigt, eigentlich hätte sie nicht spüren dürfen, dass ich sie sondiere.«

»Das war nicht Ihre Schuld! Sie hat doch gesagt, sie hat sich besonders ausbilden lassen, um so was zu bemerken«, entgegnete ich und versuchte, die Bilder von vorhin in meinem Kopf zu sortieren. »Haben Sie irgendwas von dem kapiert, was Sie aus ihr rausgezogen haben?«

»Eins ist klar, sie war dort und hat die Arenakämpfe beobachtet, anscheinend auch gewettet und gespeist«, meinte mein Lehrer. »Auch deinem Namen bin ich begegnet. Wer war der Tigerhai, dessen Bild sie im Kopf hatte, warst du das?«

Peinlicherweise konnte ich nicht wissen, ob ich das gewesen war oder mein Bruder. Als Hai hatte ich keine – wie man so schön sagt – »unveränderlichen Kennzeichen«.

»Also kurz gesagt, reicht das nicht für eine Verurteilung vor dem Rat?«, fragte Mr Clearwater.

Mein Verwandlungslehrer schüttelte den Kopf. »Dafür hätten wir zweifelsfrei in ihren Gedanken lesen müssen, dass sie wusste, dass mindestens ein Wandler in diesem Netzkäfig war und dass ihr das egal war.«

Wir waren alle enttäuscht, aber ich wahrscheinlich am meisten. Ich biss mir auf die Lippe, um mich davon abzulenken und nicht vor Wut die Faust gegen die Autoscheibe zu knallen.

Mr Clearwaters Handy klingelte. Als er sah, wer dran war, ging er ran und stellte laut.

»Eine unglaubliche Frechheit war das!«, verkündete Lydia

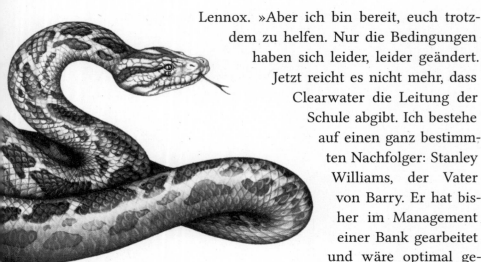

Lennox. »Aber ich bin bereit, euch trotzdem zu helfen. Nur die Bedingungen haben sich leider, leider geändert. Jetzt reicht es nicht mehr, dass Clearwater die Leitung der Schule abgibt. Ich bestehe auf einen ganz bestimmten Nachfolger: Stanley Williams, der Vater von Barry. Er hat bisher im Management einer Bank gearbeitet und wäre optimal geeignet für eure Schule, weil er für mehr Disziplin sorgen würde und ihm die Finanzen nicht ständig dermaßen entgleiten würden.«

»Ah der«, murmelte Mr García säuerlich. Ich erinnerte mich ebenfalls. Dieser Mr Williams hatte versucht, während des Sumpfschüler-Aufstandes die Kontrolle bei uns zu übernehmen. Zum Glück ohne Erfolg. Würde Mrs Lennox es diesmal schaffen, ihn uns aufzudrücken? Aber das konnte Mr Clearwater nicht machen! Er konnte nach Miss White nicht auch noch weggehen!

»Verstehe. Wir melden uns, sobald wir uns entschieden haben, Mrs Lennox«, sagte Jack Clearwater und legte auf.

Ich fühlte mich abwechselnd wütend und besorgt. »Mr Clearwater ... Sie bleiben aber doch unser Schulleiter, oder? Wir finden bestimmt eine andere Lösung, Wave freizukriegen!«

»Tiago ...«, begann Jack Clearwater vorsichtig, und da ahnte ich schon, was kommen würde. »Ich darf nicht riskieren, dass

Wave stirbt. Wenn ihm irgendwas passiert, würde ich mir das nie verzeihen.«

»Heißt das etwa, Sie *tun das wirklich, was Mrs Lennox will?*« Ich schrie ihn an und wusste, dass mich das nicht beliebt machen würde. Aber in diesem Moment war mir das egal.

»Ja, genau das heißt es«, sagte Jack Clearwater.

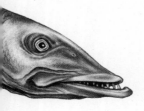

Ein Barrakuda
aus der Hölle

Vielleicht sollte ich dir erklären, warum ich es mache.« Jack Clearwater starrte geradeaus auf die Straße, seine Hände umklammerten das Lenkrad. »Als ich in deinem Alter war und noch mit meiner Mutter in den Rocky Mountains lebte, habe ich mich mit einem Wels-Wandler angefreundet, der in einem Bergsee wohnte.« Er holte tief Luft. »Eines Tages waren wir eigentlich verabredet, aber ich wollte lieber in die Bibliothek, wo ich ein paar interessante neue Bücher entdeckt hatte. So habe ich nicht mitbekommen, dass sich mein Freund in dieser Zeit versehentlich an Land verwandelt hat.«

Ich war erschüttert. »Ist er ... gestorben?«

Mein Schulleiter nickte. »Später, in Florida, bin ich mal mit einer wilden Delfinschule geschwommen und habe mich immer öfter gefragt, wie andere Wasser-Wandler klarkommen. So hatte ich die Idee, eine Schule für sie zu gründen, damit es nicht mehr zu so schrecklichen, unnötigen Unfällen kommt. Verstehst du, warum mir die Blue Reef so wichtig ist?«

»Ja«, sagte ich nur.

»Der Rat war skeptisch, ob jemand, der erst Mitte zwanzig ist, eine Schule leiten kann. Deswegen haben *wir* Schwierigkeiten mit der Finanzierung und die Clearwater High hat keine, weil sie vom Rat unterstützt wird.« Mr Clearwater seufzte. »Meine Mutter hat sich natürlich für mich und die Blue Reef eingesetzt, aber es hat nicht gereicht.«

»Bitte geben Sie nicht auf«, sagte ich.

Sobald wir die Eingangshalle der Highschool betraten, drängten sich Jasper, die Delfinclique und Juna um uns und Fragen prasselten auf mich nieder. »Was war denn los?« – »Wo ist Finny?« – »Was ist mit Mr García passiert?«

Ihr habt Finny nicht im Tierheim abgegeben, oder?, fragte Nox aus dem großen Aquarium heraus, Linus' Seepferdchen-Nachwuchs um sich geschart. Drei Miniseepferchen, für die sich ihr Vater leider nicht verantwortlich fühlte.

»Nein, und auch nicht im *Sea Adventure*«, sagte ich erschöpft, während meine beiden Lehrer in den ersten Stock verschwanden. Weil mich niemand gebeten hatte, irgendwas geheim zu halten, berichtete ich den anderen, was passiert war. Erschrockene Stille folgte, dann redeten alle durcheinander.

»Der arme Wave!«, sagte Shari.

»Hoffentlich bekommt Finny nicht zu viel Stress.« Blue sah besorgt aus.

»Das meint die Lennox nich' ernst, oder?«, empörte sich Jasper.

Wie ernst sie es meinte, fanden wir sehr bald heraus. Und zwar gleich am nächsten Morgen.

»Bitte alle Schüler und Lehrer in die Eingangshalle«, hörte ich Jack Clearwater nach dem Frühstück durchsagen. Kurz darauf war es dort gedrängt voll. Auch Finny, die ziemlich blass wirkte, war da; ihr Vater hatte sie gestern Nacht zurückgebracht.

Betroffen sahen wir unseren jungen Schulleiter mit den hellblonden Haaren und den freundlichen, manchmal ein bisschen verträumten Augen die Treppe herunterkommen. Er hatte seine Stadtklamotten – Hemd und Jeans – an und trug Rucksack und Koffer.

Gleichzeitig kam mit einer schicken silbergrauen Limousine auf dem Parkplatz jemand an: ein dünner blasser, unsportlich wirkender Mann mit Seitenscheitel. Nach einem kritischen Blick auf die Außenseite der Schule betrat er die Eingangshalle, warf uns Schülern einen flüchtigen Blick zu und steuerte dann die Lehrer an. »Stanley Williams«, stellte er sich vor, ohne zu lächeln. »Der neue Schulleiter.«

»Ich weiß«, sagte Jack Clearwater, ein »Herzlich willkommen« wollte ihm wohl nicht über die Lippen.

Mr García nickte dem Neuen zu. Mrs Pelagius warf Barrys Vater einen bohrenden Blick zu. Sie war gerade in ihrer Gestalt als nicht sehr große alte Frau, die ein wenig gebeugt ging und ihr silberweißes Haar in einem Pagenkopf trug. Ivy Bennett versuchte immerhin, freundlich zu sein, aber hauptsächlich wirkte sie nervös.

Bei einem schnellen Blick in die Runde stellte ich fest, dass selbst Barry sich nicht darüber zu freuen schien, dass sein Vater angekommen war. »Halt dich ein bisschen aufrechter!«, befahl der ihm auch prompt – und so laut, dass alle im Umkreis es hören konnten. »Und was für ein Hemd soll das denn sein? Schämst du dich nicht, so was in der Öffentlichkeit zu tragen?«

Ich fand Barrys Hemd sehenswert – auf einem grünen Hintergrund tummelten sich rosa Flamingos.

»Das habe ich mir selbst gekauft, Dad«, sagte Barry, er schien sich unwohl zu fühlen und kratzte sich ständig am Hals.

»Du wirst dieses Hemd sofort nach dieser Veranstaltung *wegwerfen,* ist das klar?«, zischte Mr Williams und verstummte dann glücklicherweise, denn nun begann Mr Clearwater zu den versammelten Schülern zu sprechen.

»Ihr habt vielleicht schon gehört, was passiert ist«, sagte er. »Mrs Lennox will uns nur mit Wave helfen, wenn Mr Williams mich ablöst. Seid so nett und macht ihm das Leben nicht allzu schwer, ja?«

»Aber wie lange bleiben Sie denn weg?«, rief Juna verzweifelt.

»Weiß ich noch nicht.« Jack Clearwater sah furchtbar müde aus. »Tut mir leid, Leute. Ich kann nicht anders.« Er schwang sich den Rucksack auf den Rücken und nahm seinen Koffer.

»Moment.« Farryn García umarmte ihn und Mrs Pelagius folgte seinem Beispiel.

Noemi begleitete ihn zur Tür, eine große Pantherin mit glänzend schwarzem Fell und geschmeidigen Bewegungen. Dann erst ließ sie ihn gehen und blickte ihm traurig hinterher. So wie Lucy, der es wieder besser ging und die sich für den Abschied ins Aquarium der Eingangshalle gezwängt hatte. Das war mit einer Pazifischen Riesenkrake darin richtig, richtig voll.

Fast beschwingt, ergriff nun Mr Williams das Wort. »Es ist mir eine Ehre, nun für diese Schule verantwortlich zu sein. Ab jetzt weht hier ein anderer Wind! Ist es wahr, dass ihr bisher keine Hausaufgaben hattet?«

Wir nickten vorsichtig und ahnten, was jetzt kam.

»Das geht natürlich gar nicht. Ab jetzt wird hier intensiv gelernt, nur Spitzenleistungen und Tüchtigkeit zählen. Und Geldprobleme wird diese Schule nie wieder haben, dafür werden wöchentliche Besuchertage sorgen, bei denen ihr euch in Selbstbeherrschung üben und euren vollen Einsatz für diese Schule unter Beweis stellen könnt. Ihr habt das ja das letzte

Mal richtig gut gemacht. Ihr habt Talent fürs Geldverdienen – entwickelt das weiter, Leute!«

Niemand freute sich so richtig über das Lob, vor allem, als wir hörten, dass der nächste Besuchertag schon am nächsten Donnerstag stattfinden würde und wir in unserer Freizeit dafür trainieren sollten. Eins war inzwischen klar – Lydia Lennox krempelte die Blue Reef Highschool so um, wie sie sie haben wollte. Und Barrys Vater war dabei ihre bis zum Kragen mit hohlen Worten und bescheuerten Ideen gefüllte Marionette.

In der ersten Stunde hatten wir mal wieder Verwandlung.

Und natürlich kam Chris zu spät. »Schon wieder! Das muss ich eintragen«, sagte Mr García und machte eine Notiz im Klassenbuch. Vielleicht hätte er es nicht getan, wenn er gewusst hätte, was für Folgen das haben würde.

In dieser Stunde durften wir mit Gedankenstrom-Übertragungen experimentieren – wie passend. Fast unmerklich nickten mein Verwandlungslehrer und ich uns zu und der Schatten eines Lächelns huschte über seine Lippen.

Die zweite Stunde war Kampf und Überleben. Oje.

»Jetzt bitte alle verwandeln, Kinder!«, rief Miss Bennett und klatschte zweimal. Waren wir jetzt in der Vorschule? Was kam als Nächstes, würden wir uns an den Händen nehmen und zusammen im Kreis tanzen?

In der Lagune war ein ziemliches Gedränge, als alle ins Wasser stapften. Es dauerte eine Weile, bis jeder geschafft hatte, in seine zweite Gestalt zu schlüpfen, und dann war es ganz schön eng im Flachwasser, besonders wenn man in Maras Nähe war. Aber auch Toco brauchte viel Platz, er schwamm als fetter Alligator mit angelegten Beinen umher, indem er seinen Schwanz als Paddel benutzte. Dabei rammte er fast Finny, die sich zum Ausweichen platt auf den Boden legen musste und dabei beinahe Nox erdrückt hätte. *Toco, du bist heute echt ein Reptil des Grauens*, motzte Finny, während Nox sich beschwerte: *Ich kann nichts sehen, geh runter von mir, Plattfisch!*

Barry dagegen musste ständig den Delfinen ausweichen, die aufgeregt durcheinanderwirbelten und sich mit Pfiffen und Schnarren verständigten.

»So, prima ... und jetzt bitte eine Reihe bilden«, forderte unsere neue Kampflehrerin uns auf. Als wir alle halbwegs nebeneinanderschwebten oder -schwammen, fügte sie hinzu: »So, und jetzt kämpft bitte gegen den Seawalker rechts von euch!«

Ich wandte meinen Tigerhaikörper nach rechts und fand mich Auge in Auge mit einem winzigen Seepferdchen wieder, das vor meiner Schnauze schwebte.

Das ist unfair, piepste Linus. *Kann die mir mal sagen, wie ich dich besiegen soll?*

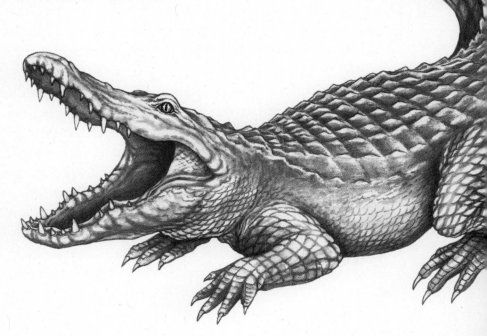

Auf die Nase hauen?, schlug ich ratlos vor.

Das kann ich natürlich versuchen. Linus war ernsthaft sauer. *Aber wenn du jetzt das Maul aufmachst, saugst du mich ein und es ist aus mit mir!*

Stimmt, musste ich zugeben.

Einigen wir uns auf unentschieden?

Okay, sagte ich.

Vielen anderen Kampfpaaren ging es ähnlich. Finny wirbelte wie ein Herbstblatt um Mara herum, die sich wie in Zeitlupe bewegte, und verpasste ihr schließlich einen Knutschfleck auf den Nacken. Zähne hatte sie ja keine. Lucy packte unsere Qualle Zelda mit zwei ihrer acht Arme und war anschließend damit beschäftigt, sie nicht zu zerquetschen. Toco und Barry fingen wieder mal an, sich zum Spaß gegenseitig eins auf die zu Schnauze geben, obwohl sie eigentlich ganz andere Kampfpartner hatten. Am Strand versuchten Jasper und Daphne-die-Möwe ziemlich hilflos, sich zu duellieren. Das sah so aus, dass Daphne auf Jaspers Rücken hockte und mit dem Schnabel auf seinen Panzer einhackte, während Jasper *Das kitzelt, das kitzelt!* rief.

Riffhai Ralph jagte die erschrockene Izzy im Kreis durch die Lagune, sodass sie immer wieder kurze Flugstrecken einlegen und übers Wasser gleiten musste. Nicht nur ich sah besorgt, dass Ralph sich allmählich in einen Fressrausch hineinsteigerte, als er immer wieder nach ihr schnappte. Schließlich schoss Chris als Seelöwe zu ihnen hinüber. *Lass sie in Ruhe,* motzte er Ralph an und glitt zwischen die beiden. *Du hast gewonnen und jetzt zisch ab, okay?*

Hey, alles cool, Alter, chill mal, gab Ralph beleidigt zurück.

Danke, Chris! Izzy ließ sich ausgepumpt auf die Wasseroberfläche fallen.

Schließlich wurde Juna im Wasser ohnmächtig, als sie schon beim ersten Angriff einen Stromschlag von Leonora abbekam.

»Bei der großen Welle!«, schrie Miss Bennett, rannte ins Wasser und verfrachtete den reglosen Falterfisch in ihren (hastig im Meer ausgespülten) Kaffeebecher. »Wo ist eure Krankenstation?«

Noah verwandelte sich, zog sich hastig eine Badehose an und rannte voraus, um ihr den Weg zu Mrs Misaki zu zeigen. Besorgt schauten wir ihnen nach.

Ich wette, die Koffeinreste machen Juna gleich wieder wach, meinte Finny.

Stimmt. Noah schwamm durch die Kaffeewolke in der Lagune und probierte. *Uäh. Ekliger Nachgeschmack.*

Diese Stunde war ungefähr so lustig wie ein Tsunami, sagte Shari genervt und düste ab in den tiefen Teil der Lagune.

Ach, ich fand's okay, ich hätte Noah fast besiegt, meinte Blue.

Weil er dich hätte gewinnen lassen!, gab Shari vom Meeresboden aus zurück und begann, ihre Muscheln in den Schnabel zu nehmen und neu zu sortieren.

Oh, meinst du wirklich? Blue tauchte auf und prustete verbrauchte Luft aus ihrem Blasloch. *Voll nett von ihm, meine Kampfnote ist nicht besonders.*

Miss Bennett tauchte nicht mehr auf, dafür zum Glück Juna, wieder quietschlebendig. *Schon krass, ich kann mich an gar nichts erinnern!,* erzählte sie, während Leonora sich tausendmal entschuldigte.

In der Pause kam unser neuer Schulleiter Stanley Williams mit dem Klassenbuch in der Hand zu uns. »Wer von euch ist Christopher Jacobsen?«

»Ich«, sagte Chris, der gerade versucht hatte, eine Palme hochzuklettern. Er hörte auf zu lachen, strich sich das schulterlange, von der Sonne ausgebleichte Haar zurück und blickte ein bisschen misstrauisch drein.

»Im Klassenbuch ist verzeichnet, dass du in den letzten zwei Wochen sieben Mal zu spät gekommen bist.« Mit finsterem Blick musterte ihn Mr Williams. »So was geht einfach nicht, junger Mann. Hiermit verweise ich dich von der Schule. Ruf deine Eltern an, dass sie dich abholen, und geh deine Koffer packen!«

Chris blieb der Mund offen stehen. Uns auch.

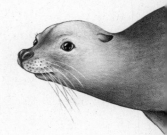

Ärger für alle

Chris sollte von der Schule fliegen? »Oh«, war das Einzige, was unserem sonst so lässigen, schlagfertigen Seelöwen einfiel.

»Bitte nicht, er wird es auch nie wieder tun!« Izzy wirkte noch entsetzter als wir anderen. »Geben Sie ihm noch eine Chance!«

»Und wer bist du?« Mr Williams strenger Blick richtete sich auf sie. »Bist du etwa das Mädchen, das schon wieder seine Schreibsachen in der Cafeteria hat liegen lassen? Jedenfalls steht *Isabel Lawrence* darauf.«

Oh ... das sah ihr ähnlich, schließlich hatte unser fliegender Fisch aus Kalifornien nicht ohne Grund den Spitznamen Dizzy Izzy, »Wirrköpfchen«. Sie tauchte grundsätzlich im falschen Arbeitsraum auf, schaffte es immer noch, sich zwischen den Hütten zu verirren, und suchte ständig ihre Sachen.

»Ähm, ja, das kann schon sein, aber ist das schlimm?« Trotzig blickte Izzy ihm in die Augen.

»Sorge einfach dafür, dass es nicht mehr vorkommt.« Mr Williams blickte eindringlich in die Runde. »Mir liegt nichts daran, euch zu quälen, ich will euch fit machen für das echte Leben, versteht ihr das? Was ihr bei mir lernt, hilft euch, auch in einem harten Arbeitsalltag zu bestehen!«

Das klang, als hätte er wenigstens ein paar gute Absichten.

Trotzdem konnte ich ihn nicht ausstehen und anscheinend ging es nicht nur mir so.

»Ich packe *nicht* meinen Koffer, ich gehe ins Meer, so wie Miss White«, presste Chris hervor. »Dieser Quallenhintern kann mich mal!«

Shari reagierte als Erste. »Heute nach der Schule Krisentreffen im Wrack?«

Wir nickten und brachten vor lauter Erschütterung kaum ein Wort heraus. Die Blue Reef Highschool ohne Chris ... nein, das ging gar nicht! Vielleicht war ich der Einzige, der wusste, warum er garantiert nicht seine Eltern anrufen würde. Seine Mutter war tot und sein Vater, der in Kalifornien lebte, vor Verzweiflung zum Alkoholiker geworden.

Der Nächste, der von unserem neuen Schulleiter eins verpasst bekam, war Ralph.

»Ey, Leute, wer hilft mir nachher beim Aufbauen der Anlage für die Party?«, fragte Ralph in der Pause. »*Wild Thing Friday*, yeah!«

Doch leider hörte ihn Mr Williams. »Was für eine Party? Ich habe keine genehmigt!«

»Aber wir dürfen jeden zweiten Freitag eine machen«, protestierte Juna, unsere Klassensprecherin.

»Ab jetzt nicht mehr«, verkündete Barrys Vater. »So was lenkt euch nur von euren Pflichten ab. Bei Gelegenheit organisiere ich für euch ein gemeinsames Kaffeetrinken mit Gesellschaftsspielen, das ist wesentlich gesünder und lehrreicher.«

»Digga!«, protestierte Ralph. »Ihren Kaffee können Sie sich in die Hose gießen!«

»Verweis für dich, Junge ... wie heißt du?«

»Kevin«, sagte Ralph. Niemand widersprach.

Mit strenger Miene notierte sich Mr Williams den Namen

und zog ab. Wütend und enttäuscht, starrten wir ihm hinterher.

Mit wutblitzenden Augen verwandelte Ralph seine Zähne und machte schnappende Bewegungen damit. An Mr Williams' Stelle hätte ich mir Sorgen gemacht. Riffhaie sind normalerweise harmlos, aber wenn sie das Gefühl haben, sie müssen ihr Revier verteidigen, können sie eklig werden.

In der Pause hatten ich, Shari und Jasper eine Arbeitsbesprechung mit der Luft-Überwachung. »Bisher haben wir noch keine Glasbodenboote gesichtet. Auch keine Boote mit Netzkäfigen, in denen Haie waren«, sagte Shelby. »Aber wir bleiben dran.«

»Könnt ihr heute Nachmittag wieder losfliegen?«, drängte Jasper.

»Ja, logisch machen wir das«, versicherte uns Maris, er wirkte bedrückt. »Aber wenn wir so eine Haikampf-Bande aufspüren, müssen wir schnell handeln. Ich bin nicht sicher, ob das mit Mr Williams geht, wenn ihr wisst, was ich meine.«

Wir nickten alle gleichzeitig.

»Wenn ihr oder Steve wirklich etwas Verdächtiges seht, sollten wir die Polizei rufen. Ich bin mir sicher, dass Finnys Vater uns anhört und ernst nimmt«, versicherte ich ihnen.

»Bestimmt. Also ich finde Mr Greyson nett«, sagte Shari. »Obwohl er Finny so viel verboten hat.«

Nach der Pause versuchte ich, mich mühsam auf Mathe und Physik zu konzentrieren. Es half ein bisschen, dass Mr García – im langärmeligen Shirt, vielleicht damit niemand seine Krallenwunden sah – so tat, als sei alles in Ordnung. »Am nächsten Dienstag gibt es zwei Ausflüge für die Erstjahresschüler«, kündigte er an. »Ich hänge heute noch eine Liste aus. Die eine Hälfte der Klasse hat einen Tiefwasserlehrgang mit mir, die andere Hälfte macht eine Riffexkursion mit Miss Bennett.«

Das klang spannend und sofort begannen Shari und ihre Delfinfreunde – die alle ganz sicher im Tiefwasser dabei sein würden –, aufgeregt darüber zu schwatzen. Dann fiel uns ein, dass Chris nicht dabei sein würde, und als auch noch Finny sagte: »Tja, ich habe leider Arrest, ich kann nicht mit«, da ging sogar den Delfinen die gute Laune flöten. Sie wussten ebenso wie ich, dass dieser neue Schulleiter jedes einzelne von Finnys Verboten auch durchsetzen würde.

Ich blieb stumm. Plötzlich hatte ich das Gefühl, dass ich dringend mal allein sein musste. So viel Shari mir auch bedeutete und so gern ich die anderen hatte.

In der Mittagspause holte ich mir ein Sandwich, ließ die von Leuten wimmelnde, laute und brütend warme Cafeteria hinter mir und wanderte den Sandstrand entlang, der fast die gleiche Farbe hatte wie Sharis Locken. Ein leichter Wind vom Meer strich über mein Gesicht. Niemand war hier und das tat gut. Schließlich war ich als Hai ein Einzelgänger.

Plötzlich wünschte ich mir, dass ich all das meinen Eltern erzählen könnte. Aber sie waren mir so furchtbar fern und ich wusste nicht mal, ob sie sich überhaupt dafür interessieren würden, was hier abging. Nein, ich würde sie nicht anrufen. Sollten *sie* sich doch mal melden und fragen, wie es mir ging!

Erst konnte ich es nicht glauben, als ich das Weinen hörte. Waren etwa nicht alle beim Mittagessen? Nein, das Geräusch kam hinter dem Bootshaus hervor und war zweifelsfrei kein jaulender Wind oder so was. Vorsichtig ging ich näher und achtete darauf, leise aufzutreten. Ich wollte denjenigen, der da weinte, nicht verschrecken.

Vorsichtig lugte ich hinter das Boothaus und sah dort eine

Frau mit langen, mit Spangen hochgesteckten braunen Haaren sitzen. Ivy Bennett! Sie hockte auf dem Boden wie ein Häufchen Seetang, hatte den Kopf in den Armen vergraben und schluchzte.

Erst wollte ich flüchten, doch es war zu spät, sie hatte mich schon gehört und den Kopf gehoben. Erschrocken versuchte sie, sich die Tränen abzuwischen und zu lächeln, aber es war sinnlos, ihr Gesicht war immer noch rot und verquollen.

»Oh, hallo, Tiago«, sagte sie. »Ich komme gleich zum Mittagessen. In fünf Minuten, okay?«

Plötzlich tat sie mir furchtbar leid. Statt abzuhauen, ging ich auf sie zu und setzte mich neben sie. »Ist nicht leicht, oder? An einer neuen Schule anzufangen?«

»Nein«, sagte sie und klang dabei furchtbar traurig. »Aber wenn es hier nicht klappt, habe ich keine Ahnung, was ich machen soll. Ich ... ich wollte ein neues Leben anfangen, verstehst du? Ich habe meine Wohnung im Norden aufgegeben, meine Möbel verkauft und bin nach Key Largo gezogen. Und jetzt läuft alles furchtbar schief hier!«

»Oje«, sagte ich betroffen.

»Die arme Juna, ich hätte sie nie diese Übung mit Leonora machen lassen dürfen. Ich bin eine schlechte Lehrerin!« Sie bekam erneut einen Weinkrampf. »Vielleicht hätte ich doch lieber in die Politik gehen sollen. Als Mädchen habe ich davon geträumt, Senatorin in Washington zu werden.« Ohne mich anzusehen, reichte mir Ivy Bennett einen zerknickten Zeitungsausschnitt. Ich glättete ihn zwischen den Fingern und betrachtete das Foto. Wow, da war Miss Bennett mit blitzenden Augen in vorderster Front bei einer Demo!

»Eigentlich unterrichte ich ja gerne, in der letzten Schule – einer für Menschen – hatte ich Spaß mit den Kindern und mit meinem Freund war noch alles prima ... ich wusste ja nicht, dass er mich damals schon ... ach, ich hatte einfach nie Glück mit Männern und wahrscheinlich werde ich nie Kinder haben! Das ist ein so furchtbar schlimmer Gedanke!« Ein neuer Tränenstrom lief ihr über das Gesicht. Verlegen versuchte sie, ihn abzuwischen. »Tut mir echt leid, Tiago, dass ich dich mit alldem belaste.«

»Was haben Sie denn damals für Fächer unterrichtet?«, wagte ich zu fragen.

»Englisch, Französisch und Gesellschaftskunde.«

»Und wie sind Sie dann hier ausgerechnet *Kampflehrerin* geworden?« Jetzt war ich wirklich neugierig.

Ivy Bennett sah aus, als würde sie sich gerne wie ein Einsiedlerkrebs in ihr Schneckenhaus zurückziehen. »Ich wollte unbedingt hierher, aber Mr Clearwater hat mir gesagt, dass nur die Position der Kampflehrerin frei ist und außerdem die Fächer Sei dein Tier und Verhalten in besonderen Fällen. Dann hab ich eben versucht, das hinzukriegen, obwohl ich nur ein Jahr lang Judo gemacht habe.«

»Verstehe«, sagte ich und biss in mein Sandwich.

»Aber jetzt erzähl mal ... du wirkst auch nicht so richtig glücklich. Was ist los?«

Bevor ich es mich versehen hatte, hatte ich ihr schon von meinen kühlen Eltern erzählt. Und wie fertig es mich machte, dass die Blue Reef Highschool wegen Mrs Lennox' Intrigen den Bach runterging. Dass ich Miss White vermisste ... und Jack Clearwater auch, obwohl er erst einen halben Tag weg war.

»Du hast es wirklich nicht leicht.« Ivy Bennett lächelte mir aufmunternd zu. »Aber vielleicht gibst du deinen Eltern noch eine Chance? Vielleicht warten sie nur auf eine Gelegenheit, dir zu helfen und dir zu zeigen, dass sie auf deiner Seite sind.«

»Meinen Sie wirklich?« Das war unwahrscheinlich – sie kannte meine Haiverwandtschaft nicht! Aber ich war zu höflich, das laut auszusprechen.

Die Strömung hilft dem, der sie aufsucht, wie die Mondfische sagen.«

»Sie können Mondfischsprache?«

»Ach, Sprachen zu lernen, fällt mir leicht, ich kann noch ein paar andere. So, wollen wir zurückgehen in die Cafeteria? Ich glaube, ich habe nun doch ein bisschen Hunger.«

Ich nicht, deshalb zog ich mich in meine Hütte zurück, aber Miss Bennett marschierte tatsächlich in Richtung der Cafeteria. Was ich sehr tapfer von ihr fand, denn eins war sicher ... dort redeten die Leute gerade über sie.

Nach der Mittagspause hatten wir Menschenkunde. Diese Stunde, die sonst Mr Clearwater gehalten hatte, übernahm Mr Williams heute persönlich. Stumm und angespannt, saßen die anderen und ich im Klassenzimmer, während er den Blick über die Schüler schweifen ließ. »Du! Steh mal auf«, sagte er zu Shari.

»Ich?«, fragte unser Delfinmädchen.

»Ja, genau du«, sagte Mr Williams. »Mal sehen, was ihr in Menschenkunde schon gelernt habt. Nicht viel, wie ich vermute, viel Gutes habe ich über euren alten Schulleiter nicht gehört. Wie nennt man den Chef dieses Landes?«

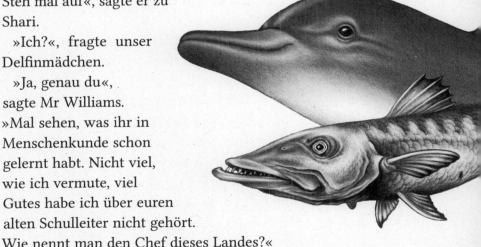

»Schwarmführer?«, riet Shari unsicher.

»Falsch – Präsident! Was muss er für Eigenschaften haben?«

»Hm, ich hab ihn schon im Fernsehen gesehen«, meinte Shari und wurde wieder etwas munterer. »Laut reden, sich mindestens einmal am Tag aufregen und richtig gut lügen?«

Das führte zu einem Wutausbruch des neuen Schulleiters, in dem es um Respekt für gewählte Staatsoberhäupter ging, den wir unbedingt noch lernen müssten. Aber er würde schon noch dafür sorgen, dass wir gute Staatsbürger werden.

Dann ging das Abfragen – das eher ein Verhör war – weiter und wurde noch schlimmer. Wieso fragte dieser Trottel die arme Shari, wie unsere Hauptstadt hieß und wer für unser Land die Gesetze machte? Sie war als Delfin aufgewachsen und erst seit drei Monaten an Land!

Aber das war Mr Williams anscheinend egal. Ich hielt es kaum aus, wie er Frage um Frage auf Shari abfeuerte, die sie nicht beantworten konnte. »Wie heißt die Währung in Japan?«

Shari war schon völlig fertig, aber sie versuchte immer noch, alles richtig zu machen. »Äh ... auch Dollar?«

»Falsch. Yen! Und in Europa?«

Ich konnte es nicht mit ansehen. So riskant es war, ich schrieb die Antwort auf meine Hand und zeigte es ihr unauffällig.

»Euro!«, verkündete Shari erleichtert.

»Richtig. Setz dich.« Williams kritzelte etwas in ein Notizbuch. »Ich will mal gnädig sein und dir keine Sechs eintragen. Immerhin hast du eine Antwort gewusst. Also eine Sechs plus.«

Fassungslos ließ sich Shari wieder auf ihren Stuhl sinken. Damit war ihre Menschenkundenote in diesem Schuljahr hinüber. Ich versuchte, ihr einen aufmunternden Blick zu schenken, doch sie ließ den Kopf hängen und sah es nicht. Blue legte ihrer besten Freundin den Arm um die Schulter.

Mr Williams bekam von Blue, Noah, Nestor und mir Blicke voll purem Hass.

Mr Williams war noch nicht fertig mit seinen Verhören. Als nächstes kam Finny dran. Sie sollte ausrechnen, wie viele Wahlmänner benötigt wurden, damit ein Kandidat Präsident werden konnte.

»Los, los, komm ans Whiteboard«, sagte Mr Williams und winkte Finny, aufzustehen.

Finny schlurfte nach vorne. Sie war in Mathe und den naturwissenschaftlichen Fächern ziemlich still, und jetzt wurde auch klar, warum. Den Tränen nahe, versuchte sie, die Zahlen zusammenzurechnen ... und schaffte es nicht.

»Schwache Leistung«, fand Mr Williams.

»Wenn Sie es genau wissen wollen, ich habe eine Rechenschwäche!« Finny schleuderte den Stift in eine Ecke.

Betroffenes Schweigen in der Klasse. Das hatten wir alle nicht gewusst, sie hatte es geschickt nicht nur vor den Lehrern, sondern auch vor uns verborgen. Wie traurig, dass die Atmosphäre in der Schule nun so vergiftet war. Mir kam der Gedanke, dass all das mit Wave angefangen hatte. Vielleicht wäre es besser gewesen, wir hätten ihn nie getroffen und er wäre einfach an unserer Schule vorbeigeschwommen. Nein, das war gemein! Er war einfach ein netter Kerl, der auf unsere Schule gehen wollte, und Seawalker mussten einander helfen.

Bei Menschen klappte das ja nicht so gut. Dann zumindest bei uns.

Ich hoffte, dass es wenigstens der anderen neuen Wandlerin, die wir entdeckt hatten, gut ging. Daisy Cousteau, genau, das war ihr Name. Würden wir jemals wieder etwas von ihr hören? Und war es ein Riesenfehler, dass wir uns gerade nicht um sie und ihre zweite Gestalt kümmerten?

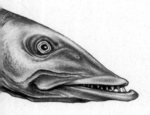

Der Plan

Das mit dem Krisentreffen war gar nicht so einfach, wie Chris feststellen musste, als er nach dem Unterricht versuchte, als Seelöwe die Bucht zu verlassen. *Schaut mal, wer hier Wache hält,* meldete er und schickte uns ein Gedankenbild von Mr Williams silbernem, stromlinienförmigem Hechtkopf, dessen Maul ihn immer mürrisch wirken ließ.

Wo willst du hin, Junge? Raus ins Meer?, fragte unser neuer Schulleiter misstrauisch.

Genau, gab Chris zurück. *Lassen Sie mich durch.*

Es wäre nicht gut für dich, ins offene Meer zu schwimmen, gab Mr Williams zurück. *Ist dir nicht klar, welche Gefahren dort lauern? Deshalb kann ich das leider nicht erlauben.*

Wie Sie wissen, gehe ich nicht mehr auf diese Schule. Das heißt praktischerweise, dass Sie mir nichts zu sagen haben. Mit einem gewaltigen Sprung setzte Chris über den Barrakuda hinweg und jagte ins offene Meer.

Mr Williams setzte seine Patrouille fort. Leider. Einem Barrakuda entgeht nicht viel von dem, was in seiner Umgebung geschieht, und pfeilschnell schwimmen kann er auch, wie ich von Barry wusste. Wie sollte Finny zum Wrack kommen? Offiziell durfte sie ja die Schule nicht verlassen.

»Ich hab's«, sagte Shari. »Blue, könntest du auf der einen Seite der Lagune, möglichst weit entfernt vom Durchgang, um

Hilfe rufen und irgendwelche komischen Bauchplatscher dazu machen? Während Williams abgelenkt ist, kannst du durchwitschen, Finny.«

»Gute Idee! Falls Williams-die-Algenpest nicht gleich zu ihr hinschwimmt, tue ich aufgeregt und drängele ein bisschen«, meinte Noah.

»Und wenn er zu schnell versucht, wieder zum Durchgang zu kommen, blocke ich ihn«, fügte ich hinzu. Die anderen grinsten, denn eins war klar, an Tigerhaizähnen traute sich keiner vorbei – ganz sicher auch kein Barrakuda.

»Hat jemand von euch Barry gesehen? Ist der im Meer bei seinem Vater?«, fragte Blue besorgt, doch wir schüttelten den Kopf.

Noah suchte den Horizont mit den Augen ab, obwohl es von hier aus nur ein grünes Mangrovengewucher mit einer Lücke dazwischen – den Durchgang – zu sehen gab. »Der sitzt bestimmt irgendwo in der Schule am Laptop und schaut YouTube-Videos. Oder er schreibt ein neues Liebesgedicht für Carmen.«

Neulich war auf geheimnisvollen Wegen eins davon an die Öffentlichkeit gekommen. Die Zeilen *Meine harte Schale bleibt nicht gleich, sondern wird ganz weich, wenn ich dich seh, oje!* waren in meinem Gedächtnis hängen geblieben, der Rest gnädigerweise nicht.

Doch wie sich herausstellte, war Mr Williams nicht das einzige Risiko. Ella hatte sich als Python im Palmhain gesonnt. Nun kroch sie als armdicke Riesenschlange züngelnd Richtung Strand. Toco hatte als Alligator am Rand des Sees herumgelegen, nun beeilte er sich, ihr auf seinen kurzen, krummen Beinen nachzulaufen.

Die beiden erreichten uns, als wir im Flachwasser standen

und uns, angefeuert von Jasper, bereit machten, uns zu verwandeln. Ausgerechnet in dem Moment, in dem wir schon die meisten Klamotten ausgezogen hatten. Man fühlt sich ein bisschen schutzlos, wenn man seinen Feinden in Unterwäsche gegenübersteht.

Na, wo wollt ihr denn hin?, fragte Ella und hob den eckigen Kopf, um uns besser beobachten zu können. *Finny, ich dachte, du hast Hausarrest?*

Finny blieb ganz cool. »Erstens zählt die Lagune zum Haus und zweitens, was geht dich das an?«

Drohend kroch Toco-der-Alligator auf sie zu. *Was fällt dir ein, so frech mit Ella zu reden, Bullentochter? Willst du eine aufs Maul?*

Was für ein Vollidiot! Was brachte ihm das eigentlich, ständig Ärger zu machen und andere Leute zu belästigen? Alligatoren, die ganz Tier waren, hatten das nicht nötig, die kümmerten sich um ihre eigenen Angelegenheiten.

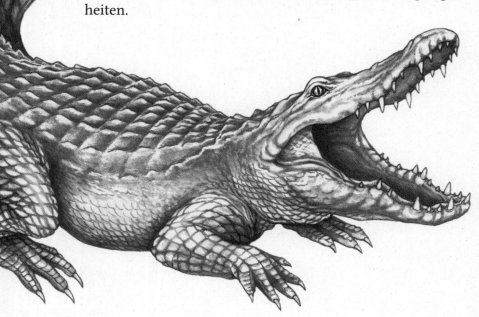

»Nein«, sagte ich und trat ihm in den Weg. »Will sie nicht.«

»Stimmt.« Lässig klappte Finny ihre Sonnenbrille zu und gab sie Jasper zusammen mit ihrem Armband zur sicheren Verwahrung. Der schaffte es, sie sich mit den Pfötchen aufzusetzen, und sah als Gürteltier mit Ray Bans ungewohnt cool aus.

Ella musterte uns noch immer. *Shari ... also ich muss sagen, als Delfin ist deine Figur eindeutig besser. Du isst gerne, was? Oder soll ich FRESSEN sagen?*

»Ja natürlich – ist doch toll, dass man hier in der Schule dreimal am Tag Beute machen kann, ohne sich anzustrengen.« Shari zuckte die Schultern und warf mir einen warnenden Blick zu. Ich wusste, was sie meinte, und versuchte, mich wieder abzuregen. Wenn ich mich in eine Prügelei – oder auch Beißerei – mit Toco verwickeln ließ, dann war ich der Nächste, der von der Schule flog.

»Jetzt mal ernsthaft«, sagte ich zu Ella und ihrem Kumpan.

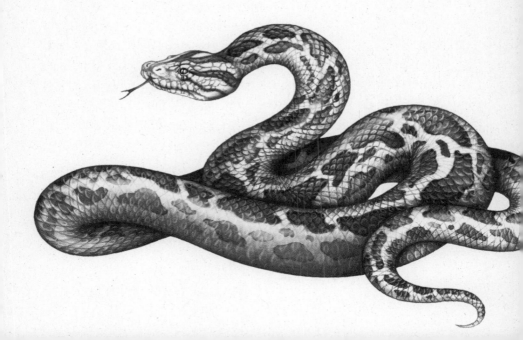

»Ihr findet diesen neuen Schulleiter nicht etwa gut, oder? Wir sollten gegen den zusammenhalten, statt uns gegenseitig fertigzumachen!«

Es kam mir so vor, als zögere Ella – nur ganz kurz. Ihre schwarze Zunge fuhr aus ihrem Maul, nahm unsere Witterung auf, zog sich wieder zurück. Doch dann entgegnete sie: *Du redest von Barrys Vater, also pass auf, was du sagst!*, und Toco kroch noch etwas näher. Gleich würde sein Panzermaul meine Schienbeine berühren. Ich war mir nicht mehr sicher, ob wir den Kampf noch vermeiden konnten, wenn er so weitermachte, denn kuschen würde ich vor ihm garantiert nicht.

Gleich trittste in meine Köttel rein, sagte Jasper.

Instinktiv wich Toco zurück und hob das Vorderbein. Der Hundekacke-Reflex.

Ein schneller Blick ging zwischen den Delfinen, Finny und mir hin und her. Dann warfen wir uns alle gleichzeitig und mit aller Kraft ins Wasser. Durch irgendein Wunder schaffte es sogar Shari, sich sofort zu verwandeln. Wir stoben davon, bevor Ella und ihr Schläger ganz kapiert hatten, was passiert war.

Alles Weitere lief so reibungslos, als hätten wir irgendwo ein Glücks-Abo abgeschlossen. Blue und Noah lockten Williams, der als Barrakuda Wache hielt, vom Durchgang weg und hängten ihn dann mit einem delfinischen Sprint Richtung Meer ab, als Finny in Sicherheit war. Während unser ungeliebter neuer Schulleiter noch irgendwas von *Was geht hier vor? Frechheit!* murmelte, waren wir schon auf halbem Weg zu unserem Wrack.

Völlig überwachsen von Korallen und Muscheln, ragte es vom Meeresgrund auf. Wir tauchten ab und schwammen durch die Einstiegsluke, dann wieder aufwärts, bis wir in den luftgefüllten Teil kamen.

Dort angekommen, erlebten wir eine Überraschung. Chris war schon da – aber nicht allein.

»Hi, Leute.« Verlegen winkte Izzy in die Runde, die nassen braunen Haare hinter die Ohren zurückgestrichen, ihren Tänzerinnenkörper in ein buntes Tuch gewickelt.

»Das ist ein geheimer Treffpunkt! Jeder muss fragen, bevor er jemanden mitbringen darf«, fuhr ich Chris an.

»Reg dich ab, Hai«, sagte Chris genervt. »Izzy ist in Ordnung, das wissen wir doch längst alle.«

»Herzlich willkommen, Izzy«, sagte Shari freundlich und schickte ein Lächeln hinterher. Dieses Lächeln, bei dem mein Herz jedes Mal zu einer feuchten Pfütze schmolz. »Jetzt lasst uns bitte besprechen, was wir gegen diesen gar nicht meerigen neuen Schulleiter machen können. Er ist erst einen Tag da und schon habe ich Lust, wieder zurück in den Ozean zu schwimmen und nie wiederzukommen!«

Ich erschrak. »Tu das nicht, bitte! Wir kriegen das hin. Wie wäre es mit einem Schulstreik?«

»Na ja, ich weiß nicht«, sagte Blue, der Noah eben galant ein Handtuch reichte.

Auch Finny hatte sich zurückverwandelt, gerade vergrub sie die Hand in unserer Snackkiste. Klar, sie hatte in der Schule ja Süßigkeitenverbot. Zum Glück sorgte Noah – dessen Eltern ein Geschäft mit Biolebensmitteln hatten – dafür, dass die Kiste immer gut gefüllt war.

»Normalerweise bin ich immer für so was, aber diesmal nicht«, meinte Finny. »Jack hat uns nicht umsonst gesagt, wir sollen uns benehmen. Wenn wir das nicht tun, schaden wir dem ganzen Wave-Befreiungsplan!«

»Wo ist Mr Clearwater überhaupt hin? Hat jemand was gehört?«, fragte ich in die Runde.

»Mrs Misaki hat gesagt, er hat sich in einem Hotel in Islamorada ein Zimmer genommen – das heißt, er ist in diesem Moment nur sechzehn Kilometer südwestlich von uns«, berichtete Chris. Erstaunt blickten wir ihn an.

»Mrs Misaki erzählt dir solche Sachen? Mir sagt sie immer nur, ich soll mir die Füße trocken wischen, bevor ich ins Sekretariat komme«, meinte ich.

»Und mir sagt sie, wenn wir Delfine ihr noch einmal einen Streich spielen, verkauft sie mich an ein Delfinarium«, erzählte Shari gut gelaunt. »Habt ihr gerochen, wie ihr Schulsekretärinnen-Preis ...«

»Shari, jetzt konzentrier dich bitte mal!« Blue runzelte die Stirn. »Hier geht es um ernste Dinge.«

»Wir könnten versuchen, ihn so auszutricksen, dass wir ein erträgliches Leben haben«, schlug Izzy vor. »Dazu müsste aber die ganze Klasse zusammenarbeiten. Wir lenken ihn ab und unterbrechen ständig, wenn er wieder so ein Verhör wie bei Shari machen will. Teilen unsere Hausaufgaben, coachen Leute, die Hilfe brauchen, bei Prüfungen und helfen ihnen beim Abschreiben.«

Das fanden wir spontan gut. »Sehr meerig. Ich rede mit Juna, die kann das organisieren, so was macht sie total gerne«, meinte ich und warf der Neuen aus Kalifornien einen anerkennenden Blick zu. Falls da wirklich was lief zwischen Chris und ihr, hatte er einen guten Geschmack! »Finny, können wir dir irgendwie helfen? Deinen Vater besänftigen oder so?«

Finny stopfte sich gerade mit der einen Hand Chips und mit der anderen Marshmallows in den Mund. Echt eklige Kombi. »Mit dem komme ich schon klar. Eigentlich ist er ja total lieb, wenn er nicht gerade zu viel getrunken hat oder denkt, dass ich auf die schiefe Bahn gerate. Ich hoffe, er versucht, Wave irgendwie zu helfen, ich habe total Angst um ihn.«

»Wenn ab jetzt alles nach Plan läuft, hilft ihm nun Lydia Lennox und die hat schon die fiesesten Verbrecher rausgeholt«, versprach ich ihr. Ob ich dabei überzeugend klang? Kaum. Ich traute dieser Python-Wandlerin nicht über den Weg. Warum sollte ich auch? Sie hatte oft genug deutlich gemacht, dass sie mich schon längst erwürgt hätte, wenn es nach ihr ginge, weil ich angeblich gemein zu ihrer Tochter war.

»Tangaroa wird uns beistehen«, sagte Noah feierlich und wir nickten. Mit einem feierlichen *Hongi* – das Ritual der Maori, bei dem sich Stirn und Nase berührten – beendeten wir das Krisentreffen.

Als wir wieder zurückgeschwommen waren zur Schule, warteten auf die anderen und mich gleich eine Menge Aufgaben. Ich musste mich an die Facharbeit über verschiedene Haiarten setzen, denn Montag früh um Viertel vor acht war Abgabe. Mir dämmerte, dass ich das ganze Wochenende durcharbeiten musste, wenn ich das schaffen wollte. Na super! Ich wünschte Mr Williams an die finsterste, schlammigste Stelle der Tiefsee. Eigentlich hatte ich vorgehabt, loszuschwimmen und Miss White suchen zu gehen. Sollte ich das trotzdem tun und ein leeres Blatt abgeben? Dann waren meine Tage an der Blue Reef High gezählt.

Rocket war natürlich enttäuscht, als ich ihn anrufen und ihm erklären musste, dass wir uns an diesem Wochenende nicht treffen konnten. »Danke noch mal für euren Einsatz neulich«, sagte ich. »Lando war der beste Darth Vader *ever* und selbst Logan war richtig gut. Jetzt weiß ich, was die Tigerzwillinge wirklich hassen!«

»Du hast nicht immer die Chance, die Hosen runterzulassen,

wenn du von ihnen gejagt wirst«, warnte mich mein Freund. »Das ist so bescheuert, dass wir uns nicht sehen. Wie soll ich euch jetzt die Minikamera geben? Und hast du mal wieder gefragt, ob die Polizei mit ihren Ermittlungen vorangekommen ist?«

»Ich rufe heute noch mal an. Kannst du zwischendurch mal vorbeikommen und uns die Ausrüstung bringen? Aber Achtung, es ist gerade ziemlich mies hier.« Ich berichtete ihm von unserem neuen Schulleiter und wie wir ihn austricksen wollten.

Rocket lachte. »Falls ihr dazu mal 'ne Ratte braucht, ruf einfach an.«

Mit ihm zu reden, hatte mich aufgeheitert, aber mich an die Facharbeit zu setzen, zog mich gleich wieder runter. Fünfzehn Seiten sollte das Ding haben. Fünfzehn!!! Der meinte das ernst, uns für die Arbeitswelt auf Leistung zu trimmen. Aber noch viel schlimmer war, dass dieser neue Schulleiter gerade dabei war, meine besten Freunde von der Schule wegzumobben. Bei meinem Wutproblem war es sowieso nur eine Frage der Zeit, bis ich auch drankam. Mein Entschluss stand fest – ich würde diese Facharbeit nicht schreiben und stattdessen das ganze Wochenende über Miss White suchen!

Als mein Handy klingelte, nahm ich es, ohne hinzuschauen, und meldete mich mit einem leicht genervten »Hallo?«.

Stille am anderen Ende. Erstaunt blickte ich auf den Bildschirm, um zu sehen, wer mich da anrief. Und stellte fest, dass die Rufnummer unterdrückt wurde.

»Hallo, Tiago«, sagte eine ruhige, weibliche Stimme. »Hier ist Alisha White.«

Der größte Fail des Jahres

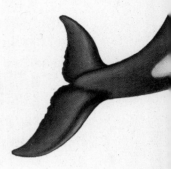

Miss White rief mich an! Es riss mich vom Stuhl hoch, was den gerade reintrippelnden Gürteltier-Jasper sofort zum Schrank flüchten ließ. Er witschte durch das runde Loch in der Schranktür und verschwand im dunklen Inneren. *Was ist? Gibt's 'n Erdbeben?*, fragte er besorgt.

Ich hatte gerade keine Zeit zum Antworten. »Miss White ... es ist toll, dass Sie ... Oh Mann, es ist so viel passiert! Wo sind Sie?«

»Es ist besser, wenn du nicht genau weißt, wo ich bin.« Miss White klang vorsichtig, aber ich hörte auch einen Hauch von Wärme in ihrer Stimme. Konnte es sein, dass sie sich ebenfalls freute, dass wir nun miteinander sprachen?

»Können Sie kommen? Hier ...« Plötzlich schnürte sich mir die Kehle zu. »Hier geht gerade alles den Bach runter. Mr Clearwater ist nicht mehr Schulleiter.«

»Was?« Sie klang ehrlich erschüttert. »Oh nein. Ist Jack etwas passiert?«

»Nicht direkt«, sagte ich und freute mich darüber, dass unser Schulleiter sie anscheinend nicht kaltließ. Knapp erzählte ich, was vorgefallen war.

Nach einem kurzen Schweigen sagte meine junge Ex-Kampflehrerin: »Aha. Heftig. Leider können wir nicht viel reden, es kann gut sein, dass dein Handy abgehört wird. Ich wollte mich nur noch mal melden und sagen, dass es mir leidtut.«

Mein Handy, abgehört? Verdattert hielt ich das Gerät von mir weg. Konnte gut sein, die Lennox kannte garantiert Leute, die so was draufhatten. Aber dann wurde mir klar, dass ich diese Chance nicht verscherzen durfte. Auch wenn jemand mithörte!

»Bitte – können Sie kommen?«, wiederholte ich. »Wir brauchen Sie hier. Egal, was Sie getan haben. Bei diesem Buckelwal-Wandler geht es um Leben und Tod.«

Ich musste nicht hinzufügen, dass es für Jack Clearwater auch um einiges ging. Sie wusste selbst, dass es ihm das Herz brechen würde, wenn jemand seine Schule zugrunde richtete.

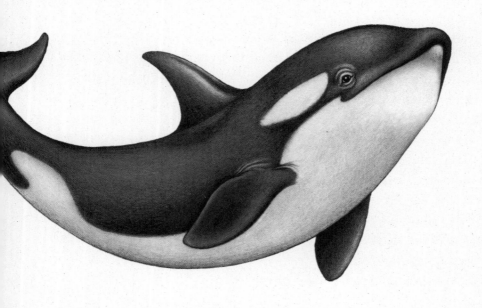

»Ich kann nichts versprechen.« Miss Whites Stimme war hart und kühl. »Aber sag mir nur kurz, ist euer Stundenplan geändert worden? Oder macht ihr weiter wie geplant?«

»Äh, bisher machen wir weiter wie geplant – wieso?«, fragte ich. Aber sie sagte nur noch »Sei vorsichtig, Tiago«, dann legte sie auf.

Was konnte sie damit gemeint haben? Ich hatte leider keine Ahnung.

»War das am Telefon wirklich die Miss White?« Jasper hatte sich aus dem Schrank herausgewagt und zurückverwandelt. Gerade setzte er seine Brille wieder auf und strahlte mich an. »Geht es ihr gut?«

»Hat sie leider nicht gesagt. Komm mit!« Ich ließ das Handy liegen – nur für den Fall, dass es wirklich gehackt worden war – und lief rüber zu Shari und Blue, die gerade ebenfalls paukten, dass ihnen das Hirn rauchte. »Weißt du zufällig, welche Delfinarten fast oder ganz ausgestorben sind?«, fragte Blue und kratzte sich an der Stirn.

»Irgendein armer Flussdelfin, glaube ich«, sagte ich. »Anderes Thema – ratet mal, wer mich gerade angerufen hat!« Sehr lange ließ ich sie aber nicht raten, ich war viel zu heiß darauf, ihnen von dem Gespräch zu erzählen.

»Oh wow, Miss White hat sich gemeldet!« Shari staunte. »Es ist ihr nicht egal, was mit uns ist.«

»Vielleicht wollte se mit dieser Frage rausfinden, ob wir die neue Kampflehrerin mögen oder nich'«, meinte Jasper.

»Glaube ich kaum, so eitel ist sie nicht«, sagte Noah nachdenklich.

Blue meinte: »Vielleicht wollte sie dir verschlüsselt etwas mitteilen, Tiago?«

»Kann sein«, sagte ich mit einem schiefen Lächeln. »Wahrscheinlich hat sie gedacht, ich wäre so schlau, dass ich es kapiere. Ist aber nicht der Fall.«

»Moment mal, Leute!« Sharis Gesicht leuchtete auf – man sah ihr immer direkt an, was sie dachte, weil sie nie gelernt hatte, sich zu verstellen. »Vielleicht meint sie den Tiefwasserlehrgang? Der ist schon lange geplant, von dem wusste sie ganz bestimmt.«

Wirklich? Ich zwang mich, die Welle der Freude ins Nichts laufen zu lassen. Noch wusste ich ja nicht, ob Shari damit recht hatte. »Du meinst, vielleicht will sie sich dort mit uns treffen?«

»Das müssen wir einfach ausprobieren«, sagte Shari und damit hatte sie absolut recht.

Leider war der Tiefwasserlehrgang erst am Dienstag. Bis dahin konnten höllenviele Sachen passieren.

Spontan entschied ich mich, die Facharbeit nun doch anzupacken. Ich wälzte stapelweise Bibliotheksbücher, forschte im Internet nach und schrieb eine Seite über Kragenhaie, die in der Tiefsee lebten und echt seltsam aussahen – mehr wie Schlangen als Haie. Dann war ein Abschnitt über Teppichhaie dran, die gefleckt wie ein Bettvorleger aussahen, den ganzen Tag auf dem Meeresboden herumlagen und auf Beute warteten, die sie schnappen konnten. Wann konnte ich endlich wieder den Teppichhai machen, ich musste dringend mal wieder einen Tag komplett chillen!

Nach mehreren Stunden Facharbeit-Tippen konnte ich nicht mehr, ich musste eine Runde schwimmen, um wieder Kraft zu sammeln. Also stürzte ich mich ins Meer, flösselte als Hai quer durch die Lagune und dann einfach geradeaus.

Aber im Meer ist selten etwas einfach. Ich war kaum eine Viertelstunde unterwegs, als ich etwas total Eigenartiges sah. Ein Stück voraus erspähte ich einen Tigerhai, der genauso aussah wie ich, sich genauso bewegte und frontal auf mich zuschwamm. Als ich mich nach rechts wandte, vollzog der Tigerhai genau das gleiche Manöver. Ich drehte nach links, der Hai mir gegenüber ebenfalls. Moment mal, gab es im Meer einen riesigen Spiegel, von dem ich nur noch nichts gehört hatte?

Dann sagte mein Spiegelbild: *Jetzt hör aber auf, mir auszuweichen, Tiago! Denkst du, ich will hier mein Revier verteidigen, oder was?*

Es war mein Bruder Steve, der als Hai im Meer lebte, weil er an Land nicht gut zurechtgekommen war. Ich freute mich, fühlte mich aber auch ziemlich dämlich. In so einem Fall tue ich meistens so, als wäre gar nichts passiert, was manchmal funktioniert und manchmal auch nicht. *Oh, hi, Steve. Cool, dich zu sehen! Was gibt's Neues von den Glasbodenbooten?*

Noch nichts, aber ich weiß, dass sie weitermachen. Steve knirschte mit den Zähnen. *In letzter Zeit habe ich drei Haie mit Harpunenwunden gesehen! Das heißt, wir müssen dranbleiben, bis wir diese Kerle auf frischer Tat ertappen.*

Die Suche aus der Luft läuft weiter, versprach ich ihm und fragte mich, ob er nur wegen der Haikämpfe hier war.

Nein, natürlich bin ich nicht nur deswegen hier, erwiderte Steve sofort, anscheinend hatte er meine Gedanken aufgefangen. *Ich mag dich, Bruderherz, hast du das nicht mitgekriegt? Und dass du mich aus diesem Netzkäfig befreit hast, vergesse ich dir nie.*

Die Anspannung sickerte aus mir heraus. *Gut, ich mag dich nämlich auch,* sagte ich und knuffte ihn zurück. *Bist du – wenn du nicht gerade Glasboote überwachst – mal wieder nach Kuba geschwommen?*

Nee, diesmal war ich kurz in Mexiko – Abwechslung muss sein.

Er seufzte. *Nur schade, dass die hübschen Mädels schreiend aus dem Wasser laufen, wenn sie mich sehen.*

In Menschengestalt hätte ich gegrinst. *Wenn die wüssten, dass du ein Herz aus Gold hast.*

Herz aus Gold? Na ja. Soll ich dir mal zeigen, was ich mit den Haikampf-Typen mache, wenn ich sie erwische?

Steve riss das Maul so weit auf, dass sich ein vorbeischwimmender Fisch fast zu Tode erschreckte und abzischte, als wäre der Teufel hinter ihm her.

Guter Plan, fand ich. *Du kannst doch bestimmt Haisprache ... kannst du unsere Artgenossen nicht warnen? Ihnen sagen, dass sie in nächster Zeit besonders vorsichtig sein sollen oder so was?*

Haie sind eigentlich meistens vorsichtig, meinte Steve. *Die meisten sind sogar richtige Schisshasen, finde ich! Ich könnte es natürlich versuchen, sie zu warnen. Aber ich fürchte, sie werden nicht kapieren, wovon ich überhaupt rede. Alles, was mit Menschen zu tun hat, ist ihnen sehr fremd.*

Aber du versuchst es?, hakte ich nach. *Du brauchst ihnen ja keine Details zu erklären.*

Okay, ich versuche es.

Während wir nebeneinander herschwammen, quatschten

wir noch über Schule, Freunde – er hatte sich mit einem jungen Muränen-Wandler angefreundet, der im Riff wohnte – und was gerade im Meer so los war. Dann musste ich leider wieder zurück, die verdammte Facharbeit wartete auf mich.

Viele Fortschritte machte ich damit aber nicht, weil kurz darauf Mr García an meine Tür klopfte. An einem Samstagabend! Normalerweise war er zu dieser Zeit bei seiner kleinen Tochter in Key West. Dass es sie gab und dass sie bei seiner geschiedenen Frau lebte, hatte Daphne neulich erst erfahren und natürlich brühwarm herumerzählt.

»Was ist?«, flüsterte ich alarmiert.

»Mrs Lennox hat zwar versprochen, dass sie Wave rausholt, aber noch hat sie nicht gezahlt«, sagte er leise, um Jasper nicht zu stören, der schon schlief. »Jack hat mich gebeten, ihn zu besuchen und zu checken, ob mit ihm alles okay ist. Ich dachte, ich nehme jemand mit, der in seinem Alter ist und der ihn kennt. Bei Shari kann ich mich nicht drauf verlassen, dass sie ihre Verwandlungen im Griff hat.«

Ich zog eine Grimasse, als ich an unseren Klassenausflug nach Miami dachte, der um ein Haar in den Abendnachrichten geendet hätte. »Bin gleich so weit«, sagte ich, streifte mir rasch eine Jeans über und wühlte in meinem Schrank nach einem sauberen Hemd. »Wie geht's Ihnen?«

Mr García schien überrascht, dass ich ihn so etwas fragte. »Geht so«, sagte er. »Hoffen wir mal, dass wir diesmal keinen Tigern begegnen.«

Wir lächelten uns zu. Was für ein lustiger Gedanke, dass er noch bis vor Kurzem unser strengster Lehrer gewesen war. Ich überlegte, ob ich ihm von Miss Whites Anruf erzählen sollte. Nein, lieber nicht, das war geheim und wir wussten ja auch nicht, was sie plante.

Auf dem Parkplatz wartete Finny auf uns, die irgendwie mitbekommen hatte, was wir vorhatten. Sie sah aus, als wäre sie gerade auf einer Beerdigung. »Ihr besucht Wave, stimmt's? Ohne mich?«

»Es würde sehr schnell rauskommen, wenn du dafür deinen Hausarrest brichst«, sagte Mr García. »Sorry.«

»Dann grüßt ihn wenigstens von mir!« Ruckartig wandte sich Finny um, sie sah schon nicht mehr, dass wir nickten. Dass wir ihren Vater grüßen sollten, hatte sie nicht gesagt ... der Arme.

Als wir in Miami ankamen, war eigentlich keine Besuchszeit, aber Finnys Vater hatte uns eine Ausnahme genehmigt. Er war auch derjenige, der uns begrüßte.

»Wie geht es Wave?«, fragte ich und versuchte, nicht sauer auf ihn zu sein. Ohne seine Einmischung hätten wir unseren Buckelwal-Wandler schon längst in Freiheit.

»Der Junge hat noch nichts gegessen, seit er bei uns ist«, brummte Nick Greyson. »Wollte nicht mal einen Schokoriegel nehmen. Wenn er damit weitermacht, müssen wir ihn in eine Klinik bringen und zwangsernähren.«

Das klang schrecklich! Mr García und ich blickten uns alarmiert an.

»Dürfen wir versuchen, ihn zu überreden, Mr Greyson?«, fragte mein Verwandlungslehrer höflich. Wir hatten in der Schule einen Umweg über die Küche gemacht und nun brachte er aus seinem Rucksack eine Kühlbox mit Sushi und eine Packung Muffins zum Vorschein.

Finnys Vater schaute sich alles gründlich an und nickte dann. »Ist okay. Hoffentlich macht das dem Jungen Appetit. Ich mag dieses rohe Fischzeug ja nicht, ein anständiger Burger ist mir lieber!«

Wir lachten pflichtschuldig.

Mr Greyson setzte sich an seinen Schreibtisch und schob dort ein paar Ausdrucke hin und her. Von oben hatte ich einen guten Blick auf seine abstehenden Ohren. »Wie hält sich Finny?«, fragte er, ohne aufzuschauen. »Ich war ein bisschen arg streng zu ihr neulich, fürchte ich. Aber es geht einfach nicht, dass sie mich hier auf meinem eigenen Revier zum Deppen macht.«

»Das wollte sie nicht«, versicherte ich ihm mit neuer Hoffnung. »Finny leidet ziemlich unter dem Hausarrest, können Sie sich das nicht noch mal überlegen?«

»Sie darf ja in eure Bucht. Dieses Mädchen liebt das Meer, wie ich es noch bei niemandem erlebt habe.« Er lachte auf. »Höchstens bei ihrer Mutter, die ist genauso. Sonst wäre sie sicher nicht Meeresbiologin geworden.«

Mr García und ich tauschten einen schnellen Blick. Wie musste es für Finny und ihre Mutter sein, mit jemandem zu leben, vor dem sie sich immer verstellen mussten? Aber wahrscheinlich ging es vielen Woodwalkern und Seawalkern genauso.

Eine Polizistin durchsuchte uns von Kopf bis Fuß, bevor wir zu Wave gelassen wurden.

Als ein anderer Officer uns die Zelle aufschloss, sahen wir sofort, dass es Wave schlecht ging. Rastlos lief er in seiner Zelle umher und wich jedes Mal erst im allerletzten Moment aus, bevor er gegen eine Wand prallte. Klar, er war geschlossene Räume nicht gewohnt und kannte nur das grenzenlose Meer.

Als Wave uns sah, wandte er sich uns ruckartig zu. »Darf ich hier raus?«

Sein Blick versuchte, in unseren Gesichtern zu forschen, aber ich wusste nicht, ob er darin etwas erkennen konnte. Viel Übung im Umgang mit Menschen hatte er ja nicht.

»Sehr bald«, versuchte ihn Mr García zu beruhigen. »Wir

haben schon alles vorbereitet, aber ein bisschen dauert es leider noch.«

Es tat mir in der Seele weh, wie die Hoffnung aus seinen Augen verschwand. »Wo ist das Mädchen mit den blauen Haaren? Finny?«

»Leider hat ihr Vater verboten, dass sie die Schule verlässt, aber sie lässt dich grüßen.« Ich versuchte es mit einem aufmunternden Lächeln, das wahrscheinlich so hohl ausfiel wie eine leere Chipspackung. »Wir haben dir was mitgebracht.« Ich hielt ihm einen Muffin entgegen.

Wave warf nur einen flüchtigen Blick darauf.

»Oder wie wäre es mit frischem Fisch?« Mr García holte das Sushi heraus und schwenkte es unter Waves Nase.

»Gerade nicht«, sagte Wave.

Iss das gefälligst, sonst weisen sie dich ins Krankenhaus ein und stecken dir eine Nadel mit einem Schlauch daran in den Arm, wollte ich ihn anschreien. Vielleicht spürte Mr García meine Gedanken, denn er wandte sich mir zu. »Mach dir nicht zu viele Sorgen, Buckelwale können sehr lange ohne Nahrung ...«

Erschrocken starrte ich ihn an. Mr García zuckte zusammen, als ihm klar wurde, was er gesagt hatte. Wir wandten uns beide zu Wave um, hofften, dass das Wort ihn nicht getriggert hatte, dass er vor seinem inneren Auge nicht gerade seine zweite Gestalt sah.

Doch als wir wahrnahmen, wie ein Zittern durch seinen Körper lief, wurde mir klar, dass genau das eingetreten war, was wir befürchtet hatten. Mit zwei Schritten war Mr García bei Wave, packte ihn bei den Schultern, blickte ihm in die Augen. »Du bist ein Mensch, zwei Beine, Füße, zwei Arme!«

Mit zusammengebissenen Zähnen kämpfte Wave gegen die Verwandlung an, doch schon verschwanden seine geballten

Fäuste, seine Arme begannen zu wachsen, wechselten die Farbe zu Schiefergrau. Als er versuchte, sich umzuwenden, erwischte mich eine dieser immer noch wachsenden Armflossen mit voller Breitseite und klatschte mich gegen die Wand. Ich prallte ab, landete auf dem Boden und fand mich mit der Nase neben einem Paar fischig riechender Flipflops wieder. Obwohl Wave noch längst nicht seine Walgröße hatte, fühlte es sich schon an, als hätte mich jemand mit einem Bagger zusammen in ein Zimmer gesperrt.

»Wave! Wo ist dein Foto?« Ich durchwühlte sein Bettzeug und den Rest der Zelle nach dem laminierten Bild seiner Menschengestalt, das wir ihm mitgebracht hatten.

Weiß ich nicht!, schrie Wave zurück. Mit menschlicher Stimme konnte er schon nicht mehr sprechen, sein Gesicht verformte sich, wurde zu einer länglichen Schnauze, die gegen die Tür knallte. Jeden Moment würde einer der Cops reinkommen, um zu schauen, was es hier für einen Aufruhr gab. Aber das war gerade nicht unser größtes Problem.

»Das Ding ist nicht da, ich finde nichts!«, schrie ich zu Mr García hinüber und bekam mal wieder Schluckauf vor Angst.

»Such weiter!«, brüllte er. »Ich versuche, es ihm direkt in den Kopf zu schicken.«

Er ließ Wave los und wurde einen Moment lang ganz still, konzentrierte sich auf den Jungen. Seine Gedanken waren so laut, dass sogar ich sie hören konnte. *Ruhig, ganz ruhig. Schau genau hin. Das bist du!* Das Bild von Waves Menschengestalt flutete mir in den Kopf, erfüllte mich mit solcher Kraft, dass ich mich nicht gewundert hätte, wenn ich mich plötzlich in diesen Jungen mit den dunkelbraunen Augen und langen Haaren verwandelt hätte.

Zum Glück war nicht ich es, der sich verwandelte.

Als zwei Cops hereinstürmten – darunter Nick Greyson – hockten wir alle drei völlig ausgepowert auf dem Boden. In erster Gestalt!

»Was war das für ein Krach? Hat der Junge Sie angegriffen?«, fragte Finnys Vater grimmig.

»Nein, nein, Tiago ist umgekippt und gegen die Tür geknallt – der Kreislauf«, behauptete Farryn García. Das erklärte leider nicht wirklich die Delle in der Tür oder die Tatsache, dass wir alle drei angeschlagen wirkten. Aber da es keine Kameras in den Zellen gab, konnten sie es hoffentlich nicht widerlegen. Schwankend stand Mr García auf und reichte mir eine Hand, um mich hochzuziehen.

»Brauchst du einen Arzt?«, fragte der Officer mich, während Greyson verkündete: »Auf jeden Fall müssen Sie beide jetzt gehen, der Besuch ist beendet.«

Wir nickten, ich brachte immer noch kein Wort heraus. Ohne uns abzusprechen, umarmten Mr García und ich Wave und hielten ihn fest.

»Gib nicht auf«, flüsterte ich ihm zu. »Halt noch ein bisschen durch – bitte!«

»Ich bin stolz auf dich, nicht jeder hätte so eine Rückverwandlung geschafft«, raunte Mr García Wave ins Ohr.

Dann mussten wir gehen.

Nick Greyson war nicht entgangen, wie mies es dem jungen Gefangenen ging. »Können Sie nicht seine Eltern auftreiben, García?«, fragte er. »Vielleicht tun die ihm gut. Außerdem sollten wir den Jungen sowieso an sie übergeben, wenn die Kaution da ist.«

Seine Eltern? Oje. Natürlich hatten wir keine Ahnung, wo die herumschwammen. »Wir versuchen unser Bestes«, versprach mein Verwandlungslehrer.

Kaum saßen wir im Auto, sagte Farryn García: »Bei der großen Welle, das war wirklich ein gigantischer Fail von mir! Wäre es zu viel verlangt, dass du Jack nichts davon erzählst? Und am besten auch Finny nicht, die redet sonst nie wieder ein Wort mit mir.«

»Könnte sein. Ja, das war wirklich ein fieser Versprecher.« Ich atmete tief durch, versuchte abzuschütteln, was wir gerade erlebt hatten. »Ich dachte wirklich, es ist aus.«

»Also, was ist?« Mr García blickte mich von der Seite an. »Aber ich verpasse dir nicht etwa eine Eins in Physik, damit du dichthältst ...«

»Ach, eine Eins in Verwandlung würde ich auch nehmen«, frotzelte ich und genehmigte mir einen Muffin. »Das vorhin hätte genauso gut mir passieren können. Aber niemand außer Ihnen hätte geschafft, ihn aus dieser halben Verwandlung zurückzubringen.«

»Kann sein«, brummte er und wir wussten beide, dass wir nie wieder darüber sprechen würden.

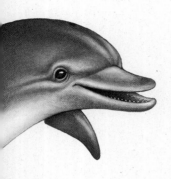

Alle für eine

Ich schuftete bis Sonntagabend, um die Facharbeit über Hai-Arten pünktlich fertigzubekommen. Als ich völlig erschöpft zum Hauptgebäude schlurfte, um mein Werk dem neuen Schulleiter ins Fach zu legen, hörte ich jemanden schluchzen. Schon wieder! Wie sich herausstellte, war es diesmal Mara, die zusammengesackt und heulend in einem der Cafeteria-Boote hockte.

»Bei der großen Welle, was ist denn?«, fragte Shari, die gerade vorbeikam.

»Ich soll fünfzehn Seiten über Mangroven schreiben, aber das schaffe ich nie!« Ströme von Tränen rannen über Maras gutmütiges Gesicht. »Ganze drei Seiten habe ich erst!«

Shari kletterte sofort zu ihr ins Boot und nahm sie in den Arm.

»Oje.« Besorgt blickte ich sie an. Bei unseren bisherigen Lehrern hatte Mara immer eine Verlängerung bekommen, aber ich ahnte, dass es damit nun vorbei war.

Immer mehr zufällig vorbeikommende Schüler fanden sich ein und wollten wissen, was los war. Shari, Finny, Izzy und ich blickten uns an. Ich ahnte, dass die anderen ebenso an unseren Plan dachten, gegen unseren neuen Schulleiter zusammenzuhalten. »Wir helfen dir«, flüsterte Izzy Mara zu, ihre Augen blitzten. »Wenn jeder von uns zwei Seiten schreibt, ist das Ding ruck, zuck fertig.«

»Wer schreibt hier was für wen?«

Wir zuckten zusammen. Still und leise war Miss Bennett hinter uns aufgetaucht und watete durch die Cafeteria. Wie viel hatte sie gehört?

Als unsere Lehrerin sah, dass Mara weinte, kletterte sie ebenfalls ins blau-weiß gestrichene Boot und legte ihr den Arm um die Schultern. »Wo drückt denn die Flosse?«

Als Mara ihr das Ganze erklärt hatte, nickte Miss Bennett. »Ah. Nicht so wahrscheinlich, dass dir Williams eine Verlängerung gibt, oder?« Sie blickte uns an. »Und deshalb wollt ihr die Facharbeit nun für Mara schreiben, stimmt's?«

Ich erstarrte. Mist! Also hatte sie alles gehört!

Schließlich war es Juna, die ganz zaghaft nickte.

»Prima«, sagte Miss Bennett entschlossen. »Und ich lese Korrektur. Wäre doch gelacht, wenn wir die Arbeit nicht bis morgen früh fertigkriegen würden.«

»Ich schaffe dieses verdammte Drecksding auch nicht«, brummte Toco verlegen. Ella und Barry – sogar der Sohn des neuen Schulleiters! – waren sofort an seiner Seite.

»Kriegen wir hin«, versprach ihm Ella und klopfte ihm tröstend auf die Schulter.

Wie sich herausstellte, brauchten auch Shari – die bisher nur vier Seiten in den Computer diktiert hatte –, Zelda und Daphne Hilfe. Noah, Blue und Leonora waren mit ihrer Arbeit schon fertig und konnten sich dafür zur Verfügung stellen. Juna und Olivia übernahmen es, Lucy, Noemi und Nox zu helfen, die ihnen ihre Aufsätze diktierten. Miss Bennett half uns bis in die Nacht hinein mit der Rechtschreibung, damit Mr Williams seinen Rotstift gar nicht erst zücken musste.

Montagfrüh war ich bestimmt nicht der Einzige, der sich ein bisschen fertig fühlte, aber auf dem Schreibtisch des Direktors lagen Kante an Kante, nach neuem Papier und Druckertoner riechend, sämtliche fälligen Facharbeiten.

»Na also – geht doch, wenn ihr euch ein bisschen anstrengt«, sagte Mr Williams und klang fast freundlich dabei.

»Den Feind einlullen« war ein Teil des Plans. Also zwangen wir uns zu einem freundlichen Lächeln und Nicken.

Aber nun richtete sich der Blick unseres neuen Schulleiters auf Noemi, die in ihrer Panthergestalt auf einem der Schultische lag. »Du heißt Noemi, richtig? Hast du inzwischen lesen und schreiben gelernt?«

Klappt schon ganz gut, antwortete Noemi stolz und schleckte sich die Vorderpfote. *Ich kann schon meinen Namen schreiben. Den hab ich mit den Krallen schon in vier Palmen geritzt und in die Schuppentür!*

»Das reicht nicht.« Mr Williams' Stimme war nüchtern. »Es ist offensichtlich, dass du in dieser Klasse nicht mithalten kannst – deine Facharbeit war viel zu kurz. Außerdem gehörst du nicht hierhin, du bist eine Schwarzer Jaguar, deine Heimat ist Südamerika!« Unser neuer Schulleiter wirkte sehr zufrieden mit sich. »Ich habe schon mit einer Woodwalker-Grundschule in Costa Rica gesprochen, die dich aufnehmen könnte. Der Flug geht am Mittwoch, die Tiertransportbox habe ich schon bestellt.«

Noemi fauchte ihn an. *Was? Das will ich nicht! Ich bin hier daheim, nicht in einem fremden Land!*

»Das stimmt«, wagte Juna einzuwenden. »Nur weil ihre Vorfahren irgendwann mal aus ...«

Mr Williams beachtete sie kein bisschen, fiel ihr einfach ins Wort. »Was fällt dir ein, mich anzufauchen, Pantherin? Raus!« Sein Zeigefinger deutete zur Tür.

Unsere Pantherin dachte nicht daran, dem Befehl zu folgen. Stattdessen ging sie mit ruhiger Würde auf ihn zu, hob den Kopf und blickte ihm in die Augen. *Sie gehören nicht in eine Schule*, sagte sie sehr entschieden. *Weil Sie nämlich Jugendliche gar nicht mögen. Spielen Sie lieber irgendwo mit Zahlen, dort, wo Sie niemandem schaden können.*

Mit diesen Worten drehte sich unsere Pantherin um und ging nach draußen.

Geschockte Gesichter und aufgeregtes Gemurmel in unserer Klasse.

Shari meldete sich zu Wort: »Mr Williams, Noemi holt durch ihre Nachhilfe irre schnell auf. In einem fremden Land, wo sie niemanden kennt, würde sie sich …«

»Schluss! Der Unterricht geht weiter!«

Bisher hatte ich mich immer mit dem Gedanken beruhigt, dass Jack Clearwater ganz sicher zurückkommen würde, sobald diese Krise mit Wave beendet war. Aber konnten wir Noemi wirklich aus Südamerika zurückholen, wenn sie erst mal dort war? Und dann flüsterte Jasper mir in der Pause zu: »Im ersten Stock vor dem Büro stehen ein paar Bilder von Mr Clearwater im Flur! Gerade packt irgendein Kerl sie ein.«

Mir wurde ganz anders. Ich lief durch die Aula und stürmte die Treppe hoch. Es stimmte. »Was ist mit diesen Bildern?«, fragte ich den Kerl.

»Ich soll sie abholen, jemand in Key West hat sie gekauft«, sagte der Arbeiter.

»Aber …«, stammelte ich. Es waren zwei Aquarelle, die Mr Clearwater selbst gemalt hatte, eins zeigte einen Weißkopf-

Seeadler, der gerade die Flügel ausstreckte, um auf einem Ast zu landen. Das andere eine Unterwasserlandschaft an unserem Hausriff. Beide waren richtig toll.

»Wieso darf die denn jemand kaufen?«, fragte ich betroffen.

Gerade kam Mr Williams aus seinem neuen Büro und marschierte an mir vorbei. Er hatte gehört, was ich gesagt hatte. »Alle Gegenstände in diesem Gebäude gehören der Schule, können also veräußert werden«, informierte er uns knapp. »Ganz offensichtlich braucht die Blue Reef High Geld, da ist es nur logisch, wenn unnötige Wertgegenstände veräußert werden.«

Hilflos mussten ich und Jasper mit ansehen, wie die Bilder abtransportiert wurden.

»Ich hab gesehen, wie er versucht hat, in die Wohnung von Mr Clearwater im ersten Stock zu kommen, kannste dir das vorstellen?«, flüsterte mir Jasper zu. »Aber es war abgeschlossen. Williams hat im Schloss rumgestochert und dabei geflucht.«

»Oh Mann«, ächzte ich. »Vielleicht will er die Wohnung auch noch ausräumen und Mr Clearwater all seine Sachen vor die Tür stellen.«

»Das lassen wir nicht zu!« Jasper streckte die Brust raus.

Ich war mir da nicht so sicher, schließlich hatten wir das mit den Bildern nicht verhindern können. »Glaubst du wirklich, wir kriegen es mit, wenn während des Unterrichts ein Möbelwagen vorfährt?«

So trostlos war die Lage, als am Nachmittag ein Gast auf dem Parkplatz auftauchte.

»Das sind Unbekannte«, warnte uns Daphne. »Und ich glaube, es ist ein Mensch dabei!« Sie rannte los, um den Menschenalarm zu drücken. Sofort war in der Schule die Hölle los, Polly tauchte als Alligator im Süßwasserteich unter, halb verwandelte Schüler zogen sich hastig an, Leute rannten durch die Gegend, Noemi zog sich aufs Dach zurück und Zelda fiel fast in Ohnmacht vor Aufregung. Jasper war so durcheinander, dass er einfach Gürteltier blieb.

Neugierig gingen ich, Shari und Blue – alle gerade in Menschengestalt – zum Parkplatz ... und sahen, wie eine Frau einen Rollstuhl aus einem Kombi auslud und auseinanderklappte. Ein zierliches Mädchen mit braunen Locken und vielen Sommersprossen ging mühsam auf Krücken zum Rollstuhl und setzte sich hinein. Daisy Cousteau!

»Oh, hi, wie schön, dass du da bist«, sagte Shari begeistert.

»Und es ist euch auch wirklich recht, dass ich hier bin?« Ein bisschen scheu blickte Daisy sich um, ihre Hände ruhten auf den metallenen Greifrädern, mit denen sie ihren Rollstuhl voranbewegen konnte. »Ich hätte jetzt eigentlich Schwimmtherapie, aber ich habe Beth überzeugt, dass wir das auch hier machen können.«

»Sie ist richtig gut darin, Leute zu überreden.« Ihre Betreuerin lächelte.

»Na klar ist uns das recht. Toll, dass du es geschafft hast«, sagte ich.

Normalerweise hätten wir sie erst mal zu unserem Schulleiter gebracht. Aber das kam diesmal natürlich nicht infrage, sonst zischte unser Gast gleich wieder ab. Zum Glück war Mr Williams gerade in die Stadt gefahren, um irgendetwas zu erledigen. Leider war auch unser Verwandlungslehrer gerade nicht da – Mr García machte mit den Zweitjahresleuten einen Ausflug ans Riff. Das war blöd, denn wir mussten dringend herausfinden, welche zweite Gestalt Daisy hatte.

»Wo leben denn eure Delfine?«, fragte Daisy. »Cool, dass ihr auch ein zahmes Gürteltier habt! Darf ich es streicheln?«

Klar, mach nur, erwiderte Jasper und Daisy stutzte. »Hast du eben was gesagt, Tiago?«

»Ja äh, gesagt habe ich: ›Klar, mach nur‹«, stammelte ich. Daisy beugte sich herab, soweit es ging, und tätschelte meinen Gürteltierfreund, der extra Männchen machte, damit sie an ihn herankam.

Das ging alles arg schnell. Es war eigentlich nicht der Plan gewesen, ihr schon nach fünf Minuten und vor ihrer Betreuerin zu erklären, dass sie sich verwandeln und Kopfgespräche führen konnte. Und wie sollten wir das mit den Delfinen machen? Einer von ihnen stand noch voll angezogen neben mir und die anderen ließen sich gerade in Olivias Hütte irgendein Computerspiel zeigen.

Ich tauschte einen Blick mit meiner besten Freundin.

»Moment, ich gebe eben den Delfinen Bescheid, dass du kommst«, sagte Shari und ging mit schnellen Schritten los. Wahrscheinlich flogen gleich hinter irgendeiner Palme Klamotten durch die Gegend, wenn unsere Delfinclique sich verwandelte und in die Lagune stürzte.

Zum Glück hatte Juna mitbekommen, was abging; unsere Klassensprecherin, die einen Kopf kleiner war als ich, wandte sich mit einem Eins-a-Gastgeberinnenlächeln an Daisys Helferin. »Wollen Sie vielleicht in der Aula einen Kaffee trinken, während Tiago Daisy die Schule zeigt? Wir passen gut auf sie auf, wir haben ein halbes Dutzend Schwimmlehrer hier!«

Seit wann waren Haie, Rochen und Delfine Schwimmlehrer? Aber das Argument schien die Therapeutin zu überzeugen. »Gerne. Kommst du auch wirklich zurecht, Daisy?«

»Jaja, logisch, bis gleich!« Ohne sich noch einmal umzuschauen, rollte Daisy los in Richtung Meer.

Ich bedankte mich mit einem Blick bei Juna und klemmte

mir die Krücken unter den Arm, die die Betreuerin mir reichte. »Moment! Warte, Daisy!«, rief ich. Sie war *wirklich* scharf darauf, mit den Delfinen zu schwimmen. Aber die hatten wahrscheinlich noch blonde Locken und Füße statt Flossen.

Um Zeit zu gewinnen, zeigte ich Daisy erst mal das Schulgelände – durch das man zum Glück gut mit einem Rollstuhl durchkam – und meine Hütte. Dort bewunderte Daisy meine neusten Zeichnungen, besonders die von einem Schwarzdelfin im Sprung. »Du kannst echt gut zeichnen. Ist das ein Tigerhai?« Sie deutete auf eins meiner Selbstporträts.

»Äh, ja.« Verlegen scharrte ich mit den bloßen Füßen im Sand. »Magst du Haie?«

»Na ja, sie sind wichtig fürs Ökosystem, aber mögen ist ein bisschen viel gesagt.« Daisy lachte. »Gibt es denn jemanden, der Haie wirklich mag?«

Jasper schmetterte ihr ein geistiges *Ja!* entgegen.

Verwirrt blickte Daisy auf Jasper herab, dann zu mir hoch. »Bist du ein Bauchredner oder so was? Oder habt ihr hier ein sprechendes Gürteltier?« Sie musste über ihren eigenen Witz lachen.

»Haha, ja, wir haben hier so einige sprechende Tiere.« Ich warf Jasper einen scharfen Blick zu und flüsterte ihm ein *Kannst du bitte mal die Klappe halten?* in den Kopf.

Hä? Meinste, ich darf dich nich' mehr verteidigen? Jasper war immer noch empört. *Aber was ist, wenn sie noch mehr gemeine Dinge zu dir sagt?*

Sie war nicht gemein, sondern ehrlich, das ist ein Unterschied, schoss ich zurück und sagte zu Daisy: »Kannst du dir vorstellen, dass manche Leute ein Geheimnis haben? Ein Geheimnis, von dem sie selbst nichts wissen?«

Daisy sah mich ratlos an. »Sprichst du oft in Rätseln?«

»Äh ... nein, eher nicht«, antwortete ich.

Weil ich zum Glück nun ein wortloses Wir-sind-bereit-Signal von den Delfinen empfing, zeigte ich Daisy den Weg runter zur Lagune. Leider gab es hier keine geteerten Wege mehr und prompt blieben die Räder ihres Rollis im lockeren Sand stecken.

»Einfach sitzen bleiben.« Wie aus dem Nichts tauchte Toco neben uns auf, packte den Rollstuhl und machte ihn mit einem kräftigen Ruck wieder flott.

»Oh, hi, Toco, hab mich schon gefragt, ob du auch da bist«, begrüßte ihn Daisy.

Toco schaffte ein Lächeln und grunzte irgendwas. Dafür, dass er nicht viel Übung im Nettsein hatte, schlug er sich ziemlich gut.

Doch es lohnte sich nicht wirklich, denn als Daisy unsere drei Delfine sah, vergaß sie alles andere. Ihr Gesicht leuchtete auf, als hätte jemand ihr gerade gesagt, dass sie im Lotto gewonnen hatte. »Ooooh ... ihr habt ja ganz unterschiedliche Arten! Ist das wirklich ein Blau-Weißer Delfin? So einen habe ich bisher nur in Büchern gesehen!«

Praktischerweise trug Daisy ein Kleid und darunter einen Badeanzug. Sie streifte sich das Kleid über den Kopf und ließ sich dann von mir die Krücken geben. »Wie heißen die drei denn? Darf ich wirklich mit ihnen ins Wasser?«

Ich stellte ihr unsere Delfinschüler vor. Doch Daisy zögerte noch, ins Meer zu gehen. »Habt ihr Quallen hier?« Sie klang nervös, was ich sehr gut verstehen konnte. Die meisten Leute hätten, wenn sie von einer Qualle so schwer verletzt worden wären, nie wieder einen Zeh ins Wasser gesteckt!

Zum Glück sah ich Zelda gerade im Palmhain chillen. »Nicht im Wasser«, sagte ich.

»Wo denn sonst, auf den Bäumen vielleicht?«, fragte Daisy und seufzte tief. »Meine Eltern killen mich, wenn sie das jemals herausfinden!« Sie humpelte ein paar Schritte weiter, bis kleine Wellen ihre Füße umspülten.

»Wie fühlst du dich?«, fragte ich gespannt, weil ich mich gut erinnern konnte, wie mein Körper auf das Meerwasser reagiert hatte. »So als ob du gar nicht mehr rauswolltest?«

Noch wussten wir nicht, ob sie überhaupt ein Seawalker war. Was war, wenn sie sich als Ameise, Landschildkröte oder Hamster erwies und sich mitten im Meer versehentlich verwandelte? Konnten Hamster schwimmen? Bei einer Landschildkröte war der Fall klar, die würde untergehen wie ein Stein. Ich hatte keine Ahnung, ob wir so ein Tier schnell genug retten konnten, bevor es ertrank. Machten wir hier gerade einen furchtbaren Fehler?

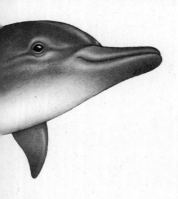

Der Styropor-Zwischenfall

Raus? Wieso sollte ich rauswollen?«, jubelte Daisy und watete ins hüfttiefe Wasser, wo unsere Delfine sie neugierig umringten. »Das ist so cool!«

Shari bewegte den grauen Kopf auf und ab und scannte Daisys Körper mit Ultraschall-Knacklauten, Blue hielt dem Mädchen die Rückenflosse hin und Noah stupste sie sanft mit der Schnauze an. Ich merkte, dass die drei sich geradezu überirdisch beherrschen mussten, um nicht drauflos zu plappern.

»Ich glaube, die wollen spielen.« Daisy war hin und weg. Sie ließ die Hand über Sharis glatten, festen Rücken gleiten, während Noah sie unternehmungslustig umkreiste.

»Das glaube ich auch«, sagte ich trocken, denn unsere drei Delfin-Wandler liebten Action aller Art.

»Aber tue ich ihnen nicht weh, wenn ich die Rückenflosse packe?«

»Na ja, du solltest nicht versuchen, sie *auszureißen*«, gab ich zurück. Doch die Frage hatte sich sowieso erledigt, denn Blue hatte Daisy die Rückenflosse schon in die Hand geschoben und zog sie behutsam durch die Lagune, während Shari neben ihr schwamm. Daisy jubelte. Noah hatte währenddessen entschieden, dass es Zeit für eine Runde Akrobatik war, er holte unter Wasser Anlauf, drehte in der Luft einen Salto und ließ sich klatschend wieder zurückfallen. Sämtliche Zuschauer in der Nähe trieften.

Und, wie war ich?, fragte Noah.

Na ja, den hast du schon mal besser hinbekommen, meinte Blue.

Klappe!, rief ich erschrocken.

Aber der Schaden war schon angerichtet. Als Daisy nach einer halben Stunde wieder an Land zurückschwamm – ihre Arme waren zum Glück kräftig –, blickte sie mir direkt in die Augen. »Du kannst mir ruhig sagen, was hier gespielt wird, Tiago«, sagte sie.

»Oh ... äh ...« Warum nur war Mr García nicht da? Wir hätten einen Verwandlungslehrer jetzt echt gut gebrauchen können!

Leider kam stattdessen Mr Williams runter zum Strand marschiert. Mist, warum hatte er nicht noch ein bisschen länger in der Stadt bleiben können? »Was geht hier vor?«

»Wir haben einen Gast, ein Mädchen aus der Key Largo Highschool«, sagte ich und versuchte, so zu klingen, als würde so was jeden Tag mindestens zweimal vorkommen. »Sie heißt ...«

»Es interessiert mich nicht, wie sie heißt.« Mr Williams klang eisig, während er Daisy fixierte. »Wer hat dir erlaubt herzukommen? Sieht das hier so aus wie eine Ferienanlage, in die jeder reinspazieren darf? Oder vielleicht wie ein öffentlicher Park? Am Donnerstag haben wir einen Besuchertag, da kannst du gerne zurückkommen. Es kostet allerdings Eintritt.«

Oh nein! Und das, nachdem ihr Besuch so gut begonnen hatte! Doch wenn er gedacht hatte, dass er Daisy einschüchtern konnte, hatte er sich getäuscht. Kämpferisch starrte sie allerdings nicht ihn, dafür aber den Kaffeebecher aus Styropor an, den Mr Williams in der Hand hielt und aus dem es dampfte. »Wussten Sie schon, dass es fünfzig Jahre dauert, bis so ein blöder Becher sich im Meer zersetzt, und dass seine Reste dann als Mikroplastik alles verseuchen?«

»Du versuchst allen Ernstes, *mich* zu belehren?«, fragte Mr Williams. »Das ist eine bodenlose Unverschämtheit!«

Shari stieß einen langen, wütenden Pfiff aus. Verständnislos blickte Daisy mich an, ihre Augen fragten mich wortlos, warum wir Infomaterial zum Schutz der Meere in ihrer Schule vorbeigebracht hatten, wenn wir selbst so schlechte Vorbilder waren.

»Es tut mir schrecklich leid«, war alles, was mir einfiel. »Das ist nicht unser richtiger Schulleiter, das ist nur ...«

Williams blickte drein, als könne er nicht glauben, was er hörte. »Unglaublich! Verweis für dich, Tiago Anderson.«

Ich freute mich nicht wirklich darüber, dass unser neuer Schulleiter es schon geschafft hatte, sich meinen Namen zu merken.

Am liebsten wäre ich abgehauen, zurück zu meiner Hütte, wo mich alle Leute in Ruhe ließen. Aber das ging nicht, ich konnte Daisy jetzt nicht allein lassen mit diesem Bankmanager, der sich als unser Chef aufspielte.

Dann wurde mir klar, dass wir nicht mehr allein waren. Eine weitere Besucherin war auf dem Weg aufgetaucht. Eine schlanke, hochgewachsene Frau mit kurzen weißen Haaren und einer leicht gebogenen Nase. Sie trug ein schlichtes Kleid, das genau die Farbe des Sommerhimmels hatte. War das eine Besucherin? Aber sie ging so zielstrebig, als wäre sie schon mal hier gewesen ... und kam genau auf uns zu.

Stanley Williams runzelte die Stirn. »Noch mehr Besucher? Was ist denn heute los?«, murmelte er und hob die Stimme, um zu rufen: »Hallo? Entschuldigen Sie! Verlassen Sie sofort dieses Gelände, hier ist bis zum Donnerstag ›Betreten verboten‹!«

»Für Menschen schon«, sagte die Frau und musterte unseren neuen Schulleiter mit einem Laserblick. »Behandeln Sie mögliche neue Schüler immer so wie dieses Mädchen? Falls ja, dann sind Sie absolut ungeeignet für Ihren momentanen Posten. Wie wäre es mit etwas ganz gewöhnlicher Höflichkeit?«

Und das war erst der Anfang. Fasziniert erlebten wir mit, wie die fremde Frau Mr Williams nach allen Regeln der Kunst zusammenfaltete.

»W-wer sind Sie eigentlich?«, fragte ein deutlich kleiner wirkender Stanley Williams schließlich. »Und woher wissen Sie, wie ich heiße?«

»Mein Name ist Lissa Clearwater«, kam zur Antwort und ich hatte einen Aha-Moment. Das war also die Mutter unseres bisherigen Schulleiters, die die Clearwater High in den Rocky Mountains führte! Carag, der Pumajunge, hatte mir von ihr erzählt. »Ich habe gehört, dass es hier gewisse Probleme gibt. Hören Sie mir genau zu, Mr Williams: Wenn Sie es wagen, dieser Schule zu schaden, werde ich höchstpersönlich dafür sorgen, dass Sie sich vor dem Rat dafür verantworten müssen. Und dann werden Ihre Verbündeten in Miami Sie schneller fallen lassen, als Sie ›Blue Reef‹ sagen können.«

»Es ... es ist ...« Mr Williams war nicht mehr zornesrot, sondern blass. Er drehte sich um und stelzte davon, wahrscheinlich um sich in Jack Clearwaters Büro zu verkriechen (das der im Gegensatz zu seinem Apartment leider nicht abgeschlossen hatte).

»Wow«, rief Daisy. »Was war das denn?«

»*Das* war ein sehr cooler Auftritt – danke!«, sagte ich und

Lissa Clearwater lächelte mir zu. »Hallo, Tiago. Carag hat mir schon viel von dir erzählt. Ich hoffe, wir können dich mal bei uns in Wyoming begrüßen?«

Ich stammelte irgendwas. Nachdem Jacks Mutter auch Jasper und unsere Delfinclique begrüßt hatte, wandte sie sich an Daisy. »Entschuldige den rauen Empfang«, meinte sie und lächelte ihr zu. »Mit dem Styroporbecher hattest du übrigens absolut recht.«

»Das hier ist keine normale Schule, oder?« Daisy hatte sich in ihren Rollstuhl zurückgehievt. »Erklärt mir bitte jemand, wer ihr seid und warum ich hier Stimmen in meinem Kopf höre?«

Du kannst uns in deinen Gedanken hören, weil du eine von uns bist, sagte Lissa Clearwater sanft ... und ließ aus ihren Armen Federn sprießen. Daisys Augen wurden groß. »Eine von euch? Aber was ...?«

Gestaltwandler, ergänzte Shari, die sich als Delfin im kaum kniehohen Wasser fläzte. *Ich weiß es auch noch nicht lange, aber glaub mir, es ist einfach meerig!*

Finny kam als Rochen aus den Tiefen der Lagune herangeflattert, ein dunkler Umriss unter den Wellen. *Genau. Wenn du Glück hast, bist du nicht ganz so platt wie ich.*

»Puh.« Daisy blies sich eine Locke aus der Stirn. »Das ist echt schräg.«

Am Anfang ist es schwer zu glauben, ich weiß, sagte Lissa Clearwater ... und verwandelte sich in einen Weißkopf-Seeadler. Ihr Kleid schwebte zu Boden, als sie die Schwingen ausstreckte und auf eine der Hütten flog.

»Und woher weiß ich, was *ich* bin? Ein Fisch, ein Vogel, ein ... Gürteltier ...« Daisy sah aus, als wüsste sie nicht genau, ob sie lachen oder weinen sollte.

Ihre Betreuerin, die sich inzwischen von ihrem Kaffee losgerissen hatte, verhinderte beides. Sie tauchte aus der Richtung des Hauptgebäudes auf und tippte auf ihre Uhr. »Daisy! Wir müssen los, sonst … oh, schau mal, ein Adler!«

»Ich weiß«, sagte Daisy und blickte ihrer Therapeutin fest in die Augen. »Beth. Wir müssen noch mal herkommen. So bald wie möglich.«

»Ja? Müssen wir das?« Beth schmunzelte. »Leider haben deine Eltern da noch ein Wörtchen mitzureden. Aber ich versuche, was zu drehen. Dann will ich aber zuschauen, was du hier machst, okay?«

In ziemlich vielen Augenpaaren konnte sie ein wortloses *Nein* lesen, was sie etwas zu verunsichern schien.

»Vielleicht«, wich Daisy aus und wehrte Tocos Hilfe ab, als sie ihren Rollstuhl vom Strand auf den Weg zurückmanövrierte. »Tschüss, Leute. Danke schon mal.« Mit einem breiten Lächeln winkte sie den Delfinen zu. »Ihr wart einfach unglaublich!«

Oh danke – sind wir!, scholl es von Noah zurück, Bescheidenheit war noch nie seine Stärke gewesen. Unsere Delfine machten in der Lagune einen Kopfstand, um Daisy mit den Schwanzflossen zuwinken zu können.

Erst als unsere beiden ungewöhnlichen Gäste wieder weg waren – Lissa Clearwater wollte wahrscheinlich so schnell wie möglich zu ihrem Sohn –, fiel mir ein, dass wir am Dienstag den Tiefwasserlehrgang hatten. Würde der Dienstag auch der Tag sein, an dem ich Miss White wiedersehen würde? Ich musste es schaffen, sie an unsere Schule zurückzuholen – wir brauchten sie dringender denn je!

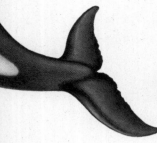

Blinder Passagier

Als ich am Dienstagfrüh am Lehrerzimmer vorbeiging, hörte ich, wie Mr García mit der Polizeistation telefonierte. »Ist inzwischen die Kaution für Wave da?«

Er hatte laut gestellt – wahrscheinlich für die anderen Lehrer –, sodass ich auch die Antwort mitbekam. »Die Hälfte schon, der Rest wird sicher bald eintreffen. Kommen Sie am besten morgen mit den Eltern des Jungen in unsere Station, dann können wir ihn in ihre Obhut geben.«

»Klingt gut, danke. Von uns kommt heute wieder jemand, der ihn besucht«, sagte mein Verwandlungslehrer und legte anscheinend auf.

Die Eltern! Wo sollten wir bloß Waves Eltern herbekommen? Und ich fragte mich auch, wieso das mit dem Geld so lange dauerte. Verzögerte die Lennox die Zahlung absichtlich, vielleicht weil sie noch wütend war wegen der Sondierung?

Als ich Farryn García wieder sprechen hörte, klang er leicht verzweifelt. »Mrs Misaki, könnten Sie sich vorstellen, sich als seine Mutter auszugeben? Uns andere Lehrer kennen die Cops leider schon.«

»Aber Mr García, wo denken Sie denn hin! Ich kann doch nicht die Polizei anlügen!«

»Schon gut«, brummte mein Verwandlungslehrer.

»Aber *ich* könnte doch …« Die Stimme von Miss Bennett.

»Das ist lieb von Ihnen, aber Sie sind zu jung.«

»Wie wäre es mit einem Rundruf bei den Eltern unserer Schüler?«, meinte Miss Bennett.

Unser Verwandlungslehrer runzelte die Stirn. »Zu riskant, dadurch könnte was durchsickern zu Lydia Lennox.«

Miss Monk, die Seeanemone aus dem Aquarium in der Eingangshalle, meldete sich zu Wort. *Guten Morgen allerseits – wer hat eigentlich in Auftrag gegeben, dass hier gerade Handwerker alle Schlösser austauschen?*

Mr García stieß einen Fluch aus und schoss aus dem Lehrerzimmer. Als er mich sah, meinte er hastig: »Ab zur Lagune, Tiago. Wir schwimmen gleich los zum Tiefwasserlehrgang.«

»Miss White war doch angeblich mal Kopfgeldjägerin, oder?«, sprudelte ich hervor. »Falls das stimmt, dann ist sie doch Profi darin, Leute – vor allem Wandler – aufzuspüren. Bestimmt könnte sie ...«

»Siehst du hier irgendwo eine Miss White?«, fuhr Mr García mich an. Seine Laune war nicht die beste.

Das schreckte weder mich noch Finny, die wie aus dem Nichts neben uns aufgetaucht war. »Wer besucht heute Wave?«, fragte sie.

»Jack. Der war auch schon am Sonntag da.« Mein Lehrer hastete an mir vorbei die Treppe hinunter in die Eingangshalle und ich hörte nur noch: »Wie bitte, was soll das heißen: ›Sie sind schon fertig‹? Wer hat Ihnen denn den Auftrag erteilt? ... Und wer hat den neuen Schlüssel? ... Was, es gibt nur einen und den hat Mr Williams? Meinen Sie das *ernst*?«

Oje. Anscheinend war unser schrecklicher neuer Schulleiter uns einen Schritt voraus.

Ich schwang meinen Hintern runter zur Lagune.

Meinst du, sie will sich wirklich mit uns treffen?, fragte Shari, als wir als Delfin und Hai darauf warteten, dass sich auch die anderen verwandelten. *Miss White, meine ich.*

Ich weiß nicht, vielleicht hat sie am Telefon auch was ganz anderes gemeint, sagte ich nur, während ich den tausend Gerüchen im Wasser nachspürte. *Iiih, jemand hat nicht riffsichere Sonnencreme benutzt, bevor er ins Meer gegangen ist!*

Bestimmt der Quallenfurz Mr Williams, sagte Ralph.

Wir waren sieben Leute beim Lehrgang. Mit dabei waren Lucy – der es wieder gut ging, die aber an der Oberfläche bleiben sollte –, außerdem Izzy, Ralph, Barry, die drei Delfine und ich. Eigentlich hatte auch Mara mitkommen sollen, aber sie hatte behauptet, sie hätte furchtbare Flossenschmerzen. Finny dagegen durfte wegen ihres Arrests nicht mit und vergrub die Hände in den Taschen ihrer Shorts, als sie uns bei der Verwandlung zuschaute. »Bestimmt werdet ihr ganz viel Spaß haben, während ich hier versauere und mit den Zweitjahresschülern Spanischvokabeln pauken muss!«

Was heißt versauern?, fragte Shari interessiert.

»Dass man Zitronensaft trinken muss«, behauptete Finny. »Eine ganze Kanne oder sogar zwei!«

Das Mitgefühl der Delfine hielt ungefähr drei Sekunden lang an, dann lieferten sie sich eine wilde, fröhliche Jagd durch die Lagune und vergaßen dabei alles andere.

Unser Lehrer gab das Signal zum Losschwimmen. *Bitte bleibt zusammen, auch wenn ihr irgendwas Appetitliches seht,* schärfte uns Mr García ein, der als Großer Tümmler voranschwamm. *Und merkt euch den Weg, es wird euer Job sein, uns wieder zurückzubringen. Achtet darauf, wo die Sonne steht, wie das Wasser schmeckt, wie ihr das Magnetfeld der Erde wahrnehmt.*

Meinst du das Gefühl, welche Richtung stimmt? Lucy schoss voran wie eine Rakete. *Haben Zweiarme das auch?*

Nee, die brauchen dafür einen Kompass, meinte Barry. *Aber es ist der Hit, wie supergut sich Carmen auch als Mensch zurechtfindet!*

Ein Dokumentarfilmer hätte sensationelle Bilder von Haien und Delfinen machen können, die absolut gleichzeitig die Augen verdrehen.

Obwohl Mr García in zweiter Gestalt Shari sehr ähnlich sah, konnte ich die beiden gut auseinanderhalten. Auf seiner grauen Haut zeichneten sich an verschiedenen Stellen helle Striche ab – Shari hatte davon auch ein paar, aber deutlich weniger.

Was sind das eigentlich für, äh, Markierungen?, fragte ich ihn.

Narben, erwiderte Shari an seiner Stelle und schwamm mit geschmeidigen Bewegungen neben mich. *Solche Spuren bleiben für immer und immer.*

Mr García seufzte. *Siehst du die Narbe auf meiner rechten Flanke? Die stammt von einem wilden Delfin. Er dachte, ich wollte ihn herausfordern, und hat mir die Zähne über die Seite gezogen.*

Oh, sagte ich. Als ich näher schwamm, um Sharis Narben genauer zu betrachten, registrierte meine hochempfindliche Nase seltsamerweise nicht nur Delfingeruch, sondern auch nasses Fell. Moment mal ...

Sekunden später schoss Chris auf uns zu, wendete mit einer eleganten Bewegung seiner Brustflossen und umkreiste uns. *Hi, Leute. Na, das ist aber ein Zufall, dass ihr auch hier seid!,* sagte er scheinheilig. *Ist doch okay, wenn ich mitkomme, oder?*

Natürlich, sagte Mr García und verlor kein Wort darüber,

dass Chris offiziell nicht mehr auf unsere Schule ging. *Wie geht's dir? Wir haben deine Sachen erst mal in einen Karton geräumt und in den Schuppen gestellt.*

Ihr dürft meine Aquaman-Comics lesen, aber wehe, ihr macht sie nass, sagte Chris.

Wir beobachteten nicht ihn, sondern Barry. Würde er das an seinen Vater petzen?

Aquaman ist doch Dreck, Thor *und* Hellboy *sind viel besser,* sagte er nur. *Wenn ich mal einen Hund habe, nenne ich ihn Thor.*

Cool, Alter – ein Tier, das sich ein Tier hält, kicherte Ralph. *Glaubst du wirklich, dein Vater erlaubt dir einen Hund?*

Er hat schon Ja gesagt, behauptete Barry. *Mein Vater kann auch nett sein, wenn er gerade mal nicht seine Pflicht im Kopf hat, und außerdem mag er Hunde.*

Na ja, Seehunde eher nicht, meinte Chris nur.

Wir schwammen weiter und weiter, aus dem flachen Küstenbereich hinaus ins offene Meer. Klar und tiefblau war es hier, Lichtspeere tanzten durchs Wasser und ließen leuchtende Muster über unsere Haut wabern.

Sieht zwar hübsch aus, aber Blau ist im Meer die Farbe der Wüste, erklärte Mr García. *Hier gibt es nur ganz wenige Nährstoffe und viel weniger Organismen als an der Küste. Wer hier überleben will, hat es nicht leicht.*

Stimmt, kein Fisch weit und breit. Chris klang enttäuscht, ich konnte seinen Magen knurren hören. Anscheinend ersetzten die Touristenhappen, die er sich hin und wieder holte, die Mahlzeiten in der Cafeteria nicht wirklich.

Sag mal, gibt es etwas an deinem Vater, das du magst? Blue versuchte, Barry in ein Gespräch zu verwickeln.

Als er versucht hat, mir Baseball beizubringen, war er echt geduldig, brummte Barry. *Außerdem kann er toll mathemati-*

sche Formeln erklären. Großzügig ist er auch – wenn ich eine gute Note geschrieben habe, gehen wir immer zusammen ein Eis essen.

Immerhin! Während ich Barry zuhörte, hielt ich Ausschau nach Miss White, doch weit und breit war kein Schwertwal in Sicht. Nur eine einsame Motorjacht zog vorbei, wir hörten ihr Motorengeräusch näher kommen.

Ein bisschen unheimlich war es schon, dass man den Meeresboden nicht mehr sehen konnte, aber nach meiner Tieftaucherfahrung mit Blue und Lucy fand ich es nicht mehr ganz so schlimm. Mr García erklärte gerade, dass viele große Meerestiere allein weite Strecken durch den Ozean wanderten, aber sich jedes Jahr an bestimmten Orten zur Partnersuche trafen, als mich etwas am Bauch kitzelte.

Blue lachte auf. *Schaut mal, Tiago hat einen neuen Freund!*

Ich konnte nicht an mir herabschauen, aber Shari schickte mir ein geistiges Bild. Es war nicht wirklich ein neuer Freund, eher ein blinder Passagier. Er hatte sich mit einer Art Saugnapf an meinen Bauch geheftet und ließ sich von mir mitziehen. *He, was soll das – zieh ab!*, schimpfte ich das immerhin unterarmlange Vieh aus, was es natürlich überhaupt nicht interessierte.

Ein Schiffshalter, erklärte uns Mr García amüsiert. *Fast jeder größere Fisch hat einen oder mehrere. Man wird sie leider ohne Hilfe nicht los. Angeblich gewöhnt man sich an sie.*

Ich will mich aber nicht daran gewöhnen, ein Taxi zu sein, beschwerte ich mich. *Kann den mal jemand abpflücken oder auffressen oder so was?*

Nachdem die Delfine sich ausgiebig über mich und den Saugfisch lustig gemacht haben, erbarmte sich Noah, teilverwandelte seine Arme und griff das lästige Biest am Schwanz.

Leider saugte es sich daraufhin so fest, dass er es nicht abrupfen konnte.

Probier es mal mit Durchkitzeln, empfahl ihm Izzy und probierte es gleich selbst. Aber erst, als Blue dem blinden Passagier einen Finger in die Kiemen steckte, gab der auf und schwamm beleidigt davon. Beinahe hätte er sich Mr García als neues Transportmittel ausgesucht, doch der wich aus und schoss so schnell voran, dass der Schiffshalter zurückblieb. Sofort suchte er sich Blue als neues Ziel aus, quiekend floh sie ebenfalls.

Ihr seid aber leicht ablenkbar – ein wilder Orca hätte euch jetzt verspeist, dröhnte plötzlich eine Stimme durch unsere Köpfe. *Ich bin hinter dem Motorboot hergeschwommen, sodass ihr mich nicht kommen hören konntet. Ein alter Trick.*

Es war eine vertraute Stimme, die ich viel zu lange nicht mehr gehört hatte!

Miss White!, jubelte ich und Mr García klang ebenfalls erfreut, als wir uns der riesigen schwarz-weißen Gestalt des Orcas zuwandten. *Alisha, was machst du denn hier?*

Ich ..., begann unsere ehemalige Kampflehrerin, doch plötzlich versagte ihr die Stimme. *Es tut mir leid, ich wollte euch nicht stören auf eurem Ausflug.*

Vielleicht weil wir uns so gut kannten, spürte ich ihre Einsamkeit, sie wehte in meinen Kopf wie der bittere Duft einer Giftblume. Doch schon nach einer Sekunde bemerkte sie es und schirmte sich besser ab.

Ach Blödsinn, fühlt sich jemand gestört? Chris umkreiste Miss White übermütig, was er bei einem wilden Orca nicht lange überlebt hätte. Obwohl ich gehört hatte, dass manche Schwertwale nur Fisch fraßen und keine Säugetiere.

Wir haben Sie wirklich vermisst, sagte Noah, schwamm neben ihr und achtete nicht darauf, dass er gerade den Schiffshalter abbekommen hatte.

Er behielt ihn sowieso nicht lange. Der Schiffshalter warf einen Blick auf Miss White, entschied sich für das deutlich größere Transportmittel und schwamm zu ihr hinüber.

Bitte kommen Sie mit uns zurück, bettelte Shari, doch ich spürte, dass Miss White noch zögerte. Auch Ralph und Barry warteten ab, beide hatten noch nichts gesagt.

Plötzlich erinnerte ich mich an Miss Whites Gedanken, die ich während des Hurrikans gespürt hatte, ihre Zweifel und Selbstvorwürfe. *Egal, was Sie früher waren und was Sie eigentlich gelernt haben, Sie sind eine gute Lehrerin geworden*, sagte ich und schwamm ebenfalls an ihre Seite. *Erklären Sie uns einfach, was genau Sie getan haben und warum. Die meisten werden es verstehen und die anderen sollen eben den Mund halten!*

Genau. Noah schoss um uns herum wie ein wild gewordenes Badewannenspielzeug. *Tangaroa wird Ihnen beistehen. Er ist ein Gott, der versteht und verzeiht!*

Miss White seufzte. *Ich fürchte, Menschen verzeihen nicht so leicht wie Götter. Farryn, was meinst du?*

Komm mit zurück, Alisha, sagte Mr García sofort.

Okay. Erst mal zum Reden, danach sehen wir weiter. Das Orca-Weibchen, mehr als dreimal so groß wie unsere Delfine, schwamm neben uns. Ich war unglaublich erleichtert. Jetzt würde alles gut werden. Bestimmt.

Blue schien sich auch zu freuen. Hier im tiefen Wasser wirkte sie ausgeglichen, ganz bei sich. Hier war sie daheim. *Ist es in Ordnung, wenn ich ein Stück vorauskundschafte?*, fragte sie und Mr García erlaubte es.

Kurz darauf schwamm Blue aufgeregt und mit Höchstgeschwindigkeit zu uns zurück. *Hab was entdeckt,* berichtete sie. *Kommt schnell mit, sonst ist es zu spät!*

Gespannt stoben wir ihr hinterher.

Sehr feurig!

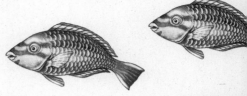
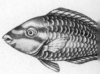

Schon aus der Entfernung hörte ich, dass im Meer vor uns ordentlich was los war. Ich hörte ein Zischen, Schnappen und etwas, was wie Schläge klang. Was in aller Welt konnte das sein?

Ein Köderball, antwortete Mr García. *Ich hatte gehofft, ich könnte euch einen zeigen.*

Was das war, sah ich kurz darauf selbst. Es war ein riesiger Schwarm silberner Fischchen, der in der blauen Weite wirkte wie eine sich ständig verändernde, flirrende Wolke. Der Schwarm hatte den Appetit vieler Meerestiere geweckt. Von oben schossen Wasservögel mit angelegten Flügeln ins Wasser wie gefiederte Raketen – daher die Schläge! – und schnappten sich Fischchen. Sie flatterten unter Wasser sogar mit den Flügeln, um tiefer zu kommen. Aufgeregte Haie zischten um den Schwarm herum und stießen immer wieder hinein, um sich den Magen zu füllen. Auch Delfine nahmen am Festmahl teil, und unglaublich schnelle, torpedoförmige Raubfische, die gierig in den Schwarm hinein- und wieder hinausjagten. Es war echt krass – erst diese blaue Leere und dann hier so ein Getümmel.

Es ist übrigens ein Sardellenschwarm und die Jäger sind unter anderem Thunfische, erklärte Mr García, er wirkte beunruhigt. *Die Vögel sind Tölpel, aber nicht ungeschickt, sondern Meister im Sturzflug. Izzy, halt dich unter meiner Brustflosse, damit die dich nicht schnappen.*

Okay, sagte Izzy eingeschüchtert und flitzte zu ihm hin. Überall schossen die Tölpel zu uns herunter wie weiße Pfeile und schnappten sich Beute.

Das reicht nicht, Farryn, antwortete Miss White. *Besser ist, Izzy schwimmt sofort zurück zur Schule. Wer geleitet sie hin?*

Ich, sagte Ralph blitzschnell. Die beiden, Riffhai und fliegender Fisch, waren ein ziemlich ungleiches Paar, als sie davonjagten – möglichst schnell möglichst weit weg von dem Köderball. Nun konnten wir uns wieder auf das Spektakel vor uns konzentrieren.

Achtet mal darauf, wie geschickt unsere Hai- und Delfinkollegen den Schwarm immer wieder zu einer Kugel zusammentreiben und an die Wasseroberfläche drängen, meinte Mr García. *Dort kann man die Fische dann leicht schnappen.*

Wie entscheiden die Fische eigentlich, wo sie hinschwimmen?, fragte ich neugierig. *Einen Anführer gibt es im Schwarm nicht, oder?*

Stimmt, meinte Miss White. *Jeder Fisch kann spontan eine bestimmte Bewegung vormachen, und alle anderen bewegen sich gleichzeitig mit ihm. Wandler, die Schwarmfische sind, nutzen das manchmal aus und lassen die anderen machen, was SIE wollen.*

Shari konnte kaum noch die Flossen still halten. *Jaja, wusste ich schon – wann dürfen wir endlich mitmachen?*

Am besten gleich! Lucy hatte sich neben uns ausgebreitet wie ein geöffneter Regenschirm und tastete mit ihren rötlich braunen Armen in Richtung des Schwarms.

Oh ja, bitte!, bettelte ich mit. In meiner Menschengestalt hätte ich mich niemals in dieses Raubfisch-Mega-Event hineingetraut, aber heute war ich zum Glück ein Tigerhai.

Mr García lachte. *Guten Appetit und viel Spaß! Aber passt auf, dass ihr nicht versehentlich gebissen werdet, hier hat jeder nur noch sein Fresschen im Kopf.*

Ich auch – Snack-Time!, jubelte Chris und stürzte sich in den Schwarm. Ich folgte ihm mit Höchstgeschwindigkeit. Es war wirklich genial – man musste nur in den Schwarm schwimmen und um sich schnappen, dann hatte man schon drei oder vier Leckerchen zwischen den Zähnen hängen. Niemand versuchte, uns zu verjagen, oder schien etwas dagegen zu haben, dass wir mitmachten. Es war genug für alle da.

Auch unsere Lehrer schlugen sich den Bauch voll. Respektvoll wichen die Haie, Delfine und Thunfische aus, als Miss White daherkam – als Schwertwal war sie die Königin hier!

Nur die Sardellen taten mir ein bisschen leid. Als wir und die anderen Jäger schließlich abzogen, war der Schwarm deutlich kleiner als zuvor und stattdessen flirrte ein Schneegestöber glitzernder einzelner Schuppen durchs Wasser. Kurz dachte ich darüber nach, warum wir als ganz normal akzeptierten, dass gerade all diese kleinen Fische gestorben waren, aber wir uns darüber aufregten, wenn Gladiatorentaucher Haie harpunierten. Wahrscheinlich war der Unterschied, dass das eine Natur war – große Fische mussten irgendetwas fressen – und das andere die sinnlose Grausamkeit von Menschen.

Es war jedenfalls ein supergenialer Klassenausflug gewesen. Blue wirkte satt und zufrieden, Shari schwärmte nonstop davon, wie meerig der Ausflug bisher gewesen war. Und Noah meinte: *Mhmm, das war lecker. Sind diese Fischchen immer hier und können wir morgen noch mal herkommen?*

Vergiss es, informierte ihn Miss White. *Fische können wegschwimmen, weißt du? Man muss viel Glück haben, um so einen Schwarm zu finden.*

Ich musste wieder einmal an Wave denken. Als Buckelwal hätte er diese Fischchen mit ein paar Riesenschlucken eingeschlürft. Wie ging es ihm als Mensch jetzt? Hatte er Hunger, war er einsam? Wann bekamen wir ihn endlich raus? Seit seiner Beinaheverwandlung am Wochenende hatte ich noch mehr Angst um ihn.

Nach ein paar Übungen und Lektionen zu Tieren des offenen Ozeans sagte Mr García ausgerechnet zu Noah: *So, jetzt führ uns mal heim zur Schule!* Wir wussten natürlich, warum er drankam – nach dem Hurrikan hatte sich unser Freund gründlich im Meer verirrt.

Aber diesmal gelang es ihm, uns zurückzuführen. Müde und zufrieden, schwammen wir am späten Nachmittag in die Lagune. Izzy war anscheinend gut wieder heimgekommen, sie hatte es sich mit einem Buch in der Hängematte zwischen zwei Palmen gemütlich gemacht. Chris war nirgends in Sicht, klar, er durfte nicht mehr hier sein.

Auch die andere Hälfte der Klasse war von ihrem Ausflug zurück und staunte unsere junge Ex-Kampflehrerin an. Die verwandelte sich, ließ sich ein Handtuch zuwerfen und stapfte ungerührt aus dem Wasser an den Strand, durch ihre sportliche Figur sah sie dadurch aus wie ein Bond-Girl. Der Schiffshalter wirkte verdutzt. Er klebte nun an ihrem Oberschenkel und kapierte sicher nicht, warum er plötzlich an der Luft war. Im letzten Moment ließ er sich fallen und schwamm davon.

Finny lachte sich kaputt, als sie es sah. »Angeln für Anfänger! Lernen wir das noch im Kampfunterricht, Miss White?«

»Nein. Man muss dabei nicht kämpfen.« Miss White lächelte ihr zu, dann wandte sie sich wieder an Mr García und ihre Miene wurde angespannt. »Wo ist Jack? Ich will als Erstes mit ihm reden.«

Farryn García erklärte ihr, in welchem Hotel sie unseren Ex-Schulleiter finden konnte. Dann ging er seine Autoschlüssel holen und gab sie ihr. Schon war Miss White wieder weg. Ich konnte gut verstehen, dass sie erst mal unter vier Augen mit Mr Clearwater sprechen wollte, und drückte beide Daumen, dass sie das hinbekamen.

Während wir uns anzogen, sah ich verdutzt, dass Handwerker sich auf dem Dach der Schule zu schaffen machten. Es sah völlig anders aus als vorher, überall ragten fies aussehende Metallstacheln hoch, wie man sie anbringt, damit sich an einem Haus keine Tauben niederlassen. Na toll.

Ich ließ den Blick schweifen. Am Strand loderte in einem Kreis aus Steinen ein Lagerfeuer. Ich freute mich, als ich sah, dass Rocket mal wieder vorbeigekommen war und schon mit Finny und ein paar anderen in respektvollem Abstand am Feuer saß. Wir klatschten uns ab. »Was Süßes gefällig?«, fragte

Rocket, öffnete eine Kühlbox und holte ein Eis am Stiel heraus. »Ich hab was mitgebracht und gebe 'ne Runde aus.«

»Äh ... nett von dir, aber ...«, sagte ich, während sich Schüler um Rocket drängten und ungefähr dreißig Hände nach einem Eis grapschten. Das Gedränge kam mir vom Köderball sehr bekannt vor.

»Wer mag, kann sich auch ein Würstchen oder ein paar Garnelen grillen«, verkündete Miss Bennett, manche Schüler fingen schon an, sich Stöcke zurechtzuschnitzen.

»Wenn ich auch nur eine winzige Garnele esse, kommt sie zusammen mit tausend Sardellen wieder heraus«, stöhnte Shari und wir anderen nickten heftig.

Olivia, Juna und Zelda schwatzten miteinander, Daphne erzählte Polly und Tino – den Neuen aus dem Sumpf – eine Geschichte über Menschen, Noemi lag schnurrend auf der Seite und Leonora hatte ihre Gitarre geholt und zupfte darauf herum. Es waren wohl alle dankbar, dass nach der ausgefallenen Party mal wieder ein bisschen was los war.

Rocket hatte wie versprochen die Minikamera mitgebracht und wir montierten sie testweise auf dem Rücken von Maris-dem-Albatros. »Jetzt können wir einwandfreie Beweise sammeln, mit denen auch die Polizei etwas anfangen kann«, jubelte ich. »Aber natürlich nur, wenn du damit fliegen kannst, Maris.«

Drückt ein bisschen, aber nicht viel, meinte Maris, flog eine Runde und filmte uns aus der Luft, wie wir am Strand hockten. *Ich nehm das Ding ab jetzt immer zu Erkundungsflügen mit.*

»Sehr cool, du bist ein Spitzen-Albatros«, lobte ich ihn. »Jetzt müssen wir nur noch die Haikampfveranstalter auf frischer Tat ertappen!«

Schließlich kam auch Mr Williams hinzu und setzte sich ein

Stück von uns entfernt in den Sand. Er zog sein Jackett aus und krempelte sein Hemd bis zu den Ellenbogen auf, vielleicht wollte er locker wirken. Interessiert registrierte ich, dass Barrys Vater ein dunkelblaues Barrakuda-Tattoo auf dem Unterarm hatte. Wir warfen ihm misstrauische Blicke von der Seite zu, während er selbstzufrieden in die Runde lächelte und begann, auf seinem Handy Nachrichten zu beantworten.

Endgültig dahin war die gute Stimmung, als Finny angestrengt in die Flammen starrte und schließlich sagte: »He, Leute. Was ist das eigentlich, das da brennt?«

Auch andere blickten nun forschend ins Feuer. Dann japste Juna: »Oh nein, das ist doch Jacks Adler-Sitzstange!«

»Und das daneben, ist das nicht diese Treibholz-Skulptur, die in seinem Büro stand?« Finny sprang auf, versuchte, das brennende Holz aus dem Feuer zu angeln, und wich mit einem Fluch zurück.

»Was? Das sind die Sachen von Mr Clearwater?«, rief Izzy.

Ivy Bennett und ein paar andere rannten los, um Löschwasser zu holen. Leider mussten sie dazu ins Bootshaus, weil wir hier am Strand keine Eimer hatten. Beunruhigt standen wir ums Feuer herum.

»Gib mir den Stock!«, rief Olivia. »Vielleicht können wir noch was davon aus dem Feuer holen!«

»Also die Sitzstange ist jedenfalls hinüber.« Ella starrte höchst interessiert in die Flammen.

Mr García kam herangestapft, er trug wie wir nur Badeshorts. »Williams! Was haben Sie *getan*?«

Stanley Williams lächelte nur. »Ich verbrenne Müll. Schließlich lautet mein Auftrag, in dieser Schule aufzuräumen.«

»Sie mieser Treibnetzfischer!« Auch Mrs Pelagius war inzwischen hinzugekommen, als kleine, gebeugte Frau mit einem von vielen Falten durchzogenen Gesicht. »Dazu hatten Sie kein Recht.«

Doch Mr García fluchte nicht nur. Ich spürte, wie er sich konzentrierte, und dann stieß er einen so starken Fernruf aus, dass mir fast der Kopf platzte.

Es dauerte keine zehn Minuten, bis ich erleichtert sah, dass eine Weißkopf-Seeadlerin über den Palmhain schwebte und zur Landung ansetzte. Sie musste sowieso in der Gegend gewesen sein, sonst hätte sie es nie so schnell geschafft. Nach wenigen Augenblicken hatte Miss Clearwater erfasst, was los war.

Habe ich Sie nicht gewarnt, Mr Williams? Ihre Gedankenstimme klang schneidend. *Gehe ich recht in der Annahme, dass weder Sie noch Mrs Lennox meinem Sohn den Schaden ersetzen werden?*

»Das ist richtig.« Stanley Williams hatte ein breites Grinsen aufgesetzt.

Dann finde ich eine uralte Form der Gerechtigkeit angemessen – Auge um Auge, Zahn um Zahn.

Bevor irgendeiner von uns reagieren konnte, war der Adler schon auf unseren neuen Schulleiter zugeflogen und ergriff sein Handy mit den Klauen.

Reiner Tisch

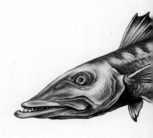

Kaum hatte Lissa Clearwater in ihrer Adlergestalt das Handy von Mr Williams erbeutet, wendete sie und schlug mit den Flügeln, um Höhe zu gewinnen. Dann ließ sie das Gerät, das sie in den Klauen getragen hatte, mitten ins Lagerfeuer fallen.

»Nein!«, brüllte Mr Williams, sprang hoch und rannte aufs Feuer zu. Dort gab es inzwischen eine Funkenexplosion, die wir aus sicherer Entfernung bewunderten.

»Lithium-Ionen-Akkus brennen echt gut«, sagte Rocket anerkennend. Das mit dem Löschen hatten sich Izzy und die anderen Eimerträger gerade anders überlegt.

Statt davonzufliegen, hatte Miss Clearwater nur gewendet. Sie landete auf Mr Williams' Jackett, dessen Besitzer gerade in mehreren Metern Entfernung herumstolperte, durchsuchte es mit dem Schnabel und holte eine Brieftasche daraus hervor. Seelenruhig nahm sie es in die Klauen und hob wieder ab.

Gespannt beobachteten wir, was geschah. Auch Mr Williams schien klar zu sein, was gleich sehr wahrscheinlich passieren würde. Mit wildem Blick hielt er an, kehrte um, raste zu seinen Sachen zurück und sprang hoch, um den startenden Adler zu packen. Zum Glück hatte er anscheinend nie Basketball gespielt, jedenfalls kam er nicht weit vom Boden weg. Seine Hände grapschten ins Leere, er stürzte und landete mit dem Hintern im Sand. Die Brieftasche trudelte in die Flammen.

»Löschwasser! Schnell!«, blökte Mr Williams und stürzte mit ausgestreckten Händen zum Ort des Geschehens. *Los, brenn schon,* forderte ich die Brieftasche auf, die noch nicht Feuer gefangen hatte.

»Kommt sofort«, sagte Finny und stellte ihm ein Bein, als er an ihr vorbeilief. Unser neuer Schulleiter bremste mit dem Gesicht im Sand. Ganz zufällig stieß Ralph gegen die beiden Wassereimer, sodass sie umkippten und ihr Inhalt am Strand versickerte. Erst jetzt kam mir die Idee, dass man eigentlich auch Sand aufs Feuer werfen konnte, um es zu löschen. Zum Glück fiel das niemand anderem ein, auch nicht Barry und seinem Vater. Die Verzögerung gab der Brieftasche die nötige Zeit, um ordentlich anzuschmoren. Toco stocherte mit dem Stock daran herum, sodass sie aufklappte und wir bewundern konnten, wie malerisch die Kreditkarten schmolzen und der Rest des Inhalts in Rauch aufging.

»Die Dollars brennen nicht so gut.« Rocket klang ein wenig enttäuscht.

»Was erwartest du?«, fragte Finny. »Solche Lappen können halt keinen Raketenstart hinlegen.«

Ich sah, dass Mr Williams auch ein Familienfoto inklusive Barry mit sich herumgetragen hatte, und verstummte betroffen. Plötzlich tat er mir leid. Barry saß schweigend neben Carmen am Feuer und sah aus, als sei ihm das alles todpeinlich.

»Es tut mir echt leid«, sagte er und sein Vater brüllte: »Das gehört sich auch so, dass du zu mir hältst!«

Er war der Einzige, der nicht gemerkt hatte, dass Barry das zu Carmen gesagt hatte. Mit blutunterlaufenen Augen starrte Stanley Williams in die Runde und wir grinsten ihm ins Gesicht. Selten hatte ich jemanden gesehen, der so stinkwütend war. »Das werdet ihr noch bereuen!«

»Na, da sind wir aber gespannt – wollen Sie uns alle von der Schule werfen?«, fragte Finny honigsüß. »Nur zu, wir haben sowieso Lust auf ein paar Tage Ferien.«

»Wenn Mrs Lennox das erfährt, werdet ihr das büßen!«

Am Motorengeräusch hatten ich und einige andere schon gemerkt, dass der Fernruf nicht nur Miss Clearwater hergeholt hatte, sondern auch unsere ehemalige Kampflehrerin. Miss White hatte sich umgezogen; ihre schlanke, durchtrainierte Gestalt war wieder ganz in Schwarz gekleidet, ihre dunklen Haare hatte sie zu einem Pferdeschwanz gebunden. Miss White warf Mr García die Autoschlüssel zu und bedankte sich mit einem Nicken. Als sie den letzten Satz von Mr Williams hörte, warf sie ihm einen Blick zu, der bei den meisten Leuten wahrscheinlich einen Herzstillstand ausgelöst hätte.

»Nur um mal eins klarzustellen – Mrs Lennox wird erst etwas davon erfahren, wenn Wave frei ist.« In Miss Whites Stimme klirrte das Eis. »Und wenn Sie vorhaben, die Schüler büßen zu lassen ... vergessen Sie das ganz schnell wieder.«

Manche Lehrer haben Autorität und andere nicht. Vielleicht ist das angeboren, keine Ahnung. Obwohl Miss White höchstens Ende zwanzig war, hatte sie sie ganz eindeutig – mit dieser Stimme hatte sie schon eine ganze Horde Amok laufender Sumpfschüler gebändigt.

Bei Mr Williams wirkte sie ebenfalls. Der Arme, zum zweiten Mal innerhalb kurzer Zeit wurde er runtergeputzt. Aber mein Mitleid hielt sich in Grenzen, als er wortlos das Feld räumte.

Kurz darauf hörten wir das Röhren eines Motors. Oje. Der raste jetzt garantiert zurück nach Miami. Würde er die Warnung beherzigen? Oder Mrs Lennox brühwarm Bericht erstatten? Vielleicht hätten wir doch lieber machen sollen, was er verlangte. Aber wir konnten doch nicht tatenlos zusehen, wenn er dermaßen miese Dinge tat!

Nach und nach wagten wir, uns zu entspannen.

»Was meinen Sie, kommt der noch mal zurück?«, fragte Polly Mr García.

»Ich glaube nicht.« Mr García atmete tief durch. »Das war's mit Mr Williams.«

Das hieß, dieser Albtraum war vorbei! Ringsum sah ich lächelnde Gesichter. Juna und Olivia klatschten sich ab, Finny riss triumphierend die Arme hoch und sogar Ella und Toco wirkten erleichtert.

Oh toll, der Gewittermann ist weg, freute sich Noemi, deren Lieblingsplatz auf dem Dach gerade durch Taubenstacheln blockiert war. *Heißt das, ich muss nicht in dieses ferne Land?*

Keine Sorge, musst du nicht, beruhigte ich sie und Noemi legte schnurrend ihre großen Pranken um mich und schleckte mir über das Gesicht. Uäh. Sie hatte leider ziemlichen Maulgeruch.

Inzwischen hatten sämtliche Leute in der Blue Reef High – Schüler, Lehrer und Angestellte wie Joshua oder Mrs Misaki – gemerkt, dass Miss White zurückgekehrt war. Leise hatten sich alle am Strand versammelt, während das Feuer langsam herunterbrannte.

»Schätze, ich schulde euch noch was«, sagte Miss White, seufzte und setzte sich. »Die ganze Wahrheit.«

Wir nickten schweigend.

»Ich bin in einer Gruppe von Orcas aufgewachsen, die sich von Robben ernähren ... als junger Schwertwal musste ich das

Tarnen und Täuschen lernen, sonst hätte ich hungern müssen«, begann meine Lieblingslehrerin. »Meine Mutter und mein Bruder haben sich erst ab und zu verwandelt und später nur noch als Orcas gelebt. Ich wollte allerdings zur Schule gehen und bin deswegen nur nachts mit ihnen geschwommen. Irgendwann hat meine Mutter zu mir gesagt: ›Die Lachsfarmen machen die Küste kaputt und in unserer Beute sind immer mehr Giftstoffe. Wenn du mit der Schule fertig bist, such dir am besten einen ruhigen Job an Land.‹«

Meine Freunde und ich lauschten gespannt, nur Ella, Toco und Barry störten durch ihr Getuschel. Miss White ignorierte die drei.

»Nur wollte ich keinen ruhigen Job, ich wollte etwas erleben, ferne Länder sehen«, fuhr sie fort. »Also ging ich zur Marine und ließ mich dort zur Kampftaucherin ausbilden, machte Einsätze überall auf der Welt.« Beeindrucktes Gemurmel am Strand, das jedoch sofort verstummte, als Miss White weitererzählte. »Aber dann bekam ich einen Chef, der mich nicht mochte und ständig schikanierte. Irgendwann bin ich ausgerastet und habe ihm einen Kinnhaken verpasst. Dafür wurde ich natürlich gefeuert.«

Als ich ihr zuhörte, machte in meinem Kopf etwas klick. Sie war ausgerastet und hatte deswegen richtig Ärger bekommen? Das war genau mein Problem! Hatte sie mich deswegen immer besonders gefördert, brachte sie mir deswegen bei, besser mit meiner Wut umzugehen ... weil sie wusste, wie das war?

»Tja, danach fand ich keinen Job mehr. Aber es gab ein paar Woodwalker und Seawalker, die mich unterstützten, die immer für mich da waren und mich für kleinere Jobs bezahlten.« Alisha White seufzte tief. »Ich dachte, sie wären meine Freunde. Als sie mich baten, ihnen zu helfen, sagte ich Ja. Sie wollten, dass ich bestimmte Wandler für sie fand – in Nord- und Südamerika, in Europa, in Japan. Das bekam ich auch hin.«

»Wann ist Ihnen klar geworden, dass mit diesen Aufträgen etwas nicht stimmte?«, fragte Noah.

»Ziemlich bald. Ich bekam mit, dass diese Leute meine Freunde verraten oder versucht hatten, sie um Geld zu betrügen. Irgendwann merkte ich erstens, dass meine ›Freunde‹ durch illegale Geschäfte Dollars scheffelten, und zweitens, dass viele Zielpersonen spurlos verschwanden, nachdem ich sie abgeliefert hatte.«

Wieso sind Sie dann nicht einfach weggeschwommen?, fragte Lucy verständnislos. *Manche Zweiarme sind steinig im Herzen, vor denen sollte man sich vielgut verstecken.*

»Ich dachte immer noch, ich schulde diesen Leuten etwas«, versuchte Alisha White zu erklären. »Und sie hatten immer gute Geschichten parat, um zu erklären, wo meine Zielpersonen abgeblieben waren. Aber ich wollte es auch nicht so genau wissen. Schließlich bekam ich für jeden, den ich ablieferte, eine fette Prämie und mochte mein Leben so, wie es war. Außerdem war ich irgendwie stolz darauf, dass ich eine der besten in diesem Geschäft war.«

Sie war ehrlich. Das fand ich gut. Aber es gab eine Frage, die mir keine Ruhe ließ. Also stellte ich sie einfach. »Haben Sie selbst jemanden getötet?«

Alisha White zögerte nicht mit der Antwort. »Ja, habe ich. Es war ein Kopfgeldjäger, der versucht hat, mich zu töten, weil ich ihm in die Quere gekommen war. Ich war ungefähr fünf Sekunden schneller.«

»Wow«, sagte Rocket. »Klingt wie aus *Blade Runner*. Einer meiner Lieblingsfilme!«

Shari und ich blickten uns an – das, was wir gerade gehört

hatten, mussten wir erst mal verdauen. Sie hatte jemanden *getötet*. Wie gruselig! Wahrscheinlich erriet Miss White, woran wir dachten, denn sie sagte ruhig: »Ich denke noch heute oft an ihn. Lange war ich ziemlich fertig deswegen ... das könnt ihr euch bestimmt vorstellen. Aber in jenem Moment hatte ich keine Wahl. Er oder ich, so war das.«

Ich und ein paar andere nickten. *Es war Notwehr,* tröstete ich mich, aber ich wusste auch, dass ich wahrscheinlich noch oft daran denken würde.

Schon erzählte Miss White weiter. »Irgendwann bin ich ausgestiegen, habe meinen Namen geändert und bin auf die andere Seite des Kontinents gezogen. Ich wollte das alles nicht mehr. Seither habe ich keinen Job mehr für diese ›Freunde‹ erledigt. Mein Leben hier ist nicht ganz so aufregend, aber es ist viel schöner, finde ich, und Herausforderungen habe ich ja auch hier.«

Wie bitte? Sie hieß in Wirklichkeit gar nicht Alisha White? Im ersten Moment war ich geschockt. Ganz schön naiv von mir. Natürlich wechselt man den Namen, wenn man nicht gefunden werden will, ist doch klar!

»Könnt ihr mir das alles verzeihen?« Alisha stellte diese Frage an alle, die in der hereinbrechenden Dämmerung am Rand der Lagune saßen.

Ich wusste, wie viel von diesen Antworten abhing, und wagte kaum zu atmen.

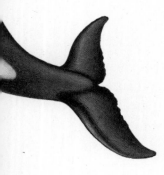

Knallhart

Würden die anderen in meiner Klasse Alisha White verzeihen – auch Ella, Toco und Barry? Musste die Entscheidung einstimmig sein?

»Also *ich* verzeihe Ihnen«, sagte Blue mit eigenartiger Stimme. »Man macht nun mal nicht alles richtig im Leben.«

»Ich auch.« Shari erhob sich, eine schlanke Silhouette im Halbdunkel. »Für meine Freunde tue ich schließlich alles. Gut, dass Sie irgendwann gemerkt haben, dass das keine echten Freunde waren. Sonst hätten die ja so was nicht von Ihnen verlangt.«

Ziemlich viele »Stimmt«-Rufe wurden laut, einer stammte von Jasper. Miss White blickte zu mir herüber, sah mich direkt an. Ich freute mich darüber, dass meine Meinung ihr anscheinend wichtig war.

»Für mich ist es okay – bitte gehen Sie nicht mehr weg«, sagte ich. Immer mehr der anderen stimmten ein. Schließlich waren es fast alle, nur meine »Freunde« rund um Ella blieben stumm. Das schien zum Glück niemandem etwas auszumachen.

Mr García war einer derjenigen, der zögerte. »Inzwischen wissen diese Leute offensichtlich, dass du hier bist und wie du heute heißt«, sagte er. »Ist das ein Risiko für uns?«

»Unwahrscheinlich. Ich habe keine offenen Rechnungen hinterlassen.«

»Wie hat Jack reagiert, als du es ihm erzählt hast?«

»Sag mir erst, was *du* darüber denkst.«

»Ich verzeihe dir«, antwortete Mr García. »Schließlich haben wir alle mal Mist gebaut. Jack hat das Gleiche gesagt, stimmt's?«

Ein knappes, wortloses Nicken war die Antwort, ihr Gesicht blieb ernst und konzentriert. Aber ihr Blick wirkte plötzlich wärmer.

Mr Garcías Handy klingelte und er ging ran. »Was? *Shit.* Ich fahre gleich hin.«

»Was ist? Es geht um Wave, stimmt's?«, fragte Finny, sie war bleich wie ein Laken.

»Ja«, sagte unser Verwandlungslehrer knapp. »Shari, Finny, Tiago, Alisha – wir fahren sofort los.«

Verblüfft blickte Finny ihn an. »Aber ich ...«

»Diesmal brauchen wir dich unbedingt. Es ist mir egal, was dein Vater dazu sagt.«

Erst im Auto kam Mr García dazu, uns Genaueres zu erklären. »Mrs Lennox ist wütend, dass ihr feiner neuer Schulleiter Gegenwind von Alisha und Miss Clearwater bekommt. Deshalb hat sie gerade den Deal aufgekündigt. Sie zieht ihr Angebot mit der Kaution zurück und vertritt Wave auch nicht mehr als Anwältin.«

»Oh ... weiß er das schon?«, fragte ich.

»Leider hat es ihm jemand gesagt und er ist dabei durchzudrehen, weil er denkt, er kann nie wieder ins Meer zurück.«

»Ach, du große Welle!«, entfuhr es Shari. Wir anderen waren einfach stumm vor Entsetzen.

Natürlich war Mr Greyson alles andere als begeistert, seine Tochter auf der Wache zu sehen. »Was genau hast du an dem Wort ›Hausarrest‹ nicht verstanden?«

Sofort hakte unser Verwandlungslehrer ein. »Es war meine Idee, Mr Greyson. Der Junge ist völlig verzweifelt und Finny ...«

»Lassen Sie mich in Ruhe mit meiner Tochter reden«, raunzte Nick Greyson. Wir hatten keine Zeit, den beiden zuzuhören, wir mussten zu Wave und ihm helfen!

Ja, es ging Wave schlecht. Er hatte noch immer eine ruhige Würde, aber ich spürte, dass er innerlich die ganze Zeit schrie. Ein Echo davon hallte in meinem Kopf wider.

»Es ist ein Rückschlag, aber keine Katastrophe, wir treiben das Geld schon noch auf«, versicherte ihm Mr García immer wieder, doch es half nichts, es kam mir vor, als würde Wave ihn kaum wahrnehmen.

»Das Meer ...«, sagte er tonlos. »Das Meer ist in mir. Ich kann es spüren. Vielleicht kann ich so dorthin kommen. Indem ich ganz tief in mich hineingehe.«

Für mich klang das ziemlich ungesund. »Wave, nein, ähm, ich glaube eher nicht, dass das gut ist. Es geht doch nichts über echtes Wasser, weißt du?«

»Du musst nur noch ein bisschen Geduld haben, ein kleines bisschen«, flehte Shari.

Finny stürmte in die Zelle und drängte uns zur Seite.

Dann umarmte sie Wave. Erleichtert sah ich, dass er langsam ebenfalls die Arme um sie schloss, er schien sich zu freuen, dass sie bei ihm war. Sein Blick war nicht mehr so fern, kehrte ins Hier und Jetzt zurück.

»Du denkst doch nicht etwa daran aufzugeben?«, schimpfte Finny ihn aus. »Das kommt überhaupt nicht infrage. Ja, es ist schwer, aber ich verzeihe dir nie, wenn du jetzt aufgibst!«

Irgendwie ging es heute ständig ums Verzeihen. Aber ganz ehrlich, es gibt schlimmere Themen.

»Darf ich mal aufs Klo?«, fragte ich den Officer, der uns die Zelle aufgeschlossen hatte.

Ich durfte. Wusste ja keiner, dass ich nur einen Ort brauchte, an dem ich allein sein konnte. Denn schon während der Fahrt nach Miami war mir immer wieder durch den Kopf gegangen, was mir Miss Bennett neulich gesagt hatte. *Vielleicht warten deine Eltern nur auf eine Gelegenheit, dir zu helfen.*

Ich setzte mich auf den geschlossenen Klodeckel, zog mein Handy hervor und drückte eine der Kurzwahlnummern. »Iris Anderson«, meldete sich eine kühle Frauenstimme. Die Stimme meiner Mutter.

»Hi, Mom«, sagte ich. Es war Absicht, dass ich sie diesmal nicht wie sonst beim Vornamen nannte. Sie sollte ganz genau mitbekommen, dass sie hier als Mutter gefragt war. »Sag mal, ihr seid doch Anwälte und ihr habt reichlich Kohle, oder?«

Halb rechnete ich damit, dass sie sofort auflegen würde. Stattdessen lachte sie. »Du bist heute so erfrischend direkt, Tiago. Was hast du für ein Problem? Übrigens sind wir gerade in den Staaten, wir könnten mal wieder bei dir vorbeikommen.«

Zum Glück war außer mir gerade niemand in der Toilette, ich konnte offen reden. Als sie hörte, dass es um einen Buckelwal-Wandler ging, lachte meine Mutter zum zweiten Mal. Das ging mir allmählich etwas an die Nieren, weil ich wusste, dass es verdammt knapp werden würde für Wave, wenn sie ihn noch länger hier drin behielten.

»Es ist nicht witzig! Er ist in einer Gefängniszelle, hat sich schon mal teilverwandelt und dreht gerade durch.« Ich schilderte ihr das Problem mit seinem Diebstahl und welche Rolle Lydia Lennox und ihre Schulleiter-Marionette in der ganzen Geschichte spielten.

Diesmal zum Glück kein Heiterkeitsausbruch. »Diese Mrs

Lennox geht mir auf die Nerven«, sagte Iris Anderson. »Leider sind wir keine Anwälte für Strafrecht und haben außerdem keine Zulassung für Florida. Aber wir kennen jemanden, der vielleicht einspringen kann. Wie viel Geld braucht ihr?«

»Zehntausend Dollar.« Mein Mund war ganz trocken, als ich es sagte. »Den Rest bezahlt der Rat.«

»Moment, lass mich kurz mit Scott reden«, kam es zurück. Endlose Sekunden vergingen.

Mit einem Klicken ging die Toilettentür auf. »Versuchst du gerade, im Klo zu tauchen?« Sharis Stimme, sie klang ehrlich interessiert. »Manchmal will ich auch dringend ins Wasser, aber *so* dringend dann auch wieder nicht ...«

»Nein, nein!«, rief ich zurück. »Alles gut. Ich komme gleich.«

»Tiago, bist du noch dran? Wir übernehmen fünftausend Dollar.«

»Danke, danke, das ist sehr cool von euch!« Ich schoss förmlich vom Klositz herunter, raste durch den gekachelten Raum und zurück zu Waves Zelle. »Mr Greyson, wie ist die Kontonummer?«

»Was?« Finnys Vater hätte vor Erstaunen beinahe seinen Kaffee verschüttet.

Ein paar Minuten später hatten meine Eltern alle nötigen Informationen ... und ich kritzelte wie manisch einen Namen und eine Telefonnummer auf irgendeinen alten

Briefumschlag aus dem Mülleimer. Der Name gehörte einer jungen menschlichen Anwältin, die gerade erst ihr Examen gemacht hatte, ein paar Autostunden weiter nördlich lebte und ein Herz für Jugendliche in Schwierigkeiten hatte.

Mein Herz raste immer noch, als ich schließlich auflegte, aber die Hoffnung kribbelte in meinem Bauch, als sei ich drauf und dran, mich teilzuverwandeln. Fünftausend Dollar schickten meine Eltern, die gleiche Summe mussten wir noch irgendwie auftreiben. Das war bestimmt irgendwie zu schaffen.

Aber auch das Gespräch selbst hatte mir gutgetan. Hatte ich den richtigen Ton gefunden, mit meinen Eltern zu reden? Hätte ich mir das nicht denken können, dass sie gerne klar und knallhart angesprochen werden wollten? Sie hatten angekündigt, mich sehr bald zu besuchen. Natürlich hatten sie nicht gesagt, dass sie sich schon freuen, das wäre zu viel verlangt gewesen. Aber sie klangen, als wären sie zumindest gespannt auf diesen neuen Tiago.

Wave beruhigte sich etwas, als er die Neuigkeiten hörte. Dann ergriff Miss White das Wort. »Erzähl mir alles über deine Eltern. Wir müssen sie herholen und dafür muss ich etwas über ihre Gewohnheiten erfahren.«

»Du tust es also? Du suchst sie?« Mr García sah sehr erleichtert aus. »Aber mehr als vierundzwanzig Stunden Zeit wirst du dafür nicht haben.«

»Ich kann sehr schnell schwimmen, wenn ich es eilig habe«, sagte Miss White und zog die Augenbrauen hoch.

Wave sprach fast zwanzig Minuten lang mit ihr, während Mr García mit der jungen Anwältin telefonierte. Dann sagte unsere Lehrerin: »Okay. Bringt mich zum Meer, ich mache mich sofort auf den Weg.«

Wir verabschiedeten uns von Wave und fuhren nach Miami

Beach, wo der Strand um diese Uhrzeit ganz den Möwen und Pelikanen, Schatzsuchern mit Metallsuchgerät und städtischen Aufräum-Trupps gehörte.

»Viel Glück«, sagte ich zu meiner Lieblingslehrerin und blickte ihr nach, als sie ins dunkle Meer hineinlief und so weit hinausschwamm, dass niemand vom Land aus ihre Verwandlung beobachten konnte. Bei der Rückfahrt saß ich hinten zwischen Finny und Shari. Das war nicht wirklich unangenehm, denn Sharis Bein berührte meins und ich konnte spüren, wie warm ihr Menschenkörper war. Ganz wunderbar warm.

»Hat dir dein Dad noch härtere Strafen aufgebrummt?«, fragte Shari unser Rochenmädchen besorgt.

Finny grinste schief. »Ja, ich hab jetzt auch noch Lieblings-T-Shirt-Verbot – alles andere war ja schon verboten. *Und* ich krieg wahrscheinlich in nächster Zeit keine Gutenachtgeschichte.«

»Dein Dad erzählt dir noch Gutenachtgeschichten?«, fragte ich fasziniert.

»Ja, wir telefonieren jeden Abend, wenn im Revier nicht gerade ultraviel los ist. Dann erzähle ich ihm, wie mein Tag war, und er erzählt mir von irgendeinem Fall, den er gerade hatte und der gut ausgegangen ist.«

Echt süß. Es würde nicht leicht werden, mit ihr zu reden und ihr zu sagen, dass sie sich keine Hoffnungen auf mich machen durfte.

»Ich leih dir *mein* Lieblings-T-Shirt«, beschloss Shari und die Mädels warfen sich quer über mich hinweg Luftküsse zu, als wäre ich gar nicht da. Sollte ich jetzt beleidigt sein oder was?

Nein, dazu war ich viel zu erleichtert.

Viel los in der Lagune

Am Dienstagabend – nach unserem Besuch bei Wave – saßen wir gerade beim Abendessen und schlangen Fisch-Tacos in uns hinein, als eine kleine Gruppe von Leuten in die Cafeteria kam. Neugierig drehten wir uns um.

Noah fiel glatt der Taco aus der Hand. »Das ist Jack!«

Ja, es war Jack Clearwater und an seiner Seite gingen Mr García und die weißhaarige Schulleiterin der Clearwater High. Alle drei lächelten. Es sprach sich blitzschnell herum, wer da eingetroffen war, und alle Schüler sprangen auf. Shari, Finny, die anderen und ich johlten und klatschten. Unser junger Ex-Ex-Schulleiter lächelte und winkte uns zu. »Guten Morgen allerseits«, sagte er. »Alles klar bei euch?«

Wir jubelten noch ein bisschen lauter.

»Mr Clearwater, dieser miese Bank-Typ hat Bilder von Ihnen verkauft«, berichtete Jasper betrübt.

»Und er hat ein paar Ihrer Sachen verbrannt!« Unsere zarte, taffe Juna war den Tränen nahe.

»Ich habe noch genug übrig – und hatte sowieso vor, ein paar neue Bilder zu malen«, beruhigte sie Jack Clearwater. »Wisst ihr, was diese Tauben-Spikes auf dem Dach sollen? Wer hilft mir, die abzureißen?«

Damit war das Abendessen beendet, zusammen mit zehn anderen Leuten stürmte ich die Treppe hoch zum ersten Stock;

dort konnte man über eine Luke hinauf aufs Dach. Noemi überholte uns alle, mit weiten Panthersprüngen jagte sie voran. Joshua holte währenddessen Werkzeug.

Natürlich schwang Carmen, unsere Profiheimwerkerin, an vorderster Front den Schraubenzieher. Auch ihr neuer Freund machte mit. Falls er Carmen dabei beeindrucken wollte, klappte das nicht. Aber Carmen war trotzdem hingerissen, sie warf ihm einen Ach-du-bist-so-süß-ungeschickt-Blick zu. »Probier es mal so«, meinte sie und demonstrierte ihm die richtige Technik.

Von Barry kam nur eine Art Knurren. Man merkte, dass es ihn runtergezogen hatte, wie sein Vater aus der Schule gejagt worden war. Er war ziemlich wortkarg seither. Zum Glück blieben Toco und Ella an seiner Seite und trösteten ihn. Ich hoffte, dass sein Vater sein Versprechen hielt und ihm den Hund schenkte.

Während ich unter der immer noch heißen Oktobersonne Stacheln abhebelte, fiel mir plötzlich auf, welcher Junge neben mir arbeitete. Ein lässiger blonder Surfertyp im ausgeblichenen T-Shirt. »Na, Tigerhai? Wann wirst du endlich hairaten?«, zog Chris mich auf.

»Geht dich nichts an«, gab ich grinsend zurück. »Darfst du wieder auf die Blue Reef gehen?«

»Ja.« Chris zog eine Grimasse. »Aber ich musste Mr Clearwater *schwören*, dass ich höchstens zweimal die Woche zu spät komme.«

»Und das kannste?« Jasper machte große Augen und lutschte an seinem Zeigefinger, der nähere Bekanntschaft mit einem Metalldorn geschlossen hatte.

»Klar kann ich das«, sagte Chris, während die neben ihm arbeitende Izzy »Neeeein!« rief. Sie meinte damit zum Glück nur ihr Werkzeug, das ihr nun schon zum zweiten Mal vom Dach gefallen war.

»Habt ihr mitbekommen, dass Williams die Vordertür abgeschlossen hat, bevor er weggefahren ist?«, fragte Nox, der ausnahmsweise mal als Mensch durch die Schule streifte. »Und er hat den einzigen Schlüssel zum neuen Schloss! Im Moment können wir durch den Vorderausgang weder raus noch rein.«

»Wenn Miss White wieder da ist, wird es damit ganz schnell vorbei sein, Alter«, verkündete Ralph, der gerade zu uns aufs Dach kletterte und sich an einen der Sonnenkollektoren lehnte. »Die knackt das Schloss in vier Komma drei Sekunden, wetten?«

Darauf wettete ich lieber nicht, weil ich das Miss White absolut zutraute.

Später am Abend, als wir an unserem Schulstrand saßen und über die vielen aufregenden Dinge quatschten, die passiert waren, gab es noch weitere gute Neuigkeiten: »Ein Geschäftsmann aus Kalifornien hat angeboten, die restlichen fünftausend Dollar Kaution für Wave zu zahlen«, verkündete Jack Clearwater, er wirkte beschwingt. »Jetzt haben wir ihn wirklich bald raus.«

»Aber ... wer ist der Typ? Warum macht er das?«, fragte ich verblüfft.

Unser Schulleiter zuckte die Schultern. »Ehrlich gesagt, ich weiß es nicht. Anscheinend hat er durch den Rat von unseren Problemen gehört. Und weil Alan Dorn selbst ein Seawalker ist, will er Wave helfen.«

»Sehr cool!«, sagte Blue. »Dann fehlen nur noch die Eltern von Wave.«

Sie fehlten nicht sehr lange. Während wir uns am Mittwochmorgen im Verwandlungsunterricht plagten – »So was geht doch gar nicht«, beklagte sich Shari, weil wir ein Körperteil nach dem anderen teilverwandeln sollten –, stürmte Enya herein, eine der Zweitjahresschülerinnen. »Draußen vor der Lagune schwimmt ein Buckelwal!«, rief sie und rannte schon weiter, wahrscheinlich um den anderen Bescheid zu geben.

Mr García wirkte ebenso neugierig wie der Rest der Klasse. »Verwandelt euch bitte zurück, dann dürft ihr schauen, was draußen los ist«, sagte er und kurz darauf drängten wir uns in Menschengestalt am Strand und glotzten nach draußen, wo aus dem Meer gerade ein meterhoher Atemstrahl aufstieg.

Eine völlig erschöpft wirkende Miss White watete aus der Lagune auf den Strand, wo schon Jack Clearwater mit einem heißen Kaffee und einem Schoko-Donut auf sie wartete. Miss White schüttete das eine hinunter und verschlang das andere. »Könnt ihr gleich mal mit dem *Zodiac* rausfahren? Sie braucht ein bisschen Hilfe bei der Verwandlung ...«

»Ich kann's noch gar nicht glauben.« Fasziniert starrte Mr Clearwater zum offenen Meer hin. »Ist sie wirklich seine Mutter? Wo hast du sie gefunden?«

»Zum Glück konnte mir Wave ein paar Tipps zu ihren üblichen Wanderrouten geben. Sie war gerade im Meer vor Grand Bahama unterwegs und zum Glück sowieso schon auf dem Weg nach Süden.«

Besorgt blickte Jack sie an. »Du bist seit gestern von hier bis Grand Bahama und zurück geschwommen? Das sind mehr als *zweihundert Meilen!*«

»Hätte ich auch geschätzt.« Miss White ließ sich auf den Sand sinken und strich sich das nasse dunkle Haar aus dem Gesicht. »Leider hab ich den Vater von Wave auf die Schnelle nicht gefunden, er schwimmt irgendwo anders herum, weil die Eltern nicht mehr zusammen sind. Reicht ein Elternteil?«

»Ja, das müsste reichen. Danke, Alisha, du warst großartig!«

Dafür bekam er ein schwaches Lächeln. »Kein Problem. Habt ihr noch so einen Donut?«

»Garantiert«, sagte ich. Während Mr García das *Zodiac* klarmachte, rannte ich los, um so viele weitere Zuckerkringel zu holen, wie ich tragen konnte.

Als ich zurückhastete, fielen mir fast die Augen aus dem Kopf. Das Buckelwal-Weibchen hatte sich durch die Lücke zwischen den Mangroven hindurchgezwängt und schwamm jetzt neben Mrs Pelagius in unserer kaum fünf Meter tiefen Lagune. Es war ein krasser Anblick, wie dieser dunkelgraue Koloss dort seine Kreise zog. Wenn sie sich ein bisschen zu heftig bewegte, setzte ihr Bauch wahrscheinlich auf dem Meeresboden auf und zermalmte dabei hoffentlich nicht Sharis Muschelsammlung.

Wo ist Wave?, rief die Wal-Wandlerin und reckte die Schnauze aus dem Wasser. *Ich bin Moon, seine Mutter, und ich will jetzt gleich meinen Sohn sehen!*

Er ist gerade nicht hier, gab Jack Clearwater zurück. *Aber wir können dich zu ihm bringen, wenn du dich verwandelst.*

Leonora und Olivia hielten schon Klamotten und Tücher bereit, in die unser Gast sich nach der Verwandlung wickeln konnte.

Obwohl Mr García Waves Mutter geduldig durch die Verwandlung führte, dauerte es fast eine halbe Stunde, bis sie schließlich als Mensch bei uns am Strand stand und mit den Fingern ihr Gesicht betastete. In erster Gestalt war Moon eine massige, freundlich dreinblickende Frau mit glatten rotblonden Haaren bis zum Po. Ich schätzte sie als nur wenig älter als unseren Schulleiter, Anfang dreißig oder so.

»Wer hat ihr denn dieses knallrote Kleid gegeben, das beißt sich schrecklich mit ihrer Haarfarbe!«, lästerte Ella, doch außer ihr interessierte das niemanden.

»Herzlich willkommen an der Blue Reef Highschool«, sagte Jack Clearwater feierlich.

»Bitte lächeln!«, rief seine Mutter Lissa und schoss ein Porträtfoto von unserem Gast. »Bis heute Nachmittag habe ich einen Pass für dich, Moon. Das ist ein Stück Papier, das bestätigt, wer du an Land bist.«

»Ich weiß nicht, was Menschen immer mit diesem Papier haben«, sagte Moon und musterte uns versammelte Schüler neugierig. »Löst sich im Wasser sowieso auf!«

»Mr Clearwater, wann können wir Wave holen?«, drängte Finny, die blass und besorgt aussah, als hätte sie letzte Nacht kaum geschlafen. »Es darf einfach nichts mehr schiefgehen!«

»Heute Nachmittag, sobald die Überweisung von Alan Dorn bei der Polizei eingegangen ist«, sagte Jack Clearwater fest. »Mit dabei sein werden Moon, Miss White, die neue Anwältin, Tiago und mit Sondergenehmigung auch Finny. Davor müssen wir ...«

»Was ist Polizei? Kann man das essen?«, fragte Moon.

»... unseren Gast noch ein bisschen coachen, fürchte ich«, fuhr unser junger Schulleiter fort und schaffte es irgendwie weiterzulächeln.

Ihr Ausweis, bitte

Das Coaching von Waves Mutter fand am Strand statt und wurde kurzerhand zu unserem heutigen Menschenkundeunterricht erklärt. Es war eine der seltsamsten Stunden, die ich bisher an der Blue Reef High erlebt hatte.

»Wenn die Polizei unser Freund und Helfer ist, wieso halten sie dann meinen Sohn gefangen?«, fragte Moon und wickelte sich das lange rotblonde Haar um die Finger.

»Das liegt daran, dass Wave einen Fehler gemacht hat«, erklärte Jack Clearwater schon zum zweiten Mal geduldig. »Finny, du spielst eine Polizistin, die Moon befragt. Los geht's.«

Unser blauhaariges Rochen-Girl baute sich hinter einer improvisierten Theke aus Holzkisten auf. Sie hatte zu diesem Anlass eine Polizistenuniform – schwarzes, kurzärmeliges Uniformhemd mit goldenem Abzeichen, dunkle Hosen, schwarze Mütze – aus unserem Verkleidungsfundus hervorgezaubert. »Guten Tag – Sie sind also Waves Mutter, Mrs O'Connor. Können Sie sich ausweisen?«

»Kann ich mich was?«, fragte Waves Mutter.

»Ihren Ausweis, bitte«, sagte Finny streng.

»Ach so, der.« Moon reichte ihr das Heftchen, das wir gerade gebastelt hatten. »Verstehen Sie, Wave ist mein erstes Kalb, ich liebe ihn sehr, und ...«

»Stopp!«, rief unser Schulleiter und atmete tief durch. »Du

sprichst nur, wenn du gefragt wirst, Moon, alles andere ist zu riskant. Und Wave ist heute dein Kind, nicht dein Kalb, ja?«

»Ja gut«, sagte Moon.

Wir hatten das alles schon zweimal geübt. Ich fragte mich allmählich, ob wir es noch schaffen würden, sie auf ihre Rolle vorzubereiten. Würde das alles die komplette Katastrophe werden? Ich machte mir furchtbare Sorgen um Wave.

»Unterschreiben Sie bitte hier, dann bringen wir Ihnen Ihren Sohn«, sagte Finny und schob ihr ein Blatt Papier hin.

»Aber gerne.« Moon wirkte voll professionell, als sie den Kuli nahm und damit etwas aufs Papier kritzelte.

»Stopp.« Diesmal war es Finny, die seufzte. »Du hältst den Kuli falsch herum, Moon. So schreibt er nicht.«

»Scheußlich kompliziert, diese Menschenwelt«, beschwerte sich die Buckelwal-Wandlerin.

»Oh ja, das ist sie.« Shari nickte mit hochgezogenen Augenbrauen. »Was meinst du, wie lange ich gebraucht habe, bis ich kapiert habe, was ein Datentarif, ein Cocktail oder ein Solarkollektor sind!«

»Gib nicht so an«, sagte Blue. »Du weißt immer noch nicht, was ein Solarkollektor ist.«

»Und ob ich das weiß, der sammelt die Sonnenstrahlen und dann ...«

»Shari! Blue! Könntet ihr bitte aufhören, Moon abzulenken?«

»Genau«, bekräftigte Finny. »Nennen Sie mir bitte Ihren derzeitigen Wohnsitz, Mrs O'Connor.«

»Blue Reef Highschool, Key Largo«, sagte Moon und lächelte stolz. Sie hatte so weiße Zähne, dass sie ihr Geld jederzeit mit Zahnpastawerbung hätte verdienen können. Kein Wunder, nie waren diese Zähne auch nur vom winzigsten Krümel Zucker berührt worden.

»Sehr gut, Moon«, sagte Jack Clearwater und wirkte, als würde er sich wieder etwas entspannen. Finny fragte sie noch nach dem – erfundenen – Geburtsdatum von Wave, das sich Moon zum Glück richtig gemerkt hatte, dann winkte unser Schulleiter mich nach vorne. »Jetzt spielt bitte Tiago die Rolle von Wave.«

Toco verkörperte den Polizisten, der mich als Wave zu seiner Mutter brachte. Er ging voll in seiner Rolle auf und packte mich so fest am Arm, dass ich dort bestimmt blaue Flecken bekommen würde. »So, Bürschchen, du bist frei. Aber wehe, du klaust noch mal was, dann buchten wir dich ein, bis du schwarz anläufst!«

Ich warf ihm einen finsteren Blick zu, um ihm zu zeigen, was ich von dieser Behandlung hielt. Wie wir es schon einmal geübt hatten, ging Moon auf mich zu und umarmte mich. »Obwohl du nicht wirklich Wave bist, freue ich mich, dich zu sehen, Sohn. Jetzt kannst du endlich aufhören, so zu tun, als wärst du ein Mensch.«

Leises Aufstöhnen aus der versammelten Klasse.

Es wurde eine sehr, sehr lange Menschenkundelektion. Zum Schluss hatten wir alles so oft geübt, dass Moon das, was sie nachher tun sollte, locker beherrschte.

Und natürlich lief es dann in Wirklichkeit ganz anders.

Während wir nach Miami fuhren, sorgte ich mich ein bisschen, dass sich Waves Mutter ungeplant verwandeln könnte – ein Buckelwal würde dieses Auto einfach *sprengen!* Doch Miss White saß neben Moon und plauderte mit ihr über die Menschenwelt, deren Gesetze und welchen Fehler Wave gemacht hatte. Natürlich hatten wir für Moon auch ein Foto ihres Menschenkörpers ausgedruckt. So kamen wir reibungslos zur Polizeistation, wo schon die neue Anwältin auf uns wartete: eine junge Frau im grauen Kostüm, die sehr tüchtig und energisch wirkte und zum Glück keinerlei Ahnung hatte, wer wir wirklich waren. Bestimmt mochte auch sie keine Haie.

»Am besten überlassen Sie mir das Reden, das ist mein Job«, sagte sie und nichts taten wir lieber.

In der Station wurden wir von Nick Greyson, der gerade seine Schicht begonnen hatte, freundlich begrüßt und Finny bekam natürlich ein Extralächeln. »Glauben Sie mir, ich bin auch froh, dass der Junge rausdarf. Ich habe nie jemanden gesehen, den es so mitgenommen hat, eingesperrt zu sein. Die anderen Kids, die wir einbuchten, leiden eher darunter, dass wir ihnen das Smartphone abnehmen!«

Wir lachten höflich. »Mein Mandant hatte nie ein Smartphone«, sagte die Anwältin spitz.

»Ja, das hab ich gemerkt«, entgegnete Nick Greyson und wandte sich an unseren Gast. »Sie sind also Waves Mutter. Die letzte Zeit war sicher nicht leicht für Sie.« Er schüttelte Moon die Hand. Das hatten wir zum Glück geübt, auch wenn man Waves Mutter immer noch anmerkte, dass sie es sehr eigenartig fand. »Ihr Junge ist in Ordnung. Sorgen Sie bitte dafür, dass er pünktlich zur Verhandlung erscheint, damit wir Ihnen die Kaution zurückerstatten können. Wäre schade, wenn das Geld verloren wäre.«

»Was?«, fragte Moon verwirrt und die neue Anwältin hakte sofort ein: »Natürlich, wir sorgen dafür. Er wird da sein und mit einem Freispruch wieder rausmarschieren, dafür sorge ich.«

»Gut«, sagte Nick Greyson. »Mrs O'Connor, geben Sie mir bitte Ihren Ausweis? Unterschreiben Sie hier.«

Moon zeigte ihren Ausweis, wie wir es geübt hatten, und malte eine Wellenlinie auf das Papier, was, wie ich fand, eine sehr passende Unterschrift war. Sehr, sehr erleichtert lächelten wir alle uns an.

Finny jubelte, als Wave zu uns gebracht wurde. Mir fiel auf, dass seine Nase gerötet war – anscheinend hatte er sich die erste Erkältung seines Lebens eingefangen –, aber über Ansteckung dachte niemand nach, er und Finny sanken in eine Umarmung. Hm, wenn ich mir das so anschaute, war es vielleicht nicht mehr nötig, mit Finny über ihre Gefühle für mich zu reden.

Aber warum beachtete dieser Buckelwal des Grauens seine *Mutter* überhaupt nicht?! Die Polizisten wirkten erstaunt, wahrscheinlich würden sie gleich misstrauisch werden. Siedend heiß fiel mir ein, dass Wave seine Mama wahrscheinlich nie in Menschengestalt gesehen hatte.

Zum Glück war ich nicht der Einzige, dem dieser Gedanke kam. Ein bisschen zu laut fragte Miss White: »Und, Wave, bist du froh, dass deine Mutter kommen konnte?«, während Moon sich mit ausgebreiteten Armen auf ihren Sohn zubewegte. Wave erkannte sie irgendwie und ließ sich von ihr drücken.

Na also. Geschafft! Es kam mir vor, als würde ich mehrere Zentimeter über dem Boden schweben vor Freude.

So rasch, dass es wahrscheinlich verdächtig wirkte, verabschiedeten wir uns. Nichts wie raus hier, bevor noch irgendetwas schiefging.

»Ciao, Dad – bis zum Wochenende!«, rief Finny und winkte ihrem Vater zu.

»Wartet, ich bring euch noch bis zum Auto«, meinte Nick Greyson.

»Ach, das ist gar nicht nötig, nein, machen Sie sich keine Umstände«, sagte Jack Clearwater.

»Schon gut, ist 'n ruhiger Abend.« Greyson trank seinen Kaffee aus, sein großer Adamsapfel wippte mit jedem Schluck. »Fängt meist erst später an, dass die Leute einander erschießen, und für die Drogendealer ist es auch zu früh. Paar Minuten Zeit hab ich.«

»Das ist nett von dir, Dad, aber wir kommen schon klar«, meinte Finny, die ebenfalls wieder nervös wurde. »Total lieb, dass ich heute kommen durfte. Ab jetzt wieder Hausarrest, kein Problem.«

»Gut – Strafe muss sein!« Greyson stand auf und rückte seinen Ausrüstungsgürtel mit Knarre, Schlagstock und Funkgerät um seine Hüften zurecht. »Bin fünf Minuten weg!«, rief er seinen Kollegen im Revier zu.

Zum Glück verabschiedete sich wenigstens die Anwältin und versprach, mit uns in Kontakt zu bleiben.

Ich war wieder total verspannt, als wir die palmenbestandene Straße entlanggingen und an drei Leuten vorbeikamen, die mit einer Kamera auf der Schulter vor dem Eingang eines Restaurants irgendeine Moderation drehten. Der Typ, der interviewt wurde, trug ein Koch-Outfit inklusive weißer Schürze, sah sehr zufrieden mit sich aus und schwafelte irgendwas über eingelegte Muscheln und Schwertfisch mit Guacamole.

Rasch gingen wir an der kleinen Gruppe vorbei, denn Kameras sind die natürlichen Feinde eines Seawalkers, der seine Verwandlung nicht ganz im Griff hat.

Noch verspannter wurde ich, als mir einfiel, dass ich vorhin ein Buch über Meere und Ozeane bemerkt hatte, das unter dem Sitz herumflog, irgendjemand aus der Blue Reef musste es dort vergessen haben. Was war, wenn Wave oder seine Mutter das sahen und es vor den Augen von Finnys Polizistenvater einen Verwandlungsunfall gab? Wahrscheinlich war ich deswegen so unfassbar blöd, meine Zähne teilzuverwandeln, damit ich mit den anderen von Kopf zu Kopf reden konnte.

Wir müssen noch das Meeresbuch wegpacken, das unter dem ..., begann ich, doch dann wandte sich Greyson mir zu. »Und du bist Tiago, richtig? Finny sagt, du machst denen in der Klasse, die andere mobben, Feuer unterm Hintern. Find ich gut. Mich haben ein paar Kids in der Grundschule so geärgert, dass ich nach Alaska auswandern wollte. Im reifen Alter von neun Jahren!«

Ohne nachzudenken, öffnete ich den Mund, um ihm zu antworten – und Nick Greysons Augen wurden groß.

Fast so groß wie meine Zähne.

Wave, Moon und die große Fischkatastrophe

Was zur Hölle ...«, begann Finnys Vater und wich vor mir und meinen teilverwandelten Zähnen zurück.

Gleichzeitig entfuhr dem armen, erkälteten Wave ein gewaltiger Nieser. Da ihm offensichtlich die Nase lief, blickte er sich ratlos nach etwas um, mit dem er sie abwischen konnte.

»Nicht!«, schrie Finny, doch da hatte Wave schon etwas gefunden – eine orange getigerte, sehr flauschig aussehende Katze. Sie hockte nichts ahnend auf einem Grundstückspfosten, an dem wir vorbeikamen.

»Ach, das wird schon ...«, sagte Wave, weiter kam er nicht. Die meisten Tiere schätzen es nicht, als Taschentuch benutzt zu werden. Die Katze überwand ihren Schreckmoment schnell, fuhr die Krallen aus und verpasste Wave das, was sie für seine gerechte Strafe hielt. Wave schrie, Moon schrie auch – wahrscheinlich, weil sie noch nie eine Katze gesehen hatte und diese hier gerade ihren Sohn angriff. Nick Greyson schrie zwar nicht, aber er konnte offensichtlich nicht fassen, was er eben in meinem Mund gesehen hatte.

Kurz, es war ein totales Chaos, und das alles, während auf der Straße langsam Autos an uns vorbeifuhren, darunter ein Polizeiwagen.

Das Fernsehteam unterbrach seinen Dreh und spähte neugierig zu uns herüber ... und es war keine drei Meter von uns entfernt!

Miss White reagierte blitzschnell. Sie ging mit langen Schritten auf die kleine Gruppe zu. »Warum geben Sie nicht einfach zu, dass ICH diese Wette gewonnen habe?«, motzte sie den Koch an. »Mein Rezept für Garnelensuppe ist viel besser als Ihres, wann sehen Sie das endlich ein?«

Selten hatte ich ein so begeistertes Fernsehteam gesehen. Sie hielten voll mit der Kamera drauf.

Dadurch bekamen sie nicht mit, dass hinter ihrem Rücken auch so einiges los war. Inzwischen hatte sich die panische, ein bisschen schleimige Katze aus Waves Händen gewunden und floh nun mit einem Riesensprung. Garantiert wollte sie auf den Boden, doch stattdessen landete sie auf Finny. Die hatte plötzlich Raubtierkrallen im Nacken und erschrak so sehr, dass sie sich in einen großen schwarzen Rochen verwandelte. Er flappte mitten auf dem Bürgersteig herum und rief *Oh nein, sorry, das tut mir so leid!* in unsere Köpfe.

Der Fahrer des Polizeiwagens bekam ebenso große Augen wie Nick Greyson vorhin. Weil er zu uns herüberglotzte, übersah er, dass das Auto vor ihm gerade bremste, und krachte ihm aufs Heck.

»Beim heiligen Gewölle«, stöhnte Jack Clearwater. »Tiago, du packst rechts an, ich links, okay?«

Unser großes Glück war, dass in der Nähe ein Springbrunnen war, der von den meisten Leuten unbeachtet vor sich hin plätscherte. Wir trampelten über Finnys Klamotten hinweg und packten den Teufelsrochen, was alles andere als leicht war, weil er sich zwar auf der Oberseite rau wie Schleifpapier anfühlte, aber auf der Bauchseite samtweich und glitschig. *Greift ruhig fest zu, ist mir egal!* Finny klang, als wäre sie den Tränen nahe. *Hat mein Dad das gesehen? Mein Dad ...*

Ja, ich fürchte, er hat es gesehen, gab Jack Clearwater grimmig zurück.

Irgendwie brachten wir es fertig, Finny zum Betonbecken zu schleifen und hineinzuschieben. *Äääh, gechlort,* meinte sie und flappte erleichtert im Wasser herum, das nicht besonders tief war. Mir wäre es als Tigerhai nur bis zur Mitte des Bauchs gegangen, aber sie war ja als Fisch praktischerweise sehr flach.

Alles okay? Kannst du atmen?, fragte ich sie besorgt. *Macht dir das Süßwasser nichts aus? Wahrscheinlich ist es wie bei mir, dass du es kurze Zeit aushalten kannnst, oder?*

Scheiße!, schrie Finny. *Was macht Wave denn jetzt?*

Mein Schulleiter und ich fuhren herum.

Das konnte ich ihr sagen, was er gerade tat. Er versuchte, über die Straße zu gehen, wahrscheinlich weil er schnellstmöglich zum Meer wollte, das nur ein paar Blocks entfernt war. Nur leider hatte der junge Buckelwal-Wandler nie gelernt, wie man sich in einer Stadt verhielt. Den Blick fest nach vorne gerichtet, überquerte er die Fahrbahn einfach irgendwo und beachtete die zwanzig Meter entfernte Ampel so wenig, als wäre sie irgendein Felsen, an dem er vorbeischwamm.

Auf der Straße waren jede Menge Autos unterwegs, schließlich befanden wir uns in Miamis Innenstadt. Mir sträubten sich die Nackenhärchen. Hatten wir den Jungen aus dem Knast geholt, nur damit er jetzt von einem Auto umgenietet wurde?

Ich raste los, rannte mit aller Kraft, um Wave rechtzeitig zu erreichen, während Jack Clearwater »Stopp! Halt an, Wave!« brüllte.

Unser Freund war vor einem weißen Subaru auf die Straße getreten. Kein großes Auto, aber auch das würde Matsch aus ihm machen, wenn es ihn erwischte! Der ältere Mann am Steuer wollte noch schnell über die Ampel huschen, bevor sie umsprang. Doch dann sah er Wave und bremste im letzten Moment hupend, seine Stoßstange war nur eine halbe Armlänge von Waves Schienbeinen entfernt. Der Fahrer war nicht begeistert.

Noch weniger begeistert war er, als Waves Mutter heranstampfte, hundert Kilo geballte Kampfstimmung im knallroten Kleid. »Wie kannst du es wagen, meinem Sohn zu drohen!« Sie funkelte den Fahrer an, der auf seinem Sitz zusammenzuschrumpfen schien.

Er hupte noch mal, wahrscheinlich weil er hoffte, damit dieses Duo aus der Hölle wegzuscheuchen. Klappte nicht. Noch wütender als zuvor packte Moon seine vordere Stoßstange mit beiden Händen, spannte alle Muskeln an ... und hob den Subaru hoch. Seine Vorderreifen schwebten mehrere Zentimeter über der Straße. Wow!

»Danke, Mom – nett von dir«, sagte ihr Buckelwalsohn, während ich ihn am Arm packte und auf den Bürgersteig zurückzog.

Leider hatte das Fernsehteam nun doch mitbekommen, dass hier irgendetwas sehr Filmreifes vor sich ging. Der Moderator und sein Kameramann hasteten herbei, die Ausrüstung noch auf der Schulter – wie viel von unserem Chaos hatten die schon gefilmt?

»Das ist eindeutig nicht mein Tag«, stöhnte Jack Clearwater. Gleich zwei Leute aus unserer Blue-Reef-Gruppe machten sich daran, das Team aufzuhalten. Finny bekam ihre Chance, als die beiden Medienleute an »ihrem« Springbrunnen vorbeihasteten. Sie raste im Kreis, um Schwung zu holen, und warf sich dann nach oben. Wie ein fliegender Teppich sauste sie durch die Luft und landete auf dem Kopf des Moderators. *Meisterhaftes Timing, aber hoffentlich hast du ihn nicht erschlagen,* meinte ich, während der Reporter etwas gurgelte, was wie »Hilfe! Ich werde ermordet!« klang.

Da er reden konnte, war er nicht schwer verletzt – gut.

Mit ebenso perfektem Timing stellte Miss White dem zweiten Mann ein Bein, als er an ihr vorbeilaufen wollte, die Kamera starr auf Moon und das Auto gerichtet. Beide – Mann und Kamera – legten eine kurze Flugstrecke ein. Nur in einem Fall endete die auf dem Asphalt. Mit ihren Reflexen, die besser waren als bei jedem Menschen, fing Miss White die schwere Kamera aus der Luft und federte dabei leicht in den Knien ab.

»Oh, Sie sind ein Engel, großartig, wie haben Sie das geschafft?«, gab der Kameramann von sich und rappelte sich, weitere Dankesworte stammelnd, auf.

»Keine Ahnung, ich war halt zur richtigen Zeit am richtigen Ort.« Lächelnd übergab ihm Miss White sein Gerät und sofort untersuchte der Mann es, er konnte kaum fassen, dass es keinen Kratzer abbekommen hatte.

Es hat Nachteile, wenn so ein Tumult inklusive Auffahrunfall nur wenige Meter von einer Polizeistation stattfindet. Inzwischen waren auch die Cops darauf aufmerksam geworden, dass vor ihrer Tür irgendetwas abging, und mindestens ein Dutzend uniformierte Beamte strömten auf die Straße. Bevor wir ein weiteres Wort sagen oder irgendetwas erklären konnten, waren wir umringt und starrten in die Läufe gezückter Dienstwaffen.

»Hände hinter den Kopf«, raunzte eine Polizistin mich an und ich hatte es ziemlich eilig damit, ihrem Befehl zu folgen. Dafür musste ich leider Wave loslassen, aber der wollte sowieso nur helfen, Finny wieder in ihr Becken zu verfrachten.

»Moment, Amy, der Junge ist einer von den Guten.« Nick Greyson war inzwischen wieder fähig zu sprechen. »Alles okay, hier gab's nur einen kleinen Unfall. Nichts passiert, Leute, ich kümmere mich drum!«

Amy erkannte ihn, nickte und entspannte sich. Aber Finnys Vater musste sein Sprüchlein noch ziemlich oft wiederholen, bis alle sich wieder beruhigt hatten.

»Was ist überhaupt los hier, Nick?«, fragte ein Kollege und hakte die Daumen in seinen Gürtel. »Sind das Dreharbeiten für 'nen Film oder was?«

»Nee, hier ist nur ein Tiertransport schiefgegangen«, versicherte ihm Finnys Vater, denn schon beugten sich einige der Polizisten staunend über das Becken des Springbrunnens, in dem Finny wieder friedlich mit den Flossen wedelte.

Tiertransport? Wie krass, er war bereit, für uns zu lügen – aber ich wusste, dass das dicke Ende noch kam!

Da die Story »Rochen in Springbrunnen« nicht ganz so ergiebig war, zog das Kamerateam ab. Als bis auf Finnys Vater auch alle Polizisten in ihre Station zurückgeschlendert waren, wagte ich langsam, wieder durchzuatmen. Ab und zu warf ich einen Seitenblick auf Nick Greyson, der nicht aufhören konnte, auf den Rochen zu starren. Oje. Das würde ein schwieriges Gespräch werden.

Jack Clearwater war noch immer blass. »Ich muss dem Rat Bescheid geben, dass hier möglicherweise eine Verwandlung gefilmt worden ist«, sagte er und zog sein Handy hervor. »Moment, ich ...«

Unsere Kampflehrerin legte ihm die Hand auf den Arm. »Alles easy, Jack.«

»Alles easy?! Das war unglaubliches Pech, dass ausgerechnet hier und heute ...«

»Ich hab ihnen die Speicherkarte aus der Kamera gezogen«, sagte Alisha White, zauberte mit flinken Fingern die Karte hervor und steckte sie Jack in die Brusttasche seines Hemdes.

Ich musste lächeln. *So* musste eine Kampflehrerin sein, ganz genau so!

Langsam nahm das Gesicht unseres Schulleiters wieder seine normale Farbe an. »Dann lasst uns jetzt bitte Wave ins Meer zurückbringen«, sagte Mr Clearwater. Sein Blick schweifte zu Finnys Polizistenvater. »Danach ... reden wir.«

»Oh ja, das werden wir«, knurrte Nick Greyson.

Angeln verboten

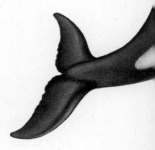

Du schwimmst weg, nicht wahr?« Finny und Wave standen sich am Strand gegenüber, Moon und wir hielten uns ein Stück abseits. Oh Mann, ich wurde neidisch, wenn ich sah, wie die beiden sich anschauten! Wave blickte unserem Rochenmädchen in die Augen, hob eine Hand und legte sie auf Finnys Wange, während Finny ihren Zeigefinger über seine Stirn, seine Nase, sein Kinn gleiten ließ. »Ja, ich muss zurück ins Meer ... aber ich komme wieder. Wenn ich darf.«

»Es wäre uns eine Ehre, wenn du hin und wieder zu Besuch kommen würdest«, mischte sich Jack Clearwater mit gedämpfter Stimme ein. »Du könntest Einzelstunden im offenen Meer oder in der Lagune bekommen. Bitte kommt zur Verhandlung zurück, ja? Sonst verlieren wir das Geld, das uns geborgt wurde. In drei Wochen musst du vor Gericht.«

»Ich werde da sein«, sagte Wave schlicht. »Danke für alles. Ihr habt viel für mich getan. Und dabei war alles meine Schuld.«

Er küsste Finny auf die Lippen, ganz ruhig und selbstverständlich. Dann drehte er sich um und watete ins Meer hinein, gefolgt von seiner Mutter. Beide zogen ihre Sachen aus und warfen sie auf den Sand.

Mit gerunzelter Stirn beobachtete Nick Greyson die beiden. »Was haben die vor?«

»Abwarten«, sagte Mr Clearwater und lächelte.

Da es allmählich dunkel wurde, verzogen sich auch die letzten vereinzelten Badegäste. Während die Sonne am Himmel hing wie eine Orange, die nur aufs Pflücken wartete, und der Himmel sich zu einem kitschigen Rosagelb färbte, beobachtete ich, wie unsere beiden Gäste als Menschen ins tiefere Wasser hinausschwammen. Keine Sekunde lang ließ ich sie aus den Augen, damit ich nicht den Moment verpasste, in dem sie sich verwandelten.

Da! Es war so weit! Wir sahen, wie eine riesige Brustflosse die Meeresoberfläche durchbrach und einen Moment lang in der Luft pendelte – ein Abschiedswinken. Wasser strömte von einem dunklen Rücken und dann erhoben sich zwei Schwanzflossen über die Wellen, als die beiden Wale tauchten.

Ich warf Nick Greyson einen schnellen Seitenblick zu. Ihm hing die Kinnlade runter. »Wo kommen auf einmal die Buckelwale her?«, fragte er. »Das sind doch nicht etwa ...«

»Doch«, sagte Finny. »Und ihr habt ihn an Land gefangen gehalten!«

Nick Greyson wandte sich an uns und musterte jeden von uns mit durchdringendem Blick. »Erklärt mir das bitte mal jemand? Und zwar jetzt gleich? Finny, willst du damit sagen, dass es wirklich ... dass du ein ...«

»Genau, Dad.« Von irgendwoher nahm Finny die Kraft, ihrem Vater in die Augen zu blicken. »Es gibt Gestaltwandler. Ich bin auch einer – und stolz darauf.«

»Also bist du ... kein Mensch.« Nick Greysons Stimme war schneidend und Finny schluckte, ich merkte, dass sie die Tränen zurückhalten musste. Sie schaute zu uns hinüber, bat uns wortlos, in der Nähe zu bleiben, ihr beizustehen.

»Wir sind alle keine«, erklärte Jack Clearwater ruhig. »Wahrscheinlich ist das erst mal ein Schock für Sie, aber Finny ist immer noch Ihre Tochter. Sie ist ein Mensch plus ein paar Eigenschaften, die Sie bisher nicht kannten, Mr Greyson.«

»Und was für welche!«, knurrte Greyson und blickte mich an. »Du bist ein Hai, Junge, stimmt's?«

»Äh, ja«, antwortete ich. »Tigerhai, genauer gesagt.«

»Kein Zweifel möglich bei diesen Zähnen! Ich wäre beinahe ohnmächtig umgefallen und all meine Kollegen hätten sich noch wochenlang über mich lustig gemacht.«

»Tut mir leid, Sir.«

Nick Greyson seufzte tief und dann ging er auf Finny zu, blickte sie prüfend von Kopf bis Fuß an. »Du bist also ein Rochen, Honey. Jetzt kann ich mir denken, warum du früher in Tränen ausgebrochen bist, wenn ich angeln gehen wollte. Wegen dir habe ich Billard angefangen!«

»Das ist cool, Dad.« Das kam von Herzen. »Billard ist *viel* besser, als hilflose Fische aus dem Wasser zu ziehen. Meine fünf Punkte Vorsprung holst du schon noch ein!«

Ich wusste, dass die beiden über den Berg waren, als Finnys Vater lächelte. Nur leider verdunstete dieses Lächeln noch schneller als eine Pfütze in der vollen Florida-Sommersonne. »Was ist mit deiner Meeresbiologen-Mom? Mit meiner Jane?«

»Walhai«, sagte Finny.

»Ein Walhai! Nicht dein Ernst? Sind das nicht die, die dreizehn Meter groß werden können?«

»Äh, doch. Sie ist allerdings nur neun Meter lang, die Weibchen sind etwas kleiner.«

»Ach. Und wann wolltet ihr mir das eigentlich alles erzählen?«

Finny war schon immer sehr ehrlich gewesen. »Eigentlich nie.«

Das steckte er ziemlich gut weg. Wahrscheinlich war ihm klar, dass er es sowieso nicht geglaubt hätte.

Ich war nicht überrascht, als Nick Greyson sich an unseren jungen Schulleiter wandte und sagte: »Ich nehme meine Tochter erst mal mit, wir müssen das daheim diskutieren. Hoffe, Sie verstehen das.«

»Natürlich. Kommen Sie gut nach Hause.« Jack Clearwater streckte ihm die Hand hin. Wir hielten alle ein klein wenig die Luft an, aber Finnys Vater zögerte nur kurz und ergriff sie. »Darf ich fragen, was …«

»Weißkopf-Seeadler«, sagte Mr Clearwater.

»Orca«, sagte Miss White.

»Sie ist der coolste Schwertwal, den es gibt, Dad«, sagte Finny und bekam dafür ein schiefes Lächeln von Miss White. Dann machten wir uns alle auf den Weg. Auf dem Rückweg setzten wir Miss White bei ihrem schwarzen BMW ab, den sie bei einem Bekannten in Miami untergestellt hatte, dann fuhren wir mit den zwei Autos zurück zur Schule.

Das Glück darüber, dass es Wave und Finny gut ging, fühlte sich an, als hätte mir jemand flüssiges Gold in die Adern gepumpt. Aber jedes Mal, wenn ich an Shari dachte, packte mich eine riesengroße Sehnsucht. Würde sie da sein, wenn wir zur Blue Reef zurückkamen, oder war sie schon mit Noah und Blue hinausgeschwommen, um draußen im Meer zu übernachten, wie sie es oft und gerne taten?

Wenn ich nur einen einzigen Wunsch im Leben frei gehabt hätte, dann diesen. Dass sie da sein würde, dass sie auf mich gewartet hätte und mich genauso anschaute wie Finny vorhin Wave.

Ich war so fertig, dass ich einschlief, kaum dass wir losgefahren waren. Zack, weg. Vollkoma.

Als ich aufwachte, lag eine Hand auf meiner Schulter. Sharis Hand. Mit einem Lächeln blickte mein Delfinmädchen mir ins Gesicht. »Schön, dass ihr zurück seid! Miss White hat gesagt, vielleicht ist es besser, wenn jemand dich aufweckt und daran hindert, im Auto zu übernachten.«

»Bist du nicht ins Meer geschwommen?«, fragte ich und blinzelte ins Mondlicht.

»Nein, ich wollte auf dich warten«, sagte Shari. »Ich hab mich schon darauf gefreut, dass du zurückkommst, weißt du?«

Das musste ein Traum sein. Ja, ganz eindeutig. Ich schlief noch.

»Was ist denn mit dir los?«, fragte Shari erschrocken.

Mir flossen gerade die Augen über. Keine Ahnung, wieso. Wie grauenhaft peinlich, vor allem, weil ich anscheinend doch wach war! Schnell wischte ich die blöden Tränen mit dem Handrücken ab.

»War alles ganz schön heftig, diese Sache mit Wave, was?« Shari zog mich aus dem Auto und zwang mich mehr oder weniger, sie zu umarmen. »Bei der großen Welle, du bist ja völlig fertig. Komm, ich bring dich zu deiner Hütte.«

Sie legte sich einen meiner Arme über die Schulter und beförderte mich in Richtung Schulstrand. Mit der Ferse kickte ich die Autotür hinter mir zu, abzuschließen brauchte man hier nicht. Wer hier versuchte, etwas zu klauen, wurde von einem Alligator gebissen. Ein Schild am Zaun wies darauf hin.

»Hast du schon gewusst, dass sich Finny in Wave verliebt hat?«, fragte ich.

»Ja, das hab ich gemerkt«, meinte Shari. »Ich gönne es ihr, Wave ist wirklich ein sehr meeriger Seawalker.«

Oh Mann. Klar, ich gönnte es Finny auch, aber *das* hatte ich jetzt nicht hören wollen.

Shari lächelte noch breiter, wahrscheinlich hatte man mir eben die Gedanken vom Gesicht ablesen können. »Aber nicht so meerig wie du, klar?«

Da tat ich es einfach. Ich löste mich aus ihrem Griff, stellte mich ihr gegenüber und fragte sie: »Magst du mich?«

»Und ob ich dich mag, du bissiges Meerestier. Man könnte sogar sagen, dass ich dich liebe. Obwohl man sich die Haut aufschürft, wenn man dich anfasst.«

Hatte ich richtig gehört? Hatte sie eben wirklich gesagt, dass sie mich liebte? Ja, hatte sie! Ich ließ mich von ihr zu meiner Hütte schleppen, bekam noch einen Kuss – leider nur auf die Stirn – und sank mit einem seligen Lächeln auf meine Koje.

»Was ist los?«, fragte Jasper, der auf dem unteren Bett gerade ein Kreuzworträtsel löste, das er schon dreimal gemacht und wieder ausradiert hatte.

»Liebe ist schön«, sagte ich.

Dann ging ich Zähne putzen.

Krasse Nachrichten

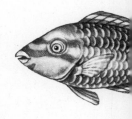

Der nächste Tag – ein Donnerstag – war unglaublich toll. Jedenfalls für Shari, mich und den Rest der Klasse. Der Besuchertag war abgesagt worden, damit wir uns auf den Unterricht konzentrieren konnten. Shari und ich saßen ganz nah nebeneinander, so nah, dass sich unsere Arme berührten. Wir lachten auch über den blödesten Witz, schauten uns ständig an und fütterten uns in der Cafeteria gegenseitig mit Fischhäppchen. Die anderen wechselten vielsagende Blicke.

Ah, ein Turtelfin und ein Romantik-Hai, kommentierte das Nox, der gerade zwischen den Tisch-Booten herumschwamm. *Und, wann küsst ihr euch?*

Ruhe da oder ich hole den Kescher, sagte ich und musste dann leider lachen.

Oh, bitte nicht, ich hab schon total Angst, mir zittern die Flossen!, gab Nox zurück und führte das gleich mal vor. Dann schwamm er mir nach, als ich zum Buffet watete, und zwickte mich mit dem Schnabel in den großen Zeh.

»Au! Willst du Haifutter werden oder was?«

Nox lachte nur. Er hatte wie die meisten anderen in der Blue Reef keine Angst mehr vor mir.

Auch meine Klassenkameraden waren happy, weil Waves Rettung geglückt war und sowohl Mr Clearwater als auch Miss White wieder unterrichteten. Gespannt beobachteten wir die beiden und versuchten zu raten, wie es zwischen ihnen stand. Es war ein gutes Zeichen, dass die beiden zusammen auf dem Dach saßen und bis weit in die Nacht hinein redeten.

Sie haben ausgemacht, dass sie morgen Abend essen gehen!, berichtete Noemi. *Das heißt, er hat ihr verziehen, oder?*

Shari, Blue, Jasper und ein paar andere Leute jubelten.

»Hast du etwa gelauscht?« Finny ließ ihre Sonnenbrille auf die Nase gleiten, setzte ihre beste Polizistentochter-Miene auf und wackelte mahnend mit dem Zeigefinger.

Noemi senkte den Kopf und ließ die Tasthaare hängen. *Ja, hab ich.*

Finny lächelte, und ihre blaugrauen Augen blickten verschmitzt drein. »Hätte ich natürlich auch gemacht. Aber du hast die besseren Öhrchen.«

Auch Lissa Clearwater wirkte sehr zufrieden, dass es ihrem Sohn und seiner Schule wieder gut ging. Ich sah sie am Lehrertisch sitzen und fröhlich mit den anderen plaudern. Anscheinend hatte sie noch nicht vor, in die Rocky Mountains zurückzukehren.

Nur zwei Leute waren nicht glücklich. In der Mittagspause schaute Steve in unserer Lagune vorbei – und er hatte Neuigkeiten.

Mehrere der Glasbodenboote haben ihre Liegeplätze verlassen, ich kann sie nicht alle kontrollieren, meldete er mir gefrustet. Das hatte ich fast befürchtet.

Ich ging Maris suchen. »Du fliegst doch weiter mit der Kamera herum, oder?«, fragte ich ihn und berichtete, was Steve mir erzählt hatte.

Er nickte. »Klar. Gestern bin ich runtergesegelt bis zum Sugarloaf Key. Shelby und ich bleiben dran.«

Steve verabschiedete sich wieder, um weiter entlang der Keys Patrouille zu schwimmen.

Auch Miss Bennett wirkte bedrückt. Am Ende der Mittagspause bekam ich mit, wie sie blass und gefasst hochging zu Mr Clearwaters Büro. Shari und ich spitzten die Ohren. »Den Unterricht in Kampf und Überleben heute Nachmittag wird vermutlich Miss White halten, nehme ich an?«, fragte sie ihn. »So wie ich das sehe, brauchen Sie mich nicht mehr.«

»Ich fürchte nicht.« Mr Clearwater klang verlegen. »Es tut mir wirklich leid, dass Sie extra hergezogen sind und ...«

»Kein Problem, ich verstehe schon. Dann gehe ich wohl mal meine Sachen packen.«

Als ich und Shari hochrannten, nahmen wir zwei Stufen auf einmal. »Mr Clearwater, Sie machen einen Fehler!«, sprudelte ich hervor.

Die meisten Lehrer finden es nicht gerade prickelnd, wenn man ihnen so was sagt, aber Mr Clearwater zuckte mit keiner Wimper. »Möchtest du das vielleicht erklären, Tiago?«, fragte er stattdessen.

»Sie kann verschiedene Tiersprachen – stimmt doch, oder, Miss Bennett?«, fragte ich unsere Igelfisch-Lehrerin aufgeregt. »Wir könnten das als neues Fach brauchen.«

»Außerdem hat sie Sei dein Tier wirklich gut unterrichtet, vielleicht könnte sie das Miss White abnehmen«, mischte sich Shari ein.

Ich war wieder dran. »Von Politik hat sie auch Ahnung, wie wäre es mal mit Gesellschaftskunde an der Blue Reef?«

»Hm.« Unser Schulleiter musterte Miss Bennett mit ganz neuem Blick. »Stimmt das mit den Tiersprachen?«

»Na ja, ich kann verschiedene Fischsprachen ... wenn das etwas hilft ...«

»Ja, das hilft«, sagte Jack Clearwater. »Setzen Sie sich bitte noch mal ... und ihr beiden habt bestimmt noch etwas anderes zu tun, oder?« Mit einer Handbewegung scheuchte er Shari und mich raus. Miss Bennett schickte uns einen dankbaren Blick hinterher.

Der Freitag war ebenso toll. Rocket war zur Nachhilfe gekommen und nach dem Unterricht schwammen Shari, Blue, Noah zum Bahia Honda Beach – dem schönsten Strand der Gegend –, um dort abzuhängen. Rocket und ich ließen uns als Menschen an der Rückenflosse mitziehen. Mein Freund lachte über das ganze Gesicht. »He, das ist fast so cool, wie im Kennedy Space Center im Space-Shuttle-Cockpit zu sitzen!«

»Gib zu, dass es besser ist«, sagte ich.

»Ja okay, es ist besser«, gab Rocket zu und rief dann freudig »Yeeeeah!«, als Blue mit ihm zusammen einen Sprint einlegte.

Als wir angekommen waren, verschlechterte sich unsere Laune etwas.

Leider völlig überfüllt, sagte Noah enttäuscht und legte eine Tauchstrecke ein. Man sah den weißen Sand kaum vor lauter Handtüchern und im türkisfarbenen, nicht sehr tiefen Wasser planschten ganze Legionen von Leuten. *Wollen wir lieber woandershin?*

»Nicht nötig – Moment«, sagte ich, schwamm näher ans Ufer heran, verwandelte mich und streckte die Rückenflosse über die Oberfläche. Ein paar Minuten später hatten wir jede Menge Platz.

Das war cool, danke, sagte Blue zu mir und wir tobten im Wasser herum, bis uns die Energie ausging.

Es wurmte mich nur, dass wir auch in dieser Woche keinen weiteren Hinweis darauf gefunden hatten, wo wieder Arenakämpfe stattfanden. Wenn mein Bruder Steve recht hatte, dann liefen diese scheußlichen Veranstaltungen weiter. Kein Wunder, mit Wetten auf Tierkämpfe ließ sich viel Geld machen. Das würden sie nicht aufgeben, nur weil die Polizei ihnen einmal auf die Finger geklopft hatte.

Als Johnny mich und Rocket am frühen Abend abholte, um uns heim nach Miami zu transportieren, freute ich mich auf ein ruhiges Wochenende mit Rocket und wusste, dass ich Shari in diesen zwei Tagen schrecklich vermissen würde.

Dann klingelte mein Handy. Es war Shelby, unsere Brandseeschwalbe. »Maris hat die Kerle im Meer südlich vom Big Pine Key gesichtet! Dort, wo man es vom Highway aus nicht bemerkt. Ein anderes Schiff und ein paar kleinere Boote und Jachten, sie haben schon Netzkäfige aufgebaut mit drei großen Haien drin. Einer davon ist wahrscheinlich ein Tigerhai, meint Maris.«

Ich schwankte irgendwo zwischen *Yeah!* und *Oh nein.* Ein Tigerhai, sie hatten auch einen Tigerhai gefangen ... konnte das Steve sein? Mein Magen fühlte sich an, als hätte ihn jemand tiefgefroren. Selbst wenn er es nicht war, wir mussten diese Tiere befreien, bevor die Veranstalter sie zum Kämpfen zwangen.

»Hat er Mrs Lennox an Bord gesehen?« Meine Hand krampfte sich um das Gerät, das ich inzwischen laut gestellt hatte.

»Für Maris schienen da erst nur Männer an Bord zu sein, die irgendwas vorbereiteten«, sagte Shelby. »Aber dann hat er eine Frau entdeckt, auf die Miss Lennox' Beschreibung passsen könnte. Sie hat den Männern Anweisungen gegeben.«

Darüber, was das bedeutete, sprach ich lieber nicht, ich hatte das mit der Millionen-Dollar-Klage noch sehr frisch im Hinterkopf.

»Wir kommen sofort«, versprach ich. »Sag Mr Clearwater, Mr García und Miss White Bescheid!«

»Die sind alle drei nicht da.« Shelbys Stimme klang verunsichert. »Mr Clearwater bringt seine Mutter zum Flughafen und Miss White ist mitgefahren. Mr García besucht seine kleine Tochter.«

Oh nein, auch das noch. Was für ein mieses Timing!

»Versuch, sie zu erreichen, sie müssen die Polizei rufen. Ist irgendjemand da, mit dem du schon mal losfahren könntest?«

»Äh, ja ... Mrs Misaki«, meinte Shelby. Unsere schlecht gelaunte Schulsekretärin, in zweiter Gestalt Muräne, kutschierte uns nicht selten auch durch die Gegend. »Ich frage sie gleich, ob sie mich fahren kann. Vielleicht kommt noch jemand mit, der gut kämpfen kann ...« Verblüfft hörte ich, wie zwei Mädchen stritten, jemand rief »He!«, dann war plötzlich jemand anderes in der Leitung. Ella. »Ich fahre auch mit, nur dass du Bescheid weißt, Tiago«, blaffte sie mich an und ich war froh, dass ich eben am Telefon nichts Fieses über ihre Mutter gesagt hatte. Das hätte sie garantiert weitererzählt.

»Äh, bist du sicher?«, war das Einzige, was mir dazu einfiel.

»Natürlich bin ich sicher. Wir treffen uns am Big Pine Key, klar?«

Ich war alles andere als sicher, ob das eine gute Idee war. War Ella überhaupt auf unserer Seite? Vielleicht ging es ihr nur darum, ihre Mutter vor uns zu warnen und zu verhindern, dass die bei dieser widerlichen Tierkampfaktion geschnappt wurde!

»Nimm dein Handy mit – diesmal brauchen wir Beweisfotos«, sagte ich.

»Na gut«, antwortete sie und legte auf. Würde sie es tatsächlich machen? Keine Ahnung. Hätte *ich* es gemacht, wenn ich rausgefunden hätte, dass *Johnny* irgendein krummes Ding am Laufen hatte? Noch weniger Ahnung.

Genau dieser Johnny, der zum Glück deutlich netter war als Mrs Lennox, hatte alles mitgehört. »Wird ein bisschen dauern, bis wir am Big Pine Key sind, fürchte ich«, knurrte er. Wir waren gerade auf dem schmalen Highway zwischen Miami und Key Largo, der mitten durch die Everglades führte.

Mein ganzer Körper kribbelte vor Aufregung. »Aber wir müssen da jetzt *sofort* hin!«

»Falls du nicht zufällig irgendwelche Superkräfte hast, von denen ich bisher nichts weiß, dann brauchen wir *mindestens* eine Stunde. Ella wird vor uns ankommen.«

Am liebsten hätte ich auf den Sitz eingeprügelt, meine Haizähne ins Armaturenbrett geschlagen.

»Wehe«, sagte Johnny, der es natürlich merkte. Und inzwischen hatte ich genug Selbstbeherrschung, dass ich es tatsächlich nicht tat.

Ich hatte mich so sehr darauf verlassen, dass Miss White alles in Ordnung bringen würde! Und nun war sie nicht da und ich musste es irgendwie ohne sie schaffen.

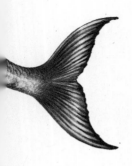

Zweimal King Kong

Wenn man es eilig hat, dann dehnt sich die Zeit manchmal zu Kaugummi. Jede Minute fühlt sich an wie zehn. Es war inzwischen früher Abend. Waren die Taucher schon im Wasser, schossen sie schon mit Harpunen auf meine armen Artgenossen, um sie zum Angriff zu reizen? Und was machten Ella und Mrs Misaki dort am Big Pine Key?

Johnny brach sämtliche Verkehrsregeln, als er über den Highway 1 nach Südwesten raste, aber zum Glück hielten uns keine Cops an.

Endlich, Big Pine Key! Wir fuhren so nah wie möglich an den Ort heran, den Shelby mir beschrieben hatte, und stellten das Auto am Rand eines Sträßchens ab, das zu einem verlassenen, von einigen wenigen Palmen und Gebüsch bewachsenen Küstenabschnitt führte. *Maris?*, flüsterte ich in Gedanken und versuchte mit aller Kraft, mich auf unseren Albatros-Wandler zu fokussieren, damit niemand anderes mich hörte. *Bist du da?*

Ich musste ein paarmal rufen, dann kam endlich eine Antwort – schwach, wie aus weiter Ferne. *Ja, allerdings über dem offenen Meer. Ella hat gesagt, ich soll mich ein Stück entfernt halten, damit ich nicht auffalle. Schließlich gibt's hier nicht viele Albatrosse. Außerdem könnten die Kerle die Kamera auf meinem Rücken sehen.*

Ich biss mir auf die Lippe. Natürlich, das stimmte, aber es klang trotzdem verdächtig nach Ella-Sabotage. Schließlich brauchten wir Kamerabilder als Beweismittel!

»Komisch, dass hier nur so wenige Autos parken«, flüsterte Rocket, der nichts von unserem Austausch mitbekommen hatte. »Der weiße Pick-up ist von eurer Schule, oder?«

»Genau.« Ich peilte die Lage, doch zu sehen waren unsere Leute nirgendwo. Dann musterte ich Rocket und zischte ihm zu: »Du kannst dich schon mal ausziehen. Oder willst du, dass man dich sogar vom Weltraum aus sieht, wenn wir uns Richtung Meer schleichen?«

»Das ist meine Lieblingsfarbe, Mann!« Rocket blickte auf sein neon-orangefarbenes Shirt hinunter.

Ich verdrehte die Augen. »Ja und? Interessiert das gerade irgendwen?«

Ohne weiteren Protest verstaute Rocket sein Outfit im Auto, dann schlichen er und Johnny (der zum Glück ein grünes Hemd trug) durchs Gebüsch. Ich warf mich auf den Bauch, denn auf dem Boden war ich durch mein sandfarbenes T-Shirt gut getarnt, und robbte profihaft hinterher.

Dass wir vorsichtig gewesen waren, zahlte sich aus. Nach ein paar Metern machte Rocket uns aufgeregte Zeichen und legte sich neben mich auf den Boden. »Da sind zwei Leute«, hauchte er mir ins Ohr. »Frag mich nicht, woher ich das weiß ... ich glaube, ich hab sie gewittert oder so was.«

»Kann gut sein«, wisperte ich zurück und schaute mich vorsichtig um.

Ich hörte ihre Stimmen, noch bevor ich sie sah. Sie unterhielten sich leise, nur hin und wieder ein Wort. Leider standen die beiden genau zwischen uns und dem Meer und es sah so aus, als sei das Absicht. Als ich den Kopf ein wenig hob, sah ich die beiden auch durch die Blätter hindurch. Die Typen – beide ungefähr Mitte zwanzig – hatten Muskeln, die von vielen Stunden in Fitnessstudios erzählten. Bei einem von ihnen beulte sich das Hemd unter der Achsel verdächtig aus. Knarre im Schulterholster, ziemlich eindeutig. Der andere trug ein Funkgerät am Gürtel.

Rocket, Johnny und ich tauschten einen besorgten Blick. Wie sollten wir an diesen beiden Wächtern vorbeikommen? Hier tatenlos rumzuliegen, bis die Polizei aufkreuzte, kam nicht infrage, vielleicht waren die gefangenen Haie bis dahin schon schwer verletzt!

Durch das Blattwerk konnte ich das Glasbodenschiff sehen, das weiter draußen vor Anker lag. Kein Wunder, dass wir hier Schwierigkeiten hatten, denn diesmal war von den Veranstaltern anscheinend die Parole »Anreise übers Wasser« ausgegeben worden. Schon zehn Boote, hauptsächlich weiß lackierte, schicke Sportflitzer, schaukelten auf einer Seite des zweistöckigen, weiß lackierten Glasbodenschiffs auf den Wellen. Es wirkte nicht so luxuriös wie das Ding, das sie letztes Mal verwendet hatten, eher wie ein Ausflugsdampfer für Touristen. Dafür sprachen auch die vielen gepolsterten Bänke an Bord. Ein paar Leute standen auf dem mittleren Deck herum, von dem aus man in den Rumpf hinunterklettern und die Ereignisse unter der Wasserlinie beobachten konnte. Aber auch, wenn ich die Augen zusammenkniff, konnte ich nicht erkennen, ob Ella und Mrs Misaki darunter waren.

Wir waren schon so nah dran ... aber näher kamen wir nicht, denn beide Wächter behielten die Umgebung wachsam im Auge. Allerdings starrten sie auch immer wieder verstohlen auf ihre Handys, wir hörten das elektronische Düdeln eines Games. Obwohl Johnny uns einen warnenden Blick zuwarf, krochen Rocket und ich in ihre Richtung, sodass wir hören konnten, was die beiden redeten.

»Oh, Mann, das ist mein vorletztes Leben.«

»Mach dir nicht ins Hemd, den Level schaffst du.«

»Nicht, wenn mich wieder dieser Zombie erwischt!«

Während ich noch rätselte, welches Game das sein könnte, zischte mir Rocket ins Ohr: »Ich lenke die beiden ab und ihr schleicht hinter ihrem Rücken vorbei!«

Noch während wir ihn anglotzten – Johnny alarmiert, ich skeptisch –, kroch Rocket rückwärts, bis er außer Sicht war. Dann kam er zurück, nun schlenderte er ganz locker und nicht besonders leise in Richtung Strand.

Die daddelnden Wächter schalteten sofort um auf Wachsamkeit.

»Hi, Leute – unser Navi hat den Geist aufgegeben«, sagte Rocket. »Das hier ist der No Name Key, oder?«

Beide Kerle schauten misstrauisch drein, doch der eine begann zu antworten. »Nein, das hier ist ...« Sein Handy gab wieder diesen Düdelton von sich.

»Oh, hey, ihr spielt auch *Zombieworld?*«, fragte Rocket erfreut. »Mich hat's immer im fünften Level gebrettert, bis ich diesen coolen Trick entdeckt habe ...«

»Welchen denn?« Der Wächter mit der Knarre trat neugierig einen Schritt näher.

»Warte, ich zeig's euch ... und kennt ihr das Easter Egg, das der Programmierer im Level acht versteckt hat?«

Schon waren die drei tief in ein Fachgespräch vertieft. Genial!

Johnny und ich schlichen los. Na also, läuft, dachte ich, denn die Typen drehten uns den Rücken zu und mit jedem Schritt kamen wir dem Wasser und unserem Ziel näher.

Dann trat ich auf einen Zweig.

Sofort zuckten die Köpfe der beiden Männer hoch. Ich wollte losrennen, doch Johnny ahnte wohl, dass wir keine Chance hatten, er warf mir einen warnenden Blick zu und nahm eine entspannte Haltung ein. »Hübsches Fleckchen«, sagte er zu mir. »Und, Picknickpause hier oder lieber woanders?«

Die beiden Typen marschierten auf uns zu und packten uns. Sie waren so nah, dass sogar ich mit meinem unterentwickelten Gespür fühlen konnte, dass sie keine Wandler waren.

»He, seit wann darf man hier nicht mehr an den Strand?«, protestierte ich, denn Johnny hatte recht, die Harmlose-Touristen-Nummer war vermutlich das Einzige, das uns jetzt retten konnte. »Tut uns leid, falls wir in ein Schutzgebiet reingelatscht sind.«

Die beiden Wächter tauschten einen Blick, aus dem ich nicht schlau wurde. Aber immerhin ließ der eine Typ Johnny los. Mich hielt der andere weiterhin mit beiden Händen gepackt.

»Gehört ihr drei zusammen?«, fragte der eine Kerl und blickte sich nach Rocket um. Doch er sah ihn ebenso wenig wie ich.

»Wo ist denn der Junge von vorhin?«, fragte der andere Wächter.

»Anscheinend abgezogen. Ohne Hose. Echt schräg.« Mit spitzen Fingern hob einer der beiden Typen die Shorts hoch, die ich vor wenigen Minuten noch an Rockets Hintern gesehen hatte.

Mir dämmerte, was passiert war, und gleich darauf entdeckte ich den dazugehörigen Hintern – jetzt ein paar Nummern kleiner – unter einem Busch in der Nähe. *Toller Zufall: Mr García hat mich heute schnelle Verwandlungen üben lassen,* berichtete Rocket. *Aber mit dir hätte er besser mal pirschen trainiert, du klingst wie ein verdammtes Nashorn!*

Kannst du uns irgendwie rauspauken?, fragte ich ihn verzweifelt und spähte hinaus zu dem Schiff der Täter. Auf dem Deck tat sich irgendwas. Zwei Leute in Neoprenanzügen sprangen über die Bordwand ins Wasser ... oh nein, die Gladiatorentaucher machten sich bereit!

Rauspauken?, fragte Rocket. *Äh, hallo, ich bin gerade eine ordinäre Wanderratte und die beiden sehen aus wie Klone von King Kong! Von ihrer Knarre mal ganz abgesehen.*

Ich wandte ein: *Du hast dich schon mal mit zwei Tigerinnen angelegt und überlebt.*

Ja, ich weiß. Da war ich wohl vorübergehend größenwahnsinnig, kam es zurück.

»Besser, wir melden das Mrs Lennox – soll die Chefin entscheiden, was wir tun sollen«, sagte der eine Wächter. Er hielt mich nur noch mit einer Hand gepackt und nestelte mit der anderen Hand sein Funkgerät vom Gürtel.

Nein, nein, nein! Lydia Lennox durfte noch nicht wissen, dass wir hier waren! Jetzt war klar, dass sie viel mehr als nur die Anwältin der Gangster war.

Wer denkt, dass er einen Tigerhai mit nur einer Hand festhalten kann, hat eindeutig nicht genug Naturdokus geschaut. Ich rammte den Typen mit aller Kraft und warf mich gleich darauf nach hinten. Verblüfft ließ der Kerl mich los, stolperte und verlor das Gleichgewicht. Leider war der Busch, in den er fiel, genau der, in dem sich Rocket versteckt hatte.

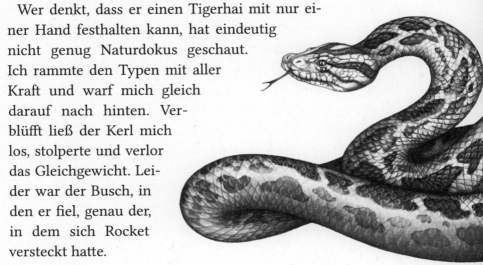

Momente bevor der Kerl den Strauch inklusive Ratte plattmachte, schoss mein Freund unter den Blättern hervor. *Na also, geht doch! Jetzt nichts wie weg hier.*

Ich sah, wie Johnnys Faust das Kinn des zweiten Wächters traf. Doch der war anscheinend Härteres gewohnt, er taumelte nur ein paar Schritte zurück und griff dann mit kalter Wut unter sein Hemd. Anscheinend trug er wirklich eine Waffe!

Im Zickzack rasten Johnny und ich Richtung Meer, es waren nur noch ein paar Meter bis dorthin. Endlich hatten wir es erreicht, eine Welle durchtränkte meine Sneakers. Aber noch waren wir nicht in Sicherheit. »Viel zu flach hier!«, rief Johnny. »Los, los, wir müssen noch weiter raus, bis wir losschwimmen können.«

Hastig schaute ich mich um, während ich spritzend durchs schienbeintiefe Wasser rannte. Einer der beiden Kerle hetzte uns nach ... und der andere zielte mit einer schwarzen Knarre auf uns. Mir blieb die Luft weg. Wenn die beiden nichts dagegen hatten, Leute in den Rücken zu schießen, dann waren wir für sie Eins-a-Zielscheiben.

Ich lenk den mit dem Schießeisen ab!, rief Rocket und ich sah, wie er über den Boden huschte.

Wie denn? Du bist nur eine Ratte, wie du eben so schön gesagt hast!

Eben, antwortete Rocket.

Ich watete weiter, so schnell ich konnte. Aber wer so was schon mal versucht hat, weiß, dass *Waten* und *schnell* leider zwei Begriffe sind, die nicht zusammenpassen. Ich hatte schon Albträume, in denen ich besser vorangekommen war.

Aber dann hörte ich erleichtert, wie der zweite Wächter aufbrüllte. »Irgend so ein Vieh kriecht gerade mein Hosenbein hoch! Aaaah!«

Super Idee. Ich hoffte, Rocket biss ihm auf dem Weg nach oben in ein paar empfindliche Körperteile. Kurz darauf war der zweite Typ dran und ließ vor lauter Panik das Funkgerät in eine Pfütze fallen, während er mit beiden Händen versuchte, Rocket aus seiner Jeans zu schütteln.

Weiter so, genial!, jubelte ich meinem Freund zu.

Endlich war das Wasser tief genug, dass wir untertauchen konnten.

»Runter!«, gurgelte Johnny, sein Gesicht war schon gefleckt wie von einer richtig fiesen Hautkrankheit. Ich tauchte, strampelte mich mit angehaltenem Atem aus meinen Klamotten und stellte mir meine Haigestalt vor. Ein starkes Kribbeln durchlief mich ...

Wartet auf mich! Rockets Stimme klang ein bisschen quiekig.

Endlich wieder ein Hai. Aber es war noch immer so flach, dass ich kaum einen Meter Wasser unter den Brustflossen hatte. Rasch ging ich tiefer, um vor Kugeln sicher zu sein, und Seegras kitzelte meinen Bauch. *Was meinst du mit Warten?*, erwiderte ich. *Ratten gehören nicht ins Meer und ...*

WARTE gefälligst, ich hab dir eben den verdammten Hintern gerettet!

Eigentlich hatten wir es eilig, wir mussten sofort zu diesem Schiff. Aber Rocket war erstens mein Freund und zweitens hatte er recht.

Schau mal, brummte der Juwelen-Zackenbarsch neben mir und glotzte nach oben.

Direkt über mir paddelte eine kleine Nagetiergestalt. Ich tauchte unter Rocket hoch und er brachte es fertig, sich mit den Pfötchen an meine Rückenflosse zu klammern. Ratten sind echt zäh.

So schnell wir konnten, schwammen wir auf das Schiff zu.

Wir hatten drei Jobs – diese Kämpfe zu verhindern, Beweise zu sammeln ... und am Leben zu bleiben! Der dritte Job war vermutlich der schwierigste.

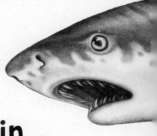

Netze, Delfine und ein Schal des Grauens

Als Erstes tauchten wir unter die »geparkten« Boote, damit uns von oben niemand sah, und Rocket kletterte an Bord. *Ich versuche, auf das Hauptschiff zu kommen,* flüsterte er. *Drückt mir die Daumen, dass keiner mich sieht.*

Sehen wir so aus, als hätten wir gerade Daumen?, gab ich zurück.

Wenn du was Interessantes siehst, schick uns einen Gedankenstrom, wisperte Johnny in Rockets Richtung, aber so, dass ich mithören konnte.

Äh, wie geht das noch mal?, kam es zurück.

Wenn du's nicht genau weißt, dann bewahrst du besser Gedankenstille, sagte Johnny. *Wir dürfen nicht riskieren, dass die Lennox dich hört.*

Ich musste wissen, was an Bord vorging, und vor allem, was Ella und Mrs Lennox dort machten. Doch erst musste ich abchecken, wie es den gefangenen Haien – einem Tigerhai, den ich nicht kannte, einem Bullenhai und einem Zitronenhai – ging.

Kurz gesagt, nicht gut. Als ich Blut im Wasser schmeckte, wusste ich, dass schon einer von ihnen getroffen war: ein Zitronenhai – um so was zu erkennen, war die Facharbeit immerhin nützlich gewesen. Während die Gäste an Bord den Kampf durch die großen Unterwasserfenster des Schiffs beobachteten, auch diesmal mit Sektgläsern in den Händen, erledigte ein Taucher im schwarzen Neoprenanzug die Drecksarbeit. Er verfolgte den Hai, pikte ihn immer wieder mit einer Lanze und versuchte, ihn zum Angriff zu reizen.

Wer stattdessen angriff, war ich. Ich schlug mit der Schwanzflosse, um zu beschleunigen, und drückte meine Schnauze gegen die nachgiebigen Käfigwände, von denen der Gladiatortaucher nicht weit entfernt war. Wirbelte noch mehr Wasser auf, drückte noch fester. Machte eine Riesendelle in diese Maschenwand.

Der Taucher erschrak furchtbar, als mein Maul ihn am Rücken berührte. Große Wolken von Luftblasen blubberten aus seinem Mund nach oben, als er herumfuhr. Der arme Zitronenhai nutzte die Gelegenheit, um in eine entfernte Ecke des Käfigs zu flüchten.

Inzwischen hatten Johnny und Rocket die Lage an der Oberfläche gepeilt.

Mrs Misaki steht an Deck und streitet sich mit jemandem herum, vielleicht dem Kapitän, berichtete mein Erziehungsberechtigter.

Mrs Misaki? Wie ist die denn aufs Schiff gelangt – geschwommen?, fragte ich, doch dann bemerkte ich schon unser schwarzes Schlauchboot, das *Zodiac,* das beim Glasbodenschiff längsseits gegangen war. Der Boden trug einen Stern mit weißer Farbe, damit wir es auch von unten erkannten, wenn wir gerade in zweiter Gestalt unterwegs waren.

Ich konnte durch Johnnys Gedanken mithören, was gesprochen wurde.

»Was fällt Ihnen ein, mich hier festzuhalten!«, tobte Mrs

Misaki. »Geben Sie mir mein Handy zurück! Und hören Sie sofort auf, hier Meerestiere zu quälen, Sie grober Klotz!!«

»Wir führen hier ein wissenschaftliches Experiment durch, Lady. Alles genehmigt.«

»Das glaube ich Ihnen keine Sekunde lang! Wo ist Ihre Genehmigung?« Kurz darauf ging es weiter: »Das da? Was ist das denn für ein mieser Wisch! Das hat doch irgendeine zwielichtige Anwältin für Sie fabriziert! Ich glaube, ich weiß sogar, wie die heißt!« Und Ella? Die sah ich gerade hinter den Unterwasserfenstern auftauchen – neben ihrer Mutter. Doch keine der beiden wirkte richtig glücklich. Ich konnte zwar kein Wort verstehen, sah aber, dass Ella mit Lydia Lennox diskutierte. Da war ein handfester Streit im Gange. Ein paar Leute hörten interessiert zu, auch wenn die meisten eher das Hai-Taucher-Duell beobachteten, das durch mich deutlich spannender geworden war.

Ich sah, wie das Handy Ellas Tasche ausbeulte. Sie hatte es dabei, benutzte es aber nicht. Das durfte doch echt nicht wahr sein! Wenn sie sich nur ein bisschen Mühe gegeben hätte, hätte sie jede Menge Beweise sammeln können. Wetten, es war zu spät, bis endlich die Polizei aufkreuzte? Carl Bittergreen, den Mafia-Boss, sah ich nirgendwo, obwohl ich nach ihm Ausschau hielt. Vielleicht war er oben an Deck?

Der Taucher hatte keine Lust, sich von mir ins Handwerk pfuschen zu lassen. Er tauchte kurz ab und ließ sich eine zweite Druckluftharpune geben. Die schien nicht für den Zitronenhai gedacht zu sein, er ignorierte das Tier ... und schwamm in meine Richtung.

Mir wurde klar, dass er mich mit dem Ding auch durch die Maschen des Käfigs treffen konnte, und wendete blitzartig.

Tiago! Da bist du ja! Ich hab mir schon Sorgen gemacht. Eine heitere Stimme, die ich so gut kannte ... und die mir einen eisigen Schreck ins Herz jagte. Shari glitt geschmeidig auf mich zu, das Delfinmaul wie immer zu einem Lächeln gebogen. Ihre Pfiffe hallten durchs Wasser. *Blue und Noah suchen leider in der falschen Richtung nach ...*

Weg da! Ich rammte sie zur Seite, ganz kurz, bevor die Harpune dort vorbeizischte, wo sie eben noch gewesen war.

Die Gäste des Haikampfs standen mit großen Augen vor den Unterwasserfenstern, kein Mund stand mehr still. Waren sie wenigstens froh, dass Shari nicht getroffen worden war? Bestimmt. Niemand wollte, dass hier ein Delfin verletzt wurde. Sterben sollten heute nur Tiere, die sowieso niemand mochte.

Aber solche Tiere konnten sich auch wehren. Ich sah, dass Lydia Lennox sich dem Fenster zugewandt hatte und mich anstarrte. Ihre Lippen waren zusammengepresst, ihr Blick eisig. *Tiago. Hätte ich mir ja denken können. Du tauchst immer dort auf, wo du unerwünscht bist.*

Ach? Ich dachte, die Leute hier wollen Haie sehen? Absichtlich schwamm ich ganz nah an den Glasscheiben vorbei, damit ich ihr in die Augen schauen konnte. Inzwischen war mir klar, dass sie keine normale Zuschauerin war. Schon wandte sich wieder jemand von der Besatzung an sie, fragte etwas. Andere Mitarbeiter standen neben ihr, warteten auf Anweisungen oder berichteten ihr irgendwas.

Bitte, Ella, kannst du das filmen?, flüsterte ich. Noch bevor Ella den Kopf schüttelte, wusste ich, dass es sinnlos war.

Ich hatte erwartet, dass Ella sich abwenden oder weiter mit ihrer Mutter diskutieren würde. Doch die redete gerade mit einem Besatzungsmitglied. Ella reagierte sofort. Sie legte eine Hand gegen die Scheibe und starrte eindringlich zu mir nach draußen. *Es tut mir leid, Tiago, ich konnte es ihr nicht ausreden!*

Sie hat geahnt, dass du kommen würdest. Besser, ihr haut ab, so schnell ihr könnt!

Was meinst du damit?, fragte ich zurück. *Was konntest du ihr nicht ausreden?*

Der Taucher hatte seine Harpune an der Leine wieder zu sich zurückgezogen und machte sich bereit für den nächsten Schuss. Wachsam behielt ich ihn im Auge, während Shari und ich ganz nah nebeneinanderschwammen, so nah, dass sich unsere Brustflossen berührten. Das fühlte sich wunderbar an, aber hoffentlich passierte ihr hier nichts! Währenddessen knipsten die miesen Gäste drauflos, wahrscheinlich gab es schon ein paar Hundert Fotos von uns beiden.

Diesmal versuchte der Taucher nicht, mich abzuknallen, vielleicht war ihm das Risiko zu groß, Shari zu treffen und damit zur meistgehasstesten Person von ganz Florida zu werden. Stattdessen wandte er sich seelenruhig wieder dem Zitronenhai zu und hielt sich dabei weit genug von den Seiten des Netzkäfigs entfernt, sodass ich nicht mehr an ihn herankam. Der wilde Hai suchte vergeblich nach einem Fluchtweg, aber als der Taucher ihn am Schwanz packte, begann er, sich wütend zu wehren.

Shari stieß einen schrillen Pfiff aus. *Können wir denn gar nichts tun?*

Ich weiß nicht, was, antwortete ich, während die Wut in mir brodelte.

Leider waren es auch diesmal keine Taue aus Hanf, die den Käfig zusammenhielten, sondern dicke Kunststoffstränge. Die konnte ich nicht durchbeißen, ohne selbst hängen zu bleiben.

Bestimmt kommt die Polizei bald, brummte Johnny. *Sie haben ein Boot in Key West stationiert, das weiß ich.*

Bis dahin ist der Hai tot! Ich brüllte nicht ihn an, sondern eigentlich die ganze Welt, die viel zu wenig tat, um Tiere zu beschützen.

Der Taucher hob das Harpunengewehr ... und von oben plumpste etwas in den Netzkäfig. Etwas, das auf den ersten Blick wie ein Bündel Klamotten aussah. Auf den zweiten Blick sah man, dass in diesem Bündel etwas drinsteckte.

He, das ist doch Mrs Misaki! Shari zirpte und trillerte vor Aufregung wie ein halbes Orchester. Sie hing als Delfin aufrecht im Wasser und schaute zu, während ich weiterschwimmen musste, um atmen zu können.

Eine Muräne mit Spuren von violettem Lippenstift wand sich aus den Kleidern hervor und schwamm mit schlängelnden Bewegungen auf den Gladiator zu. Bevor der es sich versah, hatte er einen Schal. Gelb, gefleckt und vermutlich nicht besonders warm. Es war kein Schal, um den man ihn beneiden musste, denn das eine Ende riss gerade wenige Zentimeter von seiner Nase entfernt das zähnegespickte Maul auf.

Was fällt Ihnen ein, Sie brutaler Kerl!, donnerte Mrs Misaki, sodass es wahrscheinlich jeder Wandler im weiten Umkreis hören konnte. *Lassen Sie sofort diese Tiere und ganz besonders diese SCHÜLER in Ruhe!*

Der Taucher antwortete nicht – er war anscheinend kein Wandler. Aber die Botschaft kam trotzdem an. Panisch ließ er das Harpunengewehr fallen, packte Mrs Misaki und versuchte, sie von seinem Hals zu entfernen. Tatkräftig versuchte Mrs Misaki, ihn davon abzuhalten, was sich für den Kerl wahrscheinlich anfühlte, wie mit einem Nadelkissen zu ringen.

Unruhig schwamm Shari umher, sondierte den Netzkäfig mit schnarrenden Ultraschalllauten. *Was könnte Ella gemeint haben mit ihrer Warnung?*

Kurz darauf fanden wir es heraus.

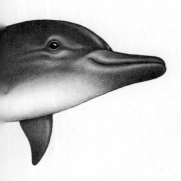

Der Schwarm

Auf den ersten Blick sahen die Barrakudas aus wie eine Wolke von Nadeln. Als sie näher kamen, eher wie silberne Schwerter im dunstigen Blau des Meeres. Immer weiter näherten sie sich uns und ich versuchte gar nicht erst, sie zu zählen. Sie waren kleiner als Mr Williams, aber dafür waren es viele, wahrscheinlich Hunderte. Ein riesiger Schwarm, eine Armee.

Sind das Jungtiere?, fragte ich Johnny, so fasziniert, dass ich fast vergaß, Angst zu haben.

Nein, diese Barrakuda-Art wird nicht größer, antwortete er. *Doch leider sind sie keine Einzelgänger wie ihre großen Verwandten …*

Was meinst du, sind Wandler dabei? Ich lauschte in mich hinein, spürte aber nichts.

Anscheinend, aber nur wenige, meinte mein Erziehungsberechtigter.

Ich wette, ich weiß, wer die hergeholt hat, stöhnte Shari, während die Barrakudas uns aus starren Augen beobachteten.

Meinst du etwa mich? Ein Raubfisch, der den anderen sehr ähnlich sah, aber doppelt so groß war und dunkle Flecken am Bauch hatte, schwamm direkt auf uns zu. *Diesmal geht es nicht um eine Schulnote, Shari, aber ich wette, du wirst auch diesmal versagen. Schließlich hast du weder die nötige Intelligenz noch die Kampfkraft.*

Aber Sie, oder was? Ich schwamm einen Scheinangriff, der ihn zu einem schnellen Ausweichen zwang.

Beleidigen Sie gerne Mädchen, Mr Williams?, fragte Johnny unseren ehemaligen Schulleiter, er klang angewidert.

Wenn sie es verdient haben, ja, kam als Antwort. *Der Junge ist ebenfalls kein großer Verlust, ich habe wenig Gutes über ihn gehört. Macht's gut, ihr drei.*

Seine Flanke blitzte im Licht silbern auf, als der große Raubfisch sich dem Schwarm zuwandte. Ich verstand nichts, als er mit den Barrakudas sprach, aber was er gesagt hatte, war ziemlich klar. Irgendetwas nach dem Motto *Schnappt euch die Beute!*

Shari! Schnell, hau ab!, schrie ich, denn ich wollte, dass wenigstens sie in Sicherheit war.

Ich bin hier und bleibe hier, gab Shari zurück und warf mir einen kampflustigen Blick zu.

Die Barrakudas schwammen die erste Attacke. Sie hatten jede Menge Zähne und schon nach Sekunden hatte ich die ersten Bisse abbekommen. Wütend schnappte ich nach rechts und links. Einen Fisch, der eindeutig kein Wandler war, zerbiss ich glatt in der Mitte, wenn auch mit schlechtem Gewissen. Dann jagte ich mitten in den Schwarm hinein, versuchte, mir noch mehr unserer Gegner zu schnappen. Doch die Fische wichen mir aus wie Quecksilber, das um mich herumfloss, es war unheimlich schwer, sie zu fassen zu bekommen.

Aber am meisten hemmte mich, dass ich mich nicht traute zuzubeißen. Was war, wenn ich dabei einen Seawalker erwischte? Auf keinen Fall wollte ich zum Mörder werden! Umgekehrt hatten die Barrakudas leider keinerlei Skrupel, *uns* fertigzumachen.

Johnny erging es am schlimmsten, er war kein schneller

Schwimmer und unsere Angreifer passten nicht in sein Maul. Die Barrakudas griffen ihn von mehreren Seiten an. *Bin gleich bei dir!*, rief ich und wollte abtauchen, um ihn zu schützen, während im selben Moment irgendein Mistkerl versuchte, mir ein Stück aus der Schwanzflosse herauszubeißen. Ich klatschte ihn weg.

Doch jemand kam mir bei Johnny zuvor.

Shari bewegte sich graziös wie eine Fechterin, als sie Barrakudas von Johnny abdrängte, quer ins Maul nahm oder mit der Schwanzflosse verdrosch. Sie drehte sich um ihre eigene Achse, schoss nach oben und unten, und das alles unglaublich präzise. Wer einmal ihre Zähne zu spüren bekommen hatte, kam nicht so schnell wieder.

Ich hörte erst mal auf, mir Sorgen um sie und Johnny zu machen, und versuchte, mich selbst freizukämpfen. Aber superschnelle Manöver waren nichts für meinen Tigerhaikörper und ich bekam immer mehr Bisse ab. Nicht alle drangen durch meine dicke Haut, aber meine Flossen taten inzwischen verdammt weh und im Wasser waren immer mehr wolkige Blutschlieren. Noch immer warfen sich uns die Barrakudas entgegen wie ein nie endender Strom von zappelndem, schnappendem Silber.

Mr Williams schaute zufrieden zu, hin und wieder sah ich ihn am Rand des Schwarms patrouillieren und seine Verbündeten anfeuern. Jedes Mal, wenn ich wütend losschoss und versuchte, ihn zu packen, wendeten dreißig pfeilförmige Raubfische alle gleichzeitig und machten vor mir die Mauer. Mein Feind gluckste amüsiert.

Mir fiel unser Tiefwasserlehrgang ein. Die Raubfische hatten den Fischschwarm nach oben gedrängt und ihn gezwungen, sich zu einer Kugel zusammenzuziehen – so hatten sie ihn unter Kontrolle bekommen!

Wir müssen versuchen, einen Köderball aus ihnen zu machen!, schrie ich Shari zu und jagte um den Schwarm herum, als wäre er eine Schafherde, die ich hüten musste.

Shari begriff sofort, schwamm unter die Barrakudas und versuchte, sie nach oben zu drängen. Doch diese Tiere waren keine panischen Schwarmfischchen, sie waren eine Armee aus silbernen Torpedos. Und wir waren nur zu zweit – wie sich herausstellte, waren das viel zu wenige Teilnehmer, um einen Köderball zu formen.

Stanley Williams erteilte einen unhörbaren Befehl und plötzlich drängten drei Dutzend Barrakudas *uns* in eine bestimmte Richtung – nach unten, zum Meeresboden. Was sollte das? Mit einem kräftigen Biss erledigte ich einen Barrakuda, von dem ich sicher war, dass er ein Fisch war, doch das beeindruckte die anderen kaum, sie stoben nur kurz einen Meter zur Seite. Dann waren schon wieder ein paar Hundert drohend blickende Raubfische über uns und zwangen uns, tiefer zu gehen.

Ich glaube, die wollen mich daran hindern, dass ich zum Atmen hochkommen kann!, rief Shari und ich war sicher, dass sie recht hatte.

Meine Delfinfreundin versuchte, die Fische über ihr aus dem Weg zu rammen, doch der Schwarm reagierte mit einem gemeinsamen Angriff. Hunderte Mäuler mit Tausenden von Nadelzähnen schnappten nach ihr. Mit einem schrillen Pfiff drehte Shari ab und tauchte wieder nach unten, wo der Schwarm uns in Ruhe ließ. Ich folgte ihr, blieb beruhigend an ihrer Seite. *Die werden das nicht ewig weitermachen,* sagte ich, glaubte aber selbst nicht daran.

Hoffentlich ... wenn ich aufgeregt bin, muss ich öfter atmen als sonst. Shari versuchte, mit einem blitzartigen Sprint seitlich an den Barrakudas vorbeizukommen. Leider waren die noch schneller, schnitten ihr den Weg ab.

Besorgt sah ich, dass Shari immer nervöser wurde. *Luft ... ich brauche Luft!*

Wir kriegen das irgendwie hin, sagte ich hilflos – was man halt so sagt, wenn man keine Ahnung hat, was man tun soll. Meine Angst um Shari legte sich wie eine dicke schwarze Gummihülle um mein Gehirn und hinderte mich komplett am Denken.

Aber dann echote wieder dieser Song in meinem Kopf, stachelte mich an. *Do you believe you can walk on water? Do you believe that you win this fight tonight?*

Einen Moment lang schmolz meine Angst weg. Ja verdammt, ich konnte diesen Kampf gewinnen – schließlich war ich eins der gefährlichsten Meerestiere überhaupt!

Wir brechen durch!, schrie ich meiner Freundin zu und spannte alle Muskeln an. Mit peitschender Schwanzflosse, mit der ich den einen oder anderen Gegner k. o. schlug, umkreiste ich Shari und biss dabei um mich, hielt unsere Feinde auf Abstand. Pfeilgerade schoss meine Delfinfreundin in dieser Schutzzone nach oben ... und durchbrach die Oberfläche! Erleichtert schnaufte Shari die Meeresluft ein, während ich sie von unten abschirmte.

Ein Problem gelöst, ein paar Hundert übrig.

Wie rasend fielen die Barrakudas über uns her, bis Mr Williams anscheinend eine kurze Pause befahl, damit sich der Schwarm sammeln konnte.

Bist du schlimm verletzt, Tiago? Diesmal war Shari es, die mich umkreiste und dabei genauer in Augenschein nahm. *Wir müssen abhauen, solange es noch geht!*

Eben hatten sich mehrere Barrakudas gleichzeitig in meine Rückenflosse verbissen und die hatte sich schon vorher angefühlt, als hätten sich eine Gruppe von irren Tätowierern daran zu schaffen gemacht. Schmerzen durchzogen meinen ganzen Körper und erschüttert sah ich, dass auch Shari verletzt war, sie blutete aus mehreren Wunden an Rücken, Schwanz und Flossen. Sofort hasste ich die Lennox und Mr Williams noch tausendmal mehr.

Ja, es hat keinen Sinn – Rückzug!, rief ich meinen Freunden zu.

Wir hatten verloren und damit gab es keine Hoffnung mehr für die drei gefangenen Haie. Die Verbrecher hatten gewonnen.

Ich hab gefilmt, was ich konnte, meldete sich Maris, der anscheinend zurückgekehrt war. *Aber von oben sieht man leider nicht viel von dem, was da unten bei euch abgeht. Seid ihr in Ordnung?*

Nicht wirklich!, rief ich zurück – immerhin, jetzt musste ich nicht mehr flüstern.

Während ich wendete, um abzuhauen, warf ich einen Blick zum Netzkäfig hinüber ... und stellte fest, dass der Taucher vor Mrs Misaki geflohen war und die Muräne sich gerade mit blitzenden schwarzen Knopfaugen durch die Maschen des Netzes wand. Oh ja, Verstärkung, die brauchten wir dringend!

Bevor es sich der große Barrakuda versah, hatte er Gesellschaft. Sehr schlecht gelaunte Gesellschaft! Mrs Misaki schwamm unserem ehemaligen Schulleiter in den Weg, wand sich mit ihrem schlangenartigen Körper um ihn herum und grub ihm die Zähne in den Rücken, um ihn festzuhalten.

Jetzt sind Sie dran, Williams – mit Ihnen habe ich noch ein paar Schuppen zu rupfen!, kreischte Mrs Misaki. *Sie haben meine Kaffeemaschine verstellt! Meine Akten umorganisiert! Und meinen Preis für die beste Schulsekretärin weggeworfen! Das – werde – ich – Ihnen – niemals – verzeihen!*

Zu jedem Wort gab es einen kräftigen Biss gratis dazu. Fasziniert beobachtete das alles der Barrakudaschwarm.

Ihr Preis hat entsetzlich gestunken!, protestierte Mr Williams hilflos.

Was geht Sie das an, was in unserer Schule wie riecht!, tobte unsere Schulsekretärin. *Nimm dies! Und dies, Mistkerl!*

Mr Williams versuchte, mit Barrakudatempo wegzuschießen, doch immer wieder schnappte die Muräne nach ihm, hielt ihn mit den Zähnen fest und hinderte ihn an der Flucht. *Übrigens, die Rechnung für alles, was Sie bei uns beschädigt oder zerstört haben, habe ich schon an Ihr Büro geschickt! 3.250 Dollar und 66 Cent inklusive Mehrwertsteuer!*

Dann ließ sie ihn los. Eine Millisekunde später sahen wir unseren ehemaligen Schulleiter nur noch von hinten. Er düste in Rekordgeschwindigkeit ab und es sah nicht so aus, als würde er noch mal wiederkommen. Der Schwarm der kleineren Barrakudas verlor sofort das Interesse an uns und folgte ihm. Kurz darauf war das Meer wieder blau und friedlich wie zuvor.

Bei der großen Strömung!, rief Shari.

Das wollte ich auch gerade sagen, schnaufte ich.

He, Leute, die Polizei ist unterwegs, wir können sie schon sehen, meldete uns Maris aus der Luft. *Aber das Schiff fährt schon die Maschinen hoch. Die könnten es noch schaffen abzuhauen ...*

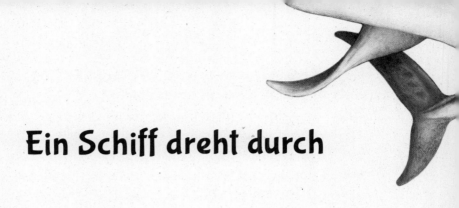

Ein Schiff dreht durch

Die Gangster durften es nicht schaffen abzuhauen – diesmal nicht! Sofort tauchten Shari, Johnny und ich auf, um uns die Sache genauer anzusehen.

Über uns hing der Rumpf des Glasbodenschiffs, daneben sahen wir die dunklen Umrisse der anderen Jachten und Motorboote. Auch von denen machten sich schon ein paar aus dem Staub, ich sah, wie ihre starken Außenborder das Wasser zu einem weißen Wirbel durchquirlten. Maschinenlärm pulsierte durchs Meer.

Keine Panik, das Polizeiboot wird ihnen den Weg abschneiden, beruhigte uns Johnny. Doch als wir die Oberfläche erreichten, sahen wir verblüfft, dass kein Polizeiboot in Sicht war. Nur zwei Streifenwagen, die an Land vorgefahren waren. Gerade waren ein paar Beamte dabei, auszusteigen und zu den Booten hinüberzustarren.

Was soll das? Die haben doch keine Chance, hier irgendjemanden zu verhaften, regte sich Johnny auf. *Hinschwimmen werden sie in voller Uniform garantiert nicht.*

Shari klatschte empört mit der Schwanzflosse aufs Wasser und bei mir bahnte sich ein Wutanfall der Extraklasse an. *Sind die denn alle bescheuert? Die dürfen die Lennox nicht davonkommen lassen!*

Mit einem Gefühl, als hätte ich ein Kilo Pfeffer gegessen, beobachtete ich, wie die beiden großen Propeller am Heck des Glasbodenschiffs zu wirbeln begannen.

Aber das Ding fuhr nicht aufs offene Meer zu.

Stattdessen drehte es durch.

Es bewegte sich Richtung Küste, bremste ab, versuchte zu wenden und krachte stattdessen in ein mit Mangroven bewachsenes Inselchen. Nachdem es dort jede Menge Zweige geknickt hatte, fuhr es nach links und stieß mit einem schicken blau lackierten Rennboot zusammen, das gerade so richtig beschleunigen wollte. Das fiel danach leider aus. Mit einer Riesendelle im Rumpf sollte man lieber Schritttempo fahren.

Noch einmal drehte sich das Glasbodenschiff und diesmal musste eins der kleineren Fahrzeuge dran glauben. Schräg hing es im Meer, als hätte es sich am falschen Sprit besoffen, während die schick gekleideten Leute darin übereinanderfielen.

Chaos! Überall Leute, die fluchten, wild gestikulierten, Anweisungen schrien oder über Bord plumpsten. Staunend beobachteten die Polizisten, wie das Schiff vor ihnen herummanövrierte und mit seinen Positionslichtern blinkte, als wäre es ein Disco-Kahn.

Was bei allen sieben Weltmeeren ..., begann Johnny, doch Rockets Gedankenstimme unterbrach ihn. *Hübsch, was? Ich hab bei der Steueranlage ein paar Kabel vertauscht. Rechts und links, Schub nach vorne und nach hinten. Und so weiter.*

Hammer-Idee! Shari und ich genossen den Anblick aus vollen Zügen.

Aber was war, wenn der Kapitän kapierte, was passiert war, und es fertigbrachte, sich darauf einzustellen? Dann konnte er es doch noch schaffen.

Nein, konnte er nicht. Denn gerade war im Meer jenseits

von uns ein sehr, sehr großes Hindernis aufgetaucht, das den Booten den Weg abschnitt und dem großen Schiff den Weg zum offenen Meer blockierte. Ich sah einen dunkelgrauen Rücken und die dunstige Wolke, als das Geschöpf ausatmete. Ein Buckelwal hatte sich in die flachen Küstengewässer der Keys gewagt. Und nicht irgendeiner, wie sich herausstellte.

Hallo, Leute – alles wässrig?, begrüßte uns Wave.

Aber hallo, antwortete ich. Als der Kapitän seinen nächsten Versuch startete davonzukommen, fuhr er nämlich mit viel Schwung rückwärts ... und setzte sein Schiff zehn Meter vom Strand entfernt auf Grund. Schlammiges Wasser wirbelte auf, als er vergeblich versuchte, es wieder flottzumachen.

Grinsend wateten die Polizisten los, um es zu entern und sich wahrscheinlich erst mal den Bootsführerschein zeigen zu lassen. Danach würden sie garantiert die Harpunen der Taucher beschlagnahmen und sich die Namen der Gäste notieren, denen das hoffentlich sehr peinlich war. An einer unauffälligen Stelle sprang eine kleine graubraune Ratte über Bord und paddelte an Land, was außer mir niemand bemerkte.

Maris, hast du das alles gefilmt?, rief ich nach oben.

Alles drauf, bestätigte unser Albatros. *Könnte man gleich so auf YouTube stellen!*

Das war leider nicht der Sinn der Sache. Wir brauchten Beweise! Hatten wir diesmal genug gesammelt? Hoffentlich.

Johnny teilverwandelte sich, um die Netzkäfige öffnen zu können, und die drei gefangenen Haie kapierten schnell, dass sie frei waren. Ohne einen einzigen Blick zurück hauten sie ab, obwohl das Wasser immer noch sehr appetitlich nach Blut roch.

Während Shari schaute, ob mit Rocket alles in Ordnung war, schwamm ich kurz neben Wave, der gerade ausprobierte, was passierte, wenn man ein kleines Motorboot mit Haikampf-Zuschauern mit der Schnauze anstupste. Was passierte, war: a) Im Inneren wurde es laut, b) Wasser schwappte hinein.

Hast du dich wieder erholt?, fragte ich ihn.

Ja – ich bin zurückgekommen, um euch was zu sagen, meinte er. *Im Gefängnis durfte ich manchmal mit den anderen Leuten dort zusammen essen und hab zugehört, was die so reden.*

Und? Noch war ich gut gelaunt.

Zwei von ihnen waren auch Wandler, keine Ahnung, was für welche. Der eine hat damit geprahlt, dass Woodwalker und Seawalker die besten Verbrechen begehen, weil sie mehr können als Menschen.

Oh, sagte ich betroffen.

Bist du ganz sicher?, fragte Johnny nach.

Ja. Und am praktischsten, hat der andere gesagt, seien diese Kids von dieser komischen Schule in Key Largo.

Dazu fiel auch Johnny nichts ein und mir auch nur ein *WAS?*. Es gab nur eine Schule für Wandler in Florida, und zwar unsere. Die war in Key Largo. Keine Verwechslung möglich.

Keine Ahnung, was das bedeuten sollte, meinte Wave, der inzwischen das Interesse an den Booten verloren hatte. *Dachte, ich sag's euch mal. Nur zur Sicherheit. Schwimm gut, schwimm weit!*

Mit einem lässigen Heben der Brustflosse machte er sich wieder auf den Weg.

Sollten wir überprüfen, sagte Johnny.

Ich war ziemlich durcheinander. *... und den Lehrern erzählen?*

Vielleicht besser erst mal nachforschen, meinte mein Erziehungsberechtigter.

Dann war es allmählich Zeit, dass wir uns an einer versteckten Stelle verwandelten. Es war ein bisschen kompliziert, an unsere Klamotten heranzukommen und ins Auto zu klettern, ohne dass auch wir von der Polizei befragt wurden, aber irgendwie klappte es. Ausgepowert, aber zufrieden, kehrten wir in die Blue Reef Highschool zurück und ließen uns dort von Miss White, Jack Clearwater und seiner Mutter, die beide kurz vor dem Flughafen umgekehrt waren, verarzten. Noah und Blue umarmten Shari und mich so fest, dass sie uns fast erdrückten, und berührten unsere Nasen im *hongi*-Gruß. Blue war den Tränen nahe. »Wir haben dich an der falschen Stelle gesucht – wie gut, dass ihr halbwegs okay seid.«

Wir hinkten zum Anlegesteg, als wir einen Bootsmotor hörten. Mrs Misaki saß allein im *Zodiac;* sie sah in ihrem gelben Kleid fast genauso aus wie zuvor, nur ihre Hochsteckfrisur zierten ein paar Salzkrüstchen. Als wäre nichts passiert, kletterte sie auf den Anlegesteg, während wir ihr halfen, das Schlauchboot festzumachen.

»Sie waren einfach meerig, Mrs Misaki«, schwärmte Shari.

»Ohne Sie hätten wir diese Barrakudas nicht geschafft«, bekräftigte ich. »Sie sind wirklich die beste Schulsekretärin in Südflorida!«

»Lieb von euch.« Mrs Misakis Lächeln sah ein bisschen aus wie ein Zähnefletschen, vielleicht war die Muräne noch stark in ihr, wie die Leute in *Star Wars* garantiert gesagt hätten. »Aber wer hat denn diese schlampigen Verbände gemacht – furchtbar!«

»Ich«, gab Lissa Clearwater zu. »Wir haben eine eigene Krankenschwester in der Schule, deshalb bin ich außer Übung.«

»Die sitzen viel zu locker! Los, los, ab in die Krankenstation, das verbinden wir jetzt mal alles neu.«

»Viel Spaß«, wünschte uns Rocket grinsend.

Kurz darauf hatten wir wunderschöne blütenweiße Verbände ... die genauso aussahen wie die vorher.

Während wir darauf warteten, dass Ella eintrudelte, sichteten wir in Mr Clearwaters Büro die Aufnahmen, die Maris gemacht hatte. Meine bandagierten Hände zitterten vor Aufregung, als ich dabei half, die Daten auf den Laptop der Schule zu überspielen. Schließlich schubste mich Rocket weg, nachdem ich zweimal mit steifen Fingern danebengetippt hatte, und übernahm das Ganze selbst.

Wir beugten uns alle gespannt vor, als Bilder über den Schirm zu flimmern begannen.

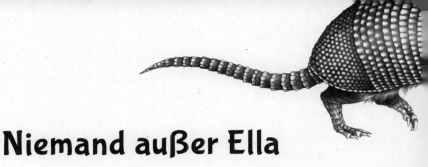

Niemand außer Ella

»Das ist richtig gutes Zeug«, sagte Jasper ehrfürchtig, während er auf den Bildschirm des Laptops starrte.

Auf dem Film sah man deutlich die drei Haie in den Netzkäfigen und wie der Taucher mit Harpune auf einen von ihnen zuschwamm, während gut gelaunte Zuschauer alles beobachteten.

»Es ist jedenfalls eindeutig, was da gelaufen ist«, meinte Miss Clearwater und Miss White nickte grimmig.

Inzwischen war auch Mr García zur kleinen »Filmvorführung« hinzugekommen und hatte sich erklären lassen, was Shari, Johnny und ich erlebt hatten.

»Unglaublich«, sagte er wütend. »Ich zeige diesen Stanley Williams sofort beim Rat an. Das war gefährliche Körperverletzung – mindestens! – und wir haben reichlich Zeugen diesmal, auch erwachsene.« Er nickte Onkel Johnny zu. Dann ließ er nachdenklich den Blick über die Gäste an Bord schweifen. »Na, so was, da sind ein paar Promis dabei. Ich glaube, das Material gebe ich gleich mal einem Bekannten von mir weiter, der beim *Miami Herald* arbeitet.«

»Gute Idee«, sagte unser Schulleiter. »Du könntest behaupten, eine Drohne hat den Film aufgenommen.«

Auch Mrs Lennox war kurz an Deck zu sehen, doch dann sahen wir sie misstrauisch hochblicken und im Bauch des Schiffs verschwinden. Wahrscheinlich hatte sie Maris bemerkt und gecheckt, dass er spionierte.

»Kein echter Beweis gegen sie«, sagte ich knapp und die Enttäuschung schmeckte gallebitter. »Das heißt, sie kann sich wieder rausreden. Obwohl diesmal eindeutig sie das Ganze geleitet hat, die Wächter haben sie immerhin ›Chefin‹ genannt. Mr Bittergreen war gar nicht da. Wahrscheinlich haben die beiden sich die Gewinne geteilt.«

»Du meinst wirklich, sie *arbeitet mit* in seiner Verbrecherorganisation?« Shari hatte ganz große, erschrockene Augen.

»Sieht fast so aus, oder?«, antwortete Miss White.

»Wenn Ella gefilmt hätte ...«, meinte ich verbittert. Die anderen sagten nichts dazu, aber ich sah ihnen am Gesicht an, dass sie das Gleiche dachten.

Jemand klopfte an. Es war Barry, wie sich herausstellte. Er blickte sehr erleichtert drein, als er sah, dass Shari und ich noch lebten.

»Wusstet du, was dein Dad vorhat?«, fragte ich ihn, während die Wut in meinem Inneren tobte wie ein kleiner, eingesperrter Teufel, der ganz dringend rauswollte. Aber Miss White stand neben mir, stärkte mir wortlos den Rücken. Ich würde es schaffen, nicht auszurasten, ganz sicher.

»Nicht genau.« Barrys Stimme hatte jede Betonung verloren. »Aber er hat mich gefragt, ob ich bei einer Verteidigungsaktion mitmachen würde. Ich hab Nein gesagt. Mein Vater hat hier so viel Mist gebaut, ich habe im Moment überhaupt keine Lust, etwas für ihn zu machen.«

»Gut«, sagte Mr Clearwater nur. »Damit hast du dir eindeutig Ärger erspart.«

»Was ist denn genau passiert?«, wollte Barry wissen.

»Ein Schwarm Barrakudas hat uns daran gehindert, einen

Hai zu befreien.« Ich hob meine verbundenen Hände, die noch vor Kurzem Flossen gewesen waren.

»Wow, cool«, sagte Barry und grinste – mein Freund war er immer noch nicht.

»Raus!«, schnauzte Miss White ihn an und unser Barrakudamitschüler zog ab.

Es dauerte noch eine weitere Stunde, bis unsere Python-Wandlerin Ella eintrudelte – ein Motorboot setzte sie bei uns an einem der Anlegestege ab und entfernte sich dann gleich wieder. Am Steg erwartete sie schon ein kleines Empfangskomitee. »Kommst du bitte in mein Büro, Ella?«, bat sie Mr Clearwater.

»Muss das sein, ich bin total müde und …«

Miss White bedachte sie mit einem stahlharten Blick und Ella hörte auf zu diskutieren. Im Büro legte unsere junge Kampflehrerin sofort mit den Fragen los. »Deine Mutter hat diese Kämpfe diesmal geleitet, oder?«

»Woher soll ich das denn wissen?« Ellas Miene war trotzig.

»Du hast mit ihr diskutiert«, stieß ich hervor.

»Ja und? Da ging es um mein Taschengeld.«

Das nahm ihr natürlich keiner ab.

»Mrs Misaki hat gesagt, du hast dein Handy dabeigehabt. Hast du damit was aufgenommen?«

»Nö … so viel gab's schließlich auch nicht zu sehen.« Ellas Blick wandte sich mir zu. »Nur Tiago, der sich mal wieder zum Deppen gemacht hat.«

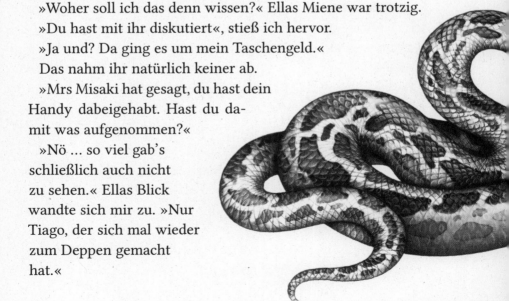

Miss White und Shari warfen mir einen besorgten Blick zu. Natürlich befürchteten die beiden Sorgen, dass ich gleich hochgehen würde wie eine Ladung TNT.

Aber sie hätten sich keine Sorgen machen müssen. Ich war viel zu verblüfft.

Manchmal spürt man, wenn jemand die Wahrheit sagt. Und manchmal hat man das deutliche Gefühl, das Gegenteil ist der Fall.

Ella hatte uns gerade angelogen.

Aber mir war klar, dass sie in diesem Raum, vor all diesen Leuten, wahrscheinlich nie zugeben würde, was sie wirklich gesagt und getan hatte. Ich musste jemanden, dem sie vertraute, dazu bringen, dass er mit ihr sprach!

Mir fiel sogar jemand ein. »Sorry, muss kurz wohin«, entschuldigte ich mich. Kaum war ich draußen aus Mr Clearwaters Büro, rannte ich los ... und machte mich auf die Suche nach Carmen.

Natürlich war sie mit Barry und Toco zusammen. »Äh, kann ich dich kurz sprechen, Carmen?«, fragte ich, während die beiden anderen mich düster musterten.

»Wieso?«

Besonders freundlich klang das nicht. »Hai-Angelegenheiten«, erklärte ich.

Carmen seufzte, nickte und ließ sich von mir in ein leeres Klassenzimmer führen, wo ich ihr alles erklärte.

»Ich soll Barry sagen, er soll Ella sagen, sie soll ihm sagen, ob sie wirklich keine Aufnahmen gemacht hat?«, wiederholte unsere Hammerhai-Wandlerin.

»Bitte«, sagte ich.

Ich hatte vieles erwartet, aber nicht das sofortige »Na gut« von Carmen. Sie lächelte sogar ein kleines bisschen. »Mach ich. Immerhin hast du geholfen, mich aus meiner Hütte zu schleppen. Du weißt schon. Bei meiner Verwandlungspanne in der Nacht. Dafür hattest du noch was gut. Jetzt aber nicht mehr, klar?«

»Klar«, sagte ich. »Und könnte ich vielleicht dabei zuhören? Du weißt schon, wenn Barry Ella fragt?«

»Sonst noch was? Soll ich dir noch ein Date mit einem Albino-Walhai besorgen?«

Ich zuckte mit keiner Wimper. »Wenn du das schaffst? Ich mag Walhaie.«

»Boah, du nervst«, sagte Carmen.

Zufrieden ging ich zurück zu den anderen, ohne ihnen zu verraten, was ich gerade in Bewegung gesetzt hatte.

Carmen hielt ihr Versprechen und überredete Barry. Kurze Zeit später war es so weit. Inzwischen war es tiefste Nacht und Johnny schlief in einer der Gästehütten, weil er so spät nicht mehr losfahren wollte nach Miami. Ich lag im Gestrüpp, das den Süßwassersee umgab und fühlte, wie sumpfiges Wasser langsam meine Klamotten durchtränkte. Ungefähr drei Dutzend Moskitos zeigten ein ungesundes Interesse an meinen Waden. Aber ich rührte mich keinen Millimeter, denn gerade kamen die richtig interessanten Sachen zur Sprache.

»Hast du gewusst, dass deine Mutter da sein würde?«, brummte Toco. »Hat sie dich vielleicht sogar eingeladen, bei diesem Haiklatschen dabei zu sein?«

»Hat sie nicht, aber ich hab mir schon gedacht, dass sie da sein würde.« Ella klang nicht besonders gut gelaunt. »Ich hab ihr erklärt, dass solche Kämpfe total daneben sind. Aber sie hat's leider gar nicht eingesehen und mich gefragt, was ich meine, woher die Kohle für mein Gucci-Täschchen kommen würde.«

»Blöd«, beklagte sich Toco.

»Ja! Besonders weil sie mir letztes Mal beteuert hat, sie wäre nur zufällig auf dem Schiff gewesen. Das war einfach nicht wahr!« Mürrisch zerpflückte Ella ein Blatt.

»Sag mal ... hast du nicht doch ein paar Fotos gemacht?«, fragte Barry wie vereinbart.

»Hab ich nicht. Die hätten mich sofort an Land geschafft und ich hätte nicht mehr mit Mom reden können. ABER ...« Ella grinste. »Ich hab an meinem Handy in meiner Tasche den Knopf der Aufnahme-App gedrückt. Das Bild ist natürlich die ganze Zeit schwarz, aber man hört uns sehr gut reden.«

Schockiertes Schweigen bei ihren Freunden, lautloser Jubel bei mir. Ich hatte richtig geraten!

»Was willst du machen?«, fragte Barry, er klang beeindruckt. »Damit zur Polizei gehen?«

»Ich hab echt lange drüber nachgedacht«, berichtete Ella. »Nein, zu den Bullen gehe ich nicht. Sondern woandershin.«

Ein Traum wird wahr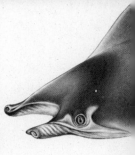

»**U**nd? Zu wem wirst du gehen mit der Tonaufnahme von deiner Mutter?« Toco hielt es vor Spannung kaum noch aus.

»Zu meiner Mom«, sagte Ella. »Die kann ruhig wissen, dass ich die Aufnahme habe. Ich will, dass sie mit diesem Scheiß aufhört. Ja, ich mag Tiago auch nicht, aber das mit diesen Tauchern und den Harpunen ist wirklich ekelhaft.«

Wow. Ich war tief beeindruckt. Ella sammelte so schnell Sympathiepunkte, dass ich kaum mit dem Registrieren nachkam.

»Krasse Idee«, murmelte Barry. »Vielleicht sollte ich meinen Vater auch mal erpressen. Damit er deiner Mom nicht jeden bescheuerten Wunsch von den Lippen abliest.«

Ella grinste. »Mach das. Ist 'n Versuch wert. Ich find gut, dass du nicht mehr versuchst, es ihm recht zu machen.«

Zum Glück gingen sie und ihre Kumpane bald darauf ins Bett. Sehr viel später, als wirklich niemand mehr wach war in unserer Süßwasserzone, stand ich sumpfverschmiert und zerstochen auf und ging direkt unter die Dusche in unserer Hütte. Mit Klamotten.

In meinem Kopf waren jede Menge schwarze Gedanken, die auch tausend Liter Wasser nicht weggespült hätten. Waren meine Eltern so viel besser als die von Barry und Ella? Immerhin hatten sie sich vierzehn Jahre lang nicht bei mir gemeldet und mit ihrer kühlen Art kam ich immer noch nicht klar.

Immerhin war es nett gewesen, dass sie uns mit Waves Kaution ausgeholfen hatten. Ob sie ihr Versprechen halten und mich besuchen würden? Eins war klar, ich würde sie nicht erpressen, damit sie sich mit mir trafen!

Am nächsten Morgen frühstückten alle Schüler, die übers Wochenende in der Schule blieben, als sei überhaupt nichts passiert. Das fühlte sich irgendwie seltsam an. Immerhin waren Shari, Johnny und ich in wirklich ernster Gefahr gewesen.

Ella wirkte entspannt, war aber ziemlich blass. Ob sie schon mit ihrer Mutter gesprochen hatte? Ohne mich zu beachten, ging unser Python-Girl mit ihrem gefüllten Teller an mir vorbei.

»Danke«, sagte ich zu ihr.

Ella hob den Kopf, ihre grünen Augen musterten mich finster. »Wofür?«

»Du weißt, warum«, meinte ich.

Sie sagte nichts, doch ihr Gesichtsausdruck wurde etwas entspannter ... aber auch trauriger, weil sie garantiert an die bittere Diskussion mit ihrer Mutter dachte.

Wir nickten uns zu, dann ging ich zu Johnny hinüber, der am Lehrertisch saß; wir wollten zusammen mit Rocket endlich aufbrechen nach Miami. Shari schlenderte neben mir her. Ihre Delfinfreunde waren übers Wochenende bei Noahs Eltern, nur Shari hatte – Sensation! – gesagt, dass sie lieber bei mir bleiben wollte. Jedes Mal, wenn ich daran dachte, war ich auf Wolke zehn. Mindestens.

Es klingelte an der Eingangstür der Schule. Verblüfft hörten alle auf zu essen. Mr Clearwater ließ den Löffel sinken, den er gerade in sein Porridge mit braunem Zucker hatte tauchen wollen. Er und seine Mutter tauschten einen Blick. »Erwartest du einen Gast?«

Unser Schulleiter schüttelte den Kopf, stand auf und ging durch die Aula zur Tür.

Eine Art Blitz aus Freude und Hoffnung durchzuckte mich. Vielleicht waren das meine Eltern, die nur vergessen hatten, Bescheid zu sagen?

Ich war so ein Depp. Was sollte diese blöde Hoffnung jedes Mal? Sie waren es natürlich nicht. Total überraschend. Zum Glück war es auch nicht Lydia Lennox. Hätte ja sein können.

Dafür war es ein anderer besonderer Gast, mit dem Jack Clearwater zurückkam. Ich erkannte das Mädchen mit den dunklen Locken und den Sommersprossen sofort und schickte ihr ein Willkommenslächeln. Es war Daisy Cousteau, die wir auf der Highschool kennengelernt hatten. Erleichtert sah ich, dass es ihr gut zu gehen schien, sie war sonniger Laune. Also keine ungeplante Verwandlung, bei der sie irgendwo als Fisch auf einem Teppich gelandet war. Gott sei Dank!

Daisy sah fröhlich, aber auch sehr entschlossen aus, als sie mit beiden Händen die Räder ihres Rollstuhls voranbewegte. Zum Glück war sie diesmal ohne Betreuerin gekommen.

Als sie Shari und mich bemerkte, lächelte sie uns zu. »Hi, schön, euch wiederzusehen! Sorry, ich konnte nicht früher kommen, meine Mutter ist eine unglaubliche Klette. Habt ihr jetzt Zeit, um mir zu helfen ... äh ... oder hab ich das alles nur geträumt?« Sie blickte Lissa Clearwater an. »Es ist so krass, in meinem Traum haben Sie sich in einen Adler verwandelt!«

Miss Clearwater warf den anderen Lehrern einen Ich-übernehm-das-Blick zu. »Zeit zu sehen, in was *du* dich verwandeln kannst.«

»Es war also nicht ...«

»Nein. Komm, wir gehen an den Strand, für den Fall, dass

deine zweite Gestalt dringend ins Wasser muss. Shari, Tiago und Toco, kommt ihr?«

Toco – der die Wochenenden fast immer in der Schule verbrachte – sprang auf, als hätte er auf Sprungfedern gesessen. Ohne einen Blick zu seinen Kumpels begleitete er uns zum Strand. Es war ein bisschen mühsam für Daisy, sich mit dem Rollstuhl durch den Sand zu bewegen, und ich sah, wie sie sich auf die Lippe biss, während sie sich abmühte. »Darf ich?«, fragte Toco und streckte die Hand nach den Griffen an der Rückseite des Rollstuhls aus.

»Na gut, danke«, gab Daisy nach und Toco schob sie an.

Lissa Clearwater ließ uns nah zum Wasser gehen, Shari watete sogar bis zur Hüfte ins Meer hinein und schien nicht mal zu bemerken, dass ihr Shorts und T-Shirt klatschnass am Körper hingen. »Was jetzt? Soll sie jetzt einen Tieratlas durchschauen oder so was?«, fragte Daisy gespannt.

»Später vielleicht.« Lissa studierte Daisys Gesicht, betrachtete ihre feinknochigen Hände, musterte ihre ganze Gestalt. »Hast du schon mal ein Kribbeln gespürt, als du ein bestimmtes Tier gesehen hast?«

»Klar, schon oft«, sagte Daisy und wir holten überrascht Luft. »Es kribbelt fast immer in mir, wenn ich mit Mom und Dad am Meer bin ... ich dachte sogar schon, ich bin irgendwie allergisch gegen die Salzluft oder so was!«

Jacks Mutter stutzte. »Überall am Meer? Oder nur hier in Florida?«

»Oh stimmt ... als wir mal zusammen in Irland am Meer waren, habe ich das nicht gespürt.« Daisy überlegte. »Komisch, oder? Woran kann das liegen?«

Vielleicht war sie in zweiter Gestalt ein Fisch, den es nur hier in Florida gab? Ich hoffte so sehr, dass sie dann trotzdem schwimmen konnte. Irgendwie.

»Ich habe schon einen Verdacht.« Lissa lächelte verschmitzt und wandte sich an mich. »Welche Tiere sieht man besonders häufig, wenn man in diesem schönen Staat an den Strand geht?«

»Möwen«, sagte ich sofort. Die waren überall und kackten überallhin. Gerade saßen fünf davon (Daphne nicht mitgezählt) auf dem Dach unseres Bootshauses.

»Pelikane«, sagte Shari und deutete auf einen großen grauen Vogel mit langem Schnabel, der auf einem Pfosten unseres Anlegestegs hockte. Zwei andere schaukelten gerade gemütlich auf dem Wasser unserer Lagune.

Daisy wirkte auf einmal wie eine gespannte Bogenseite. So extrem aufgeregt, wie ich sie noch nie gesehen hatte. »Ihr meint, ich könnte ... ein Vogel sein? Aber dann könnte ich ja vielleicht ...«

»Ja«, brummte Toco, und in seinen Augen war die gleiche gespannte Erwartung.

»Schau dir erst mal die Möwen an«, bat Lissa Clearwater unseren Gast, doch Daisy schüttelte schnell den Kopf. »Kein Kribbeln.«

Dann die Pelikane. Daisy strahlte über das ganze Gesicht, sie atmete schneller, ihre Wangen waren gerötet. »Ja«, sagte sie nur.

Wir wagten noch nicht, begeistert zu sein. Dafür war es zu früh.

»Konzentrier dich auf deine Arme, stell dir vor, es wären Schwingen.« Lissas Stimme klang ruhig und eindringlich, fast hypnotisch. »Es sind große graue Flügel, breit und kräftig. Wenn du damit in die Luft greifst, tragen sie dich nach oben ...«

Daisy schloss die Augen und streckte die Arme aus. Nie hatte ich mich über Federn so gefreut wie über die, die nun aus ihren Händen und an den Außenseiten ihrer Arme sprossen. Eine halbe Stunde später startete Daisy Cousteau zu ihrem ersten Flug. Mühelos glitt sie über die Lagune und ihr lautloser Jubel füllte unsere Köpfe.

Titelseite

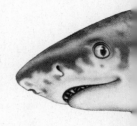

Ein Pelikan war Daisy also! Das war die perfekte zweite Gestalt für sie. Statt zu laufen, konnte sie fliegen. Starten und landen konnte sie auf dem Bauch. Nur als sie versuchte, auf einem Pfahl zu landen wie die anderen Pelikane, landete sie zappelnd im Wasser. *Okay, ich hab's kapiert, meine Beine funktionieren auch als Pelikan nicht,* brummte Daisy, hockte sich aufs Wasser und ließ sich treiben.

Mit den Füßen voranpaddeln kannst du also auch nicht, meinte Miss Clearwater. *Versuch mal, dich mithilfe von Wind und Strömung dorthin zu bewegen, wo du hinwillst.*

Schnell hatte Daisy den Bogen aus. Nun verwandelte sich auch Lissa Clearwater und zeigte ihr als Weißkopf-Seeadler, wie man senkrecht ins Meer hinabstieß, um sich einen Snack zu holen. *Ein eingebauter Einkaufsbeutel, wie cool ist das denn!,* rief Daisy, als ein glückloser Fisch in ihrem Kehlsack zappelte.

Shari, Toco und ich vergaßen die Zeit, während wir auf dem Strand hockten und den beiden zusahen.

Erst viel später konnte Miss Clearwater Daisy überreden, ihre neue Freiheit wieder aufzugeben und in den Rollstuhl zurückzukehren. Ich hätte auch keine Lust gehabt, mich wieder in dieses Ding zu hocken.

»Oje, schon Mittag?« Es klang nicht ganz so deutlich, als Daisy es aussprach, weil sie gerade halb Pelikan und halb

Mensch war. Beinahe wäre ihr Rolli umgekippt, als sie flatternd versuchte, sich wieder darin niederzulassen. »Ich muss zurück, sonst denken meine Eltern, ich wäre tot oder entführt worden oder so was ...«

Als sie wieder im Rollstuhl saß, wirkte sie noch immer überglücklich, aber ich sah, dass ihr etwas Sorgen machte. »Alles okay?«, fragte Shari.

»Wie soll ich das nur Mom und Dad beibringen?« Daisy seufzte. »Ich meine, hallo? Haben euch eure Eltern geglaubt, was ihr seid?«

»Ja – wir sind eine bissige Familie«, sagte ich trocken.

»Meine Eltern sind noch delfinischer als ich«, versicherte ihr Shari.

»Allesamt Gürteltiere!« Jasper reckte stolz das Kinn.

»Vielleicht könnte Jack mal mit deinen Eltern reden«, schlug Lissa Clearwater vor.

Aufgewühlt verließ uns Daisy und ich hoffte, dass wir sie bald wiedersehen würden und sie irgendwann auf die Blue Reef Highschool gehen durfte.

»Es ist nicht so, dass wir es eilig hätten – aber wann schwingst du endlich deinen Hintern zum Auto?«, rief Rocket.

»Moment«, sagte ich und drückte Shari an mich. »Bis Montag. Es könnte sein, dass ich dich bis dahin ziemlich vermisse.«

Es fühlte sich supermutig an, das zu sagen. Meine Belohnung war zwar kein Kuss, aber immerhin ein Lächeln und eine schöne, feste Umarmung. »Für einen Hai hast du echt viele Gefühle«, meinte Shari und blickte mich so neugierig an wie eine Forscherin, die gerade ein seltenes Exemplar entdeckt hat. Nur hatte dieses Exemplar bestimmt keinen so seltsamen Gesichtsausdruck wie ich gerade.

»Oh sorry, das war nicht sehr nett, oder?«, fügte Shari

hinzu. »Was ich eigentlich sagen wollte, du wirst mir auch fehlen!«

Kurz darauf flog Lissa Clearwater zurück zu ihrer eigenen Schule in den Rocky Mountains. Sie hatte sich nun doch entschlossen, auf eigenen Schwingen zurückzufliegen, obwohl es ein weiter Weg war. Sie bekam einen großen Schlussapplaus von uns allen; ohne sie hätten wir es nicht geschafft, diese Krise zu meistern.

Ich machte mich auf den Weg nach Miami. Den Rest des Wochenendes verbrachte ich mit Rocket damit, in seinem nach Kleber stinkenden Zimmer ein aus gefühlt zehn Millionen Teilen bestehendes Raumschiff zusammenzusetzen, mit seiner Oma Sally in einem Feinkostladen stinkenden französischen Käse zu probieren und mir mit Johnny Tischtennisduelle im Garten von Sallys Haus zu liefern. Das war eine nette Abwechslung zu dem, was ich in letzter Zeit so alles getan hatte.

Den großen Knall gab es dann am Montag.

Es gab ihn nicht, als Miss White morgens laufen ging, wie sie es vor ihrem Verschwinden immer getan hatte, oder als Jasper sich versehentlich unter unserer Schranktür einklemmte. Es gab ihn auch nicht, als Finny von ihren Eltern abgeliefert wurde. Im Gegenteil, alle drei wirkten fröhlich und drückten sich zum Abschied. Mit federnden Schritten stürmte Finny herein. »Alle versöhnt! Wir hatten ein supergeniales Wochenende im Meer inklusive Rochen und Walhai! Jetzt, wo alle Bescheid wissen, kommen meine Eltern viel besser miteinander klar, hab ich den Eindruck.«

»Sehr cool«, sagte ich und lächelte ihr zu.

»Das habt ihr wirklich gut gemacht, Leute«, lobte Nick Greyson und klopfte mir und Shari auf die Schultern. »Wir haben übrigens begonnen, entlang der Küste mit Drohnen zu patrouillieren, um solche Arenakämpfe sofort zu entdecken und zu bekämpfen, wenn irgendwo Vorbereitungen getroffen werden. Und ich und meine Kollegen setzen uns dafür ein, dass es strengere Strafen für solche Tierquälereien gibt. Wir haben übrigens Anhaltspunkte, dass Bittergreen und seine Leute mit tatkräftiger Hilfe der Lennox ein ganzes Wett-Imperium betreiben, man kann auf Pferde, auf Boxer, auf Autorennen und alles Mögliche andere setzen. Die Haikämpfe sind nur eine Sparte.«

»Aha«, meinte ich. »Was war mit dieser angeblichen Genehmigung, die die Veranstalter der Haikämpfe hatten?«

»Das war natürlich Bullshit, den diese Lydia Lennox für sich und ihre kriminellen Kumpel fabriziert hat«, berichtete Finnys Vater. »Damit hätten sie Haie erforschen dürfen, aber das haben sie ja offensichtlich nicht getan. Keine Sorge, diese Pseudogenehmigung bewahrt diese Kerle nicht vor Strafe.«

»Danke, Mr Greyson«, sagte Shari feierlich und Finny umarmte ihren Dad gleich noch mal.

Es gab den großen Knall erst, als wir uns ins blau-weiße Tisch-Boot gesetzt hatten. Erst hörten wir einen Wagen draußen auf dem Parkplatz brutal bremsen. Dann stieß jemand die Eingangstüren auf, ohne sich die Mühe zu machen zu klingeln. Es war Lydia Lennox. Sie trug ein weißes Businesskostüm mit türkisfarbener Bluse, eine Perlenkette und hochhackige Pumps. Die schleuderte sie von sich, watete so energisch durch die Cafeteria, dass sie eine Bugwelle bekam, und knallte eine Zeitung auf den Lehrertisch.

»Wer war das?«, donnerte Mrs Lennox.

Nur Miss Bennett sah eingeschüchtert aus. Mr Clearwater hob die Augenbrauen, Mr García verschränkte die Arme und Miss White setzte den Blick auf, mit dem sie schwierige Schüler zu ungefähr einem Drittel ihrer Größe schrumpfte.

Ganz gemächlich hob Mr Clearwater die Zeitung auf – es war ein *Miami Herald* – und betrachtete die Titelseite und das Foto darauf, das aus unserem Albatros-Video stammte. »Knackige Überschrift.«

Wir reckten die Hälse. »*Blutiges Spektakel! Bekannter Fernsehmoderator wettet auf illegale Tierkämpfe*«, entzifferte Juna, die am nächsten dran war. »*Auch weitere prominente Bürger ergötzen sich an Vorführungen, bei denen angeblich schon Tiere zu Tode gequält wurden. Gestern war keiner von ihnen für eine Stellungnahme zu erreichen ...*«

Wow. Ich konnte mir den Shitstorm schon vorstellen.

»Warst du das, Dreckshai?« Mrs Lennox funkelte mich an und mir blieb fast das Herz stehen, weil ich an die Millionen-Dollar-Klage dachte.

»Nein, ich«, mischte sich mein Verwandlungslehrer ein. »Ich habe mir erlaubt, einem Journalistenfreund einen kleinen Tipp zu geben.«

»Hat es nicht gereicht, dass das verdammte Schiff einen Totalschaden davontrug und außerdem beschlagnahmt worden ist?«, giftete Ellas Mutter ihn und Mr Clearwater an. »Auf all diesen Kosten bleiben wir sitzen, und dazu noch dieser Umsatzeinbruch!«

Sie versuchte nicht mal, so zu tun, als hätte sie mit den Kämpfen nichts zu tun. Interessant – sie hatte von »wir« gesprochen. Vermutlich waren Bittergreen und sie ein Team.

Finny grinste. »Klingt toll«, sagte sie. »Wünsche ans Universum funktionieren also doch! Ich hab mir nämlich gewünscht, dass sich kein Kunde mehr zu Ihnen verirrt.«

Mir ging etwas ganz Ähnliches durch den Kopf, also begann ich zu applaudieren ... und immer mehr Schüler stimmten ein. Ella applaudierte nicht mit, schwieg aber mürrisch, statt ihre Mutter zu verteidigen. Dafür bekam sie statt der gewohnten Luftküsschen einen harten Blick, der nichts Gutes verhieß. »Wir sprechen uns noch, junge Dame – wirklich unglaublich, wie du dich gerade mir gegenüber verhältst!«, zischte Lydia Lennox, watete zum Eingang, zerrte sich die Pumps zurück an die Füße und stürmte hinaus. Anscheinend hatte Ella sie tatsächlich mit der Tonaufnahme erpresst.

»Übrigens habe ich Nachricht vom Rat bekommen«, sagte Farryn García in die Stille hinein. »Mr Williams wird mindestens drei Monate in einem Aquarium bekommen, das der Rat als Gefängnis betreibt. Ohne Bewährung, weil er schon öfter negativ aufgefallen ist.«

Diesmal fiel der Applaus doppelt so laut aus.

Eine bissige Familie

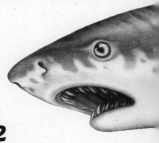

Wenn jemand hinausstürmt, ist er normalerweise weg. Doch diesmal erklang kein Geräusch von Reifen, die sich in Kies wühlten. War Mrs Lennox etwa noch da und warum? Da sich meine Freunde gerade am Buffet einen Nachschlag holten, gingen Jasper und ich auf Erkundung.

»Moment mal«, japste ich, als ich sah, was auf dem Parkplatz vor sich ging.

Mrs Lennox unterhielt sich dort mit zwei Leuten, die mir sehr, sehr bekannt vorkamen. Eine schlanke, elegant gekleidete Frau mit ebenholzfarbener Haut und – das konnte ich sogar von hier aus erkennen – strahlend blauen Augen. Und einem hochgewachsenen hellhäutigen Mann mit leicht angegrautem Haar, der mit Jackett und Hemd aussah wie ein Manager aus einem großen Unternehmen in Downtown.

Meine Eltern! Sie hatten ihr Versprechen gehalten, sie waren hier!

Ja, ich freute mich – und gleichzeitig hatte ich Schiss, dass wieder irgendetwas schiefgehen würde zwischen uns.

Die Zeit, in der sie sich mit Ellas Mutter unterhielten, kam mir endlos vor. Verstanden die sich etwa?! Aber dann nickten sie sich zu, ohne sich die Hand zu geben, und meine Eltern gingen in Richtung Schule, während Mrs Lennox zu ihrem SUV marschierte und abdüste.

»Besser, du redest allein mit denen«, sagte Jasper und verdrückte sich.

Dann standen wir uns gegenüber, Iris Anderson, Scott Anderson und ich.

»Hallo, Tiago«, sagte mein Vater freundlich und von Iris bekam ich ein Begrüßungslächeln, was sich ziemlich gut anfühlte.

Immerhin, wir waren uns nicht mehr ganz so fremd wie bei unserer ersten Begegnung.

»Hi«, antwortete ich. »Kanntet ihr die Lennox schon?«

»Was für eine unangenehme Frau«, sagte meine Mutter. »Stimmt es, dass sie im organisierten Verbrechen mit drinhängt und deutlich mehr ist als nur die Anwältin von Bittergreen?«

»Wenn ich darüber spekuliere, dann verklagt sie mich auf eine Million Dollar, hat sie gesagt.«

Zwei Paar Augenbrauen hoben sich. »Na ja, wir sind Anwälte, wir würden es bestimmt schaffen, das vom Tisch zu fegen«, meinte Scott. »Also mach dir keine Sorgen.«

Auf einmal fühlte ich mich leicht, ganz wunderbar leicht. Ich war nicht allein in diesem Kampf und war es nie gewesen.

»Okay«, sagte ich und konnte in dem Moment nicht anders, als meine Eltern anzulächeln. »Mit Wave ist es übrigens prima gelaufen, wir haben ihn freibekommen. Danke, dass ihr mitgeholfen habt.«

»Wer hat den Rest der Kaution bezahlt?«, fragte meine Mutter interessiert.

Ich durchwühlte mein Gedächtnis. Treffer.

»Ein Typ namens Alan Dorn«, berichtete ich. »Wir kennen ihn nicht, aber er ist anscheinend ein reicher Seawalker, den der Rat auf unser Problem aufmerksam gemacht hat.«

»Eigenartig«, meinte Scott. »Und ihr wisst wirklich nichts über ihn?«

»Leider nein.« Ich zuckte die Schultern. »Außer dass er in Kalifornien wohnt. Google hat nichts ausgespuckt, nur dass ihm eine Import-Export-Firma gehört.«

Während wir redeten, gingen wir langsam auf die Schule zu. Ich war hin- und hergerissen. Eigentlich war die Mittagspause vorbei, wir hatten noch einige Stunden Unterricht, aber ich konnte doch jetzt nicht weg!

»Wartet ihr einen Moment?«, bat ich meine Eltern, rannte in die Cafeteria, steuerte den Lehrertisch an, an dem auch Mr Clearwater saß, und sprudelte hervor: »Meine Eltern sind da, ich weiß nicht, wie lange sie bleiben können ...«

Mr García, Miss White und unser Schulleiter tauschten einen Blick. »Du bist für den Rest des Tages entschuldigt, Tiago«, sagte Jack Clearwater.

»Oh cool, danke!«, rief ich und raste zurück.

Ich fühlte mich wieder ein bisschen eingeschüchtert, als wir zusammen hinunter zum Strand gingen. So wie Mrs Lennox trug auch meine Mutter hochhackige Schuhe, sie ging darin wie ein Model. Doch dann zog Iris die Schuhe aus, um barfuß weiterzuschlendern, und Scott schlug vor: »Wie wäre es, wenn wir eine Runde zusammen schwimmen?«

»Gute Idee«, sagte ich. Das Meer war es, das uns verband.

Hätte irgendjemand uns gesehen, er hätte sich wahrscheinlich gewundert – zwei Tigerhaie und ein Blauhai mit tiefblauem Rücken und spitzer Schnauze, die friedlich nebeneinander herschwammen. Hätte mein Bruder Steve sich noch dazugesellt, wären wir sogar drei Tigerhaie gewesen – der Albtraum eines jeden Schwimmers! Aber ich hatte keine Ahnung, wo er gerade herumzog.

Wir haben gehört, dass du diesen Haikämpfen ein Ende bereitet hast, sagte Iris. *Gut gemacht. Scheußliche Sache, solche Duelle.*

Es fühlte sich richtig gut an, dass sie das sagte. Wie die beste Medizin der Welt.

Wir waren zu dritt, allein hätte ich es nicht geschafft, wandte ich ein.

Ich zeigte ihnen das Riff, dann unser Wrack, das sie sehr meerig fanden und ausgiebig umkreisten, und die Stelle, wo ich mich auf der Suche nach Shari in diesem fiesen Geisternetz verfangen hatte. Und das Wunder geschah, sie interessierten sich für alles.

Es kam mir allerdings ziemlich schräg vor, dass mitten im offenen Meer ein Tigerhai den anderen *Wie läuft's in der Schule?* fragte.

Jetzt wieder gut, seit wir unseren richtigen Schulleiter und unsere Kampflehrerin zurückhaben, erzählte ich und dann musste ich natürlich alles berichten, was in der Blue Reef Highschool in letzter Zeit so alles abgegangen war.

Meine Eltern lachten über die schmelzenden Kreditkarten. *Die Clearwaters können bei Bedarf echt hart drauf sein,* meinte meine Mutter und es klang anerkennend. Wie nebenbei schnappte sie sich einen vorbeischwimmenden Fisch und verschlang ihn mit zwei Bissen. Das erinnerte mich daran, dass Blauhaie auch Menschen gefährlich werden konnten.

Ich war in Versuchung, ihnen irgendwie zu beweisen, wie hart ich drauf sein konnte, aber dann dachte ich an das Desaster vom letzten Mal und ließ es sein. Vor ihnen anzugeben, hatte nicht funktioniert. Vielleicht sollte ich einfach ich selbst sein und das machen, was ich sowieso tat?

Es war ein schöner Ausflug und doch war ich froh, als wir

zurück waren und meine Eltern nach dem Abendessen wieder abzogen.

»Du bist immer noch angespannt, was? Wenn du mit ihnen zusammen bist?«, meinte Noah.

»Ja. Und ich denke noch viel zu oft daran, was für einen Eindruck ich auf sie mache.« Ich seufzte.

»Das wird schon noch«, versuchte Blue, mich zu trösten. »Cool, dass sie dich gelobt haben!«

Ja, das war cool gewesen. Gerade weil ich mich nicht gegen die Haikämpfe eingesetzt hatte, um sie zu beeindrucken, ich hatte dabei eher an Steve gedacht.

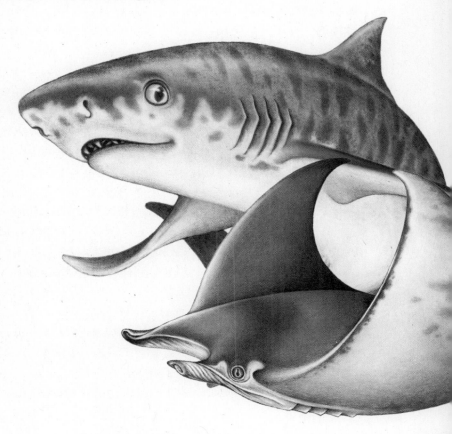

Nach dem Essen sagte ich Tschüss zu Jasper und meinen anderen Freunden, um noch ein bisschen vor meiner Hütte zu sitzen und zu zeichnen – ich hatte ein paar Barrakuda-Motive im Kopf, die förmlich danach schrien, auf Papier gebannt zu werden.

Doch jemand fing mich ab, noch bevor ich meine Hütte erreichte.

Finny!

»Ich wollte schon länger mit dir sprechen«, sagte sie.

»Oh echt?« Ich lächelte schief.

Gemeinsam wanderten wir durch den Palmhain und ich wusste mal wieder nicht, was ich sagen sollte. Zum Glück war es Finny, die den Anfang machte. »Du hast vielleicht gemerkt, dass du mir gefällst …« Sie grinste mich an.

»Schon ein bisschen«, gab ich zu.

»Aber das mit Wave war wie ein Blitzschlag. Ganz anders. Ich wollte dir nur sagen, dass ich es toll finde, dass wir befreundet sind. Da muss sich gar nichts ändern.«

»Ja, finde ich auch!«, antwortete ich erleichtert und dann umarmten wir uns kurz, bevor ich mich – diesmal allein – wieder auf den Weg zu meiner Hütte machte.

Aber keine Chance auf ein ruhiges Zeichenstündchen. Diesmal war es Shari, die auf mich zuschlenderte. Natürlich schlug mein Herz schneller, so wie immer, wenn ich sie sah.

»Und, wie wär's, wenn wir mal wieder zum Wrack schwimmen?«, fragte Shari und trat von einem Menschenfuß auf den anderen – war sie etwa nervös?

Ich war es auch, denn so wie es klang, wollte sie keine Freunde fragen, ob sie mitkommen wollten. Hieß das etwa, wir würden ALLEIN dort sein? Oh, mein Gott. Ich konnte fast fühlen, wie meine Herzklappen flatterten. Oder waren das diese

Schmetterlinge im Bauch, von denen in Romanen die Rede war?

»Klar gerne«, sagte ich. Am besten, wir schlichen uns mehr oder weniger weg, es war ja auch ein bisschen peinlich, wenn alle von unserm »Date« erfuhren.

Doch dann kamen Blue und Noah den Strand entlang. »Hi, Leute – ich schwimme mit Tiago zum Wrack, damit wir ein bisschen allein sein können!«, kündigte Shari fröhlich an und gab ihnen ihre Drei-Flossen-Kette zum Aufbewahren.

Nein, ich wollte nicht im Boden versinken, ich stehe nicht so auf Treibsand. Aber es war knapp.

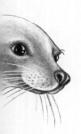

Ganz schön klebrig

Blue und Noah verzogen keine Miene, als Shari ankündigte, dass wir zum Wrack schwimmen wollten.

Dafür aber Chris. Er blickte besorgt drein, als er uns zu zweit zum Meer gehen sah. Ich fing einen Blick auf, der ziemlich eindeutig sagte: *Denk bloß nicht, dass ich so leicht aufgebe ...*

Obwohl ich ihn sonst sehr mochte, wandte ich mich diesmal ab, ohne ihn zu grüßen. Shari hatte sich entschieden – Pech für ihn, das musste er akzeptieren!

Wir verwandelten uns in der Lagune und irgendwie war nun alles in Ordnung. Ich war nicht länger ein planloser, verlegener Teenager, sondern ein Tigerhai, dem niemand etwas anhaben konnte. Und mit Shari zu schwimmen, fühlte sich wunderbar vertraut an. Hin und wieder blickte ich verstohlen zu ihr hinüber. Zum Glück waren von dem Kampf nur sehr kleine, punktförmige Narben auf ihrer Delfinhaut geblieben.

Es war ein bedeckter, regnerischer Tag und das Meer nicht so sonnendurchflutet, wie ich es mochte, aber egal. Wir tauchten hinunter zum Wrack, verwandelten uns mit mehr oder weniger Schwierigkeiten, kletterten in den luftgefüllten Bereich, zogen uns was an und warfen uns auf die bunten Gummikissen.

Oh Mann! Es gab so viel, was ich ihr sagen wollte, aber ich brachte nichts davon heraus. Also fragte ich: »Wie wär's mit einem Snack?«, und fischte eine Tüte Chips aus dem Regal.

»Sind noch Jelly Beans da?«, erkundigte sich Shari und die Antwort lautete Ja, Noah hatte für Nachschub gesorgt. Die feuchte Luft hier unten hatte ihnen allerdings nicht gutgetan. »Egal – sie kleben nicht so sehr wie die Eingeweide von Seegurken, also guten Appetit!«

»Woher weißt du, wie die Eingeweide von Seegurken sich anfühlen? Fresst ihr die etwa?« Seegurken sahen aus wie sandpanierte Gummischläuche und taten nichts anderes, als auf dem Meeresboden herumzuliegen.

»Nee, nee, die schmecken nicht. Sie schleudern ihre Eingeweide heraus, wenn sie sich angegriffen fühlen. Das Zeug wächst tatsächlich in ihnen nach.«

Krasse Verteidigungstaktik!

»Sag mal, was meinen eigentlich deine Eltern dazu, dass wir jetzt zusammen sind?«, fragte ich Shari. »Immerhin bin ich ein Tigerhai ...«

»Ach, die haben sich nur ganz kurz aufgeregt«, berichtete meine Delfinfreundin. »Ich habe ihnen klargemacht, dass das meine Entscheidung ist.«

»Cool«, sagte ich erleichtert.

Wir futterten und quatschten über das Meer, unsere Lehrer und alles, was passiert war, bis Shari mich plötzlich wieder so neugierig ansah. Oje ... das war ihr Ich-erforsche-die-Menschen-Blick – was kam jetzt?

»Sag mal, Tiago ...«, fing sie an.

»Ja?« Oh nein, ich bekam Schluckauf, ausgerechnet jetzt!

Shari musste lachen. »Wenn du dieses Hicksen machst, klingst du ein bisschen wie ein Seelöwe, der andere aus seinem Revier scheuchen will.«

»Äh, ach so, echt jetzt.« Das musste sie von Chris wissen, andere Seelöwen gab es in der Gegend nicht. Grr. Aber komischerweise half es, dass sie den Schluckauf witzig fand. Dadurch hörte es auf, peinlich zu sein, und ich lachte einfach mit. Fünf Minuten und einen Becher Limo später war das Hicksen weg.

»Was wolltest du denn fragen?«, meinte ich und Shari legte los: »Also, ich weiß ja aus dem Meer, was Delfine machen, die sich mögen. Aber was machen Menschen? Soll ich schlechte Gedichte für dich schreiben, so wie Barry an Carmen?«

Ich prustete vor Lachen Limo über die Kissen. Das hieß, wir mussten erst mal putzen, damit die nächsten Wrack-Besucher nicht festklebten. Dann fragte ich: »Was machen denn Delfine? Mit denen kenne *ich* mich nicht so aus.«

»Wenn zwei Delfine gute Freunde oder verliebt sind, schwimmen sie oft so, dass sie gleichzeitig zum Atmen hochkommen«, erklärte Shari. »Es fühlt sich so verbunden an, gleichzeitig zu atmen!«

»Hm, wir könnten es versuchen.« Einen Moment lang lauschte ich auf Sharis Atemzüge und versuchte, meine darauf abzustimmen. Nach nicht mal einer Minute gab ich auf. Zu anstrengend!

»Okay, das ist nicht so gut ... in Menschengestalt schnauft man ja die ganze Zeit. Ziemlich seltsam!« Shari überlegte. »Außerdem schwimmen Delfingefährten oft nebeneinander und manchmal auch so, dass sich ihre Flossen berühren.«

Wir sagten nichts mehr. Meine Hand bewegte sich auf ihre zu und ihre Hand kroch trippelnd wie eine Krabbe zu meiner hin. Dann verschränkten sich unsere Finger und ein Strom von Wärme floss zwischen uns.

»Wow«, sagte ich und blickte in Sharis fröhliche haselnussbraune Augen.

»Genau.« Shari lächelte mich an.

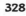

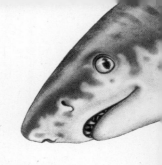

»Stell dir vor, ich wäre nie an die Blue Reef High gekommen oder Mrs Lennox wäre es gelungen, mich von der Schule zu verbannen – ist das nicht ein absolut schrecklicher Gedanke?« Auf meinem nackten Arm bildete sich eine Gänsehaut.

»Das wird sie nicht schaffen«, sagte Shari. »Wenn du dich weiterhin so gut im Griff hast wie in letzter Zeit.«

Ja, sie hatte recht, Mrs Lennox würde es wieder versuchen. Aber nun war Miss White wieder da und ich hatte dazugelernt. »Ich werde ein Tigerhai sein, der seine Kraft kennt und damit umzugehen weiß«, sagte ich feierlich. »Und der für ein ganz bestimmtes Delfinmädchen durch die tiefste Tiefsee schwimmen würde.« Shari grinste und verlegen fügte ich hinzu: »Na ja, okay, bis zweihundert Meter oder so.«

Darauf stießen wir gleich mal mit einem Becher Limo an.

Danksagung

Wieder einmal danke ich meinem Sohn und Juniorlektor Robin, außerdem Christian und meinen Testleserinnen Sonja, Anna Brünner, Hedi Magdalena Schmidt, Karen Ellermann, Christian Seiss sowie meiner unentbehrlichen Testleserin, Assistentin und Website-Moderatorin Sabine Hirsekorn.

Kurz erzähle ich euch, wie Daisy entstanden ist. Diese Figur haben Joy Spemann, die selbst im Rollstuhl sitzt, und ich zusammen entwickelt, was großen Spaß gemacht hat. Danke für dieses wunderbare Mädchen, Joy!

Ich bedanke mich auch bei Markus Frorath, Emma Fiszel, Corinna Schwetz und Johanna W., die bei meiner Versteigerung für die Aktionsgemeinschaft Artenschutz e.V. mitgemacht haben und dadurch helfen, Meeresschildkröten zu schützen! Das findet auch Mrs Pelagius richtig gut.

Natürlich danke ich wie immer auch Stefanie Letschert vom Arena Verlag, die mich super betreut, und meinem Lektor Frank Griesheimer, obwohl er doch tatsächlich gedacht hat, Miss White wäre eine Frau mittleren Alters. Aber dafür hatte er auch diesmal wieder tolle Vorschläge parat, was ich noch an der Geschichte ändern sollte, um sie besser zu machen. Ein großes Dankeschön auch an meine Agenten Gerd F. Rumler und Martina Kuscheck, bei denen ich oft das Gefühl habe, dass sie 24/7 – also buchstäblich rund um die Uhr – für mich da sind!

Und nicht zuletzt ein ganz großes Dankeschön an euch Fans, weil ihr so hinreißend mitfiebert und meine Bücher so liebt. Euch verdanke ich, dass die Seawalkers sich regelmäßig auf der Bestsellerliste tummeln dürfen. Also sage ich Danke, und zwar dir – genau, dich meine ich, denn schließlich liest du doch gerade dieses Buch, oder?

PS: Das, was Tiago Shari schenkt, ist übrigens eine »Beaus Stachelschnecke«.

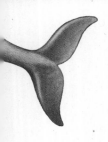

10 Dinge,
die du für das Meer tun kannst

Katja Brandis, Autorin von *Seawalkers* (katja-brandis.de)

1. **Verwende weniger Plastik!** Denn viele Plastikgegenstände landen leider im Meer, sogar bei uns in Europa, und richten dort Schaden an. Gegenstände, die du im Alltag brauchst, müssen nicht unbedingt aus Plastik sein, natürliche Materialien halten länger und schaden der Umwelt weniger!

2. **Clever einkaufen.** Wenn du shoppen gehst, nimm Stoffbeutel, einen Rucksack oder einen Korb mit, dann brauchst du keine Plastiktüten. Es ist zwar schwierig, beim Einkauf Plastikverpackungen zu vermeiden. Aber du könntest zum Beispiel die Getränke für deine nächste Party in Mehrweg- statt Einwegflaschen besorgen. Du könntest Produkte bevorzugen, die es in Glas oder Papierverpackungen gibt. Und deine Familie könnte Obst und Gemüse lose oder in mitgebrachten Netzen kaufen.

3. **Sammle Müll an Flussufern.** Habt ihr vielleicht einen Bach oder Fluss bei euch in der Nähe? Frag doch mal deinen Lehrer, ob ihr nicht gemeinsam mit der ganzen Klasse oder Schule den an den Ufern herumliegenden Abfall beseitigen könnt! Denn Plastikmüll und anderer Dreck, der in die Flüsse gerät, wird meist irgendwann ins Meer gespült.

4. **Iss weniger Fisch.** Leider sind riesige Fischereiflotten fast überall dabei, die Ozeane leer zu fischen, und Fischzuchtanlagen an der Küste verdrecken das Meer. Deshalb iss lieber etwas seltener Fisch oder bitte deine Eltern, nur noch Bio-Garnelen oder Fisch mit MSC-Siegel zu kaufen. Das MSC-Siegel auf einem Fischprodukt 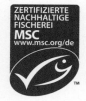 bedeutet, dass der Fisch aus einer nachhaltig arbeitenden Fischerei stammt. Iss möglichst keine großen Raubfische (Schwertfisch, Zackenbarsch, Barrakuda o. Ä.) – die sind oft im Urlaub auf den Speisekarten zu finden und dadurch bedroht.

5. **Kaufe möglichst keine Fleece-Kleidung.** Von Fleece-Pullovern lösen sich bei jeder Wäsche Tausende winziger Kunststofffasern, die von den Kläranlagen nicht herausgefiltert werden können und über die Flüsse ins Meer gelangen. Dort werden sie von Lebewesen versehentlich gefressen. Viel besser ist Kleidung aus Baumwolle oder Wolle.

6. **Kaufe im Urlaub keine Produkte aus Meeresgeschöpfen,** also Sachen, die z. B. aus Muscheln oder Korallen hergestellt wurden.

7. **Benutze nur Sonnencreme, die Gewässern nicht schadet.** »Normale« Sonnencreme enthält leider chemische Stoffe, die Riffen und Meerestieren nicht gut bekommen. Deswegen hat zum Beispiel Hawaii schon verboten, sie zu verwenden. Es gibt inzwischen speziell entwickelte Sonnencreme, du erkennst sie daran, dass z. B. »Reef safe« oder etwas Ähnliches darauf steht. In Deutschland kaufen kann man z. B. Waterlover Sun Milk von Biotherm oder Sonnencreme von Caudalie mit dem Label »Ocean Protect«. Vor Ort in tropischen Küstenländern gibt es noch viele, viele Marken mehr.

8. **Verhindere die Klimaerwärmung.** Die Klimaerwärmung lässt Korallenriffe absterben und das Meerwasser saurer werden. Um das Klima zu schützen, könntest du seltener mit dem Auto fahren und öfter das Fahrrad oder öffentliche Verkehrsmittel nehmen. Im Winter auch mal einen dicken Pulli anziehen, statt die Heizung weiter aufzudrehen. Und seltener mit dem Flugzeug Urlaub machen.

9. **Beteilige dich im Umweltschutz oder organisiere eine Spendenaktion.** Engagieren kannst du dich zum Beispiel in den Jugendgruppen von Umweltorganisationen. Und wie wäre es mal mit einer Spendenaktion für den Ozean, zum Beispiel über ein Schulfest, einen Flohmarkt oder den Verkauf selbst gemachter Produkte? Oder du könntest dir statt eines »normalen« Geburtstagsgeschenks eine Spende für den Schutz des Meeres wünschen.

10. **Gib diese Tipps weiter.** Zum Beispiel könntest du in der Schule einen Vortrag über das Thema halten oder ein Projekt zum Thema starten. Oder wie wäre es mit einem Artikel in der Schülerzeitung?

Katja Brandis
Seawalkers

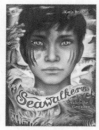

978-3-401-60612-5

Gefährliche Gestalten

Für Tiago ist es ein Schock, als er herausfindet, dass er ein Gestaltwandler ist. Und was für einer: In seiner zweiten Gestalt als Tigerhai wird er sogar von seinen Mitschülern gefürchtet. Einzig das fröhliche Delfinmädchen Shari hat keine Angst vor ihm. Doch ihre Freundschaft wird bereits beim ersten Abenteuer auf die Probe gestellt.

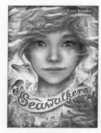

978-3-401-60613-2

Rettung für Shari

Tiago ist glücklich, dass er an der Blue Reef High bleiben darf, auch weil er in Delfinwandlerin Shari eine Freundin gefunden hat. Die kann er gut gebrauchen, denn nicht alle sind glücklich über seine Anwesenheit. Bei einem Menschenkunde-Ausflug spitzt sich die Lage zu. Als Shari in große Schwierigkeiten gerät, setzt er alles auf eine Karte, um sie zu retten.

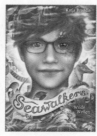

978-3-401-60527-2

Wilde Wellen

Neuerdings bevökern zahlreiche Reptilien- und Python-Wandler die Schule und sorgen für Chaos. Nun baut sich vor der Küste von Florida auch noch ein gewaltiger Hurrikan auf. Haiwandler Tiago, Delfinmädchen Shari und ihre Freunde entscheiden sich, aufs offene Meer zu fliehen. Doch sind sie dort wirklich in Sicherheit?

Arena | **Jeder Band:**
Gebunden
Auch als E-Book und als Hörbuch
bei Arena audio erhältlich
www.arena-verlag.de

Katja Brandis
Woodwalkers

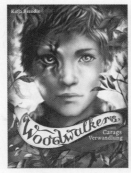 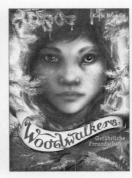 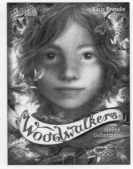

Carags Verwandlung (1)
ISBN 978-3-401-60606-4

Gefährliche Freundschaft (2)
ISBN 978-3-401-60607-1

Hollys Geheimnis (3)
ISBN 978-3-401-60608-8

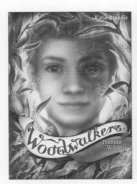 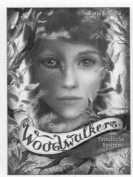 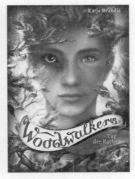

Fremde Wildnis (4)
ISBN 978-3-401-60609-5

Feindliche Spuren (5)
ISBN 978-3-401-60610-1

Tag der Rache (6)
ISBN 978-3-401-60611-8

Arena

Auch als E-Books erhältlich.
Die Hörbücher erscheinen bei Arena audio.

Jeder Band:
Gebunden
www.arena-verlag.de

Katja Brandis
Khyona

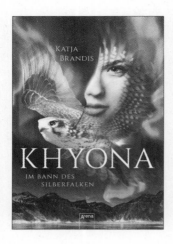 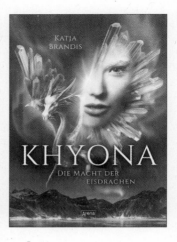

Im Bann des Silberfalken

Die Macht der Eisdrachen

Der Islandurlaub mit ihrer neuen Patchworkfamilie ist genauso anstrengend wie Kari sich das vorgestellt hat. Doch als ihr ein silberner Falke begegnet und sie ins Reich Isslar gebracht wird, verändert sich alles. Ehe Kari sich versieht, steckt sie mitten in einer magischen Welt voller Trolle, Eisdrachen und Elfen, in der Geysire über das Schicksal entscheiden und ein geheimnisvoller junger Mann über die Vulkane der Insel herrscht.

Ein Jahr ist vergangen, seitdem Kari das magische Isslar mit seinen Eisdrachen, Elfen und Vulkanen zurückgelassen hat. Doch die Sehnsucht nach dem charismatischen Andrik und die Ungewissheit darüber, wer sie ist, lassen Kari nicht los und treiben sie zurück nach Island. Doch kaum ist Kari durch das Grüne Tor nach Isslar getreten, gerät sie in einen Strudel aus Machtspielen und Intrigen.

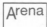

Band 1
480 Seiten • Arena Taschenbuch
ISBN 978-3-401-51192-4
Auch als E-Book erhältlich

Band 2
480 Seiten • Arena Taschenbuch
ISBN 978-3-401-51211-2
www.arena-verlag.de